Psychiatric and Mental Health
NURSING

Psychiatric and Mental Health
NURSING

RUTH ELDER | KATIE EVANS | DEBRA NIZETTE

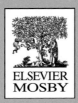

ELSEVIER
MOSBY

Sydney Edinburgh London New York Philadelphia St Louis Toronto

ELSEVIER

Mosby
is an imprint of Elsevier

Elsevier Australia
30–52 Smidmore Street, Marrickville, NSW 2204

This edition © 2005 Elsevier Australia
(a division of Reed International Books Australia Pty Ltd)
ACN 001 002 357

National Library of Australia Cataloguing-in-Publication Data

Psychiatric and mental health nursing.

Includes index.
Tertiary students.
ISBN 0 7295 3729 3.

1. Psychiatric nursing – Australia – Textbooks. 2.
Psychiatric nursing – New Zealand – Textbooks. I. Elder,
Ruth. II. Evans, Katie. III. Nizette, Debra.

616.890231

Publisher: Vaughn Curtis
Publishing editor: Meg O'Hanlon
Developmental editor: Rhiain Hull
Edited and project managed by Kay Waters
Cover and text design by Wing Ping Tong
Typeset by Sun Photoset Pty Ltd
Printed in Australia by Southwood Press

Contents

Preface

When we set out to write this book, our intention was to design a text which would be useful for all nurses, irrespective of the context of their practice, but especially so for undergraduate nursing students. We invited colleagues teaching and working in mental health to contribute from the breadth of their expertise, and we wrote specifically for an Australian and New Zealand readership, addressing topics such as local legislation and policy—topics absent from the overseas texts on which we have traditionally relied.

The text is divided into four parts. Briefly, Part 1 explores broad areas such as the history of mental illness and mental health care, the nurse, contexts of practice and the politico–legal implications of practice. Part 2 aims to contextualise practice, examining theories about mental health and wellness across the lifespan and within societies and cultures, as well as exploring crisis, loss and assessment issues. Part 3 develops a better understanding of the major mental illnesses, examines DSM-IV-TR diagnoses, interventions and effective treatments, and examines the client's experience of mental illness. Part 4 focuses on psychopharmacology and therapeutic skill development for practice, and applies skills to clinical situations.

Chapters begin with key points, key terms and learning outcomes, and conclude with questions and exercises to facilitate teaching and learning. Critical thinking challenges, class engagement activities, nurses' stories, case studies and research briefs encourage an active awareness of the complex issues related to mental health and illness.

Most chapters incorporate 'nurse's story' vignettes, illustrating the knowledge possessed by practising psychiatric mental health nurses, and to give students insight into the world of practice. We editors were hospital-trained and we fear that much of the concentrated, practical and interpersonal skills and knowledge that enhanced our own training could be lost as the nursing workforce ages and leaves the profession. Contributions from nurses working in clinical and management roles as well as nurse academics communicate skills in counselling, assessment, interviewing, history taking and a range of interventions.

This text acknowledges the importance of a client-focused approach and supports a holistic philosophy of practice. This holistic approach assists the beginning practitioner to understand that mental wellness is a concept that balances mental illness, and that mental illness is caused by a complex web of circumstances. A healthy society requires that mental health needs are acknowledged and services developed to enhance the existing protective factors in our communities.

We hope that this text will have a wide appeal because of its practical approach and the support it offers students and teachers as well as all practitioners working with those who have a mental health problem. In an environment where technical and professional evolution is continuous and inevitable, we wanted above all to stress the importance of a personal and humane approach to psychiatric mental health nursing practice.

Ruth Elder, Katie Evans, Debra Nizette, July 2004

Contributors

Murray Bardwell
RN, RPN, DipAppSc, BN, MNSt
Lecturer in Nursing
Australian Catholic University, Ballarat, Vic

Pat Barkway
RN, BA, MSc(PHC)
Associate Dean (International)
Senior Lecturer Mental Health Nursing
School of Nursing and Midwifery
Flinders University, Adelaide, SA

Jan Barling
RN, DipAppSc, BA, MN, MRCNA, FANZCMHN
Lecturer, Mental Health Nursing
School of Nursing and Health Care Practices
Southern Cross University, Lismore, NSW

Christina Bobrowski
RN, BA(Hons)
Lecturer, School of Nursing
University of Tasmania, Launceston, Tas

Pat Bradley
ANZCMHN, MRCNA, MAAQHC, RGN, RPN, DipAppSc(Nursing),
GradDip Health Education
Nurse Educator, Top End Mental Health Service
Casuarina, NT

Norma Cloonan
RN, BA(Soc Wel)
Clinical Nurse Consultant for Dual Diagnosis
Intellectual Disability and Mental Illness
South Western Sydney Area Health Service, NSW

Janette Curtis
RN, BA, DipPubHlth, PhD, MANZCMHN, MRCNA
Deputy Head Nursing, Coordinator Mental Health
Nursing Programs
University of Wollongong, Wollongong, NSW

Ruth De Souza
GradDip Adv Nurs Practice (Counselling), MA(Hons), RCpN
Program Coordinator, Mental Health Support Work
School of Health and Communities Studies
Unitec, Auckland, New Zealand

Ruth Elder
RN, BA(Hons), PhD
Lecturer, School of Nursing
Queensland University of Technology, Brisbane, Qld

Stephen Elsom
RN, BA, MNJ, MHN, FANZCMHN
Senior Lecturer, Faculty of Medicine, Nursing and
Health Sciences
Monash University, Melbourne, Vic

Katie Evans
RPN, BA, MLitSt, PhD, FANZCMHN
Lecturer and Convenor of the Postgraduate Mental
Health Program
School of Nursing, Griffith University, Brisbane, Qld

Gerry Farrell
RN, PhD, FANZCMHN,
Professor and Head of School, Tasmanian School
of Nursing
University of Tasmania, Launceston, Tas

Kim Foster
RN, RPN, DipAppSc, BN, MA, PhD candidate (Griffith)
Senior Lecturer and Director Undergraduate Studies
(External), School of Nursing Sciences
James Cook University, Cairns, Qld

Michael Groome
RN, BA(Psychology/Sociology), MSc
Lecturer, School of Nursing,
Australian Catholic University—National, Vic

Charles Harmon
RN, DipTeach(Nursing), BHS(Nursing), MN, FANZCMHN
Lecturer, School of Nursing and Midwifery,
Faculty of Health, University of Newcastle, Newcastle,
NSW

Kristin Henderson
RN, RM, RPN, DipApp Nurse Ed, BNursing, GradDipScComm,
MHlthSc
Team Leader, Child and Family Therapy Unit
Royal Children's Hospital Brisbane, Brisbane, Qld

Sue Henderson
RN (Psychiatric Nurse), BAppScNur
Lecturer, School of Nursing
Monash University, Melbourne, Vic

Jan Horsfall
RPN, BA(Hons), MA(Hons), PhD
(Ret) formerly University of Western Sydney,
Sydney, NSW

Debra Jackson
RN, PhD
Associate Professor, School of Nursing, Family and
Community Health
College of Social and Health Sciences
University of Western Sydney, Sydney, NSW

Lauretta Luck
BA(Psych) (NSW), MA(Psych) (USyd), RN, MRCNA
Deputy Head of School / Clinical Director
Senior Lecturer, School of Nursing Sciences
James Cook University, Cairns, Qld

Jem Masters
RN (RGN, RSCN, RMN, UK), GradDip Nurs Mgmt, Manager
of Management (Public Sector, Health), FANZCMHN
Director of Operations, Infant, Child and Adolescent
Mental Health Services, Macarthur Health
Service, Sydney, NSW

Phillip Maude
RN, PhD, MNurs(Res), BHSci, Dip MHN WASON, FANZCMHN
Coordinator, Higher Degrees and Research
School of Nursing, The University of Melbourne
Manager Psychiatric Education and Research,
The Alfred, Melbourne, Vic

Paul Morrison
BA(Hons), PhD, PGCE, GradDip Counselling, RMN, RGN,
AFBPS CPsychol MAPS
Professor, Department of Nursing
School of Health Sciences, University of Canberra,
Canberra, ACT

Wendy Moyle
RN, DipAppSci, BN, MHSc, PhD
Associate Professor and Postgraduate Programs
Coordinator
School of Nursing, Griffith University, Brisbane, Qld

Eimear Muir-Cochrane
BSc(Hons), RN, RPN, GradDip Adult Education, MN Studies, PhD
Associate Professor, School of Nursing and Midwifery,
Division of Health
Sciences, University of South Australia, SA

Deb Nizette
RN, Endorsed MHN, DipAppSc(Nurse Ed), BAppSc Nursing,
MNSt, FANZCMHN, FRCNA
Lecturer, School of Nursing
Australian Catholic University McAuley, Banyo,
Brisbane, Qld

Anthony J O'Brien
RGN, RPN, BA, MPhil(Hons)
Senior Lecturer, Mental Health Nursing
School of Nursing, University Of Auckland
Auckland, New Zealand

Louise O'Brien
RN, BA, PhD
Senior Lecturer, School of Nursing Family and
Community Health
University of Western Sydney, Sydney, NSW

Elaine Painter
BA(Nurs Sc), M Primary Health Care, RN, MHN
Clinical Nurse Consultant, Eating Disorders
Outreach Services
Royal Brisbane Hospital, Brisbane, Qld

Christine Palmer
RGON, RPN, DipAppSc(Nurse Ed), BAppSc(Nursing), MN
Formerly Massey University, New Zealand

Philip Petrie
MEdStud, BN, RN
Deputy Chief Executive Officer of The Centre
(BHCCA Inc), Bankstown, NSW

Fran Sanders
BA(Anthropology), MSPD (Master Social Planning & Development)
Lecturer, School of Nursing
Queensland University of Technology, Brisbane, Qld

Irvin Savage
RN, BA Health Science (Health Promotion)
Private consultant

Vicki Stanton
RPN, RMRN, BASocWel, MASocSc, GradDipPubHlth,
GradCertMgmt, FANZCMHN
Manager, Central Australian Mental Health Service
Department of Health and Community Services, NT

J Richard Taylor
RN, RPN, BEd, MEd
Lecturer, School of Nursing
Australian Catholic University, Melbourne

Barbara Tooth
RN, RM, BA(Hons), PhD
Visiting Senior Fellow, Illawarra Institute of
Mental Health
The University of Wollongong, Wollongong, NSW

Kim Usher
DNE, DHS, BA, MNursS, PhD, RN, RPN, RMRN
Associate Professor and Head, School of Nursing
Sciences,
James Cook University, Townsville

Tim Wand
DASNurs, GradDip MHNurs, MNurs
Mental Health Nurse Practitioner
Emergency Department, Royal Prince Alfred Hospital
Sydney, NSW

Pam Wood
RN, RPN, BANurs, RenalCert, GradDipEd
Course Coordinator for Interstate Students, Lecturer,
School of Health Sciences
Charles Darwin University, NT

Reviewers

Jan Allan
RN (Cert Gen, Cert Psych), DNE, BA(Soc Sci), MEdAdmin, EdD
Formerly Head, School of Nursing and Health Science
Charles Sturt University, Bathurst, NSW

Cally Berryman
PhD, Med, BN (Community Health), RN
Lecturer, Coordinator, Substance Abuse Studies
(Research and Honours), School of Nursing
and Midwifery
Victoria University, Melbourne, Vic

Julie Bradshaw
RN, RPN, BHlthSc, MNurs(Hons)
Lecturer, School of Nursing and Health Studies
Central Queensland University, Rockhampton, Qld

Michael Clinton
PhD, MSc, BA(Hons), BA, RMN, SRN, RN FETeachCert, RCNT,
PGCertEd, RNT
School of Public Health, Curtin University, Perth, WA

Ruth De Souza
Graduate Diploma in Advanced Nursing Practice (Counselling),
MA(Hons), RCpN
Program Coordinator, Mental Health Support Work
School of Health and Communities Studies
Unitec, Auckland, New Zealand

Barbara Fiveash
RN, RPN, RSCN, DNE, BHlthSc, MN, PhD
Senior Psychiatric Nurse, Adult Mental Health
Mildura Health Service, Mildura, Vic

Paul Morrison
BA(Hons) PhD, PGCE GradDip Counselling, RMN RGN AFBPS
CPsychol MAPS
Professor, Department of Nursing,
School of Health Sciences, University of Canberra,
Canberra, ACT

Erina Morrison-Ngatai
RCpN, BHScN, PGradCert Mental Health Nursing
Lecturer, Mental Health Nursing
School of Health Sciences
Massey University, Palmerston North, New Zealand

Ian Munro
RPN, RN, BAppSc (CHN), MN(Admin), PhD
Lecturer, School of Nursing
Deakin University, Melbourne, Vic

Anthony Welch
PhD, MEd, BEd, GradDip Counselling, DipAppSc(NEd), RN, RPN
Senior Lecturer, Program Leader, Bachelor of Nursing
RMIT University, Melbourne, Vic

Edward White
PhD, MSc(SocPol), MSc(SocRes), PGCEA, RMN, DipCPN, RNT,
FANZCMHN, FCN
Director of Research and Professor of Mental Health
Nursing
University of Technology, Sydney, NSW

Acknowledgements

Every attempt has been made to trace and acknowledge copyright, but in some cases this may not have been possible. The publisher apologises for any accidental infringements and would welcome any information to redress the situation.

Box 4.2, World Health Organization 2001, Mental Health, New Understanding, New Hope, WHO, Geneva. Online: http//www.who.int/whr2001/2001/ main/en/chapter4/Box 5.1. Rights of the Mentally Ill. Reproduced with permission.

Figs 4.2 & 4.3, Ministry of Health 1997, Moving forward: The national plan for more and better mental health services. Reproduced with permission from the New Zealand Ministry of Health.

Box 5.3, Mental Health Commission 2001, Recovery competencies for New Zealand mental health workers, Wellington: Mental Health Commission

Table 5.1, p 19, text extract and p 75, Box 5.5, Australian and New Zealand College of Mental Health Nurses (ANZCMHN) 1995, Standards of practice for mental health nursing in Australia, Greenacres: ANZCMHN; 1995 Standards of practice for mental health nursing in New Zealand, Greenacres: ANZCMHN. Reproduced with permission.

Fig 7.1, Ivey A & Ivey M 2003, *Intentional Interviewing and Counselling: Facilitating Client Development in a Multicultural Society* (5th edn), Thompson Brooks/Cole, Pacific Grove, CA. Copyright Brooks/Cole Publishing, a division of Thompson Learning.

Questionnaire, Parry G 1990, *Coping with Crises*, British Psychological Society in association with Routledge, London.

Box 10.3, *Treatment Protocol Project 2000, Management of Mental Disorders*, Vol. 1 (3rd edn), World Health Organization, Collaborating Centre for Mental Health And Substance Abuse, Sydney. Copyright Australasian Medical Publishing Company.

Fig 10.1, Nursing physical assessment form, New South Wales Health 2001, *NSW Mental Health Outcome and Assessment Training (MH-OAT) Facilitator's Manual*, NSW Health, Sydney. Reproduced with permission.

Table 10.3, Narayan MC 2003, Cultural Assessment Checklist, *Home Health Care Nurse*, 21(9): 611–18. Reproduced with permission from Mary Narayan, MSN, RN, CS, CTN.

Table 10.4, New South Wales Health 2001, *NSW Mental Health Outcome and Assessment Training (MH-OAT) Facilitator's Manual*, NSW Health, Sydney, Overhead 44, reproduced with permission.

Box 10.6, reprinted with permission from the *Diagnostic and Statistical Manual of Mental Disorders*, 4th edn, text revision. Copyright 2000 American Psychiatric Association.

Box 11.1, Hamer BA 1998, Assessing mental status in persons with mental retardation, *Journal of Psychosocial Nursing & Mental Health Services*, 35(5), pp 27–31. Copyright Beth Hamer RN, BA, MS, CPMHN (C). Reproduced with permission.

Figs 17.1, 17.2 & 17.3, Australian Bureau of Statistics 1998, *Mental Health and Wellbeing: Profile of Adults, Australia, 1997*, ABS, Canberra. ABS data used with permission from the Australian Bureau of Statistics (www.abs.gov.au).

Figs 17.4 & 17.5, Australian Bureau of Statistics 1998, *Mental Health and Wellbeing: Profile of Adults, Australia, 1997*, ABS, Canberra. ABS data used with permission from the Australian Bureau of Statistics (www.abs.gov.au).

Box 17.1, reprinted with permission from the *Diagnostic and Statistical Manual of Mental Disorders*, 4th edn, text revision. Copyright 2000 American Psychiatric Association.

Extract (p 271) from *Who's Afraid of Agorophobia?* by Neville A 1986, published by Arrow Books, London. Used with permission of the Random House Group Limited.

Table 17.3, Rapee RM 1998, *Overcoming Shyness and Social Phobia: A Step-by-Step Guide* (2nd edn), Lifestyle Press, Killara, NSW. Reproduced with permission.

Box 12.1, *Diagnostic and Statistical Manual of Mental Disorders*, 4th edn, text revision. Copyright 2000 American Psychiatric Association.

Box 15.1, *Diagnostic and Statistical Manual of Mental Disorders*, 4th edn, text revision. Copyright 2000 American Psychiatric Association.

Boxes 15.2 & 15.3, *Diagnostic and Statistical Manual of Mental Disorders*, 4th edn, text revision. Copyright 2000 American Psychiatric Association.

Table 16.1, adapted from *Diagnostic and Statistical Manual of Mental Disorders*, 4th edn, text revision. Copyright 2000 American Psychiatric Association.

Case study (p 272), Rapee RM 2001, *Overcoming Shyness and Social Phobia: A Step by Step Guide* (2nd edn), Lifestyle Press, Killara NSW, p xiii.

PART

1

Preparing for Psychiatric Mental Health Nursing

The Effective Nurse

*Debra Jackson and
Louise O'Brien*

KEY POINTS

- Mental health nursing is a challenging and stimulating area of practice that requires synthesis of knowledge from a range of disciplines.
- The development of therapeutic relationships is the key to effective mental health nursing.
- Mental health nurses and clients together develop therapeutic alliances as a milieu for growth and recovery.
- Self-awareness, insight and reflexivity are fundamental skills for mental health nursing.
- Mental health nursing requires sustained and close engagement with people in highly charged situations and this can lead to stress and burnout.
- Burnout syndrome has three elements—emotional exhaustion, depersonalisation and reduced personal accomplishment.
- Mental health nurses are required to develop therapeutic alliances while maintaining clear professional boundaries.
- Supportive collegial relationships can enhance the skills and confidence of mental health nurses at all stages of their careers.

LEARNING OUTCOMES

The material in this chapter will assist you to:
- describe the nursing skills needed to care for the spiritual needs of clients
- describe the three components of empathy
- define self-awareness, and describe a strategy for developing self-awareness
- discuss the three phases of reflection
- list the factors that contribute to stress and burnout in nursing
- explain strategies for managing stress and avoiding burnout
- explain the importance of maintaining professional boundaries
- describe the benefits of mentoring and preceptoring.

KEY TERMS

- burnout
- burnout syndrome
- caring
- clinical supervision
- empathy
- ethics
- evidence-based practice
- healing
- hope
- mentoring
- preceptoring
- professional boundaries
- recover
- reflection
- reflective practices
- self
- self-awareness
- self-disclosure
- spirituality
- stress
- therapeutic alliance

INTRODUCTION
Mental health nursing is one of the most interesting and challenging areas of nursing practice, and requires a fusion of all your professional knowledge, clinical and interpersonal skills and experiences. Although nurses in all settings care for the mental health and wellbeing of the patients and clients in their care, those patients or clients with acute or chronic mental illnesses have complex and perhaps long-term needs. Patients or clients with chronic mental illness often engage in frequent and regular encounters with the health-care system. The long-term and cyclic nature of some mental illnesses means that the therapeutic relationships between mental health nurses and their clients can last for long periods. They can also vary in intensity as clients move along a continuum between periods of high dependence at one end (in acute phases when they are experiencing symptoms of their illness) and independence at the other (when their symptoms are less troublesome or their mental illness resolved).

Skilful mental health nursing requires more than a sound knowledge of human physiology, psychology, psychiatry and pharmacology. In order to practise effectively, nurses working in mental health need to be open-minded and reflective, and to have developed an understanding of esoteric concepts such as spirituality and hope. They also need to understand the nature and boundaries of professional and therapeutic relationships. Personal qualities such as responsiveness, self-awareness and insight are also essential. This chapter introduces some of the concepts and issues that are fundamental to the provision of effective and safe mental health nursing practice.

CARING
Caring is widely considered to be central to nursing theory and practice, and is frequently cited as a reason for choosing a nursing career (Jackson & Borbasi 2000; Wilkes & Wallis 1993). Although 'caring' is a word that is used widely in the nursing and health-care literature, as a concept it is ill defined. It is also controversial, and as you engage with the literature you will find that there are arguments for and against nursing adopting the concept of caring as the cornerstone of the discipline. Most of these arguments are concerned with:
- the gendered nature of caring (Speedy 2000)
- the care/cure debate (Jackson & Borbasi 2000)
- the 'fit' of a concept like caring in a discipline that is dominated by scientific biomedical discourses (Dunlop 1986)
- the inherent conflict between the concept of caring, and the economic rationalism and social privilege that control the provision of health services (Jackson & Raftos 1997; Jackson & Borbasi 2000)
- concerns with the dichotomy of *professional* nurse caring (what nurses do) and *informal* caring (the caring available to people through their own social networks and personal relationships) (Jackson & Borbasi 2000).

Nurse scholars have invested much time and energy in trying to explain what it is that makes nurse caring special or different from informal caring and from the caring provided by other professionals (i.e. medical practitioners). There have also been many attempts to find a 'fit' between caring as a construct, and the biomedically dominated and economically driven health-care sectors within which nursing is situated.

From a mental health perspective there are even more issues to consider in relation to nurse caring. For example, there are special issues associated with caring for consumers who are compelled (perhaps unwillingly) to accept professional care under one of the Mental Health Acts (see Ch 4 for mental health legislation). Historically, mental health nursing has been associated with custodial care and control. Godin (2000) captures the current dilemma of mental health nurses when he raises questions about the *dis*-ease between the caring and coercive roles that mental health nurses assume. Godin positions caring as 'clean' and constructs the coercive control elements of mental health nursing (a term he uses for forced treatment, community orders and so on) as 'dirty' (Godin 2000, p 1396). While Godin's argument is particularly focused on clients and nurses in the community, many of the issues he raises (related to forced administration of medication, seclusion and detention) are relevant to nurses in the inpatient setting as well. The absolute vulnerability of clients who can be detained against their will and subjected to various treatments that they may vigorously and robustly resist, means that elements of the caring role such as patient advocacy are absolutely critical to skilful and compassionate mental health nursing practice.

HOPE AND SPIRITUALITY
There is still much we don't know about recovery, healing and how people manage chronic health problems. Why do some people pull through a disease, while others succumb? How is it that some people seem to cope very well with even very invasive treatments, while others suffer terribly? How do some people with chronic mental illnesses function well in the community, while others are in and out of hospital in a revolving-door syndrome? We know that factors such as personality, resilience, social support, general health and access to acceptable (to the client) health services all play a crucial role in client outcomes (see Ch 2 for more on consumers, recovery, rehabilitation and resilience). But the importance and value of concepts such as hope, and the role it plays in the lives of clients and their families, are areas of increasing interest. There is growing recognition of the concept of hope and its relationship to health, wellbeing and recovery from illness or traumatic life events.

'Hope' is a taken-for-granted term and although it is seen a lot in the literature, it is seldom clearly defined. We know it is a complex and multidimensional variable that has optimistic and anticipatory dimensions and involves looking ahead to the future. Daly, Jackson & Davidson (1999, p 43) refer to hope as 'a positive source of power' that individuals can find and foster. Their findings suggest that hope arises from suffering, adversity or misfortune of some sort (Daly et al. 1999). After undertaking a concept analysis of hope, Stephenson (1991, p 1459) defined it as 'a process of anticipation that involves the interaction of thinking, acting, feeling and relating, and is directed toward a future fulfilment that is personally meaningful'.

In the literature, the concept of hope is consistently associated with spirituality and the belief systems that individuals hold (Daly et al. 1999). For example, Daly et al. (1999) describe a theme they named as 'having faith in the primacy of a higher power' (p 42), to capture the idea that spirituality is central to the meanings that can be drawn from major life events. Of course, spirituality does not only refer to religious issues. Goddard (1995) differentiates *metaphysical* spirituality, which she says focuses on the notion of God or a higher power, from *existential* spirituality, which relates to values, beliefs, ideologies and philosophies that provide individuals with guidance and direction throughout their lives. Furthermore, she states that spirituality is a way of understanding and making meaning of life, and is apparent in commonplace as well as unusual circumstances (Goddard 1995).

Concepts like hope and spirituality have tended to sit uneasily in a clinical world dominated by a biomedical scientific world view (Crawford, Nolan & Brown 1998). The biomedical model values things that can be seen, measured and quantified. Although they can be felt, hope and spirituality cannot be seen, touched or smelt and cannot always be clearly articulated, and so occupy what Crawford et al. (1998, p 214) term 'an embarrassed silence'. However, if we recognise that spirituality underpins the meanings that people make of illness and other life events, and that hope is a variable that has healing potential, then we cannot ignore the importance of spirituality in practice. Indeed, Thompson (2002) reinforces the importance of recognising and responding to the spiritual care needs of clients, and calls for nurses to include spiritual care as a crucial aspect of holistic client care.

So, this leads us to the question: What skills do we need if we are to care for the spiritual needs of our patients and clients? The short answer is that we need to develop effective interpersonal skills. Being open to the belief systems of other people, active listening, being alert to the cues that tell us the things that matter to a person, self-awareness, spiritual awareness and reflective skills are considered crucial in the provision of spiritual care (Greasley, Chiu & Gartland 2001; Thompson 2002).

CRITICAL THINKING CHALLENGE 1.1

Colleen is a 37-year-old Aboriginal woman who has a two-week history of becoming increasingly disorganised, thought-disordered, agitated and distressed. She reports hearing voices, and finds this very upsetting. She states that these voices are calling out to her and telling her things. While admitting Colleen to the ward you note that she is visibly distressed, appears to have difficulty concentrating and sometimes makes seemingly inappropriate responses to your questions, while at other times her responses are appropriate.

Colleen has no previous history of psychotic illness, though she does have a history of alcohol-related problems. She discloses that she has been drinking more than usual over the past month. Colleen tells you that her mother and uncle died two years ago in a car accident, and that her husband died of a heart attack six weeks ago.

- What are the main issues here?
- How might Colleen's recent social history be related to her current health status?
- How could the nurse respond to Colleen's distress?

THERAPEUTIC USE OF SELF

Therapeutic relationships are the central activity of mental health nursing. They are the foundation upon which all other activities are based. Mental health nursing is thus firstly an interpersonal process that uses self as the means of developing and sustaining nurse–client relationships. Therapeutic use of self involves using aspects of your personality, background, life skills and knowledge to develop a connection with a person who has a mental health problem or illness. We intentionally and consciously draw on our ways of establishing human connectedness in our encounters with clients. The process is based on genuine interest in understanding who the client is and how they have come to be in their current situation.

The purpose of using self therapeutically is to establish a therapeutic alliance with the client. Clients in mental health services may not only be suffering from frightening symptoms or perhaps overwhelming mood changes, or out-of-control thoughts and feelings; they also suffer from alienation and isolation. Clients may be fearful of talking to others about their symptoms or difficulties because they fear being rejected and seen as 'crazy', or they may have had experiences of rejection because of their mental illness that make it difficult for them to form relationships. Studies of clients' experiences of mental health services repeatedly provide evidence that being understood and listened to in a thoughtful, sensitive manner confirms their humanity and provides hope for their future (Lally 1989; Leete 1987; Ruocchio 1999).

In the process of using self therapeutically, the nurse develops a dialogue with the client in order to understand their predicament. Clients need to feel safe enough to disclose personal, difficult and distressing information. It is in the way in which the nurse can convey genuine interest, concern and desire to understand the client that a therapeutic alliance can be established. How the nurse relates, and what prior understandings she or he brings to the encounter, will affect this relationship.

Heifner (1993) used the term 'positive connectedness' to describe the therapeutic alliance that develops between clients and nurses in psychiatric settings. Heifner describes a relationship that develops from initial contact, to the revelation of vulnerability by the client, leading to a high investment by the nurse in the client, and the recognition of a common humanity with the client and feelings of reciprocity that result in connectedness between the client and the nurse. Both nurses and clients view such connectedness positively in terms of health outcomes for the client.

Therapeutic use of self is embedded in the theoretical frameworks of the interactionist nursing theorists Peplau, Travelbee, and Patterson & Zderad (Meleis 1997), who locate the focus of nursing in nurse–patient interactions and relationships. These theorists define health and illness as part of the human experience, and the goals of nursing as developing human potential to find meaning in the experience (Meleis 1997, p 190). They stress the importance of self as a therapeutic agent.

Empathy and therapeutic use of self

The ability to empathise with clients is positively linked with the ability to develop therapeutic relationships. Studies have consistently shown that clients value empathic nurses highly (Forchuk & Reynolds 2001; Geanellos 2002; O'Brien 2000, 2001). Empathy is not merely a feeling of understanding and compassion for the client. Empathy, as used in the therapeutic relationship, has a number of components. First, empathy involves an attempt to understand the client's predicament and the meanings that the client attributes to their situation. This means that the nurse makes a conscious attempt to discuss with the client their current and past experiences and the feelings and meanings that are associated with these experiences. Secondly, the nurse verbalises the understanding that she or he has developed, to the client. The understanding that the nurse has of the client's situation will be at best tentative; we can never really know what life is like for another. However, the process of seeking to understand, and of conveying to the client the desire to understand, creates the opportunity for further exploration in a safe relationship. In addition, maintaining the stance of trying to understand rather than making assumptions averts the tendency to make judgments about clients and their behaviour. The third component of empathy is the client's validation of the nurse's understanding. One of the most important aspects of the development of the therapeutic relationship through empathic understanding is that the nurse can convey to the client his or her desire to understand. This level of empathic attunement allows the client to participate in identifying those aspects of their illness and health-care experience that are problematic.

Evidence-based practice and therapeutic alliance

The value of a therapeutic alliance, developed through therapeutic use of self, has been clearly identified from the perspective of nurses and clients in qualitative studies in Australia (Geanellos 2002; O'Brien 2000, 2001; Walsh 1999) and in the United Kingdom (Graham 2001). In the United States, Forchuk et al. (1998) and Forchuk & Reynolds (2001) demonstrated that the provision of continued therapeutic relationships with nurses was linked with a reduction in admission rates and an improved quality of life for patients discharged from hospital.

SELF-AWARENESS

The process of understanding others begins with understanding the self (see also Ch 2). 'Self' is a concept that describes the core of our personality. We use the concept of self when we want to convey our uniqueness as a human being. The self has consistent attributes that pervade the way we live in and experience the world. It is awareness of these attributes of self that can enhance the

ETHICAL DILEMMA

You are caring for Jack, a 22-year-old male with bipolar disorder who had been admitted to the acute care unit during a manic episode. In addition to his bipolar disorder, Jack is hepatitis B positive. He has been scheduled under the Mental Health Act, and is currently being nursed with several other scheduled patients in a close observation area. Jack is observed attempting to initiate sexual activity with a couple of female patients. There is a 'no sex' policy in the unit and Jack has been reminded of this on several occasions. However, Jack tells you that he intends to form sexual relationships with some of the female patients.

Questions

1 What could the nurse do? List the options available.
2 Identify the potential risks and benefits of each option you have identified.
3 What ethical principles need to be considered?

way we relate to others. A strong sense of self allows us to develop resilience in dealing with the difficulties and complexities of human communication and experience. Self-awareness is about knowing how you are going to respond to specific situations, about knowing your values, attitudes and biases towards people and situations, about knowing how your human needs might manifest in your work.

The purpose of being self-aware is to know those things in our background and way of relating that might affect how we relate to clients. The way we view people is always subjective. The lens through which we look at the world is always our own. Although there can be no true objectivity, knowledge of the things that impinge on our subjective view of the world allows us to identify how they influence our thinking.

Nurses need to be aware of the belief systems and values that arise from their cultural, social and family backgrounds. Everyone develops biases that affect the way they view other peoples' behaviour. Behaviour that is understandable to one nurse might not be understandable to another. However, the self is not static but constantly evolving and sensitive to experience. We bring values, biases and beliefs to nursing and to our relationships with clients, and in turn those relationships offer the opportunity for self-development. It is through the process of self-reflection and the examination of particular experiences that nurses can learn.

Work in the mental health area requires the ability to listen to, respond to and empathise with people from a range of backgrounds. Unexamined belief systems can become obstacles to the development of a therapeutic alliance with a client. Lack of self-awareness can cause nurses to respond to a client's distress and behaviour in ways that may not be helpful. It may cause nurses to use their power coercively in the belief that this is best for the client. Lack of self-awareness can lead to nurses being overly concerned, refusing to allow the client choice or overwhelming them with advice, in an attempt to protect them. Alternatively, nurses may avoid contact with particular clients, or fail to respond to distress.

REFLECTION

Reflection is 'a process of consciously examining what has occurred in terms of thoughts, feelings and actions against underlying beliefs, assumptions and knowledge as well as against the backdrop (i.e. the context or the stage) in which specific practice has occurred' (Kim 1999, p 1207). Reflection allows nurses to examine both their practice (actions) and the accompanying cognitions (thoughts) and affective meanings (feelings) in relation to values, biases and knowledge and in relation to the context in which the situation occurred. The purpose of reflection is to increase self-awareness, as well as to develop a conscious knowledge base for practice. Johns (2001, p 241) suggests that

the purpose of reflection is to 'surface contradiction between what [the nurse] intends to achieve within any situation and the way she [sic] actually practices'.

Developing reflective practices

Most models of reflection involve three phases (Greenwood 1998; Johns 2001; Kim 1999).

1 In the *descriptive phase*, nurses create descriptive narratives of specific clinical situations. The narratives include descriptions of actions, thoughts and feelings as well as descriptions of the situation and factors surrounding the situation. This process increases the nurse's ability to include self, and the context as well as the specific client and health problem, in their understanding of the clinical experience. To some extent nurses do this in verbal handovers or in discussion about specific events. In these situations, however, nurses tend to be selective about their responses and the contextual factors.

2 The *reflective phase* involves the comparison of the narrative with the nurse's beliefs, biases and knowledge. This involves the identification of the nurse's knowledge base, as well as values and belief systems. This allows for identification of gaps in knowledge, as well as previously unexamined beliefs about the client, the situation or the role and intentions of the nurse. The potential for further development of knowledge, clinical skills and self-awareness is enhanced by the reflective process.

3 The *critical/emancipatory phase* allows the nurse to identify differences between intentions and actions, thoughts/feelings and espoused values, values and practice, client needs and the nurse's actions. This phase allows for self-critique, learning and change. It also allows for the development of greater understanding of the influence of the context on the nurse's actions.

PROFESSIONAL BOUNDARIES

Professional nursing boundaries are invisible yet powerful lines that mark the territory of the nurse (see also Ch 2). Professional boundaries define a role, and allow the nurse to say, 'This is what I do. This is the purpose of my presence here.' Professional boundaries are important in all areas of health care, but in mental health nursing they have an increased importance due to the nature of the work of mental health nurses and the vulnerability of the client population. Over time there has been a decrease in formal divisions between staff and clients in mental health services, with the encouragement of friendliness and collaborative partnerships (Brown, Crawford & Darongkamas 2000). Mental health nurses have to be able to maintain professional boundaries while simultaneously developing close therapeutic relationships with clients based on empathy and positive connectedness. While many of the interactions and interventions of mental health nurses may appear social in nature (e.g. playing table tennis, cards or volleyball, going for a walk or having a coffee with a client), it is the therapeutic intent and the conscious awareness of the purpose of the relationship that put them within the professional role. It is when interventions and interactions lose their therapeutic intent and are instead primarily for the benefit of the nurse that professional boundaries begin to be breached.

Professional boundaries are maintained by the nurse having a clear understanding of his or her therapeutic role, being able to reflect on therapeutic interactions, and being able to document and narrate his or her interventions. Maintaining professional boundaries is always the responsibility of the nurse.

Self-disclosure

Mental health nurses use self-disclosure as a way of developing therapeutic relationships with clients. Many of the relationships that nurses have with clients are very long-term, either by repeated admissions to hospital or by continued contact in community settings. In a study of nurse–client relationships between community mental health nurses and clients with long-term mental illness, nurses described the use of self-disclosure. 'The nurses used their own experiences of living a life to: be seen as ordinary people; be credible; illustrate aspects of being-in-the world; allow the clients to identify with them; and to normalise the client's fears and difficulties' (O'Brien 2000, p 188). The clients described the nurse as 'a friend—but different . . . not like other friends' (O'Brien 2001). The clients were able to identify that the therapeutic relationship was different even though they knew things about the nurse's life (O'Brien 2001, p 180). Similarly, Geanellos (2002) noted in a study of adolescent mental health nursing that there was a close relationship between nurses and the adolescent clients. Participants in her study commented that the nurse 'was more like a person than a nurse' (Geanellos 2002, p 178).

However, self-disclosure should be used consciously and carefully. The boundary issue is not whether disclosure occurs or does not occur. The issue is the nature of the disclosure and whether the nurse burdens the client with his or her personal problems (Gutheil & Gabbard 1998). The decision about what to disclose to clients about your life needs to be made in advance. In the above studies these experienced nurse clinicians were able to use their own life experience to relate in ways that were beneficial to clients without overburdening them. Experienced clinicians, in these studies, also made decisions about what to share with clients according to the length of the relationship and what the client could use productively.

STRESS AND BURNOUT
Stress
(See also anxiety disorders in Ch 17, crisis and loss in Ch 9, and therapeutic interventions in Ch 23.)
Stress is a physiological response to any stressor or demand (Cohen 2000) and a fact of life for everyone. When a person experiences a stressor, their homeostasis is disturbed and their body activates a stress response. Any foundational anatomy and physiology textbook can provide you with details of the stress response. For the purposes of this book it is enough to understand that the stress response involves the release of substances into the blood that cause a range of physiological changes including changes to heart rate, blood pressure and the gastrointestinal tract. Prolonged stress can be harmful and can have a negative effect on physical and mental health.

Stress can be experienced as negative (*distress*) or positive (*eustress*). A stressful event can have a positive effect, because it can be a catalyst for a person to make changes such as learning new skills, or a stimulant to some sort of positive action (Thorpe & Barski 2001). Individuals can respond differently to the same stressor. For example, you and a friend might need to travel from

---

ETHICAL DILEMMA: Professional boundaries

You are a newly graduated nurse working in an acute psychiatric inpatient unit. One evening you admit a 21-year-old woman (Kellie) to the ward for nursing care. Kellie has been in a car accident and has several compound fractures to her right leg. She is in traction and so is to be nursed in bed. She has been admitted to the psychiatric ward because she has a history of paranoid schizophrenia. Though she is currently stable from a mental health perspective, she has been admitted to the unit because the orthopaedic ward staff felt they could not give her adequate care.

Kellie settles into the ward well, and passes her time with knitting, watching television and enjoying the company of visitors and other inpatients in the unit. After a few days, when you are on afternoon shift, you notice that one of your colleagues is sitting at Kellie's bedside. On reflection you realise that this colleague has been spending quite a bit of time with Kellie since she has been admitted, even staying and chatting to her well after the end of shift. At about 7 pm you approach the colleague (who should have gone off at 3.45 on completion of the morning shift) to ask if they know Kellie personally. The colleague replies, 'No, not personally, but we get on pretty well and my ex-girlfriend was a schizophrenic too'.

Questions

1 What are the main issues here?
2 Are any ethical issues involved? If so, what are they?
3 What could you do in this situation?

Darwin to Bathurst Island, and the only means of travel available is a light aircraft. You might find the thought of flying in a light aircraft stressful and anxiety-provoking, but your friend might find it exhilarating and exciting. Both you and your friend are experiencing stress reactions, but are experiencing them very differently.

Like other professions that involve close and sustained engagement with people, nursing is innately stressful (Coffey & Coleman 2001). Mental health nurses frequently encounter situations that are tense and unpredictable, and these factors are known to increase stress levels (McGowan 2001). In addition, therapeutic relationships can last for considerable periods of time and can be incredibly challenging at times. It is very important, then, to learn to monitor and manage your own stress, because unchecked stress can become chronic, and can result in burnout syndrome (Melchior et al. 1996).

Burnout syndrome

'Burnout' and 'stress' are words that are often seen together, because one (stress) is seen as a precursor to the other (burnout). However, stress is a feature of life and, when managed properly, does not lead to burnout. Unlike stress, which has some positive features (it can be a catalyst for effecting positive change such as learning a new skill), burnout has no positive aspects, for the person experiencing it or for those around them. 'Burnout' is a term that was first seen in the literature in the mid-to-late 1970s, and it is widely considered to be a contributing factor to the current worldwide nursing shortage (Haddad 2002).

Burnout is used to describe a pattern of emotional exhaustion, depersonalisation and decreased personal accomplishment—together these three components are sometimes called 'burnout syndrome' (Melchior et al. 1996). While the effects of emotional exhaustion will vary from person to person, feelings of depression, irritability, a sense that you have nothing more to give, and of being emotionally overwhelmed by work are commonly described (Barling 2001; Haddad 2002). Depersonalisation can lead to unkind, indifferent, uninterested, deprecating, belittling and/or distant responses to clients (Barling 2001; Haddad 2002). It is not difficult to imagine how distressing it would be for a client to be nursed by someone who responded to them and their situation in a cold and unfeeling way rather than with the warmth, caring, empathy and respect we ourselves would wish for if we were sick and needing care. The third element of burnout syndrome—reduced personal accomplishment—describes feelings of ineffectiveness, ineptitude, low satisfaction and a perceived lack of success in work (Barling 2001).

It can be seen that burnout syndrome is an undesirable state, not only because of the detrimental influence it has on nurse–patient interaction, but also because of the negative effects on the affected nurse and his or her immediate colleagues. It has also been associated with diminished work performance, increased staff turnover and misuse of drugs and alcohol (Ewers et al. 2002). From the perspective of the affected person, there is nothing worse than going to work when you feel unhappy and distressed. Working with colleagues who are irritable, depressed and exhausted adds to everyone's stress. When people are experiencing emotional exhaustion and reduced personal accomplishment it is difficult for them to work effectively as a team member. They may find they are too lacking in creative energy to perform properly in some areas. For example, irritability might compromise a nurse's ability to mentor and support a novice or inexperienced nurse effectively.

Nurses are considered to be particularly susceptible to developing burnout syndrome because of the nature of nursing work, which involves a high level of close contact with people who are often in emotionally charged situations (such as when they or a loved one are experiencing sickness, pain, anxiety or exhaustion) as well as factors such as lack of autonomy and high workload, which are also common hallmarks of the nursing workplace (Jackson, Clare & Mannix 2002). Mental health nursing involves long periods of working in intensely stressful situations, which may be exacerbated by the environment (e.g. secured areas), and the literature suggests that these factors make burnout an issue of particular concern to mental health nurses (Melchoir et al. 1996; Ewers et al. 2002). The task for nurses, therefore, is to develop strategies to avoid getting burnout syndrome. Haddad (2002) positions burnout syndrome as an ethical issue in nursing, and considers that all nurses have a moral imperative to reduce burnout by taking active steps to avoid burnout in themselves.

Avoiding burnout syndrome

Burnout syndrome has been repeatedly linked to the current shortage of nurses and so there have been many research studies and published research reports on ways in which nurses can reduce burnout syndrome or avoid getting it. Most of these reports acknowledge two main areas that can be manipulated to avoid burnout: aspects of the individual nurse; and the environment in which the nurse works. It is important that we each learn to know ourselves and our limitations. In nursing we are often encouraged to develop reflective skills, and these are very helpful in learning to understand ourselves and our own responses to stressors (Thorpe & Barski 2001). If we are aware that we are becoming moody, irritable, short-tempered, or that we are not feeling empathetic towards clients, then this can be an indication that it is time to step back and reflect on the situation (Haddad 2002). Most health-care facilities in Australia and New Zealand provide a range of measures to assist staff, and these include debriefing, counselling and other measures.

It is important to extend the same care to ourselves that we offer to those in our care. Nursing is a high-stress profession and therefore it is necessary to be active in managing stress. Though it can be difficult to fit leisure activities around shift work and study, it is important to maintain a balanced and healthy lifestyle, and take the time to participate in enjoyable leisure activities. Continuing to learn and develop skills can also be effective. Ewers et al. (2002) undertook a study to see if psychosocial intervention training affected the levels of burnout in forensic mental health nurses. Their findings suggested that staff undergoing intervention training showed a significant decrease in burnout rates. Though individuals can do things to reduce their risk of burnout, institutional practices are strongly implicated in nurses' susceptibility to burnout syndrome, and Haddad (2002) clearly positions burnout as a systemic problem rather than an individual one. Therefore it is also important to ensure that institutions and managers adopt policies and practices that support nurses rather than contribute to stress and burnout.

PROFESSIONAL SUPPORTIVE RELATIONSHIPS
Clinical supervision
Clinical supervision is a process that focuses on the clinical work of the nurse. It provides an arena where the nurse can reflect with another experienced clinician on their clinical interactions and interventions. Fowler & Chevannes (1998) note that there is a high degree of compatibility between reflective practice and clinical supervision. Johns (2001) suggests that the success of reflective practice in creating change depends on the relationship between practitioner and supervisor. The purpose of clinical supervision is professional support, education and professional development, and enhancement of the quality of clinical practice (Mullarkey, Keeley & Playle 2001).

Clinical supervision is not limited to review of case work or of actions, but provides an opportunity for nurses to reflect upon the subjective experience of their work (Rafferty 2000). In order to develop the nurse's capacity for empathy, acceptance, nurturing and honest reflection, the clinical supervisor needs to be able to model these capacities in their relationship with the supervisee.

Preceptorship and mentoring
Preceptorship and mentoring are two different models for professional relationships that can be developed between nurses. A *preceptoring* relationship is usually based in the clinical area. When you are new to an area, such as when you are a student taking part in clinical learning, or a new graduate entering the workforce, or a new employee in a clinical setting, you will often be allocated a preceptor. The preceptor will generally be a nurse with considerable experience in a particular clinical environment, and will usually have completed specialised in-service training to prepare for the preceptoring role. They will understand the difficulties and challenges facing people who are new to the area, and they will assist you to develop skills and confidence, and will facilitate your becoming part of the team in the particular area (Freiburger 2002). You will remain under the guidance of the preceptor for a set period of time or until you feel confident to take your place as a fully independent and functioning member of the team. Preceptors tend to be attached to wards or units, so when you go to a new area you will likely be working with a different preceptor.

Mentors have many roles, but the core of mentoring is a partnership between two people that generates mutual learning as well as positive growth and development. Mentors are usually chosen because of their personal qualities and the achievements they have made. Unlike a preceptoring relationship, a mentoring relationship is not mediated through employment in a particular ward or unit. Rather, it is a long-term relationship that continues throughout a

---

NURSE'S STORY: Clinical supervision

Marietta is working in an acute inpatient unit. She has two years' experience. She arrives at clinical supervision saying that she feels angry with one of her clients, a young woman with a diagnosis of depression who self-harms. She had spent considerable time with the client in the preceding days, and felt that she had developed a good relationship with her. Last night after she had gone home, the client had cut her arms with a razor blade. Today the client is belligerent, appearing to take delight in having 'fooled' the nurses. Marietta says that the other staff have reinforced her belief that she was 'sucked in' and she is now confused about how to proceed with this client.

The supervisor asks Marietta to tell in detail the story of what happened. She then asks Marietta to outline her feelings about, and knowledge of, the client before and after the

incident. The supervisor listens attentively and empathically, encouraging further exploration of the incident and Marietta's feelings about it. Marietta admits to feeling guilty, and is concerned that she may have said or done something to provoke the incident. Together they consider how the client might have been feeling and what possible triggers to self-harm might have existed. They go on to consider what Marietta saw as important in developing the relationship with the client. The supervisor suggests some reading that Marietta can undertake to increase her understanding of self-harm-related behaviours. Together they identify what might be the goals of nursing interventions with this client. Marietta resolves to talk to the client about how the client was feeling last night and what provoked the self-harm incident.

career or for as long as the parties want it to, and is sustained through changes of employment. Mentoring helps people to grow and develop and reach their potential. Both preceptoring and mentoring provide additional avenues for debriefing and feedback that can help in dealing effectively with confusing or upsetting incidents.

As with all relationships, certain qualities are needed by both parties, including commitment, honesty, integrity and effective interpersonal skills. Mentors and preceptors need additional skills, such as problem-solving, clinical currency and expertise (in the case of preceptors or clinical mentors), appropriate scholarly, administrative or research expertise, the ability to provide constructive criticism and other feedback, understanding of professional boundaries and relationships, and the ability to maintain confidentiality where appropriate.

CONCLUSION

This chapter has introduced some of the core concepts and ideas that shape and inform mental health nursing practice. To be effective and therapeutic in caring for others, nurses must understand such concepts as caring, hope and spirituality. Stress and burnout are hazards for nurses and others in the caring professions and therefore nurses must learn to recognise and manage their own stress. Therapeutic relationships lie at the heart of mental health nursing, and a clear understanding of professional boundaries is crucial to the development and ongoing sustainability of such relationships.

Mental health nursing is an exciting and challenging area of nursing practice. Effective mental health nursing requires the culmination of all your skills as well as your professional and life experiences, and it offers a stimulating and rewarding career path. As we strive to meet the complex needs of diverse communities and provide care within increasingly restrictive economic environments, there are many challenges before us. Developing positive personal qualities such as self-awareness, and fostering productive and supportive collegial relationships, will help us to meet the challenges that lie ahead.

EXERCISE FOR CLASS ENGAGEMENT

An effective way of developing self-awareness is the use of questioning. To raise your awareness of some important issues, ask yourself the following questions, then discuss your responses with other members of your group or class.

■ What kinds of values do I hold important as a framework for living? Where do these values come from? How do they inform my understanding of what it is to be a person in this world?

■ How has my family of origin influenced how I view the world? What values did my family hold as important? What do I see as important in family life?

■ What do I know about why I choose to be a nurse?

■ What are the pervading social attitudes towards people in mental distress or with mental illness? What are my beliefs about people in mental distress or with mental illness?

■ What experiences have I had that influence how I feel about people with mental illness?

REFERENCES

Barling J 2001, Drowning not waving: burnout and mental health nursing, *Contemporary Nurse*, 11(2/3), pp 247–59.

Brown B, Crawford P & Darongkamas J 2000, Blurred roles and permeable boundaries: the experience of multidisciplinary working in community mental health, *Health and Social Care in the Community*, 8(6), pp 425–35.

Coffey M & Coleman M 2001, The relationship between support and stress in forensic community mental health nursing, *Journal of Advanced Nursing*, 34(3), pp 397–407.

Cohen J 2000, Stress and mental health: a biobehavioral perspective, *Issues in Mental Health Nursing*, 21(2), pp 285–302.

Crawford P, Nolan P & Brown B 1998, Ministering to madness: the narratives of people who have left religious orders to work in the caring professions, *Journal of Advanced Nursing*, 28(1), pp 212–20.

Daly J, Jackson D & Davidson P 1999, The experience of hope for survivors of acute myocardial infarction, *The Australian Journal of Advanced Nursing*, 16(3), pp 38–44.

Dunlop M 1986, Is a science of caring possible?, *Journal of Advanced Nursing*, 11(3), pp 661–70.

Ewers P, Bradshaw T, McGovern J & Ewers B 2002, Does training in psychosocial interventions reduce burnout rates in forensic nursing?, *Journal of Advanced Nursing*, 37(5), pp 470–6.

Forchuk C & Reynolds W 2001, Clients' reflections on relationships with nurses: comparisons from Canada and Scotland, *Journal of Psychiatric and Mental Health Nursing*, 8, pp 45–51.

Forchuk C, Westwell J, Martin ML, Bamber-Azzopardi W, Kosterwa-Tolman D & Hux M 1998, Factors influencing movement of chronic psychiatric patients from the orientation to the working phase of the nurse–client relationship on an inpatient unit, *Perspectives in Psychiatric Care*, 34, pp 36–44.

Fowler J & Chevannes M 1998, Evaluating the efficacy of reflective practice within the context of clinical supervision, *Journal of Advanced Nursing*, 27, pp 379–82.

Freiburger O 2002, Preceptor programs: increasing student self-confidence and competency, *Nurse Educator*, 27(2), pp 58–60.

Geanellos R 2002, Transformative change of self: the unique focus of (adolescent) mental health nursing?, *International Journal of Mental Health Nursing*, 11, pp 174–85.

Goddard N 1995, 'Spirituality as integrative energy': a philosophical analysis as requisite precursor to holistic nursing practice, *Journal of Advanced Nursing*, 22(4), pp 808–15.

Godin P 2000, A dirty business: caring for people who are a nuisance or a danger, *Journal of Advanced Nursing*, 32(6), pp 1396–1402.

Graham I 2001, Seeking a clarification of meaning: a phenomenological interpretation of the craft of mental health nursing, *Journal of Psychiatric and Mental Health Nursing*, 8, pp 335–45.

Greasley P, Chiu LF & Gartland M 2001, The concept of spiritual care in mental health nursing, *Journal of Advanced Nursing*, 33(5), pp 629–37.

Greenwood J 1998, The role of reflection in single and double loop learning, *Journal of Advanced Nursing*, 27, pp 1048–53.

Gutheil TG & Gabbard GO 1998, Misuses and misunderstandings of boundary theory in clinical and regulatory settings, *American Journal of Psychiatry*, 155(3), pp 409–14.

Haddad A 2002, An ethical view of burnout, *RN*, 65(9), pp 25–6, 28.

Heifner C 1993, Positive connectedness in the psychiatric nurse–patient relationship, *Archives of Psychiatric Nursing*, 7(1), pp 11–15.

Jackson D & Borbasi S-A 2000, The caring conundrum: potential and perils for nursing. In: Daly J, Speedy S & Jackson D (eds), *Contexts of Nursing: An Introduction*, McLennan & Petty, Sydney.

Jackson D & Raftos M 1997, In uncharted waters: confronting the culture of silence in a residential care institution, *International Journal of Nursing Practice*, 3(1), pp 34–9.

Jackson D, Clare J & Mannix J 2002, Who would want to be a nurse? Violence in the workplace: a factor in recruitment and retention, *Journal of Nursing Management*, 10(1), pp 13–20.

Johns C 2001, Reflective practice: revealing the [he]art of caring, *International Journal of Nursing Practice*, 7(4), pp 237–45.

Kim HS 1999, Critical reflective inquiry for knowledge development in nursing practice, *Journal of Advanced Nursing*, 29(5), pp 1205–12.

Lally S 1989, Does being in here mean there is something wrong with me?, *Schizophrenia Bulletin*, 15(2), pp 253–65.

Leete E 1987, The treatment of schizophrenia: a patient's perspective, *Hospital and Community Psychiatry*, 38(5), pp 486–91.

McGowan B 2001, Self-reported stress and its effects on nurses, *Nursing Standard*, 15(42), pp 33–8.

Melchior M, Philipsen H, Abu-Saad HH, Halfens R, van de Berg A & Gassman P 1996, The effectiveness of primary nursing on burnout among psychiatric nurses in long-stay settings, *Journal of Advanced Nursing*, 24(4), pp 694–702.

Meleis AI 1997, *Theoretical Nursing: Development and Progress* (2nd edn), Philadelphia, New York.

Mullarkey K, Keeley P & Playle JF 2001, Multiprofessional clinical supervision: challenges for mental health nurses, *Journal of Psychiatric and Mental Health Nursing*, 8, pp 205–11.

O'Brien L 2000, Nurse–client relationships: the experience of community psychiatric nurses, *Australian and New Zealand Journal of Mental Health Nursing*, 9, pp 184–94.

O'Brien L 2001, The relationship between community psychiatric nurses and clients with severe and persistent mental illness: the client experience, *Australian and New Zealand Journal of Mental Health Nursing*, 10, pp 176–86.

Rafferty MA 2000, A conceptual model for clinical supervision in nursing and health visiting based on Winnicott's (1960) theory of parent–infant relationship, *Journal of Psychiatric and Mental Health Nursing*, 7, pp 153–61.

Ruocchio PJ 1999, The importance of psychotherapy in remission and relapse, *Psychiatric Services*, 50(6), pp 745–9.

Speedy S 2000, Gender issues in Australian nursing. In: Daly J, Speedy S & Jackson D (eds), *Contexts of Nursing: An Introduction*, McLennan & Petty, Sydney.

Stephenson C 1991, The concept of hope revisited for nursing, *Journal of Advanced Nursing*, 16, pp 1456–61.

Thompson, I 2002, Mental health and spiritual care, *Nursing Standard*, 17(9), pp 33–8.

Thorpe K & Barsky J 2001, Healing through self-reflection, *Journal of Advanced Nursing*, 35(5), pp 760–8.

Walsh K 1999, Shared humanity and the psychiatric nurse–patient encounter, *Australian and New Zealand Journal of Mental Health Nursing*, 8, pp 2–8.

Wilkes L & Wallis M 1993, The five Cs of caring: the lived experience of student nurses, *Australian Journal of Advanced Nursing*, 11(1), pp 19–25.

CHAPTER

2

The **Context** of **Practice**

Vicki Stanton and Barbara Tooth

KEY POINTS

- Mental health nursing practice is primarily influenced by the attitudes, values and beliefs of the nurse.
- Theories about mental health and mental health practice can influence a nurse's attitudes, values and beliefs.
- The ability to think critically and develop self-awareness are therefore central to nursing practice.
- Nurses are continually drawing on an ever-changing knowledge base and responding to the influence of this in their practice.
- The recovery approach provides the guiding principles for all mental health practice.
- The ultimate goal of mental health practice is to value the worth and facilitate the capacity of all persons to be active participants in society, and to provide the necessary range of resources that will help them to meet this goal.

LEARNING OUTCOMES

The material in this chapter will assist you to:
- demonstrate an understanding of the role of your attitudes, values and beliefs as a key factor in how you work with people, and of the role of theories in this process
- explain the rationale for the shift in knowledge base towards holistic and strengths-based practice
- appreciate the value of reflective practice and continually developing self-awareness
- identify the reasons for a consumer focus being the basis for mental health practice
- provide a rationale for the current preference for recovery-orientated practice
- describe the principles of recovery-orientated practice
- understand the interrelationship between individuals, the broader community, various services and policies and how the components complement each other in facilitating recovery-orientated practice.

KEY TERMS

- community
- consumers
- dualism
- health and wellness
- holism
- multidisciplinary teams
- non-government organisations
- participation and empowerment
- partnerships
- professional boundaries
- recovery
- rehabilitation
- self-help
- stigma
- strengths

INTRODUCTION

This chapter discusses some of the fundamental concepts and principles underlying what nurses do when they work with people, particularly people with mental health needs. It builds on the previous chapter by reinforcing the importance of reflection in order for nurses to become competent practitioners, and it provides a context for the chapters that follow.

To make sense of mental health nursing practice requires an understanding of the factors that can influence it. These include mental health policy, current theories about the various aspects of mental health, and the attitudes, values and beliefs that guide our thinking. People's thinking changes over time and this is determined by the experiences they have had and by changes in thinking about what constitutes appropriate practice. In mental health in the past few decades, the rate of change in thinking about practice has been significant. This chapter addresses some of the major shifts in thinking that influence our understanding of *what* mental health nursing practice entails, the rationale behind *why* it is approached in this way, *how* it is actually put into practice, and the settings *where* nurses are likely to practise.

It can be tempting to think that mental health nursing is a discrete area of practice of little value to the general nurse, but this is far from the truth. The fundamental concepts and principles underlying mental health nursing are considered so important to general practice that they have been incorporated into undergraduate nursing courses in Australia and New Zealand. The comprehensive course is intended to provide a holistic approach to nursing care and a basis for later specialist practice.

THE RELATIONSHIP BETWEEN THEORY AND PRACTICE

To begin to make sense of professional nursing practice requires an understanding of the relationship between theory and practice.

What is a theory?

Theories provide the rationale for the actions that guide our practice.

- A theory is a set of constructs, hypotheses, principles and propositions about a specific phenomenon.
- A theory is not a statement of fact, nor is it the whole truth, but more a partial truth that hopefully will lead to the development and understanding of something that is better than that which currently exists.
- Theories can be either *formal* (written with detailed support and presented to others in the field) or *informal* (residing in people's conscious or subconscious thoughts).
- Theories generate hypotheses about specific phenomena that can be tested to determine the theory's usefulness, predictive ability or 'fit'.

The last point is important to understand because theories can be revised, built on by others or disproved as a result of applying the principles of the theory to practice and evaluating their usefulness and 'fit'. For example, theories promoting *dualism* (mind and body as separate and independent entities) had been dominant in medicine for some time but their limitations are now widely acknowledged. *Holism* (mind and body cannot be separated) now provides the best 'fit'.

The concepts of dualism and holism will be discussed later but the example illustrates the fact that theories are not static. They are time- and context-specific and tell the reader about the theorist's thoughts on a subject based on their comprehensive knowledge and experience in a specific topic at that time. Theories also give us insights into how individual theorists make sense of their world—behind every theory is the person who proposed it. Knowing something of the person's background and experience can help to put the theory into context and provide a framework for making sense of the range of theories about certain phenomena. This framework also helps to demystify theories and their role in practice.

In fact we are all theorists (albeit informal theorists). We make hypotheses (propositions to explain specific phenomena) about ourselves, others, situations and larger world events, and we make predictions about what will happen in the future based on our past life experiences. Testing these hypotheses will either support our predictions or make it clear that we need to revise them. This also holds true in nursing practice, where nurses have been found to be theorisers of their everyday practice (Cox, Hickson & Taylor 1991; Graham 2000).

Which theory best guides practice?

How do beginning practitioners determine which formal theory is most appropriate for their nursing practice? It is not a question of deciding which theory is right or wrong, but rather of appreciating that there can be a number of ways of understanding a particular phenomenon. Nursing is just one of a number of disciplines in the field of mental health. There is a general body of knowledge in mental health and each discipline draws on this to expand the understanding of practice issues. In turn there are discipline-specific theories that add to the existing body of knowledge. These various theories can complement or contradict each other, or express similar ideas, but all theories expand our understanding of specific phenomena, and each has valid points. They can provide richness and depth that is invaluable in professional practice and life in general. However, theories are time-limited, because nothing is static and change is inevitable.

Nursing theorists

A significant number of nurses have written about nursing practice, beginning with Florence Nightingale. It is only recently, however, that nurses have moved from writing about *what* they do, to writing about *how* and *why* they do it. There are now a number of nursing theorists who provide a broad range of ideas that can be overwhelming for the student nurse. It is the application of these theories to practice that determines their usefulness. To help make sense of nursing theorists, Alligood & Tomey (2002) have outlined a method of ranking the different theorists into three categories:

- *philosophies*—this category uses higher-order constructs and propositions about the nature of nursing. An example is Rogers (1970), who defines nursing as a holistic science of human nature and development.
- *conceptual models/grand theories*—these theories are more practically derived and suppose an outcome. Examples are Henderson's theory (1966), which focuses on outcomes of nursing care, and Orem's theory (1971), which establishes the notion of self-care as integral to nursing.
- *middle-range theories*—these more closely describe practice issues for nursing (McEwan & Wills 2002). Peplau's 1952 theory (reprinted in 1988) focuses on therapeutic interpersonal processes in the nurse–client relationship, and has been very influential in mental health nursing.

As mentioned previously, theories reflect the theorist's world view at the time of writing. So a comparison of Florence Nightingale with a recent nursing theorist would demonstrate the constantly evolving nature of theory within a dynamic social context and in response to reflections on nursing practice. Theorists have contributed to the body of knowledge that describes nursing practice, leading to improvements in the discipline of nursing.

Incorporating theory into practice

How then do beginning practitioners make sense of what they read and incorporate this into their practice? This requires the ability to:

- think critically
- continually develop self-awareness
- identify your values, beliefs and attitudes and appreciate their origin
- modify your values, beliefs and attitudes
- tolerate and even embrace ambiguity
- be an *active* participant in the quest for knowledge.

The ability to think critically about what you read and what you do is essential. Critical thinking is an ongoing process that requires an open mind on a whole range of views. Just as important as the ability to think critically is the awareness that we are more likely to favour those theories that provide the 'best fit' with our already developed world view. We do this to alleviate the anxiety

we will experience if we choose a theory that is inconsistent with our already established thoughts. It is a normal subconscious process. This is an important concept to understand in the lifelong activity of becoming more self-aware.

The requirement to be self-aware and to think critically about the basis for your practice can be frustrating for beginning practitioners because there is no clear step-by-step 'cookbook'. Understandably, when nursing students, undergraduate and postgraduate, come into a course they want to be told what it is they need to learn and do in this new area so they can be effective and feel competent. From our experience it is not uncommon for students to want to collect a 'bag of skills' to prepare them for everyday practice. Nurses want to know what they can *do* to people so they can feel competent and alleviate the ambiguity about their practice. Students can become impatient and disgruntled if these skills are not given up front, and the course can be seen as 'airy fairy' or even useless. This is more likely to occur in students who prefer to be passive recipients rather than active participants in their professional development.

Your attitudes, values and beliefs underlie what you do when you work with people. It is these personal informal theories that provide the foundations for practice and determine which formal theories are more appealing to you. It is only with increasing self-awareness, critical thinking and reflection that the continual process of construction and reconstruction takes place and competent professional nursing practice develops. This process takes time.

The importance of reflection

Teaching skills by themselves will not improve clinical competence or performance. This statement is supported by research. *Reflection*, a component of the critical thinking process, has been shown to affect each nurse's individual understanding of a range of practice issues (Graham 2000). Reflection has also been shown to increase nurses' awareness and clarify aspects of themselves and their role. Read & Law (1999) found that one of the strongest predictors of change in nurses' attitudes was contact with people who had experienced mental health problems. This is understandable because it is not easy to hold preconceived attitudes once you have had experience in a new area. Inevitably the knowledge gained from this personal contact will challenge previously held beliefs and lead to their revision—we are more likely to fear what we do not know.

In part, this may help explain why the more highly technical areas of nursing practice may be desirable to beginning practitioners—they do not confront nurses with their views about mental health or their own mental health issues. Mental health nursing does require examining how a person understands themselves, others and their relationships. This can be a challenging but ultimately rewarding endeavour. It may be easier to avoid addressing these issues in other areas of nursing, but these skills are fundamental to all areas of nursing requiring human interaction.

THE CONTEXT OF NURSING PRACTICE

While formal nursing theories, our informal theories and the knowledge base of other disciplines inform the knowledge base of nursing practice, the context within which nursing education and health service provision take place also influence nursing practice. After all, practice is the application of knowledge and this does not occur in a vacuum.

Putting theory into practice

The implementation of practice based on theory is not straightforward. Practice settings can be complex because they require mediation between people with different views, philosophies, beliefs and ways of interpreting what is required for effective mental health practice. Added to this is the influence of political, social, cultural and environmental constraints. (These issues are discussed in greater detail in Chs 4 to 6.) However, the current push for evidence-based practice has particular implications for mental health practice, and these are discussed here.

Demand for evidence-based practice

Within Australia and New Zealand, and indeed most of the Western world, there is a demand that only those practices that have been shown to be effective be sanctioned in the provision of health care. This is known as evidence-based practice. Although there is a valid argument for this and intuitively it makes sense, it can be problematic in the provision of truly effective and meaningful mental health care, and it raises a number of issues that warrant further discussion.

Issues for discussion

1   Evidence-based practice is based solely on observable practices validated using the scientific method—The scientific method requires that practices, their rationale and the theories behind them be clearly identified and documented. The only form of practice (treatment) that meets this criterion is that which can be observed and measured (this is known as quantitative research). The 'treatment' must then be 'tested' (this is known as empirical evidence) and this is usually done through 'randomised controlled trials'. In such studies consumers of health services are divided into two groups. The first group is known as the treatment group and, as the name suggests, they receive the treatment that is the object of the study. The second group is known as the control group—they are matched to the treatment group for factors such as age, gender and status but they do not

receive the treatment. Both groups are monitored for changes in exactly the same way, usually by various types of well-defined outcome measures. The measures for the two groups are then compared to determine whether the treatment has been effective.

Although there is a valid argument for this approach, there is an equally strong argument that intuition and tacit knowledge (unspoken knowledge), which are ignored by the scientific method, are invaluable in improving the quality of mental health care and nursing care in particular. For example, the nature of the interactions between nurses and the people with whom they work is very important in determining outcome. This has not been comprehensively studied within nursing but it has in research on the outcomes of psychotherapy, which is very similar in nature. This research has consistently found that the 'non-specifics of psychotherapy' (genuineness, non-possessive warmth and unconditional love) are the most important in determining outcome (Hubble, Duncan & Miller 1999). These findings are important for the following reasons:

- It is not the (measurable) techniques that the professional uses, but factors to do with the nature of the relationship between professional and person, that are critical.
- In their relationships with people, professionals do use their intuition and unspoken knowledge base (tacit knowledge).
- What appears to be the key factor in determining a good outcome is the ability to use our humanness in a way that is healing.
- The above cannot be measured using the quantitative scientific method required for evidence-based practice as described above.

2   Evidence-based practice comes from the validated expert knowledge of professionals—Evidence-based practice is derived from the expert knowledge of professionals and what they believe to be important in treatment. Professionals decide what is important to study and they also devise the treatments used in research. Evidence-based practice does not come from the expert knowledge of people with the lived experience of mental distress and what works for them. Unfortunately it is all too common for people's lived experience to be discounted as unimportant because it is subjective and cannot be validated, and therefore it is omitted. Yet there is strong evidence (Roberts 2000) that valuing people's stories is essential to improving outcome, and this is the essence of the narrative approach in mental health.

3   Resolving the tension—Rather than argue for the benefit of one approach over the other, it is more useful to acknowledge the tension between the two approaches and then move on to appreciating how they can complement one another. Roberts (2000) argues that both are needed in medicine and psychiatry because narrative practices preserve individuality, distinctiveness and context, whereas evidence-based guidelines offer a foundation for what is reliable and generally correct. It is the practitioner who needs to bridge the gap between the two approaches, to both appraise the evidence and appreciate a person's meaningful experience (Palmer 2000).

To bridge such a gap it is important for the beginning practitioner to be aware of the factors involved in becoming competent in mental health practice. The ability to think critically is important, and reflective practice helps in this process. Reflection is a personal activity. When reflection takes place in groups (reflexivity), important dialogue between nurses about what they have learned can affect the shared meaning of the group. It enables not only the development of tacit knowledge in the beginning practitioner but also its articulation by experienced nurses. Welsh & Lyons (2001) found that if nurses were asked why they performed in certain ways they were able to provide a rationale. Intuition comes with exposure to a whole range of situations and people over time, and this tacit knowledge complements nursing knowledge. It is 'increasingly evident that it is far more than just theoretical knowledge that informs the practice of expert nurses' (Crook 2001, p 4). Articulation of experienced nurses' tacit knowledge allows it to be examined and verified (Welsh & Lyons 2001). This helps validate more of what actually happens in practice and thereby complements evidence-based practice.

The following section outlines some of the major changes in thinking about mental health practice and continues the theme of providing a context for understanding nursing practice issues.

CHANGING BELIEFS ABOUT THE FOCUS OF NURSING PRACTICE
From dualism to holism
Dualism is derived from the Cartesian idea (Rene Descartes 1596–1650) that there is a mind–body duality, the body being a passive agent or vehicle with an immortal soul separate and absolutely distinct from the body. The concept of dualism has made the body the domain of medicine, and the soul or moral features (mind) of the individual the domain of religion and philosophy.

Failure to see the interdependence (holism) of the mind and body has led to the view of the body as a machine, with technical advances in science considered the necessary interest of medicine. This view suggests that only scientifically observable phenomena and technical knowledge are valued (Short, Sharman & Speedy 1994). Within this paradigm medicine, including psychiatry, has increasingly focused on the person's symptoms to the exclusion of most other things.

Dualism: issues for mental health practice
In a dualistic approach to mental health practice:
- Health professionals are taught to look for syndromes (a collection of symptoms) and to value only that which can be observed (the basis of evidence-based practice).
- The focus is on deficits within the functioning of the brain, and this objectifies the person and their problems.
- The mind is not seen as influencing the physical body and vice versa.
- Traditionally, professionals have not been taught to value the meaning of the symptom(s) for the person or to understand the impact of the symptom(s) on the person's life.

NURSE'S STORY: The limitations of dualistic practice

When the authors of this chapter began mental health nursing (in the 1970s), which at the time was undertaken predominantly in large psychiatric institutions, our tasks were to observe people's signs and symptoms and document them in the person's file so the extent of the deficits could be noted and treated by the psychiatrists. The basic aim was to alleviate symptoms, primarily through medication, so the person could return to their home environment. People often stayed within the institutions for many years. During this time, the meaning and impact of these symptoms for the person were considered irrelevant. In fact, conversations along such lines were actively discouraged because it was believed that this would make the person's condition much worse.

One of the authors has a very vivid recollection of working in a 'back ward' (a ward for people with supposedly chronic and disabling illnesses requiring long-term care over many years) where one of the patients had exhibited a fixed delusion since she was admitted at the age of seventeen. At the time she was twenty-four years old and the 'delusion' was still just as distressing. The woman believed that her stepfather was the devil; she would become highly distressed whenever he visited with her mother, and the distress continued long after he left. The staff believed it was a delusion because they perceived the stepfather to be very caring and concerned about the woman's welfare. A young female doctor new to the ward decided to take up this woman's case because the delusion had not responded to medication. She went through the woman's file since admission and found that no one had actually talked to the woman about the content of the delusion (what it meant for her). When the doctor finally asked, the woman told her that she had been sexually abused by her stepfather from a very young age, and that for her he represented the devil.

Although this is a dramatic example, it illustrates the need for holistic practice and the need to include the meaning of the experience for the person and not limit practice to the observation of signs and symptoms.

- Meaning and purpose are considered to be within the realm of the mind, subjective and therefore of no scientific value because they are difficult to measure and standardise.

This dualistic position is no longer tenable because people with lived experience of mental distress have not found the focus on symptoms and problems helpful. What helps is an understanding of the meaning people make of their experience of mental distress, and the ability to assist them in managing the impact of this on their lives (Tooth, Kalyanasundaram Glover & Momenzadeh 2003) so they can participate fully in community life (Kalyanasundaram 2002).

Holistic practice within nursing has as its main goal the healing of the whole person, recognising the importance of the interrelationships between biological, psychological, social and spiritual aspects of the individual.

Holism: issues for mental health practice

According to a holistic approach to mental health practice:

- It is meaningless to separate out the 'parts' of a person as if they were discrete entities. A fundamental tenet is that the whole is greater than the sum of its parts (for example, a person's social needs cannot be separated out for treatment, but must be considered in relation to all aspects of the person).
- Attention is paid to all aspects of the individual and the interrelationship between them.
- Holistic practice attends to the person's relationships with others, society and the greater cultural context of the community.
- Principles underlying such practice include trust, hope, respect for individual freedom and allowing people to exercise their rights as citizens.
- A person's rights include their civil, social and personal rights, including the right of choice and the 'dignity of risk'.

The significant shift in thinking away from dualism towards an acceptance of holism has brought with it a much richer nursing experience that validates the complexity of life and cultural experience. Yet even our understanding of holistic practice has changed over time. In the past decade, holistic practice was promoted under the banner of bio-psychosocial care. However, the increasing emphasis on recovery-orientated practice has outdated that concept.

The continually expanding understanding of holism affects how mental health nursing is practised. For example, services are increasingly using combinations of traditional and complementary therapies. In services for people who have experienced torture and trauma, massage and counselling are routinely provided in recognition of the impact of the deep physical and psychological wounds left on the individual.

Many people are increasingly pursuing complementary and alternative health-care options, and mental health nurses can anticipate consumer expectations of accessing a range of care options. These include treatments such as acupuncture, therapeutic touch, massage, homeopathy, imagery and spiritual healing, to name a few. Respecting the individual's right to choose what type of health care they receive, and exploring the range of available options in a way that fully informs the individual not only of options but also of their consequences, is empowering practice.

Challenges arise for the mental health nurse practising a holistic approach within the mainstream health system, as the latter is based primarily on a medical, scientific approach geared to dualistic thinking rather than holistic thinking. In many practice settings, workforce shortages and pressure within health systems may present challenges for implementing holistic practice. (These issues are discussed in greater detail in Chs 4 to 6.)

From deficits to strengths

Just as there has been a shift from dualism to holism as a result of dualism's failure to provide an adequate basis for practice, so there has been a shift from focusing on deficits to working with strengths. As we have already stated, practice that is based on the medical model focuses on identifying signs, symptoms and what the person cannot do, so that a diagnosis can be made and a treatment plan devised to redress these areas of weakness or deficit. However, people who have experienced mental distress are more interested in focusing on what they *can* do, in order to move on with their lives and to live as normally as possible within their community (Deegan 1988).

Working with strengths was first used in education and is not a new concept. Educationalists found that focusing on a person's deficit and trying to fix it was likely to make

---

NURSE'S STORY: Holistic practice within a mainstream setting

Nurses working in the inpatient mental health facility of Alice Springs Hospital are continually challenged to provide holistic mental health care to indigenous people of the Central Australian region, who comprise approximately half of all admissions. Holistic practices include the encouragement of traditional indigenous practices alongside Western medicine. The mental health nurse provides Western treatment and counselling alongside indigenous traditional healers when the family indicates that this is necessary for the wellbeing of the person. The traditional healer, or *nangkeri*, is considered a crucial part of the care provided to indigenous people to address the cultural and spiritual issues for indigenous people receiving mental health care in Central Australia.

the person feel more anxious, blocked or even immobilised—the problem would often be exacerbated rather than alleviated. The inability of the person (and the professional) to solve the problem led to a sense of failure, and a downward spiral was not uncommon.

In a deficits-based approach, when mental health professionals think there is little hope of overcoming the difficulties the person is experiencing, the problem is to protect the person from experiencing further failure. It is typically suggested to the person that they should avoid stress, for example, by stopping work or stopping study. A person's right to have the dignity of risk is taken from them. We all have the basic human right to attempt what we choose, to succeed or fail and to learn from the experience—this is how we develop and grow. In practice, nurses should not advise against a person undertaking a particular activity, but instead work with the person to explore the advantages, disadvantages and possible consequences of an action so they can make an informed choice.

The focus on a person's deficits also reinforces the notion that the problem resides within the individual. Unfortunately, it has been common to blame the person for not responding to the clinician's intervention. It is important to keep in mind the old adage that people don't fail, programs do. In these circumstances pessimism rather than optimism prevails for all concerned, with a consequent stripping of hope.

In contrast, focusing on strengths values a person's resilience, aspirations, talents, uniqueness, what the person can do and how these strengths can be mobilised and built upon to overcome current difficulties. A key therapeutic practice is reframing from a pessimistic world view to an optimistic one that instils hope. For example, the nurse would want to know what the person has done in the past to overcome life's difficulties and how they could use the strength within themselves to overcome their current problems. The nurse encourages the person to think of ways that will work for them. The nurse does not impose his or her ideas but may offer suggestions, and works with the person to explore and create options. Nurses use the knowledge gained from a variety of sources to help in this exploration. The nurse works in partnership with the person—the nurse's role is to reinforce the person's plan and remind them of it if and when they do become unwell. An illness-focused approach is based on the belief that overcoming a problem merely returns the person to the status quo. A strengths-based approach, on the other hand, is inherently person-focused, and opens up a whole range of possibilities.

Focusing on strengths does not mean that problems and the illness are ignored, but rather that problems will be taken care of in the process of healing. For example, the person would be encouraged to understand their signs of becoming unwell and to devise a plan of action they believe would work for them. For some people with severe mental health problems these plans can be formalised and are called 'advance directives'. These spell out the person's wishes in regards to treatment and who they would like to advocate on their behalf should they be mentally unable to do so. In this way a strengths focus allows the practitioner to respect the person's abilities, beliefs, values, support systems, goals, achievements and resources even when they are acutely unwell.

There is limited research comparing the outcomes of strengths-based practices and standard care. However, there is evidence that although people receiving both types of treatment improved, those receiving strengths-based practices had their symptoms reduced by half (Barry et al. 2003), spent fewer days in hospital and were more satisfied with the services they received (Bjorkman, Hansson & Sandlund 2002).

Daniel Fisher (1994), a psychiatrist with lived experience of psychiatric disability (his term) highlights the importance of a strengths focus: 'I no longer search for the sickness in myself or in those I grew up with as an explanation for my woes. Instead I search for the strengths in myself and those close to me which propel me through my version of the suffering we all share but seldom face' (Fisher 1994, p 1).

Charles Rapp has been the leader in this strengths focus in mental health practice. He has written extensively on the subject and proposed the *strengths model* (1998), whose principles underlie the practice of modern case management. (Case management is addressed in greater depth in Ch 23.) A summary of the principles of his strengths model is as follows:

- The aim of strengths-based practice is to focus on the person's strengths and not on pathology, symptoms, weaknesses, problems or deficits.
- The community (social interactions) is viewed as an oasis of resources, *not* as an obstacle to working with people. The wider community provides far more naturally occurring resources than those that can be provided by mental health teams. The emphasis is on engaging people in existing community services rather than creating disability only services.
- Interventions are based on the principle of self-determination and nothing is done without the person's approval. The person determines their care and has the same right to make mistakes and learn from them as everyone else (this has also been referred to as the 'dignity of risk').
- The relationship between the person and their case manager is primary and essential. The case manager needs to be available and with the person when the going gets tough as well as in the good times.
- Assertive outreach is preferred to other forms of intervention. This is because you can learn a lot more about a person when you see them in the context of their environment.
- People with serious mental illness continue to grow, learn and change (Rapp 1998).

NURSE'S STORY: Moving from deficits-based to strengths-based practice

Lucy, a young Aboriginal woman, was referred to me by Aboriginal health workers from the community health centre. These workers had been called to see Lucy on repeated occasions over the years since she had left the Aboriginal children's home in which she was raised. Lucy presented with many health problems and had more recently been binge drinking and engaging in self-harm behaviour—taking overdoses and cutting herself.

When I began working with Lucy it was immediately apparent that her self-esteem had been shattered. She walked with her head bowed, felt great discomfort with eye contact, felt people were judging her and that no one cared about her. Unfortunately, her experiences in the emergency department after she had self-harmed reinforced her low self-esteem, because the nursing staff in the emergency department had responded angrily to her behaviour.

Working with Lucy to identify her strengths was an extremely slow and involved process of gradual engagement, building up trust, exploring her issues of loss and trauma, and assisting her to consider options she believed could improve her mental health. One of these was searching for family members through the Aboriginal Link Up program. Throughout this process, I actively reinforced every step Lucy took that demonstrated her ability to deal with life issues without resorting to binge drinking and self-harm behaviour. Lucy was encouraged to look at healthy ways of reducing stress, and started to focus on writing and playing music, two activities that had given her great pleasure when she was younger.

Several years into this process, Lucy had located many of her family members and dealt with the issues using healthy coping mechanisms. She is now employed as a musician and has a well-developed sense of self-esteem.

The critical nursing process of enhancing strengths in people who have relied on less positive ways of coping is demonstrated in the nurse's story above.

From patient to consumer

Consistent with the shift in focus from deficits to strengths is the change in terminology from 'patient' to 'consumer'. The word 'consumer' refers to people who have the lived experience of mental distress who have received care from mental health professionals. Generally people have challenged the use of value-laden terms because they can shape the interactions that arise between people. The term 'patient' is considered too bound up with illness and the medical model, with deficits, and with the disparity in status between patient and professional. The term 'patient' also implies a more passive role, with the person being the recipient of care. The term 'client' has similar connotations to 'patient'. The term 'consumer' implies a more active role, with the person having rights, responsibility and a more equitable relationship with the care provider. 'Consumer' is currently considered acceptable to most people, although some prefer the term 'user' or 'survivor'.

Consumers are the focus of mental health practice. The Mission Statement of the Standards of Practice for Mental Health Nursing in Australia and New Zealand emphasises the primacy of focusing on consumers to reinforce this goal and identifies some ways in which it may be achieved through nursing practice:

The primary focus of care is the consumer of mental health services. Nursing works in partnership with people as health care consumers, acknowledging and valuing their personal expertise and giving a specialised form of support as they work their way through a health-related experience.

(Australian and New Zealand College of Mental Health Nurses Inc. 1995)

Labels can be harmful and can significantly influence the interactions between people with lived experience and those who work with them. Nurses are in a powerful position in being able to influence community attitudes towards people with mental distress. We need to take every opportunity to communicate in ways that combat stigma, promote people's dignity, deepen community understanding, and contribute to interactions that are empowering.

From rehabilitation to recovery

In the previous discussions on the shift from dualism to holism and from deficits to strengths, it was reasonably easy to identify the difference between the concepts. However, this is not always the case with rehabilitation and recovery. We have chosen to address rehabilitation, a component of mental health services where nurses practice, in this section because of the tendency to talk about 'rehabilitation' as if it has been replaced by 'recovery'. The concept of recovery has not replaced rehabilitation but it has changed the way it is practised.

Psychiatric *rehabilitation* is provided for people who experience severe and enduring forms of mental illness, with the primary aim of reintegrating the person back into the community. Traditionally, rehabilitation aimed to optimise functional ability by focusing on deficits in a range of areas such as social, vocational, symptom management, activities of daily living (hygiene, cooking, budgeting, travel and so on) and accommodation. Professionals, including nurses, assessed the person's deficits to determine their rehabilitation needs and the person then attended a rehabilitation service where programs (often run by nurses) would address these skills deficits. This approach to rehabilitation has been criticised (Deegan 1988) because it requires people to progress through predetermined skills-based training programs regardless of individual needs.

Deegan makes a useful distinction between recovery and rehabilitation in mental health services.

Disabled persons are not passive recipients of rehabilitation services. Rather, they experience themselves as recovering a new sense of self and of purpose within and beyond the limits of the disability . . . Rehabilitation refers to services and technologies that are made available to disabled persons so they may learn to adapt to their world. Recovery refers to the lived or real life experience of persons as they accept and overcome the challenge of disability.

(Deegan 1998, p 11)

Hence there has been a significant shift away from highly prescriptive rehabilitation programs to recovery-orientated rehabilitation. Recovery-focused rehabilitation programs emphasise consumer-directed goals and outcomes, and maximise options in the setting of the consumer's choice.

Recovery begins the moment the person develops a serious mental health problem. It is both a personal act (something the person does) and an approach (how others facilitate the process). 'Recovery' has been difficult to define but it focuses on the person being able to live well with or without the illness. The following comprehensive definition by a leading Australian psychiatrist will be used for this chapter. It clearly articulates the many facets of recovery and provides direction for how others may assist in facilitating this personal experience.

Recovery is the uniquely personal and ongoing act of reclaiming and regaining the capacity to take executive control of goal-directed living that is satisfying, purposeful and meaningful, with self-perception as a contributing citizen after one or more encounters with a mental illness, sometimes even with the limitations and challenges imposed by the illness, its treatment and personal and environmental responses to it.

(Kalyanasundaram 2002, p 5)

In practice the nurse's role is to help facilitate a person's recovery, and mental health policies provide the guiding framework for such practice. Policies are based on current theories and knowledge in the field of mental health. Hence the philosophy of care is continually being revised and updated. In practice, there can be a time lag in the implementation of policies and this appears to occur in many countries throughout the world. This delay is in part understandable because of the lengthy process of developing policies and plans, educating the workforce on their implementation, setting up the structures and then providing the necessary resources. In the fast-changing area of mental health, there has been difficulty in keeping mental health practice, including nursing practice, current. (These issues are discussed in more detail in Chs 4 to 6.)

It is important to note that there is a philosophical difference between Australia and New Zealand in the orientation of their mental health policy documents and, hence, practice. In New Zealand the need for a recovery approach in the delivery of services is emphasised strongly (Mental Health Commission 1998), whereas the recovery approach is not addressed in Australian policy documents. We are aware of a number of practitioners in Australia who are incorporating a recovery orientation into their practice, but this is not advocated in policy. We have argued in the past (Tooth & Stanton 1993) that Australia's approach to mental health care lags about ten years behind other Western countries. For example, Anthony presented recovery as the guiding vision for mental health practice in America in 1993 (Anthony 1993). Recovery is now considered the most appropriate approach to guide practice and it informs this chapter.

Recovery-orientated practice is guided by thinking about what you do when you work with people, and this is influenced by your theoretical and experiential knowledge. We highlighted the centrality of the nurse's attitudes, values and beliefs in guiding practice at the beginning of this chapter. This position is consistent with New Zealand's Recovery Competencies for Mental Health Workers (Mental Health Commission 2001), which states that recovery practices are more often couched in terms of attitudes and knowledge than in terms of behaviour or sets of skills.

Superimposed on the above is the trend to use the words 'rehabilitation' and 'recovery' interchangeably—this use of language creates additional confusion, particularly for beginning practitioners. In some instances services that have been called 'recovery orientated' continue to be based on old rehabilitation practices (Jacobson & Curtis 2000). The distinguishing features of all services will be the principles of practice that guide them and how these are implemented—that is, it will be the values, attitudes and beliefs of the service, and the professionals who make up that service, that will determine whether the practices are truly recovery orientated. According to Jacobson & Curtis (2000) this necessitates a fundamental shift towards the sharing of both power and responsibility within the therapeutic relationship. The following section briefly addresses the current principles of recovery and the consequent implications for practice. (These are discussed more fully in Chs 21 and 23.)

CRITICAL THINKING CHALLENGE 2.1

How would mental health service provision be different if it was driven by consumers and meeting consumers' needs rather than the needs of mental health professionals?

PRINCIPLES OF RECOVERY-ORIENTATED PRACTICE

In the past decade, many consumers have written their stories of recovery and experiences of care, providing the initial impetus for the recovery movement (Deegan 1988; Lovejoy 1984; Unzicker 1989) and the push for recovery-orientated practice. People who have the lived experience of severe mental distress can and do recover, and to a very large extent their stories indicate that this has occurred without the involvement of mental health professionals—and, unfortunately, in spite of it in some cases. In light of this feedback, it is time we examined our practice to determine how we can best promote recovery. Practice needs to be person-orientated and respectful of people's lived experience and expertise. The following list of principles (Onken et al. 2002) provides an excellent frame of reference for this purpose.

- The service contends with more than the person's symptoms; it is holistic.
- The service promotes individual decision-making and taking of responsibility.
- The system meets basic human needs and addresses people's problems in living.
- It empowers people to move towards self-management of their condition.
- The system is orientated towards hope and emphasises positive mental health and wellness.
- The system assists people to connect through mutual self-help.
- It focuses on positive functioning in a variety of roles, building and rebuilding positive relationships.

The document entitled 'Recovery Competencies for New Zealand Mental Health Workers' (Mental Health Commission 2001, www.mhc.govt.nz) provides indicators of how recovery can be promoted through practice in mental health settings, and we encourage you to read it. Services need to contend with more than the person's symptoms by providing holistic care; and this care must meet basic human needs and address people's problems in living. Everyone needs a home, employment, a living wage and genuine control over their life. It is important that services are orientated towards hope and emphasise positive mental health and wellness.

Onken et al. (2002) provide a useful context for understanding recovery-orientated practice. They have organised the principles into three areas: personal characteristics/aspects of recovery; the complex inter-relationship between various services, systems, policies, cultures and society (that is, recovery-orientated service provision); and the nature of the relationship between all those involved in mental health. Each of these is discussed below.

Personal characteristics/aspects of recovery

Australian research (Tooth et al. 1997), supported by international research (Onken et al. 2002; Ralph 2000; Ridgeway 2001; Toper et al. 1998), has identified personal characteristics as the most important factor in aiding recovery. Specifically, consumers identified the following as the most important factors in their recovery:

self-determination; realisation of the need to help themselves and take responsibility for their illness; finding ways to monitor and manage the symptoms of their distress; optimism and spirituality. Recovery practice must allow active participation, provide choice, give hope and, above all, allow the person to discover meaning or purpose and direction in their life (Jacobson & Curtis 2000).

To facilitate this process, nursing practice needs to promote, rather than hinder, the active taking of control and responsibility for one's life. Nursing practice empowers the person to move toward self-management of their illness by promoting individual decision-making and personal responsibility. That is, nurses need to facilitate self-help.

Facilitating self-help

Care is the basis of nursing practice, and this creates tension between doing something for someone and encouraging people to care for themselves. There are times when fostering dependency by doing tasks for the person is necessary, but in many cases it is counter-productive.

Self-help is a valuable strategy that we all employ in dealing with life's challenges. We are experts on ourselves, with our own knowledge base of how we have coped in the past and what strategies have worked for us in dealing with life crises. However, there are times when our past coping mechanisms no longer work and we need to find new ways of dealing with difficult situations. In times of crisis or personal distress, individuals can become overwhelmed and lose sight of their own capacity for problem solving. At a practical level, the role of the nurse is to *be with* the person (listen to the person to understand their concerns, fears and experience) while at the same time helping the individual to tap into their own wisdom by reminding them that they have coped in the past, and reinforcing the value of their own self-knowledge. Nurses don't need to find the answers, but they do need to encourage the process of self-help and identifying the person's strengths so they can take effective control of their life. Such practice is important in building a sense of self-control and autonomy.

Box 2.1 'Being with' a person to promote self-help

Examples of questions the nurse can use:
- Can you help me to understand what the experience of . . . means for you?
- What are you most concerned about at the moment?
- Have there been other times in your life when you have had similar feelings?
- How did you overcome these difficulties in the past?
- What do you think you need now to help with your current situation?
- What do you know about yourself that will help you in your current situation?

The list in Box 2.1 is not exhaustive but it illustrates the therapeutic use of questioning. You are encouraged to complete the class exercise on self-help at the end of this chapter.

The process of self-help can be a protracted one when individuals are faced with illness or life situations that are either outside the range of their experience, or have consequences that require significant levels of adjustment. Nurses and other health professionals have an important role in both keeping hope alive for the person and in facilitating self-help in a practical way during this time. The process of adjustment to illness may involve moving through various stages of searching for help from others, until the individual realises that they do have the capacity to help themselves. The following quote from a consumer highlights this point.

> There wasn't much I could do at the beginning. When I started, basically I had to wait and the breaks would come. Like the people would accept the fact that I'm ill and eventually, if society, say, doesn't give me the means to heal myself, then they will leave me alone anyway and then I will have the choice and the chance of helping myself out, and that is what happened.

(Tooth et al. 1997, p 33)

Self-help can also involve seeking assistance and support from other people who have had similar experiences. Self-help groups are useful in assisting people to gain support, learn coping skills, tap into resources, find out information about health-care options, and realise new expectations on the basis of meeting people in similar situations (O'Brien, Kennedy & Ballard 1999). It is important for nurses and other health professionals to be available to such groups if their presence is requested. In practice the nurse's role is one of working with the group to determine their needs and then providing the necessary support in an empowering manner.

RECOVERY-ORIENTATED SERVICE PROVISION
The community

The right to treatment in the community has been enshrined in the United Nations Principles for the Protection of Persons with Mental Illness and for the Improvement of Mental Health Policy, and endorsed within the National Mental Health Strategy in Australia (Commonwealth Department of Health and Aged Care 2002) and the Blueprint for Mental Health Services in New Zealand (Mental Health Commission 1998). These rights emphasise the 'least restrictive alternative for treatment', with a focus on autonomy and respect for cultural background.

Services need to facilitate people's active and meaningful participation in the community and it is clear from listening to consumers that there is a need to consider a broader range of options than has traditionally been available within the mental health system. In addition, people's needs change over time and therefore services must be comprehensive and flexible enough to cater for these changes. Most importantly, the options must not tie consumers to mental health services, but rather promote options within the broader community (Anthony 2000).

To assist the person in this endeavour requires services to be orientated towards recovery. In practice there is a complex interrelationship between services (government, non-government and general community), systems, policies, cultures and society. Government health services form a small but important part of the assistance people require. People are likely to also come into contact with government disability support services, welfare services (for financial support), housing services, employment

---

NURSE'S STORY: What nursing can achieve in the community

Johanna, a 26-year-old woman, had recently emigrated from Armenia with her husband Frank and six-month-old son. Johanna was experiencing her second episode of major depression with psychotic features. Her previous psychiatric treatment prior to coming to Australia had been entirely hospital based, and when community care was suggested for this second episode of depression, Frank was reluctant to take any risks until Johanna was completely well. Frank was at work during the day, they had no family or friends in Australia, and he could not take leave to care for Johanna. Therefore he felt she would be safer remaining in hospital. Johanna was afraid that if she stayed in hospital as long as she did on her previous admission, she would not bond with her son. Frank was persuaded to support the option of community care when reassured that resources were available to provide support during the day. Family care workers were identified who were available to provide support in their home during the day. A small network of women from Armenia who met at the local migrant resource centre also provided much-needed social support.

The nurse in this situation used existing local community resources to provide support. These supports enabled Johanna to remain at home with her son and facilitated her recovery. The nurse provided education to Johanna about depression, medication and early warning signs, as well as addressing issues of health and stress management. Johanna reported that this episode of depression was not as prolonged as her previous one where she was hospitalised. She felt less isolated, more in contact with family and other people, and wanted to get better because she was encouraged by the normal day-to-day activity around her. Johanna felt confident that with the support of the nurse she could explore her illness and learn how to manage it.

services, from the non-government sector through to general services provided for everyone in the broader community. Collaboration and coordination between these various players is essential. At a practice level, case management aims to ensure that this occurs, and nurses are required to use high-level skills in coordinating these services and supports across multiple agencies where there are no formalised linkages in place (Reynolds & Inglis 2001). (Case management is addressed in detail in Ch 23.)

The mental health service

Within the mental health service there are a number of settings in which a nurse may practise. The most common of these include inpatient services in general hospitals, crisis teams, community mental health teams and rehabilitation services. Nursing practice in these settings will be aimed at: alleviating symptoms and distress; controlling and resolving critical or dangerous problems; obtaining the services the person needs and wants; developing the person's skills and supports in relation to the person's goals; engaging the person in fulfilling and satisfying activities; advocating for the upholding of a person's rights; providing the people, places and things the person needs to survive (e.g. shelter, meals, health care); facilitating self-help by encouraging the person to exercise their voice and make choices in their life; and promoting a healthy lifestyle. The focus of practice in the various settings will be determined by the person's needs at the time, and these change over time.

The nurse's story on p 22 illustrates how community mental health nurses can provide a range of supports for people to achieve outcomes that are not possible within a hospital-based treatment episode.

Multidisciplinary teams

Multidisciplinary teams are considered routine in the provision of mental health care within the community. The standard mix of disciplines within mental health teams includes nurses, psychologists, psychiatrists, social workers and occupational therapists. This mix of disciplines is seen as necessary to provide a holistic approach to care. The different professional groups provide complementary approaches that honour the complexity of the consumer. Each discipline has a body of knowledge and a framework for practice that emphasises different aspects of how to work with people. The framework of each discipline involves theoretical underpinnings that shape the approaches adopted by professionals.

While there are distinct approaches to practice that arise within each discipline, there are also significant core activities of mental health work that are common to all disciplines, such as the necessity of engagement and maintaining a therapeutic alliance, assessment and care planning in collaboration with consumers and carers, and many other basic activities (Kelly, Simmons & Gregory 2002). A growing number of postgraduate mental health

programs provide core competencies to professionals from all disciplines in mental health care in an interdisciplinary framework (Rolls, Davis & Coupland 2002). Supervision within multidisciplinary teams engages all disciplines in routinely reviewing team approaches and practices, and in shared philosophies that are implemented in a collaborative way toward achievement of positive consumer outcomes (Mullarkey, Keeley & Playle 2001).

No single discipline can prepare workers with the range of knowledge and skills required for the diversity that is encompassed in mental health practice. It is necessary for all professionals to respect and understand each other's skills and orientation for working in different ways, and to work collaboratively and interdependently. The orientation and discipline of any worker should not be seen to categorise or limit the capacity of that individual to develop a broad range of practice skills within the multidisciplinary team. Consumers frequently tell us that our credentials as human beings are the most important aspect of good quality care.

Health and wellness

Consistent with the holistic approach and a recovery orientation to service provision is a focus on promoting health, wellness and a healthy lifestyle. In policy documents this is referred to as promotion and prevention of mental illness. This focus on health and wellness needs to be considered by nurses in all practice settings where they enter into partnerships for health care. These practice settings include all mental health specific programs and services, general health settings and the broader community.

Mental health and wellbeing requires attention to needs such as shelter, food, meaningful occupation, a living wage and access to community facilities. Attention must also be given to those factors in the community that place people at risk of developing mental health problems. Promotion of mental health and wellness, early intervention and the prevention of illness is a major platform of the National Action Plan for Promotion, Prevention and Early Intervention for Mental Health 2000 (Commonwealth Department of Health and Aged Care 2000). The National Action Plan suggests that partnerships between a broad range of health and community stakeholders is necessary to influence health outcomes. Risk and protective factors that are common to a number of outcomes affecting mental health can be targeted from a population approach, as well as targeted to at-risk groups and high-risk individuals (health and wellness are discussed in greater detail in Part 2).

Non-government organisations

Non-government organisations (NGOs) play a key role in the provision of support to consumers and carers affected by mental illness through direct service delivery, complementing existing mental health services, and strengthening community supports and partnerships

(Commonwealth Department of Health and Aged Care 2002). This fundamental role in providing for the range of needs of people with mental illness is crucial in achieving community integration for people with mental illness. The role of the nurse is to be aware of the range of services offered by NGOs so this knowledge can be passed on to the people with whom they work. Nurses can also work with these organisations in activities such as raising community awareness. The nurse's story below is an example of an initiative by Rotary that was instigated by a mental health nurse.

The partnership between Rotary (non-government sector), consumers, mental health professionals and community members is a good demonstration of effective collaboration. Non-government supports are provided across a range of settings including: mental health specific services such as the Richmond Fellowship, the Schizophrenia Fellowship, mental health associations; and NGOs such as the Salvation Army, and service clubs that operate at a local community level to support people with a range of special needs within their communities, such as Apex, the Lions Club and Rotary.

The range of services provided by NGOs in the mental health sector include:

- direct service provision (e.g. residential services provided through the Richmond Fellowship)
- mutual support (e.g. the Association of Relatives and Friends of the Mentally Ill (ARAFMI))
- advocacy and information
- public education (e.g. Rotary)
- community development.

Within Australia and New Zealand a considerable range of consumer organisations provide advice, advocacy, support and service delivery. Some of the major national and state NGOs focused on consumer and carer issues are listed in Box 2.2. Many other organisations operate at the local level throughout Australia and New Zealand.

Box 2.2 Consumer organisations and useful websites

- Australian Mental Health Consumer Network is a national network for mental health consumers.
- Mental Health Council of Australia (MHCA) is an independent peak national body for mental health (www.mhca.com.au).
- Sane Australia is a national charity helping people seriously affected by mental illness (www.sane.org).
- Mental Illness Fellowship of Australia Inc. (formerly Schizophrenia Services) provides counselling, support, awareness and research.
- Association of Relatives and Friends of the Mentally Ill (ARAFMI) is a support group for families and friends.
- Te Puna Web Directory is a general directory to New Zealand and Pacific websites developed by the National Library of New Zealand/Te Puna Matauranga o Aotearoa (http://tepuna.natlib.govt.nz).
- Te Puna Kokiri provides information on Te Punu Kokiri and links to other Maori-related websites (www.tpk.govt.nz).

NURSE'S STORY: Rotary Australia—increasing understanding of mental illness

Rotary Australia has embarked on a series of community forums to support increased understanding of mental illness in the community.

In 2003 the Rotary organisation in Alice Springs held a public forum on mental illness, inviting well-known consumer activist Simon Champ as guest speaker, along with a local indigenous speaker, a local psychiatrist and a young woman who has experienced mental health problems. The aim of the forum was to promote public discussion on how the community could become a more caring and inclusive place for people who experience mental health problems. Each of the invited speakers gave their ideas on what could happen within the community to enable people with mental health problems to feel more included. This was followed by a general panel discussion where presenters answered questions from the audience.

The following outcomes were achieved:
- Members of the public who attended the forum reported a greater understanding of the experience of mental illness and the role of mental health services.
- After a venting of community concerns there was a general feeling of 'we are all in this together' and a spirit of collaboration was established.
- This breaking down of barriers resulted in a 'meeting of people' that was focused on the outcome of improving mental health in the Central Australian community; the latter activity gave heart to the consumers and carers at the forum because they could see a tangible outcome.
- The forum enabled people who had concerns about their own or a family member's mental health to approach service providers and representatives of self-help groups for assistance.
- A number of community members became involved for the first time in the peak NGO—the Mental Health Association of Central Australia.
- An effective ongoing working relationship was forged between the mental health services and Rotary, with plans for ongoing collaborative activities.

RELATIONSHIPS IN MENTAL HEALTH PRACTICE

It is important for all those involved in mental health practice to focus on positive functioning in a variety of roles, building and rebuilding positive relationships. In policy this issue is addressed under the headings of partnerships, participation and empowerment.

Partnerships, participation and empowerment

The concepts of partnerships, participation and empowerment are inextricably linked. A partnership between different service providers or other stakeholder groups as well as between service provider and service recipients invites participation that hopefully leads to empowerment, not just for consumers but for all concerned.

The Alma Ata Declaration on primary health care was built on the principles of equity and justice (World Health Organization 1978) and the key component was universal access to resources that would enable people to become more self-reliant and able to exercise control over their own health. Promoting health in this way enables people and their families to participate actively in illness prevention, its management and outcome.

The shift in focus from treatment to prevention stimulated formation of the informed-consent and consumer movements. People were better educated and informed about their choices, the risks and the benefits, and were searching for meaningful interactions with service providers. This paved the way for relationships such as partnerships to promote the dynamic dialogue required for this changing focus in health care, while at the same time reducing inequities between participant groups. You are encouraged to read the article by Gallant, Beaulieu & Carnevale (2002), which provides an excellent discussion of partnerships.

People's participation in mental health care occurs individually at a therapeutic level and collectively at a systems level. Participation at an individual level can be either passive or active (Townsend 1998) and there is tension between the two. Passive participation occurs when care is given to dependent recipients; active participation occurs when people are facilitated, guided, encouraged or supported to help themselves.

At a systems level there have been international as well as national changes in policy to include participation of consumers and carers in various aspects of the mental health system. This change has occurred because it was argued that consumers and carers are more in tune with consumer needs than are trained health professionals (Townsend 1998). Change at a practice level will require a significant increase in consumer involvement.

The shift in the World Health Organization's approach to health promotion towards a focus on people taking control of their own lives naturally led to discussions on empowerment. Since then the concepts of partnership, participation and empowerment have become fundamental principles underlying mental health practice. These concepts now appear in a range of health policy and educational documents worldwide. Empowerment has been a buzzword in the past decade, particularly in the case of mental health for people who have experienced serious emotional or mental distress. However, for some the implied need to be empowered has been seen as condescending because it implies that the person does not have power in the first place. Clearly this is not the case and again highlights the need for caution in making general assumptions about the wide range of human experiences and the meaning an individual makes of these experiences.

The most common form of disempowerment occurs when there is a failure to hear people's stories of their experiences and their problems of living (Barker 2001). When health professionals ask questions purely in order to feel they have performed their professional duties, disempowerment is likely to result.

Professional boundaries

The concept of professional boundaries relates to practices for ensuring a 'safe' environment for consumers that is predictable and based on ethical practice. Boundaries in mental health practice are vital in light of the historical legacy of abuses in psychiatry, the vulnerability of many consumers of mental health services, and the potential for harm inherent in the relationship between nurse and consumer. The behaviour that most clearly constitutes a boundary violation is sexual contact between mental health professional and consumer, an unquestionably prohibited behaviour.

Many other areas within the relationship between mental health nurse and consumer may constitute problematic behaviour—this may include physical contact, gift giving, self-disclosure, and personal or social involvement, depending on the circumstances. Behaviour in any individual relationship between mental health nurse and consumer is generally not bound in a fixed or rigid way, as this might inhibit the nurse's ability to respond to different individuals in whatever way is most relevant in a given situation.

The issue of professional boundaries arises because the nature of working in mental health necessitates the development of therapeutic relationships. In a New Zealand study (O'Brien 1999), mental health nurses were found to be aware of the risk of overstepping boundaries because of the contradiction arising from minimising the professional role and 'being natural' with consumers. However, this was seen as invaluable in establishing and maintaining a relationship. Similarly, community nurses saw 'bending the rules' to meet the individual needs of the consumer as an important part of their practice (professional boundaries are discussed in more detail in Ch 5).

CONCLUSION

We encourage you to reflect on how the principles of mental health practice are fundamental to all nursing practice regardless of setting. We hope we have encouraged you to think about how you can participate more fully in your practice by developing your awareness of the complexities and realities of the context in which practice occurs. More specifically, we hope you appreciate how your attitudes, values and beliefs play a crucial role in your everyday practice.

Mental health nursing practice is also influenced by an ever-evolving knowledge base; hence the principles informed by this knowledge base continue to change and evolve. Practice is time- and context-specific, making the ability to tolerate and incorporate change vital. Consequently your thinking about your practice will be continually influenced by your developing self-awareness, your incorporation of new ideas into your practice, and your increasing professional and personal experience.

The primary focus of mental health nursing practice is the consumer and how nurses can help facilitate the consumer's recovery. Nurses can assist in this process by working in partnership with consumers to help them realise their potential and tap into a wide range of community resources and supports, of which mental health services are just one. Just as importantly, we hope you find the experience of mental health nursing as rewarding as we have.

EXERCISES FOR CLASS ENGAGEMENT

Imagine yourself in the following situations.

SCENARIO 1

You have been hospitalised with an acute medical condition. Medical advice is that you have diabetes. You are being given instructions for self-management of insulin injections and monitoring of blood sugar levels before discharge from hospital.

SCENARIO 2

You have been hospitalised after an acute episode of depression. Medical advice to you is that there is a high likelihood that you have bipolar depression. You are being given instructions on the possible side-effects of the antidepressant medication you have been prescribed, and advised that you will have to continue taking some form of medication indefinitely.

Questions

In groups of four or five, discuss your thoughts and feelings about the above scenarios. Use the following questions as discussion points. Note similarities and differences in opinion among group members as well as between the two scenarios.

- What are your immediate concerns?
- What information would you seek?
- What type of support would you wish to receive, and from whom would you wish to receive it?

- What would be the most important knowledge and skills for nurses in the different care units?
- What could your nurse do that would be helpful or unhelpful?
- What do you think will be important considerations for the rest of your life?
- Do you think you should take an active role in your present and future care?
- How could this best be achieved?

SCENARIO 3

Emily is 36 years old and married to Grant, with whom she has two sons, aged five and seven. They have recently moved to a regional centre of Australia and have no family supports. Emily is currently experiencing her second episode of bipolar disorder, and she is in the hypomanic phase of her illness. Grant is very concerned about Emily's ability to be an effective parent but he also has longer-term fears about their relationship.

Question

- How could the principles of recovery-orientated practice be used to assist Emily? Focus on aspects of the client's recovery rather than symptom management.

REFERENCES

Alligood MR & Tomey AM 2002, *Nursing Theory: Utilization and Application*, Mosby, Missouri.

Anthony WA 1993, Recovery from mental illness: the guiding vision of the mental health service system in the 1990s, *Psychosocial Rehabilitation Journal*, 16(4), pp 11–23.

Anthony WA 2000, A recovery-orientated service system: setting some system level standards, *Psychiatric Rehabilitation Journal*, 24(2), pp 159–68.

Australian and New Zealand College of Mental Health Nurses Inc. 1995, Standards of Practices for Mental Health Nursing in Australia, ANZCMHN Inc, Greenacres, South Australia.

Barker P 2001, The Tidal Model: developing an empowering person-centred approach to recovery within psychiatric and mental health nursing, *Journal of Psychiatric and Mental Health Nursing*, 8(3), pp 233–40.

Barry KL, Zeber JF, Blow FC & Valenstein M 2003, Effect of strengths model versus assertive community treatment model on participant outcomes and utilization: two-year follow-up, *Psychiatric Rehabilitation Journal*, 26(3), pp 268–78.

Bjorkman T, Hansson L & Sandlund M 2002, Outcome of case management based on strengths model compared to standard care. A randomised controlled trial, *Social Psychiatry and Psychiatric Epidemiology*, 37(4), pp 147–52.

Commonwealth Department of Health and Aged Care 2000, National Action Plan for Promotion, Prevention and Early Intervention for Mental Health, Mental Health and Special Programs Branch, Commonwealth Department of Health and Aged Care, Canberra.

Commonwealth Department of Health and Aged Care 2002, National Mental Health Report 2002: Seventh Report. Changes in Australia's Mental Health Services under the First Two Years of the Second National Mental Health Plan 1998–2000, Commonwealth of Australia, Canberra.

Cox H, Hickson P & Taylor B 1991, Exploring reflection: knowing and constructing practice. In: Gray G & Pratt R (eds), *Towards a Discipline of Nursing*, Churchill Livingstone, Melbourne.

Crook JA 2001, How do expert mental health nurses make on-the-spot clinical decisions? A review of the literature, *Journal of Psychiatric and Mental Health Nursing*, 8(1), pp 1–5.

Deegan PE 1988, Recovery: the lived experience of rehabilitation, *Psychosocial Rehabilitation Journal*, 11(4), pp 11–19.

Fisher DB 1994, Hope, humanity and voice in recovery from psychiatric disability, *Journal of the California Alliance for the Mentally Ill*, 5 (recovery issue), pp 13–15.

Gallant MH, Beaulieu MC & Carnevale FA 2002, Partnership: an analysis of the concept within the nurse–client relationship, *Journal of Advanced Nursing*, 40(2), pp 149–57.

Graham IW 2000, Reflective practice and its role in mental health nurses' practice development: a year-long study, *Journal of Psychiatric and Mental Health Nursing*, 7(22), pp 109–17.

Henderson V 1966, *The Nature of Nursing*, Macmillan, London.

Hubble MA, Duncan BL & Miller SD 1999 (eds), *The Heart and Soul of Change: What Works in Therapy*, American Psychological Association, Washington DC.

Jacobson N & Curtis L 2000, Recovery as policy in mental health services: Strategies emerging from the states, *Psychiatric Rehabilitation Journal*, 23(4), pp 333–41.

Kalyanasundaram V 2002, Recovery: An Overview (unpublished manuscript).

Kelly T, Simmons W & Gregory E 2002, Risk assessment and management: a community forensic mental health practice model, *International Journal of Mental Health Nursing*, 11(4), pp 206–13.

Lovejoy M 1984, Recovery from schizophrenia: a personal odyssey, *Hospital and Community Psychiatry*, 35(8), pp 809–12.

McEwan M & Wills EM 2002, *Theoretical Basis for Nursing*, Lippincott Williams & Wilkins, Philadelphia.

Mental Health Commission 1998, Blueprint for Mental Health Services in New Zealand, MHC, Wellington.

Mental Health Commission 2001, Recovery Competencies for New Zealand Mental Health Workers, MHC, Wellington.

Mullarkey K, Keeley P & Playle JF 2001, Multiprofessional clinical supervision: challenges for mental health nurses, *Journal of Psychiatric and Mental Health Nursing*, 8(3), pp 205–11.

O'Brien AJ 1999, Negotiating the relationship: mental health nurses' perceptions of their practice, *Australian and New Zealand Journal of Mental Health Nursing*, 8(4), pp 153–61.

O'Brien PG, Kennedy WZ & Ballard KA 1999, *Psychiatric Nursing—An Integration of Theory and Practice*, Nursing Core Series, McGraw-Hill, New York.

Onken SJ, Dumont JM, Ridgeway P, Dornan DH & Ralph R 2002, Mental Health Recovery: What Helps and What Hinders? National Technical Assistance Center for State Mental Health Planning, (NTAC), National Association for State Mental Health Program Directors (NASMHPD), Alexandria, VA.

Orem DE 1971, *Nursing: Concepts of Practice*, McGraw-Hill, New York.

Palmer R 2000, Eating disorders, *British Journal of Psychiatry*, 176, pp 197–9.

Peplau HE 1952 (repr 1988), *Interpersonal Relations in Nursing*, Macmillan Education, London.

Ralph RO 2000, Review of Recovery Literature: A Synthesis of a Sample of Recovery Literature, National Technical Assistance Center for State Mental Health Planning (NTAC), National Association for State Mental Health Program Directors (NASMHPD), Alexandria, VA.

Rapp C 1998, *The Strengths Model: Case Management with People Suffering from Severe and Persistent Mental Illness*, Oxford University Press, New York.

Read J & Law A 1999, The relationship of causal beliefs and contact with users of mental health services to attitudes to the 'mentally ill', *International Journal of Social Psychiatry*, 45(3), pp 216–29.

Reynolds A & Inglis S 2001, Effective Program Linkages. An examination of current knowledge with a particular emphasis on people with mental illness, Australian Housing and Urban Research, Swinburne, Monash Research Centre, Melbourne.

Ridgeway P 2001, ReStorying psychiatric disability: learning from first-person accounts of recovery, *Psychiatric Rehabilitation Journal*, 24(4), pp 335–43.

Roberts GA 2000, Narrative and severe mental illness: what place do stories have in an evidence-based world?, *Advances in Psychiatric Treatment*, 6, pp 432–41

Rogers ME 1970, *The Theoretical Basis of Nursing*, FA Davis, Philadelphia.

Rolls L, Davis E & Coupland K 2002, Improving serious mental illness through interprofessional education, *Journal of Psychiatric and Mental Health Nursing*, 9(3), pp 317–24.

Short SD, Sharman E & Speedy S 1994, *Sociology for Nurses: An Australian Introduction*, MacMillan, Melbourne.

Tooth B, Kalyanasundaram V & Glover H 1997, Recovery from Schizophrenia: A Consumer Perspective, Report to Health and Human Services Research and Development Grants Program, Canberra, Australia.

Tooth B, Kalyanasundaram V, Glover H & Momenzadeh S 2003, Factors consumers identify as important to recovery from schizophrenia, *Australasian Psychiatry*, 11(1), pp 70–7.

Tooth B & Stanton V 1993, The relationship between mental health nurses' attitudes to treatment and the treatment setting in which they work, *Australian Journal of Mental Health Nursing*, 2(6), pp 273–80.

Toper A, Svensson J, Borg M, Bjerke C & Kufas E 1998, Recovery from severe mental disorders: a study of turning points, International Mental Health Network Conference, Trieste, Italy.

Townsend E 1998, *Good Intentions Overruled: A Critique of Empowerment in the Routine Organisation of Mental Health Services*, University of Toronto Press, Toronto.

Unzicker R 1989, On my own: a personal journey through madness and re-emergence, *Psychosocial Rehabilitation Journal*, 13(4), pp 71–7.

Welsh I & Lyons CM 2001, Evidence-based care and the case for intuition and tacit knowledge in clinical assessment and decision making in mental health nursing practice: an empirical contribution to the debate, *Journal of Psychiatric and Mental Health Nursing*, 8(4), pp 299–305.

World Health Organization 1978, Primary Health Care. Report of the International Conference on Primary Health Care, Alma Ata, USSR, 6–12 September.

Historical Foundations

Katie Evans

KEY POINTS

- The medical writers of Greece and Rome were able to recognise and differentiate between the major categories of mental illness.
- Graeco-Roman treatment methods for mental illness were generally compassionate.
- Research into the ancient literature shows that superstition and the supernatural were less influential on views about and treatment of the mentally ill than has been popularly believed.
- The family has traditionally cared for and nursed the mentally ill members of society for most of humankind's recorded history.
- Nursing has existed as a profession since Graeco-Roman times but references to nursing as a dedicated professional activity are sparse in the ancient literature.
- For most of recorded history, the function of mental health/psychiatric nursing is not distinguished from general nursing.
- Medical and nursing practices were less sophisticated during mediaeval times.
- Graeco-Roman knowledge was kept alive during mediaeval times in monasteries and in the East, and revived during and after the Renaissance.
- The asylum developed as a response to social conditions and the emergence of new, chronic psychiatric conditions.
- Institutional care and/or hospitalisation are relatively recent alternative treatment modes.
- Historical research can reveal the truth about the antecedents of accepted conditions such as schizophrenia and hysteria.

KEY TERMS

- asylum
- doctor
- family
- gender
- Graeco-Roman
- Greece
- historical
- history
- hysteria
- mediaeval
- mental disorder
- mental illness
- midwife
- nurse
- nursing
- research
- Rome
- schizophrenia
- superstition
- witches

LEARNING OUTCOMES

The material in this chapter will assist you to:
- discern the different ways in which mental illness has been constructed in past times
- examine the ways in which literature delineates and defines mental illnesses
- understand the ways in which diverse societies adapt to their mentally ill members
- appreciate the various approaches that have been used to treat the mentally ill in the past
- critique the hypothesis that treatment has progressively improved over time
- discriminate between compassionate and inhumane nursing processes.

INTRODUCTION

This chapter examines mental disorders, the ways in which they have been regarded, and the ways in which they have been treated in past times. It traces the transition from individual family care to the emergence of organised care for the mentally ill. The consequent professionalisation of the people who treat and care for sufferers of mental disorders is described, and it will become clear that it is difficult to distinguish between the activity of nursing the physically ill and that of nursing the mentally ill when mental illness is often seen in physiological terms. We will establish what constituted a mental disorder in past times and societies, and how mental disorder was regarded, and consider how these perceptions about mental disorder differ from those of today.

Each generation and society blends new knowledge with the inherited scholarship of the past. Occasionally the progression falters, as it did during the Middle Ages when the vast scholarship of the Graeco-Roman period was for centuries barely kept alive by the diligence of monastic orders in the West, and by Eastern scholars. Fortunately, Graeco-Roman discoveries in science and medicine, literature and the arts were recovered during the Renaissance and thereafter.

The British statesman Winston Churchill believed that studying history gave the modern politician a practical advantage, saying: 'The farther back you look, the farther forward you can see'(Howells 1991, p 1). An opportunity to reflect upon the historical precedents for prevailing mental disorders, and the ways in which they have been diagnosed and treated in the past, can enhance the richness and depth of contemporary clinical practice.

Mental disorder cannot be discovered by archaeology, or by any other means than written sources, and sometimes the terminology cannot be translated exactly. It is inevitable that in the millennia covered briefly in this chapter, attitudes towards mental disorder and the mentally ill, and even mental disorders themselves, will have changed over time. Also, as with our own society and culture, attitudes towards mental disorder probably would have differed within that society or culture at any given time. Both ancient and modern ideas about mental disorder and 'madness' are contextual and shifting. Sometimes the ancient world seems remarkably familiar, but there are moments when we realise how different is the world we inhabit now. We can learn from both the differences and the similarities. The history of a discipline or profession provides a common ground from which to evaluate clinical experience. We can learn from the mistakes of the past but we can also take pride in our predecessors' achievements.

THE VALUE OF HISTORICAL ANTECEDENTS

There is an increasing tendency to discount the historical antecedents of mental disorders and their treatment, as health and medical education abandons its emphasis on the teaching of Latin and Greek. Sigmund Freud and his colleagues received a sound classical education, which included the study of Latin and Greek, legend and mythology (Richards 1991). Just as the Greek language determined the nomenclature of most body parts and diseases, it has also influenced the naming of early psychoanalytic phenomena such as *mania* and *melancholia*, *neurosis* and *psychosis*, the *ego* and the *id* and the Oedipal and Electra complexes.

Perhaps it is the need to believe that modern medical science holds the key to a better world that leads some writers to deride the achievements of the past, or to ignore them completely. However, in some cases medicine, culture and society have not improved dramatically. Sometimes the past can hold valuable lessons and precedents which have been lost and which, when rediscovered, can assist us to achieve the best possible outcome for ourselves as health-care practitioners and for our clients. Suer (1995) says that modern French psychiatry is based on ancient medicine, and traces the survival in modern psychiatric care of ancient medical terminology, psychiatric terms (e.g. mania and melancholia), theories of aetiology (airs, climates and humours) and personality types.

Nursing is a genuinely ancient career with honourable credentials. Other professions use and even invent historical precedents to assist in the glorification of their own profession. For example, psychiatry as a profession has only slowly developed in the course of the past one hundred and fifty years since the American Psychiatric Association was commenced in 1844 with only thirteen members. Yet the influential medical historian and psychoanalyst Bennett Simon boasts that what makes the medical model 'unique' is the unbroken line which joins ancient and modern practitioners (Simon 1978).

Alexander & Selesnick, in their classic and much-reprinted psychiatry text, maintain that psychiatrists and psychiatry are the culmination of an intellectual and professional evolution which began with witch doctors and philosophers, and claim that: 'the precursor of the psychiatrist was any man who tended another in pain. The story of psychiatry thus begins with the story of the first professional healer' (Alexander & Selesnick 1966, p 3). It is clear that the possession of a lengthy historical pedigree is considered an advantage for a profession. For example, occupational therapists also claim that their chosen work has ancient Graeco-Roman origins in the treatment of mental disorders (Busuttil 1992).

Some nurses have also wished to demonstrate that their profession has existed since ancient times. For example, Doona (1992) claims as 'nurses' three women from the ancient literature, Euryclea, Cilissa and Medea's nurse, but none of these characters can be said to be 'nurses' as we understand the term today. All three characters are aged women who had in their youth 'nursed' or suckled children. They would not have cared for ill or wounded patients as would their modern 'nursing' counterparts.

In the present climate, which emphasises tertiary education, research and professionalisation in nursing, if nurses were to investigate and to own their own true history, how distinguished is the lineage they might claim! Nurses do not need to invent or inflate their historical achievements in order to celebrate them and commemorate their ancient colleagues.

Mental health nurses are not well served by existing mental health nursing texts if they seek to find out more about the history of mental health care or mental disorders. One standard mental health nursing text (Fontaine 2003) entirely omits the originators of the Western medical knowledge base—the ancient Graeco-Roman medical writers—and commences its historical overview with Florence Nightingale's *The Art of Nursing*. When this omission is compared with the conspicuous interest shown in treatment modalities such as Ayurvedic medicine, shamanic healing, naturopathy, animal-assisted therapy, aromatherapy and Reiki, the reader might consider the book's focus to be excessively present-centred.

Another text makes the statement that 'Little is written about nursing in early historical accounts because the care of the sick was considered an ordinary event—it seems that it was not important enough to record' (McAthie 1999). This statement is debatable on many levels. It assumes that because no research is known to the author, none was undertaken; and it reveals a lack of awareness of the greatly enhanced 'visibility' of women in literature and society in recent years. The social context in which Western nursing takes place today has altered enormously. Today's professional nursing, undertaken outside the home in institutions removed from the family, is an exception in the historical sense compared with the millennia during which nursing was undertaken by the family and their peripheral members, neighbours, slaves and servants, or later by religious orders.

The origins of medical care are addressed by McAthie (1999, p 4) in a brief and inaccurate statement using a text written in 1938: 'Religion and medicine were united very early, with medicine men, and later physicians, becoming priests'. This chapter will illustrate how an over-simplification of this kind can be misleading. Another standard mental health nursing text provides a similarly confused and barren coverage of the centuries preceding the eighteenth century. Boyd (2002) asserts that mental disorders in the first century AD were believed to be caused by sin or demonic possession and that 'clergymen' often treated patients by exorcism, which, if unsuccessful, led to the patients' being excluded from the community or put to death. But as we will see, the Roman writer Celsus (25 BC – c. 79 AD) lived and wrote in the first century AD, and the enlightened and humane methods he advocated for the treatment of the mentally ill could as well be used to great effect today.

Brief, inaccurate and negative appraisals of the historical precedents for the treatment of mental illness are,

sadly, all too common, as is the tendency to present the past in an inappropriately ethnocentric fashion. To Boyd, the *History of Psychiatric Mental Health Nursing* is relevant mainly in the context of the United States. A similarly narrow approach is taken by Frisch (2002) and by McAthie (1999), whose table of 'Significant events in nursing in the twentieth century' addresses only events that occurred in the United States. At least McAthie mentions the importance of the Nightingale model to the development of nursing programs in the United States, but Frisch's sole mention of the 'Nightingale model' is provided with no explanation or context.

Neither does Frisch (2002) differentiate between 'primitive cultures' which confused medicine, magic and religion, and 'early civilisations' such as the Graeco-Roman, wherein the vast Hippocratic Corpus is reduced to a statement that Hippocrates attributed melancholy to an excess of black bile and believed that a cure could be effected by bloodletting. Frisch represents mental health care in the millennia preceding the eighteenth century as exclusively custodial and restricted to the confinement of lunatics who were thought to be evil, witches or heretics—a feared, criminal population.

The reverse was more often true. Having a mental disorder in past times was not necessarily an impediment to leading a productive and consequential life. Ancient societies did not acknowledge many of the manifold mental disorders which are assiduously identified and isolated today, and in some ways they were more compassionate and tolerant than many societies today. It seems that the aim of modern medical or psychiatric writers in propagating exaggeratedly negative notions about the past is to emphasise the belief that things have changed for the better, a belief which might be meaningful to the health profession, but does no justice to the past.

PAST IDEAS ABOUT MENTAL DISORDER

The terms 'mad' and 'insane' are not acceptable medical terms for mental illness today, but these general terms have in the past been used to describe a wide range of symptoms and behaviours. The Latin word *insana* means 'not of right mind' and the equivalent Greek term is *mania*. The term 'mad' is a middle-English, pre-twelfth-century word which is still used today to describe a loss of reason and judgment. Metallic mercury poisoning in the felt-hat industry produced toxic effects which gave rise to the expression 'mad as a hatter'.

The idea of 'madness' in the ancient world usually implied mania or psychotic illness. Medicine recognised and treated mainly those mental disorders which disrupted a person's normal functioning in society, or which threatened the social order. Violence, agitation or excitement, being overtly out of touch with reality, experiencing hallucinations or delusions, melancholia causing inertia and inability to carry out one's normal tasks, or epilepsy, usually succeeded in attracting medical attention. As is the case in our own society, sometimes a person was called 'mad' because their behaviour differed from the usual societal norms.

There are some issues which we can examine to help us in understanding the ways in which mental illness might have been constructed in the past. The theory of the humours was a systematic hypothesis that sought to explain why some people were susceptible to certain kinds of illness, including mental illness. The humoural theory (see below) was still being applied in the nineteenth century, and has been correctly described as the first diagnostic classification system (Mack et al. 1994). Mental illness has in the past been seen by some as a punishment from the gods or God, and we will examine the role of the supernatural, and the perceived influence of God/gods upon the minds of humankind. The survival of some mental illness across different times and cultures will also be considered with the assistance of vignettes and case studies collected from primary source literature. Finally, the different meanings of 'madness' and the mental state which it implies will be assessed.

The 'humours'

Early Greek medical texts tended on the whole to view mental disorder as a physiological illness. This is generally the case in the earliest of these, the Hippocratic Corpus (c. 469–399 BC), a collection of works that were not all written by a doctor named 'Hippocrates', but by a variety of authors. The humoural theory was based on the belief that the body contained within it four humours—blood, phlegm, yellow bile and black bile—which were produced in various organs of the body. Each humour intrinsically possessed a basic quality such as heat, cold, dryness and moistness. Disease developed when internal or external factors disturbed the balance of the humours, and the imbalance produced injurious effects such as madness. Black bile and phlegm in particular caused mental illness, and an individual might be predisposed to mental illness because of hereditary factors. These theories are explained more fully in the Hippocratic Corpus: *The Nature of Man*, *Regimen I* and *The Sacred Disease*.

Some words which are still used to describe a person's personality derive from humoural theory. The description of a person as 'phlegmatic' (cold and sluggish) retains the ancient meaning, that the person suffered from an excess of 'phlegm'. The 'melancholy' person was believed to have too much 'black bile' in their system, which led to a form of depression, and the person who could be described as 'choleric' possessed excessive yellow bile, which made them passionate and easily angered. In the 'sanguine' person, blood predominated over the other humours, and in both ancient and modern times to be sanguine is to be confident and hopeful.

Mental disorder was believed to be especially prevalent in spring and at the beginning of winter when the humours were believed to be stirred into activity by changes in the weather. Each person was believed to have been born with a constitution in which 'dryness' and 'wetness', 'fire' and 'water' were mixed. Those with a preponderance of 'dryness' and 'fire' could be intelligent but also impetuous and inclined to more agitated forms of insanity, while those in whom 'coldness' and 'water' predominated were prone to fearfulness and depression.

Some aspects of the humoural theory are of a sophistication which is perhaps not appreciated by modern critics, but in fact the four-factor theory of temperament and body function has not only survived, it has been revived in the areas of personality assessment and the prediction of vulnerability to physical disease. (Hawkins 1982; Lester 1990; Merenda 1987). Research such as that currently being undertaken into the human genome similarly seeks to find some intrinsic yet individual factor which will explain why certain people are vulnerable to specific diseases, a continuation of the same quest that originally led to the devising of the humoural theory two and a half thousand years ago.

Supernatural influences

The *Diagnostic and Statistical Manual of Mental Disorders* (DSM-IV) (American Psychiatric Association 1994, p xxiv) cautions against labelling behaviour that is based in the religious beliefs of another culture as pathological:

A clinician who is unfamiliar with the nuances of an individual's cultural frame of reference may incorrectly judge as psychopathology those normal variations in behavior, belief, or experience that are particular to the person's culture. For example, certain religious practices or beliefs … may be misdiagnosed as manifestations of a Psychotic Disorder.

It has always been difficult in practice to differentiate religiously motivated behaviour from mental disorder. Research indicates that the more the religious beliefs of others deviate from the mental health professional's beliefs, the more liable the professional is to judge the others' beliefs as mentally unhealthy (Sanderson, Vandenberg & Paese 1999). Knowing this, the mental health professional needs to recognise their potential for making judgments based on erroneous religious or cultural assumptions.

Greece and Rome

Herodotus (490–425 BC) wrote *The Histories*, the first prose work ever recorded. He is our primary source of information about Cleomenes the First of Sparta, who reigned between c. 519 BC and 490 BC, so Herodotus could interview people who actually knew Cleomenes. Cleomenes' illness illustrates both an instance of ancient mental illness which culminated in suicide, and an evaluation by Herodotus, who is personally unable to decide between a superstitious cause and a rational one for Cleomenes' madness and death. He includes contemporary opinions about the cause of Cleomenes' illness.

CASE STUDY: Cleomenes of Sparta

According to Herodotus's informants, Cleomenes could have suffered from a mild form of mental illness throughout his life, but towards the end of his life he 'went quite mad' and his family had him confined to the stocks, bound and guarded. Cleomenes' subsequent suicide is reported in some detail.

   As he was lying there, fast bound, he asked his jailer, when no one else was there, to give him a knife. At first the man, who was a serf, refused, but Cleomenes, by

threats of what he would do to him when he recovered his liberty, so frightened him that he at last consented. As soon as the knife was in his hands, Cleomenes began to mutilate himself, beginning on his shins. He sliced his flesh into strips, working upward to his thighs, and from them to his hips and sides, until he reached his belly, and while he was cutting that into strips he died.

(Herodotus, *The Histories*, vi.75)

Herodotus reports the opinions of Cleomenes' contemporaries concerning his suicide. Some Greeks said he was being punished by the gods for his impiety, but his fellow Spartans believed that 'heaven had no hand in Cleomenes' madness, but by consorting with Scythians he became a drinker of strong wine, and thence the madness came' (vi.84). The Spartans were a pragmatic people, and they were better acquainted with the man, his behaviour and the events surrounding his death. Their attribution of Cleomenes' death to prosaic, organic causes, and their specific rejection of the theory that Cleomenes' madness was divinely inflicted, is proof that mental illness was not universally believed to be the result of divine punishment.

In the case study below, Plutarch (c. 50 – c. 120 AD) relates that Alexander the Great acted upon religious convictions and advice when he put to death a person who was mentally ill, deluded and hallucinating.

Alexander the Great was harsh upon this man because he believed that if the god Serapis had instructed the man to wear Alexander's crown and robes, this could be an omen foreshadowing his own death. Perhaps it is scenarios such as this which lead many modern authors to believe that mental illness was always punished harshly, or regarded by ancient societies with superstitious dread (Blakemore 1988; Devereux 1970; Dodds 1951; Hershkowitz 1998; Parker 1983; Roccatagliata 1991; Rosen 1968; Simon 1978; Stone 1997). This position is not wholly supported by the evidence. Perhaps there was a clear line of demarcation between the medical position on mental disorder and 'popular' attitudes and beliefs.

The Greeks seem generally to have differentiated between disease-induced madness and divinely caused madness. The Hippocratic Corpus (c. 469–399 BC) states that the gods were more likely to purify and sanctify than to harm, and derides doctors who assigned a supernatural cause to epilepsy or mental disorder, denouncing them as charlatans who were at a loss because they did not know how to treat the patient and 'sheltered themselves behind superstition' (*The Sacred Disease* II–IV).

The medical term *melancholia* was used by both the Greek comic playwright Aristophanes (c. 457–385 BC) and the Greek politician Demosthenes (384–322 BC), evidence that medical terminology was in common usage by as early as the fifth century BC. In Plautus's (c. 254–184 BC) *The Menaechmi* the doctor inquires as to whether a patient's disorder was due to possession or hallucinations, indicating that although possession was a recognised 'disorder', it was clearly able to be distinguished from hallucinations by the medical profession, popular playwrights and their audiences.

The Hippocratic Corpus's disapproval of superstition was still shared by Roman society over five centuries later, when Soranus of Ephesis (98–138 AD) stated in his work on gynaecology that the best midwives were free from superstition, and did not 'overlook salutary measures on account of a dream or omen or some customary rite or vulgar superstition' (Book I.II.4).

Perhaps two different attitudes toward mental abnormality coexisted in classical antiquity: the traditional one, which was 'superstitious and magical' and attributed abnormal behaviour to supernatural intervention; and the other, which is found in the medical literature, which rejects the supernatural or the divine agency as an

---

CASE STUDY: Plutarch, *Life of Alexander*, LXXIII–LXXIV

[Alexander] was playing at ball, and when it was time to dress again, the young men who were playing with him beheld a man seated on the king's throne, in silence, wearing the royal diadem and robes. When the man was asked who he was, he was speechless for a long time; but at last he came to his senses and said that his

name was Dionysius . . . and for a long time had been in chains; but just now the god Serapis had come to him and loosed his chains and brought him to this spot, bidding him put on the robe and diadem and sit on the throne and hold his peace. On hearing this, Alexander put the man out of the way, as the seers directed . . .

explanation. Medical terms were adopted and used by the public, and they coexisted with superstitious or religious beliefs about possession and divine punishment. This would be a similar situation to that in which we might believe in both medical technology and in 'the stars' or astrology, simultaneously.

The Christian era

The spread of Christianity did not eliminate the association in some quarters of mental illness with the influence of supernatural agencies. Instead, the belief that the old pagan gods caused mental illness was translated into a belief that the devil might be at work when a person experienced hallucinations or delusions. In the late thirteenth century the Inquisition began to deal with isolated cases of supposed witchcraft involving heresy, but it was not until the fifteenth and sixteenth centuries that mass persecutions took place, involving accusations of night-flying, intercourse with the devil, transformation into animals and malicious spells. Both the sufferers from mental illness and those associated with them, or believed to have injured them, could be the objects of suspicion and ill-treatment.

By the 1630s the tide was beginning to turn against the persecution of witches, and influential writers such as Robert Filmer denounced witch-hunting. The American colonies were slow to react to European trends, and in 1692 one hundred and fifty 'witches' were tried and nineteen were hung in Salem, Massachusetts. The cause of the bizarre behaviours of the adolescent girls involved have been hypothesised by modern scholars as being due to ergot poisoning or mycotoxin (Woolf 2000), but whatever the cause, when the hysteria died down, public revulsion resulted in the annulment of the convictions and the release of those of the convicted who had survived. This event marks the virtual end of witch-hunting.

During a period of around two centuries a number of so-called 'witches' were put to death, but the figures on 'wise women' killed as witches because they were healers seem to be greatly exaggerated in some sources. Perhaps the emergence of the women's liberation movement in the 1970s and its adoption by early nursing scholars contributed to a discourse wherein women's unrecorded and uncelebrated role as healers was being explored. The persecution of witches for practising inherited healing arts seemed to offer some explanation for the failure of women to be recognised as health professionals. However, it is difficult to locate research evidence to support assertions that 'millions' of witches or 'wise women' were killed in societies which were basically illiterate. Neither is there any indication that all of the witches who were persecuted were practising healers or that all healers were persecuted as witches.

MENTAL DISORDERS FOUND IN GRAECO-ROMAN SOURCES

What follows is the result of comprehensive research into mental disorders in the ancient Greek and Roman literature (Evans 2000).

The *mood disorders* or affective disorders (see Ch 15) consisting of mania and depression, alone or in combination, were found to exist in the ancient literature, although the term *melancholia* evolved in meaning over the centuries. It by no means always meant the equivalent of 'depression', in the way it is constructed today. The most convincing and earliest conclusive instance of major depression was that suffered by the prominent Roman lawyer, statesman, philosopher and author, Marcus Tullius Cicero (106–43 BC). At his most despondent, Cicero tended to withdraw from the Roman society in which he was celebrated, and retire to the country, as his surviving letters testify. Cicero wrote to his friend Atticus on most of the days they were separated, and his copious correspondence clearly documents three diagnosable episodes of major depression. An excerpt of one of Cicero's letters is shown below.

The *anxiety disorders* (see Ch 17) as they were manifested in the ancient world have not previously been the subject of a great deal of critical attention in the modern secondary literature, but convincing examples of anxiety disorders are described in the classical texts. The case study from the Hippocratic Corpus (see overleaf) describes two ancient examples of phobic avoidance, and that which follows from Plutarch describes an instance of post-traumatic stress disorder.

Both the anxiety disorders and the *personality disorders* (see Ch 16) were acknowledged by ancient cultures to be serious, chronic mental irregularities which could influence the sufferer's life, but they were not considered to be illnesses which required treatment. A number of examples of personality disorders have been identified, but since the concept of a personality disorder is often culturally determined, particular care was taken to ensure that the subject of the case study was considered by their peers to have differed from societal norms.

CASE STUDY: Cicero, *Letters to Atticus*, Astura 9 March, 45 BC

In this lonely place I do not talk to a soul. Early in the day I hide myself in a thick, thorny wood, and don't emerge till evening. Next to yourself solitude is my best friend.

When I am alone all my conversation is with my books, but it is interrupted by fits of weeping, against which I struggle as best I can. But so far it is an unequal fight.

CASE STUDY: Hippocratic Corpus, Volume VII; *Epidemics* 5.81–2

Nicanor's affection, when he went to a drinking party, was fear of the flute girl. Whenever he heard the voice of the flute begin to play at a symposium, masses of terrors rose up. He said that he could hardly bear it when it was night, but if he heard it in the daytime he was not affected. Such symptoms persisted over a long period of time. Democles, who was with him, seemed blind and powerless of body, and could not go along a cliff, nor on to a bridge to cross a ditch of the least depth, but he could go through the ditch itself. This affected him for some time.

CASE STUDY: Plutarch, *Life of Alexander*, LXXIV.1–4

[Cassander] had only recently come to Babylon, and when he saw some Barbarians doing obeisance to Alexander, since he had been reared as a Greek and had never seen such a sight as this before, he laughed boisterously. But Alexander was enraged, and clutching him fiercely by the hair with both hands dashed his head against the wall ... Cassander's spirit was deeply penetrated and imbued with a dreadful fear of Alexander, so that many years afterwards, when he was now king of Macedonia and master of Greece, as he was walking about and surveying the statues at Delphi, the sight of an image of Alexander smote him suddenly with a shuddering and trembling from which he could scarcely recover, and made his head swim.

There was in the ancient literature evidence which affirmed that *epilepsy* was believed to be related to mental illness. Epilepsy can exhibit psychiatric sequelae, but whereas it was considered to be a mental disorder in the ancient world, it is not so regarded today. The *substance-related disorders* (see Ch 19) were, conversely, not in ancient times conceded to be mental disorders, although drunkenness might lead to socially unacceptable behaviour. Alcohol-related disorders proved to be a complex topic; examples of these disorders were located in ancient Greek and Roman literature. Indeed, although excessive alcohol consumption seems to have caused or complicated many medical conditions, ancient medical and societal opinion seemed to indicate that conditions such as alcohol abuse, dependence and withdrawal went largely unrecognised (Evans 2000).

Some *psychotic disorders* (see Ch 14) were documented and recognised as such in the ancient Graeco-Roman literature, but this author's research indicates that the full gamut of criteria which would justify a modern diagnosis of schizophrenia (early onset, hallucinations, delusions and a degree of chronicity) was not apparent anywhere in the ancient Greek and Roman texts (Evans, McGrath & Milns 2003). The reportage of symptoms for all of the major mental disorders in the ancient literature was often inadequate to satisfy modern diagnostic criteria with reference to the duration and range of symptoms.

MENTAL DISORDERS NOT FOUND IN THE ANCIENT LITERATURE

The case study of King Cleomenes of Sparta (on p 32) provided evidence that although his contemporaries might have considered Cleomenes to be chronically insane, and that he had a psychotic episode which was well documented, a diagnosis of schizophrenia could not be made. Indeed, although the anxiety disorders and major depression appear to have survived in the exact form in which they present nowadays, indicating that these disorders can be said to be stable across time and culture, schizophrenia appears not to have manifested itself in the same way, or perhaps not to have existed in classical times (Evans, McGrath & Milns 2003).

Historical perspective on schizophrenia

Michel Foucault, the French philosopher considered by many to have made a significant contribution to our understanding of the social construction of madness, commences his study with the fifteenth century (Foucault 1967). Foucault had no medical background and does not describe his subjects with sufficient clarity to allow clinical diagnoses to be made. To Foucault, 'madness' encompassed a bizarre collection of disorders: melancholia with delusional guilt, melancholy allied with mania, nymphomania, delirium, vertigo, hysterical convulsions, hysteria and hypochondria.

Some of Foucault's subjects appear to suffer from a form of chronic, lifelong 'madness' which disabled them from undertaking productive work, so they are identified with 'the indigent'. They are represented as deluded, demented and hallucinated, reduced to an animal state in which they are inured to 'hunger, heat, cold, pain' (Foucault 1967, p 74). Frequent references to the ability of the 'mad' to endure physiological hardship suggest a degree of neurological damage. Perhaps they were the victims of syphilis, which Grmek (1991) believes had emerged in Europe by then. Perhaps they suffered from chronic schizophrenia, if indeed this disorder had evolved by the late Middle Ages.

Research into the origins of schizophrenia have led some to conclude that not only has schizophrenia changed in its manifestation within the past fifty years, but that it might exhibit such different symptoms in different cultures as to cause one to question whether the diagnostic criteria refer to the same condition (Ellard 1987; Jeste et al. 1985). Other reputable researchers believe that schizophrenia appeared in recent centuries. H. Fuller Torrey and his colleagues have investigated the origins of schizophrenia, and they postulate that the disorder is the product of a genetic mutation which occurred in recent centuries. Supporting evidence has been collected of viral-associated sequences in the brains of individuals suffering from schizophrenia (Yolken et al. 1997). It has been hypothesised that urban birth, household crowding and/or the transmission of a virus from household cats could assist the spread of the virus (Torrey & Yolken 1995, 1998; Torrey, Bowler & Clark 1997).

The state of medical knowledge at present can assist in tracking the development and dissemination of new or unfamiliar diseases, but if schizophrenia emerged in a less technical and literate society, its advent would have gone undocumented. Mental illness leaves no trace on skeletal remains; it can only be traced in the surviving literature.

CRITICAL THINKING CHALLENGE 3.1

If schizophrenia were proved to be of viral origin, how would that change the way in which the disorder is regarded by society and the medical profession?

'Hysteria': a translation error

The familiar term 'hysteria' is not an ancient Greek word and does not appear in any Greek dictionary or lexicon of Greek words. A number of ancient passages which have been interpreted as referring to a mental affliction arising in the womb appear to refer only to physical gynaecological complaints. The problem resides in the translation. The evidence suggests that the translator has bestowed a modern and anachronistic meaning upon the Greek text that is not supported by the evidence (King 1993).

It is a remarkably durable belief that 'hysteria' is a feminine mental disorder which has been recognised since the days of Hippocrates. This belief confers upon hysteria a spurious respectability, whereas it was proved conclusively over a decade ago that the term 'hysteria' was invented by Littre, the French translator of the Hippocratic Corpus in the late nineteenth century. Helen King's informative scholarship will be briefly summarised, because 'hysteria' is still considered to be one of psychiatry's most celebrated apparent legacies from the ancient medical literature, and once something passes into the inherited 'knowledge' associated with a discipline, it is hard to eradicate even if it is untrue.

Since Freud 're-discovered' hysteria it seems that male therapists have been especially keen to reinforce the notion that women have always been prone to gender-specific ills,

and that men can cure them. Bennett Simon (1978) described Freud's psychoanalysis of a female patient's 'hysterical expression of the thwarted sexuality of the recently widowed young woman' and added that 'Greek doctors knew that virgins and widows were most susceptible to those diseases of the womb called "hysterical"' (Simon 1978, p 25). In fact, Simon devotes an entire chapter in his book about mental illness in ancient Greece to hysteria and social issues, commencing with the statement that 'Hysteria, the disease of the "wandering uterus" was given its name by the Greeks' (Simon 1978, p 238). The respected psychiatric textbook, Kaplan & Sadock's *Synopsis of Psychiatry*, attributes Hippocrates with having 'introduced the terms "mania" and "hysteria" as forms of mental illness in the fifth century BC' (Kaplan, Sadock & Grebb 1994). But 'hysteria' is not a Greek word, and therefore Hippocrates did not use it.

Acceptance of the fact that 'hysteria' was a mental illness typically found in women and first described in the Hippocratic Corpus is dependent upon the incorrect translation of the words *hysterike*, *hysterika* and *hysterikos*, words which translate as 'suffering in the womb'. King (1993) found that hysteria is in reality 'but a mare's nest, a spurious entity' (Gilman et al. 1993, p xi). *Hysterikos* was not considered to have connotations of mental illness in the ancient literature. The Emile Littre (1839–61) edition of the Hippocratic Corpus translates *hysterikos* as 'hysteria', in French *hysterie* (King 1993, p 7). By examining the original Greek texts, King found that Littre's chapter headings, such as 'Hysterie', have no analogies in the Greek manuscripts; Littre freely transposes the medical categories of his own time. King concludes that Littre translated the Hippocratic Corpus in the mid-nineteenth century, when the psychiatric condition 'hysteria' had begun to be a debated ideology. He expected to find hysteria in the text, and of course he found it, and composed his headings accordingly. The diagnosis was therefore made by the translator (King 1993, p 8).

It is probable that Celsus's translator, Spencer, was similarly influenced. The error was perpetuated in Spencer's 1935–38 translation of Celsus. Spencer notes for example that in *De Medicina 5.21.6* the woman's 'fits' would have been 'hysterical fits'. Similarly, Spencer appends a footnote to indicate that the *Hippocratic Corpus: Aphorisms* V 35 is 'a description of hysteria' when it is more properly translated as 'suffering from illness in the womb'. Freud collaborated with Joseph Breuer to produce *Studies in Hysteria* in 1895. If *hysterikos*, meaning in Greek 'afflicted with suffering in the womb', is translated as 'suffering from hysteria', it is clear that the translation is influenced not by the original language of the text but by the meaning which Charcot, Freud and Breuer attached to the psychiatric diagnosis of 'hysteria' in mainly female patients in the late nineteenth century (Evans 2000).

King suggests that in 'hysteria' we do not hear 'the insistent voice of a fixed entity calling across the centuries':

Nineteenth-century hysteria, a parasite in search of a history, grafts itself by name and lineage onto the centuries-old tradition of suffocation of the womb, thus making Hippocrates its adopted father. It is time that father disowned his hybrid child.

(King 1993, p 64)

Unfortunately, the parasite hysteria remains attached to Hippocrates in the minds of many, despite being conclusively disowned, because historical research is too often ignored or disregarded.

GENDER AND HEALTH CARE

In Western countries we are now used to considering nursing to be a profession suited to either gender. Indeed, psychiatric mental health nursing was predominantly the province of the male nurse since asylums were created to confine the seriously mentally ill who could not be accommodated in society before the development of neuroleptic medication in the 1950s, because males possessed an advantage in terms of strength.

In past centuries nursing was considered to be the natural province of women, an extension of the maternal, caring role, but the absence of women in the literature has made nurses and nursing difficult to trace. The classicist who wrote an early essay entitled 'Ancient Nursing' wrestles with what he sees as the absence of nurses in the ancient world: 'so little is told us of nurses and nursing. The conclusion we are tempted to draw from this silence is that the task of nursing fell to the women, whether slaves or free, of the household' (Jones 1923).

The usual attitude towards 'respectable' women in ancient male-dominated societies was conservative and patriarchal. Ancient ideas about how women should conduct themselves are encapsulated in Pericles' speech to the Athenian women in 430 BC:

Perhaps I should say a word or two on the duties of women to those among you who are now widowed . . . the greatest glory of a woman is to be least talked about by men, whether they are praising you or criticising you.

(Thucydides ii.46)

Women have traditionally been poorly educated, and little has survived of the writing that the educated few have accomplished. Most ancient authors wrote about their male, aristocratic peers, and because so much of the literary evidence from most centuries preceding the most recent two or three is limited by the writer's upper social class and male gender, much historical research cannot accurately report the incidence of any type of illness in the female gender. Where women are mentioned, whether in the medical literature, in the histories, in biographies of their menfolk, in fiction or in poetry, it is from the perspective of a male and any such account cannot be said with certainty to represent the authentic female experience.

Women usually appear in the ancient medical literature in their reproductive role, in relation to childbirth and any gynaecological disorders which might prevent or complicate childbirth. Most health problems a woman might have were attributed to the possession of a womb. The Roman poet Martial (c. 40 AD – 104 AD) records that when male doctors were called in to treat 'women's complaints' both they and their female patient's true motives were probably sexual. Note that the modern, mistaken term 'hysteria' has been used by the translator instead of the more correct translation 'pain in the womb'.

One day Leda announced to her aged husband, 'I'm suffering from hysteria. I'm sorry, but I'm told that nothing but intercourse will make me feel cheerier'.

(Martial, *The Epigrams*, 11.71)

'Leda' had been attended by female nurses, but they leave when the doctors arrive, whereupon the doctors 'hoist and prise open her legs' with the exclamation: 'Ah, serious medicine!'. The male doctors are depicted as eager to 'treat' this illness fabricated to procure the sexual services of younger lovers. In a society where medical practitioners were male, the ailments of women, being outside the experience of men, could be seen as counterfeit, even if the prevailing masculine ideas about the innate immorality of women did not intrude.

'Leda' was an upper-class woman, but in the course of their lives most women were unlikely to be treated by a male physician. In fact women probably received little medical attention that was unrelated to reproductive affairs, and they would have treated themselves and their dependants in the seclusion of the women's quarters.

CARING FOR THE MENTALLY ILL
Graeco-Roman origins of Western care

In ancient Greek and Roman times the Greek hero and god of healing, Asclepius, whose staff wound about with a snake inspired the present symbol of medicine, was commemorated by temple healing centres called 'Asclepions'. Treatment consisted of a combination of medical and priestly practices but the main ceremonial treatment practised there was the ritual of incubation (temple-sleep and the interpretation of dreams). In the Hippocratic Corpus it is said of dreams: 'For when the body is awake the soul is its servant, and is never her own mistress, but divides her attention among many things . . . but the mind never enjoys independence. But when the body is at rest, the soul administers her own household . . .' (Regimen IV, LXXXVI).

This recognition of the importance of the unconscious as expressed in dreams was surprisingly sophisticated, and the prominence given to dreams in the ancient world was not equalled until Freud's work in the area two and a half thousand years later. Yet the Asclepion was not an infallible remedy. In his play *The Wasps*, Aristophanes, the Greek writer of comedy, depicted a case of dementia which was treated initially by purification rites and a stay in the Temple of Asclepius, but the only treatment which was effective in preventing the demented patient from leaving the house was putting the house under guard and having every opening covered with netting. Graeco-Roman medical science and theory were highly sophisticated, but medical treatment was predominantly the concern of the individual, with perhaps assistance from the medical practitioner if the family was prosperous.

When he showed signs of a violent mental disturbance, Cleomenes of Sparta, who reigned between c. 519 and 490 BC, had been confined to the stocks by his family, who kept him bound and guarded. Despite this, he managed to trick the jailer into giving him the knife with which he suicided. The Roman medical writer Celsus (25 BC – before 79 AD) wrote five centuries after the time of Cleomenes, but it is clear that the kind of treatment which was considered suitable for the person who was mad and violent in Roman society had not changed a great deal in the intervening centuries. First, Celsus differentiates between the several forms of insanity:

> some among insane persons are sad, others hilarious; some are more readily controlled and rave in words only, others are rebellious and act with violence; and of these latter, some only do harm by impulse, others are artful too, and show the most complete appearance of sanity whilst seizing occasion for mischief, but they are detected by the result of their acts.

(Celsus III.18.3)

Celsus prescribed distinct interventions for the fearful, the violent, the melancholy and those who exhibited 'untimely laughter' (III.18.10). He allowed that those who 'merely rave in their talk, or who make but trifling misuse

of their hands' ought not to be constrained unnecessarily, but he recommends that it is best to fetter those who are violent 'lest they should do harm, either to themselves or to others. Anyone so fettered, although he talks rationally and pitifully when he wants his fetters removed, is not to be trusted, for that is a madman's trick' (III.18.4).

This description perfectly fits the treatment accorded to Cleomenes. The mentally ill person who was violent presented a challenge in the era before the advent of the major tranquillisers in the 1950s. There was little alternative to physical restraint as a means of preventing the violently mentally ill from harming themselves or others, and physical restraint was, as it sometimes still is, the only means of preventing harm to the person or the environment.

Yet Celsus was basically humane and he respected individual differences. He recommended that the patient not be frightened, that they be kept in an environment that was reassuring, either in the light or in the dark, whichever was the most 'quieting of the spirit' for the patient. 'It is best, therefore, to make a trial of both, and to keep that patient in the light who is afraid of darkness, and him in darkness who is frightened by light' (III.18.5). Celsus forbade restraint for any longer than was required, and recommended that the restraint be removed the moment it was unnecessary. Just as the prevention of harm to the patient or to others is still regarded as a legitimate reason for restraining a patient under the mental health legislation of many countries, including Australia, it also remains a legal requirement that restraint be alleviated as soon as is practically possible.

Celsus outlines a medley of responses that can be helpful in treating various mental disorders. The variety and sophistication of his suggested interventions can be seen as the birthplace of counselling techniques that are used in mental health nursing to this day. In the examples which follow, the patient is depressed and/or anxious. He is at home, and the simple yet effective suggestions were meant to be followed by family or friends.

> *Some need to have empty fears relieved, as was done for a wealthy man in dread of starvation, to whom pretended*

ETHICAL DILEMMA

Now that those who merely rave in their talk, or who make but trifling misuse of their hands, should be coerced with the severer forms of constraint is superfluous; but those who conduct themselves more violently it is expedient to fetter, lest they should do harm, either to themselves or to others.

(Celsus, *De Medicina*, III.18.4)

The regulation that the patient be prevented from harming themselves or others is still regarded as a legitimate reason for restraining a patient under most mental health legislation. Celsus forbade restraint for any longer than was strictly

necessary, saying: '[sometimes] there is nothing else to do but restrain the patient, but when circumstances permit, relief must be given with haste'.

(III.18.6)

Question

Is physical restraint too primitive a treatment for the mentally ill client who is violent? The forced ingestion of tranquillisers is often seen as a more humane alternative. Is chemical restraint a more humane or less humane alternative to physical restraint?

legacies were from time to time announced ... in others, melancholy thoughts are to be dissipated, for which purpose music, cymbals, and noises are of use ... More often, however, the patient is to be agreed with rather than opposed, and his mind slowly and imperceptibly is to be turned from the irrational talk to something better.

(Celsus, *De Medicina*, III.18.10–12)

Reassurance was clearly used to good effect, and it is interesting that the invention of good news to enhance hopefulness was not considered unethical if it was effective. The patient was to be entertained, distracted and amused. Other suggestions included reading to the patient, games and storytelling 'especially by those with which the patient was wont to be attracted when sane', and praising any work the patient was able to produce. People who the patient liked and esteemed were urged to eat with them to stimulate their appetite and to 'gently reprove his depression as being without cause' (Celsus, *De Medicina*, III.18.18).

In 331 AD, around seven centuries after the Hippocratic Corpus was written, and two and a half centuries after Celsus wrote, the Roman emperor Constantine the Great decreed that the Church should take responsibility for the care of the sick after a plague (perhaps anthrax) devastated the Roman Empire. The first public hospital in Europe was founded by a Roman woman, Fabiola, at Ostia near Rome in 390 AD. Europe has had a strong tradition of health care by religious orders which has continued across the centuries since that time.

Eastern medical care

It is Ceylon which holds the honour of establishing the world's first hospital in 437 BC. At around the same time one-third of the population of Athens died of the plague (typhus or smallpox) without the benefit of organised medical assistance. The first public hospitals in India were founded in 256 BC, and the medicines used were supplied by the ruler (Mellersh 1999).

The Indian public hospital system had developed upon egalitarian principles and by 400 AD it offered free treatment to all regardless of wealth or rank. Indian hospitals had become the benchmark, and the idea was transferred to China, although in China hospitals were usually only available to the fee-paying elite. After 430 AD when the rebellious Christian sect, the Nestorians, had been exiled from Constantinople, taking Greek medical texts with them, India and Persia used the texts to make independent medical and scientific progress (Mellersh 1999).

After the fall of the Roman Empire, the Greek and Roman medical texts survived, having been copied and kept by religious orders in the West. This knowledge was both adopted and enhanced by the Eastern scholars; by 660 AD, Indian physicians had developed sophisticated bladder and digestive tract surgery. In the ninth century a hospital was established in Baghdad which by the tenth century had become the largest medical faculty in the

world, with twenty-four physicians. Whereas Western medicine and health care stagnated until around the twelfth century, Muslim, Japanese and Chinese scholars developed extensive surgical, anatomical and pharmacological expertise (Mellersh 1999).

Western developments

The East retained its scientific ascendancy as the Catholic faith gained control in Europe. Access to health care in Europe in the Middle Ages was limited to that provided by religious orders at hospices which could care for those few in society who did not have family to provide services for them. The Christian church was instrumental in forestalling some forms of medical research by forbidding practices such as the mutilation of the dead. This tended to hamper the training of medical personnel, the study of anatomy and eventually surgical interventions of most sorts.

Indian physicians had developed sophisticated bladder and digestive tract surgery at much the same time as the Hotel Dieu was opened in Paris (660 AD). The Hotel Dieu was technically a hospital but was more concerned with treating the patient's soul than their ailments. In the fifteenth and sixteenth centuries the Renaissance had reawakened European scholarship and engendered advances in many fields, including health care. Flamel had established fourteen new hospitals in Paris, St Thomas's hospital had been established in London, and universities proliferated throughout Europe (Mellersh 1999).

As time progressed, society changed and the health-care needs of the population changed too. During the eighteenth and nineteenth centuries the Industrial Revolution caused rural societies to be disrupted due to many of their inhabitants deserting their rural homelands to seek work in the factories and manufacturing towns, thereby removing themselves from the traditional sources of societal and family health care. This coincided with an apparent upsurge of schizophrenia in industrialised societies. Schizophrenia appears not to have existed in the ancient Greek or Roman worlds (Evans et al. 2003) and some researchers postulate that it evolved comparatively recently, sometime in the seventeenth century (Jeste et al. 1985), causing a crisis in the evolving health-care systems and demanding the creation of new solutions.

The asylum

Chronically ill and displaced populations required the creation of institutions which could cater for their needs. For some time little distinction was made between the mentally ill and other persons unable to exist independently in society. The dissolution of the monasteries in England in 1536 had restricted funding of hospitals by the Church, but previous to this many early hospitals and carers had been allied with the Church. The mentally ill were confined with others most in need of care and detention: lepers, criminals, the indigent, the unemployed and the ill. Perhaps a vestige of the confusion this caused between mental illness, indigence and wickedness can be found in the stigmatising view of the mentally ill which has persisted to this day in some societies.

By 1400 Bethlehem Hospital in London ('Bedlam') was devoted to the treatment, or more correctly the confinement, of the mentally ill, and in 1851 Colney Hatch in London was built, the largest lunatic asylum in Europe. It was desperately needed. At this time there were in the United Kingdom alone some 3579 'lunatics' in public asylums, 2559 in the 139 licensed houses devoted to the treatment of mental illness, and 8000 more in workhouses or at home. The asylums were characterised as 'warehouses for the unwanted', the aged, destitute vagrants, alcoholics and syphilitics. Europe and the United States followed suit (Mellersh 1999).

Custodial care was for a long time the only option if a mental disorder followed a chronic, disabling course in the absence of modern psychotropic medications, which were only developed less than five decades ago. Macalpine & Hunter investigated the alleged mental disorder of King George III, which they attribute to the medical condition porphyria (Macalpine & Hunter 1969). It is clear that some of the methods of treating perceived mental disorder had not altered significantly in the two millennia since Hippocrates. The King was cupped, bled, and dosed with emetics and purgatives, secluded from family and friends, and physically restrained for the protection of himself and others (Macalpine & Hunter 1969).

CRITICAL THINKING CHALLENGE 3.2

- What would be some of the disadvantages, difficulties and changes for the client, the family and for society if the mentally ill were cared for by the family?
- What would be the advantages for the client and for society if the family was solely responsible for the care of the mentally ill?

DOCTORS AND NURSES

The amount of medical knowledge that existed in ancient times could be learned by an educated person of average intelligence. The concept of role specialisation in health care was less developed in the pre-modern eras, and the amateur was not sharply distinguished from the professional. Even where roles such as 'doctor', 'nurse' or 'midwife' existed, their areas of expertise would be quite different from what they are now. For example, the midwife could be employed for the birth by wealthier families, but she relied upon family members for assistance,

and handed the baby to wet nurses, who assumed the care of the infant.

Furthermore, it is impossible to distinguish between psychiatric mental health nurses and general nurses until relatively modern times, because the distinction between disorders of the mind and disorders of the body is of relatively recent origin. In this respect, ancient nursing was more holistic than it is today, when the distinctions between the disciplines appear to be stressed more than the similarities.

Ancient Greece and Rome

There were instances noted as early as Homer (c. eighth century BC) of systematic nursing of patients. The *Iliad* (c. 800 BC), which describes the Trojan War, depicts the wounded as being removed to tents dedicated to healing, and tended mainly by captured slave women under the direction of Greek surgeons, although on the battlefield the 'nurses' were more often men attached to the military force.

The Roman writer Celsus is an important source for the history of medicine, but it is doubtful that Celsus was a practising physician. The philosophers Plato and Aristotle, amongst others, wrote about medical subjects although they had no formal medical training. The Greeks formalised scientific medical training at recognised medical schools such as Cos, Cnidos and later Alexandria. The early Greek doctor had no special status but, like a craftsman, he travelled from town to town and most probably employed his pupils as nurses. There was no form of licensure, but pupils were bound by an agreement: the *Hippocratic Oath* is one early form of private contract (Hornblower & Spawforth 1996).

In the Hippocratic Corpus it appears that in the absence of the doctor the patient was attended to by family members, slaves or medical students, who reported the patient's progress to the doctor. The sensitive advice from the Hippocratic Corpus (shown below) would be useful for any person who cared for an individual who was physically or mentally ill.

The Roman poet Martial (c. 40–104 AD) probably exaggerated when he said that the doctor who attended him had forty-five students with ninety hands who examined him, but there would have been some students in any case. We may assume that a great deal of the information given in the clinical histories such as the *Epidemics* is the result of their observations and those of the family or carers. The information gathered about the patient required an awareness of what was significant and what was not, which means that responsible and intelligent laypersons would have been satisfactory sources of

---

NURSE'S STORY: Hippocrates: Volume VII; *Epidemics* 6.4.7

Kindnesses to those who are ill. For example to do in a clean way his food or drink or whatever he sees, softly what he touches. Things that do no great harm and are easily got, such as cool drink where it is needed. Entrance, conversation. Position and clothing for the sick person, hair, nails, scents.

NURSE'S STORY: Celsus, *De Medicina*, Vol I, Book III, 6.6

The bath and exercise and fear and anger and any other feeling of the mind is often apt to excite the pulse; so that when the practitioner makes his first visit, the solicitude of the patient who is in doubt as to what the practitioner may think of his state, may disturb his pulse. On this account a practitioner of experience does not seize the patient's forearm with his hand, as soon as he comes, but first sits down and with a cheerful countenance asks how the patient finds himself; and if the patient has any fear, he calms him with entertaining talk, and only after that moves his hand to touch the patient. If now the sight of the practitioner makes the pulse beat, how easily may a thousand things disturb it!

---

information. The nurse's story above warns the reader of the sensitivity required when 'the practitioner' approaches the patient. The exact role of 'the practitioner' is never specified.

Mistrust of doctors was apparently widespread in ancient society. Compare the reflective and idealistic image of holistic health care conveyed in the two excerpts with the distrust the poet Martial, who was roughly contemporary with Celsus, exhibits below.

I was unwell. You hurried round, surrounded
By ninety students, Doctor.
Ninety chill, north-wind-chapped hands then pawed and
probed and pounded.
I was unwell: now I'm extremely ill.

Martial 1972, *Epigrams*, 5: IX

In the Roman-occupied lands—that is, most of what we know today as Europe, as well as North Africa and the Middle East—there existed a lively alternative culture which could be xenophobic about doctors, who were usually Greek and foreign. These people often applied and further developed traditional folk remedies in treating families and large households.

Sometimes it was the male head of the household who nursed the sick or directed their treatment. The Roman senator Marcus Cato (The 'Censor') was suspicious of Greek doctors so he wrote a book of prescriptions, recipes and regimens, and used it successfully to treat himself and his family. Plutarch says: 'By following such treatment and regimen he said he had good health himself, and kept his family in good health' (Plutarch, *Marcus Cato*, XXIII, 3–4).

Midwives and nurses
One male author who offers posterity a glimpse of those previously invisible in the literature—women, infants and a whole array of health personnel including midwives, nurses and assistants of various kinds—is Soranus of Ephesus (c. 98–138 AD), who wrote the earliest surviving text on gynaecology, building on some earlier sources that have not survived. Soranus was a renowned physician from the Greek city of Ephesus on the Mediterranean coast of what is now Turkey, who worked during the reigns of the Emperors Trajan and Hadrian. Most of the good medical schools were Greek, and their graduates travelled the world plying their trade. However, Soranus wrote for the benefit of the female midwife and for the wet nurse, who both fed the infant and treated childhood ills. Both appeared to be independent practitioners who were called in by the family when they were required.

The translation of *The Gynecology* in 1956 by Owsei Temkin, Professor Emeritus of the history of medicine and a former director of the Johns Hopkins Institute of the History of Medicine, is clearly a product of a time and culture in which the midwife had a role subordinate to that of the doctor, who made the command decisions as the natural leader of a 'medical team'. Culture-bound beliefs led Temkin to make unwarranted authorial comment about the text, in which he assumes that although the midwife herself is consistently addressed by Soranus, she must be 'working under the supervision of a physician'. This is incorrect.

The first part of *The Gynecology* (see opposite) describes the necessary attributes of a midwife, and this passage has a timeless quality. Soranus could be describing the ideal modern nurse (or nursing student) and it is significant that many of the skills she must possess, such as sympathy, reassurance and the sharing of secrets, would encourage a therapeutic relationship which would benefit the mental health of the client. Note that the midwife is required to be a female, whilst elsewhere in the work the doctor is presumed to be a male.

The ancient Greek midwife was clearly well trained. The skills she was expected to master were many, and they included many which might be considered to be traditionally medical functions, such as independent practice, diagnosis, prescribing and case management. She also selected and supervised the wet nurse, who was also skilled in treating the ailments of childhood. The translator Temkin felt that it was 'more natural' to think that *The Gynecology* was addressed to physicians, who could then 'explain' it to the midwife, but Soranus's text is clear that the physician was only called to assist the midwife in her duties if the labour had been obstructed and surgical intervention was required to extract the fetus by hooks and embryotomy (IV; III [XIX], 9 [61]).

To conceal the true role of the ancient Greek midwife as an independent professional practitioner is to remove her historical importance, while simultaneously consolidating the dominant role of the physician. The reader is furtively

NURSE'S STORY: Soranus's *Gynecology*, Book I.1.1-3: 'What persons are fit to become midwives?'

She must be literate in order to be able to comprehend the art through theory too; she must have her wits about her so that she may easily follow what is said and what is happening; she must have a good memory to retain the imparted instructions (for knowledge arises from memory of what has been grasped). She must love work in order to persevere through all vicissitudes (for a woman who wishes to acquire such vast knowledge needs manly patience). She must be respectable since people will have to trust their household and the secrets of their lives to her . . . She must not be handicapped as regards her senses since there are things which she must see, answers which she must hear when questioning, and objects which she must grasp by her sense of touch. She needs sound limbs so as not to be handicapped in the performances of her work and she must be robust, for she takes a double task upon herself during the hardship of her professional visits.

NURSE'S STORY: Soranus's *Gynecology*, Book I.II.4: 'Who are the best midwives?'

It is necessary to tell what makes the best midwives, so that on the one hand the best may recognize themselves, and on the other hand beginners may look upon them as models, and the public in time of need may know whom to summon. Now generally speaking we call a midwife faultless if she merely carries out her medical task; whereas we call her the best midwife if she goes further and in addition to her management of cases is well versed in theory . . . trained in all branches of therapy (for some cases must be treated by diet, others by surgery, while still others must be cured by drugs . . . able to prescribe hygienic regulations for her patients . . . she will be unperturbed, unafraid in danger, able to state clearly the reasons for her measures, she will bring reassurance to her patients, and be sympathetic . . . She will be well disciplined and always sober, since it is uncertain when she may be summoned to those in danger. She will have a quiet disposition, for she will have to share many secrets of life . . . she will be free from superstition so as not to overlook salutary measures on account of a dream or omen or some customary rite or vulgar superstition.

being instructed: this is the way it always has been—the midwife would be breaking with an age-old tradition should she (or he) seek more autonomy. Remarkably, Temkin's interpretation has not previously been challenged by nursing scholars, perhaps because of an indifference to the importance of historical research and inquiry in nursing.

The midwife has retained her importance in the lives of birthing women. Many centuries after Soranus, Charles Dickens incorporated the character of the nurse and midwife Sairey (or Sarah) Gamp in his novel *Martin Chuzzelwit* (1844) when the practice of nursing had begun to be reformed. In the exaggeration of her fondness for tea and strong liquor, Gamp is usually cited by nurses as an example of the type of nurse who was made obsolete by the Nightingale training system (Summers 1997).

It is possible that a society could hold respectful and ribald views of midwives simultaneously. The Roman dramatist Terence (c. 186–159 BC) wrote roughly simultaneously with Plautus, but his midwife Lesbia, summoned to attend a childbirth in *The Girl From Andros*, is a serious, sober and independent practitioner (Terence 1976). Perhaps Gamp was meant to be a caricature in the tradition of the midwives in classical Graeco-Roman writers of comedy, in much the same way as nurses are depicted in modern television dramas, films, books and advertisements in roles that run the gamut from skilful professional to scantily clad temptress.

PIONEERS AND PROFESSIONALISATION

To many nursing scholars Charles Dickens' fictional character Sarah Gamp represents the earliest, and one must say the worst, historical role model in nursing. There is an understanding that previous to that time nursing was the exclusive province of the religious orders, both male and female, or the domestic amateur, but as this chapter has demonstrated, the roots of the nursing profession extend much further back than the nineteenth century, and for most of this time it is not possible to isolate mental health nursing from general nursing. The body of knowledge contained in the ancient texts delineates a competent practitioner, technically expert, systematic, professional and well respected. St Vincent de Paul formed the association later named The Sisters of Charity in 1617, and they combined general nursing with caring for the insane. The care delivered to the mentally ill ('lunatics') in asylums was harsh—indeed, if the asylum was overcrowded, as was often the case, the jail was considered an appropriate alternative.

It often happens that a number of advances in an area are made almost simultaneously. This was the case with nursing, and nursing the mentally ill in particular. Despite slower communication methods and transport, new ideas were shared and each advance fuelled further advances in key areas across the world. Each of the English-speaking countries has its own nursing pioneer who is credited with bettering the lot of the mentally ill.

Unusually, in the days when women were relatively constrained in what they could achieve, the pioneer general nurses were predominantly women. Nightingale incorporated both religious and feminine attributes when she called nurses 'sister', spoke of nursing as a 'vocation' and dressed nurses in the nun-like uniform and coif (Chatterton 2000). However, the establishment of the asylum system in the middle of the nineteenth century provided both the impetus for the evolution of mental health nursing as a profession distinct from general nursing (Hamblet 2000) and a different gender balance from that which applied in general nursing. Asylums also ensured that mental health nursing developed along institutional lines in both the United Kingdom and its colonies.

In the asylums, more male attendants were employed initially for their strength, although photographs of asylums in the nineteenth century clearly show female nurses, dressed in the starched general nurse's garb of the period (Chatterton 2000). Since the introduction of neuroleptic medications in the middle of the twentieth century, and with the increasing emphasis on professional qualifications, attendants became nurses, endowing this branch of the nursing profession with an enduring tradition of male practitioners.

The United States

Dorothea Lynde Dix (1802–1887) is credited with responsibility for mental health care reform in the United States. Dix was not a nurse, but a teacher who ran a Sunday school class for the inmates of the local asylum, who were kept in uncomfortable and unsanitary conditions. From the mid-1840s she successfully lobbied states in the United States and Canada for better mental health care and state-run hospitals. During the American Civil War (1861–65) Dix was appointed Superintendent of Women Nurses. The United States was among the first to recognise that confining the mentally ill to protect society from their derangement was not necessarily of benefit to the client. The first training for psychiatric nurses in the United States was organised at McLean Asylum in 1882.

The United Kingdom

In the United Kingdom, Florence Nightingale (1820–1910) is usually credited with being the trailblazer for modern nursing, although Elizabeth Fry opened the first institute for the training of Protestant nurses in London. Accounts of the originality of Nightingale's work also tend to ignore the fact that she initially spent time in the Lutheran deaconess facility at Kaiserwerth, Germany, which was itself a product of the centuries-old European tradition of religious nursing.

In 1854 Florence Nightingale collected and trained a force of nurses to tend the English troops who were involved in the Crimean War, in Turkey. English troops in Scutari died more frequently from diseases due to unsanitary conditions than from battle wounds. The Nightingale School for Nurses was established in 1860 at the historic St Thomas's Hospital in London (founded in 1215 AD) but she had already published *Notes on Nursing* in 1859, which addressed much that is also relevant to the nursing of the mentally ill. Nightingale wrote 147 works in all, and she included philosophy, sanitation, administration, health and hospitals, emigration, discipline and women's rights among her range of subjects. The nurse who writes eloquently can have an enormous influence on the profession and on others.

After the Lunacy Act of 1845 the numbers of public asylums and nursing staff or attendants who worked in them burgeoned. In the asylums, both staff and patients were segregated on the basis of gender: males worked in the grounds or workshops under male attendants who were ex-army, prison warders or farmers; female patients performed domestic work indoors under female attendants or nurses (Chatterton 2000). This state of affairs continued until the shortage of suitable males during World War I led to the employment of more females, even in male wards, a trend which continued thereafter despite lower wages for women, until in 1922 at the first state registration exam, more female nurses passed ($n = 113$) than males ($n = 48$) (Chatterton 2000).

New Zealand

The first premises were provided for the care of 'lunatics' in New Zealand in 1846, and six provincial asylums were built on the British model between 1854 and 1872, staffed by ill-educated 'attendants' who were more akin to warders than nurses (O'Brien 2001). While general nursing rose in status, the asylum worker of the Victorian era in New Zealand and elsewhere shared the stigmatised status of their charges in the asylum, characterised as 'a warehouse of despondency and gloom' (Russell 1988, cited in O'Brien 2001, p 132). New Zealand and Australia have by virtue of their proximity and similar colonial histories and multicultural backgrounds shared a comparable agenda of training and professionalisation in the twentieth century.

Australia

Australia benefited from associations with both the Sisters of Charity and Florence Nightingale's work. Sydney Infirmary (later known as Sydney Hospital) was built in 1811, and was staffed not by trained nurses but by convict women, who were paid in alcohol. In 1839 five Sisters of Charity arrived in the colony to minister to the poor, and by 1857 St Vincent's Hospital was built and staffed by the Sisters of Charity. Nightingale influenced the earliest nursing care in Australia, when in 1868 the Colonial Secretary requested that Australia be sent a contingent of the new Nightingale-trained nurses. Lucy Osborn was sent from England to establish the Nightingale system of nursing, and she instituted hospital-based training for nurses in Sydney Hospital. Nurses received a nominal wage and board during training, paying for their training by working in the hospitals and providing cheap labour. This system stayed in place for nearly a century, with little real change.

In Australia, the belief that 'fresh air, space and the climate of the country would preclude madness' proved not to be the case, and it became essential for the maintenance of law and order to build and equip asylums modelled on similar establishments in the United Kingdom (Ash et al. 2001). The first 'lunatic asylum' was opened at Castle Hill in New South Wales in 1811. All the 'lunatics' in the new colony were sent there, and by 1825 this facility was over-crowded. Gladesville Hospital in Sydney was opened in 1837 to accommodate the surplus, and each State soon developed its own psychiatric services.

Although attempts were made to provide humane care, and numerous commissions and inquiries were conducted, overcrowding meant that custodial care was the usual strategy employed with the mentally ill. The medical model continued to see mental illness as an organic process, and the psychoanalytic theories initiated by Freud in the latter part of the nineteenth century and the early twentieth century were slow to be adopted in Australia.

Specialised mental health nursing education was not introduced until after 1910 when the first Nurses Registration Board was formed to oversee and regulate training. The Australian Nursing Federation was formed in 1924, but it was not until 1974 that the first Congress of Mental Health Nurses was held, which led to the for-mation of a professional organisation in 1978.

CONCLUSION

This chapter has provided an overview of the ways in which mental disorders have been experienced, treated and regarded in past eras. The disorders that have sur-vived in the same form over two and a half millennia have been examined, as have those that appear to be of more recent origin. The interpersonal skills which were used to treat mental illness have proved to be at times as refined and humane as any we would use today, but there have also been regressive episodes featuring incarceration of and brutality towards the mentally ill.

The transition from family-based care to institutional care has been outlined, and the emergence and re-emergence of mental health professionals has been described. The earliest documented role models for nurs-ing are found in the Graeco-Roman era. These women were as professional and competent as the women and men who practise today. Ancient Greek nurses displayed a measure of independence in their practice that has not been equalled until the present era.

One of the important changes that the professionali-sation of nursing wrought was that nursing became a commercial undertaking, a respectable source of employ-ment and independence for women as well as men, and an organised profession that displaced the traditional role of family members as carers for the ill. The mentally ill had been considered the responsibility of the asylum, or state-run institutions, for somewhat longer than the physically ill, but their treatment tended to be more humane and better regulated from the end of the nine-teenth century to the beginning of the modern era.

This historical account stops short of documenting the changes that have occurred since the early twentieth cen-tury. These have been so great and so many that they would require another chapter to describe them fully. Mental health/psychiatric nursing has blossomed into a skilled pro-fession. The challenges that concern a psychiatric mental health nurse, transformed in less than a century from ignorant attendant to university graduate, can be traced in Chapter 5, which deals with professional nursing issues.

EXERCISE FOR CLASS ENGAGEMENT

Discuss the following questions with your group or class members.

- What traditional remedies for illness or stress have you seen or heard used in your own family? Are they effective?
- Was there any alternative to the evolution of the asylum for the care of the mentally ill, given the numbers of sufferers?

- In what sense is the term 'hysteric' or 'hysterical' used today? Would you still find that there is a relationship with 'disorders of the womb', or perhaps the possession of a womb?
- Which aspects of mental health care in the past would you like to see incorporated into present mental health nursing practice? How would you go about doing this?

REFERENCES

Alexander FG & Selesnick ST 1966, *The History of Psychiatry: An Evaluation of Psychiatric Thought and Practice from Prehistoric Times to the Present*, Harper & Row, New York.

American Psychiatric Association 1994, *Diagnostic and Statistical Manual of Mental Disorders* (DSM-IV) (4th edn), American Psychiatric Association, Washington DC.

Aristophanes 1964, *The Wasps, The Poet and The Women, The Frogs*, tr. Barrett D, Penguin, Harmondsworth.

Ash D, Benson A, Farhall J, Fielding J, Fossey E, McKendrick J et al. 2001, Mental health services in Australia. In: Meadows G & Singh B (eds),

Mental Health in Australia, Oxford University Press, South Melbourne, pp 51–66.

Blakemore C 1988, *The Mind Machine*, BBC Books, London.

Boyd MA (ed) 2002, *Psychiatric Nursing: Contemporary Practice* (2nd edn), Lippincott, Philadelphia.

Busuttil J 1992, Psychosocial occupational therapy: from myth and misconception to multidisciplinary team member, *British Journal of Occupational Therapy*, 5512, pp 457–61.

Celsus, *De Medicina*, Vol I 1935–38, rev. 1940 & 1948, tr. Spencer WG, Loeb Classical Library, William Heinemann, London.

Celsus, *De Medicina* Vol III 1935–38, tr. Spencer WG, Loeb Classical Library, William Heinemann, London.

Chatterton C 2000, Women in mental health nursing: angels or custodians?, *International History of Nursing Journal*, Spring, 5(2), pp 11–19.

Cicero 1978, *Letters to Atticus*, tr. Shackleton Bailey DR, Penguin, Harmondsworth.

Devereux G 1970, The psychotherapy scene in Euripides' 'Bacchae', *Journal of Hellenic Studies*, XC, pp 35–48.

Dodds ER 1951, *The Greeks and the Irrational*, University of California Press, Berkeley.

Doona ME 1992, Judgment: the nurse's key to knowledge, *Journal of Professional Nursing*, Jul/Aug, 84, pp 231–8.

Ellard J 1987, Did schizophrenia exist before the eighteenth century?, *Australian and New Zealand Journal of Psychiatry*, 21(3), pp 306–14.

Evans K 2000, Representations of Mental Illness in the Classical Texts, unpublished doctoral dissertation, University of Queensland, Brisbane.

Evans K, McGrath J & Milns R 2003, Searching for schizophrenia in ancient Greek and Roman literature: a systematic review, *Acta Psychiatrica Scandanavica*, 107(5), pp 323–30.

Fontaine KL 2003, *Fontaine & Fletcher Mental Health Nursing* (5th edn), Pearson Education, Upper Saddle River, New Jersey.

Foucault M 1967 (repr. 1999), *Madness and Civilisation: a History of Insanity in the Age of Reason*, tr. Howard R, Routledge, London.

Frisch N 2002, Psychiatric nursing: evolution of a specialty. In: Frisch N & Frisch L, *Psychiatric Mental Health Nursing* (2nd edn), Delmar Thomson Learning, Albany, pp 17–25.

Gilman S, King H, Porter R, Rousseau GS & Showalter E 1993, *Hysteria Beyond Freud*, University of California Press, Berkeley.

Grmek M 1991, *Diseases in the Ancient Greek World*, tr. Muellner M & Muellner L, The Johns Hopkins University Press, Baltimore.

Hamblet C 2000, Obstacles to defining the role of the mental health nurse, *Nursing Standard*, 14(51), pp 34–7.

Hawkins DR 1982, Specificity revisited: personality profiles and behavioral issues, *Psychotherapy and Psychosomatics*, 38(1), pp 54–63.

Herodotus, *The Histories* Vol II: Books III & IV 1921, tr. Godley AD, William Heinemann, London.

Herodotus, *The Histories* Vol III: Books V–VII, 1922, tr. Godley AD, William Heinemann, London.

Hershkowitz D 1998, *The Madness of Epic: Reading Insanity from Homer to Statius*, Clarendon Press, Oxford.

Hippocrates 1923 *The Hippocratic Corpus* Vol I, tr. Jones WHS, Loeb Classical Library, William Heinemann, London.

Hippocrates 1923, *The Hippocratic Corpus* Vol II, tr. Jones WHS, Loeb Classical Library, William Heinemann, London.

Hippocrates 1931, *The Hippocratic Corpus* Vol IV, tr. Jones WHS, Loeb Classical Library, William Heinemann, London.

Hippocrates 1923, *The Hippocratic Corpus* Vol VII, tr. Smith WD, Loeb Classical Library, Harvard University Press, Cambridge Mass.

Hornblower S & Spawforth A (eds) 1996, *The Oxford Classical Dictionary* (3rd edn), Oxford University Press, New York.

Howells JG (ed.) 1991, *The Concept of Schizophrenia: Historical Perspectives*, American Psychiatric Press Inc, Washington DC.

Jeste DV, del Carmen R, Lohr JB & Wyatt RJ 1985, Did schizophrenia exist before the eighteenth century?, *Comprehensive Psychiatry*, 26(6), pp 493–503.

Jones WHS 1923, Ancient nursing. In: *Hippocrates*, Vol II, Introductory Essay IV, William Heinemann, London.

Kaplan H, Sadock B & Grebb J 1994, *Synopsis of Psychiatry* (7th edn), Williams & Wilkins, Baltimore.

King H 1993, Once upon a text. In: Gilman S, King H, Porter R, Rousseau GS & Showalter E, *Hysteria Beyond Freud*, University of California Press, Berkeley.

Lester D 1990, Galen's four temperaments and four-factor theories of personality: a comment on 'toward a four-factor theory of temperament and/or personality', *Journal of Personality Assessment*, 54(1/2), pp 423–6.

Macalpine I & Hunter R 1969, *George III and the Mad-Business*, Penguin Press, London.

Mack AH, Forman L, Brown R & Frances A 1994, A brief history of psychiatric classification: from the ancients to DSM-IV, *Psychiatric Clinics of North America*, 17(3), pp 515–23.

McAthie M 1999, The nature of contemporary nursing practice. In: Lindeman C & McAthie M (eds), *Fundamentals of Contemporary Nursing Practice*, WB Saunders, Philadelphia, pp 3–20.

Martial 1972, *The Epigrams*, tr. Michie J, Penguin Books, Harmondsworth.

Mellersh HEL 1976 (rev. 1999), *The Hutchinson Chronology of World History: the Ancient and Medieval World*, Helicon Publishing, Oxford.

Merenda PF 1987, Toward a four-factor theory of temperament and/or personality, *Journal of Personality Assessment*, 513(3), pp 367–74.

Nightingale F 1859 (repr. 1969), *Notes on Nursing: What it is and What it is not*, Dover Publications, New York.

O'Brien AJ 2001, The therapeutic relationship: historical development and contemporary significance, *Journal of Psychiatric and Mental Health Nursing*, 8(2), pp 129–37.

Parker R 1983, *Miasma: Pollution and Purification in Early Greek Religion*, Clarendon, Oxford.

Plautus 1965, *The Pot of Gold and Other Plays*, tr. Watling EF, Penguin Classics, Harmondsworth.

Plutarch 1914, *Lives*, Vol II, Themistocles and Camillus, Aristides and Cato Major, Cimon and Lucullus, tr. Perrin B, William Heinemann, London.

Richards A (ed.) 1991, Breue J & Freud S, *Studies on Hysteria*, tr. Strachey J & Strachey A, Penguin Books, Harmondsworth.

Roccatagliata G 1991, Classical concepts of schizophrenia. In: Howells GJ (ed.), *The Concept of Schizophrenia: Historical Perspectives*, American Psychiatric Press Inc, Washington DC.

Rosen G 1968, *Madness in Society: Chapters in the Historical Sociology of Mental Illness*, University of Chicago Press, Chicago.

Sanderson S, Vandenberg B & Paese P 1999, Authentic religious experience or insanity?, *Journal of Clinical Psychology*, 55(5), pp 607–16.

Simon B 1978, *Mind and Madness in Ancient Greece: the Classical Roots of Modern Psychiatry*, Cornell University Press, London.

Soranus 1956, *The Gynecology*, tr. Temkin O, The Johns Hopkins University Press, Baltimore & London.

Stone MH 1997, *Healing the Mind. A History of Psychiatry from Antiquity to the Present*, WW Norton & Co, New York.

Suer L 1995, The survival of ancient medicine in modern French psychiatry, *History of Psychiatry*, 6(24 pt 4), pp 493–501.

Summers A 1997, Sairey Gamp: generating fact from fiction, *Nursing Enquiry*, 4(1), pp 14–18.

Terence 1976, *The Comedies*, tr. Radice B, Penguin Books, Harmondsworth.

Thucydides 1954, *History of the Peloponnesian War*, tr. Warner R, Penguin Books, Harmondsworth.

Torrey EF, Bowler AE & Clark K 1997, Urban birth and residence as risk factors for psychoses: an analysis of 1880 data, *Schizophrenia Research*, 25(3), pp 169–76.

Torrey EF & Yolken RH 1995, Could schizophrenia be a viral zoonosis transmitted from house cats?, *Schizophrenia Bulletin*, 21(2), pp 167–71.

Torrey EF & Yolken, RH 1998, Is household crowding a risk factor for schizophrenia?, *Schizophrenia Research*, 29(1/2), pp 12–13.

Woolf A 2000, Witchcraft or mycotoxin? The Salem witch trials, *Journal of Toxicology: Clinical Toxicology*, 38(4), p 457.

Yolken RH, Yee F, Johnston N, Leister F, Bobo L, Jafari N et al. 1997, Molecular analyses of brains from individuals with schizophrenia—evidence of viral infections, *Schizophrenia Research*, 24(1/2), p 61.

4

The Australian and New Zealand Politico-legal Context

Eimear Muir-Cochrane,
Anthony O'Brien and Tim Wand

KEY POINTS

- An understanding of the history of the care of the mentally ill in Western cultures will help contextualise contemporary policy and legal developments.
- Many of the mentally ill live extremely disadvantaged lives.
- A sound knowledge of relevant legal and ethical issues is critical to contemporary mental health nursing.
- Mental health nurses require an understanding of current mental health policy at both a global and a local level to ensure that their practice is consistent with ongoing changes in health-care delivery.
- Mental health is one of the seven national priority areas for health in Australia.
- Mental health policy takes a population health approach.
- The Treaty of Waitangi (1840) is accorded a central place in the development of policy and recognition of the special health issues facing Maori.
- Consumer participation is necessary to improve the quality and responsiveness of mental health services.
- Most people with mental health problems are treated in the primary care setting.
- Mental health legislation is the legal framework that informs the involuntary treatment of individuals, defines their rights and ensures appropriate treatment.
- Mental health nurses play a significant role in raising mental health awareness through education, primary prevention and early intervention.

KEY TERMS

- community care
- consumer
- deinstitutionalisation
- human rights
- least-restrictive alternative
- mental health legislation
- mental health policy
- mental health prevention
- mental health promotion
- mental health standards
- mental health strategy
- partnership
- primary health care
- Treaty of Waitangi

LEARNING OUTCOMES

The material in this chapter will assist you to:
- outline the historical, social and political developments that have occurred in the development of mental health services in Australia and New Zealand
- discuss mental health policies in Australia and New Zealand
- understand the importance of mental health law in psychiatry
- discuss the tension between the controlling and caring functions of psychiatric and mental health nursing practice
- explain the shortage of mental health nurses in Australia and New Zealand.

INTRODUCTION

Nurses require a sound understanding of mental health policy and legislation in order to work effectively with clients in both community and institutional settings. Australia and New Zealand have been at the forefront of developing national strategies, policies and standards in line with the World Health Organization principles of access, equity, effectiveness and efficiency. This chapter describes each country's national policies, the historical events that have served to shape them and the institutions and concepts guiding their implementation. It traces the shift from a focus on the care and treatment of mentally ill persons to the mental health of the whole population. The role of the law in decisions about the involuntary treatment of people and the rights of people is also discussed. Also presented are examples of how nurses can work most effectively with people under often challenging circumstances to ensure their rights are protected.

HISTORICAL LANDMARKS

In order to gain a clear and critical understanding of how mental health services in Australia and New Zealand have developed, it is important to briefly explore some historical landmarks over the past five hundred years.

In the Middle Ages, individuals with mental illness were considered to be possessed, or to be witches; many were ostracised, excluded from community life or exposed to family brutality. Between the early nineteenth and late twentieth centuries, the mentally ill were frequently incarcerated in large asylums, usually for long periods, under the guise of community or individual philanthropy. People with mental illness were socially and physically excluded from 'normal' social life and frequently subjected to institutional brutality. Asylums were established in both Australia and New Zealand as part of the process of colonisation of each country (Maude 2001). Prior to the middle of the twentieth century, pharmacological treatments were extremely limited and, when used, often ineffective or dangerous. Most treatments were of a physical nature and often involved the use of restraints such as straitjackets and being subjected to cold water baths or showers.

After World War II, pharmacological treatments of varying efficacy and toxicity began to emerge—antidepressants first, then antipsychotics. These were so successful that many institutionalised clients were able to leave hospital for the first time in decades. These pharmacological treatments, in conjunction with an era of anti-psychiatry sentiment in society from the 1950s on, led to a forty-year period when liberal attitudes to the mentally ill prevailed, many psychiatric institutions closed down and people with mental illness returned to live in the community.

The closure of psychiatric hospitals is referred to as deinstitutionalisation and resulted in a decrease of 86 per cent in the number of psychiatric inpatients in Australia between the 1960s and the early 1990s (Human Rights and Equal Opportunity Commission (HREOC) 1993). Deinstitutionalisation also involved an expansion of community-based care and the relocation of inpatient psychiatric beds into general hospitals. Community-based resources included the establishment of community mental health centres and supported accommodation, with a greater emphasis on the multidisciplinary team (psychiatrists, nurses, social workers, occupational therapists and psychologists) (see Ch 21). However, community mental health resources have not kept pace with demand, and this lack of resources has resulted in an increase in the number of mentally ill people living in extremely disadvantaged circumstances. Thornicroft & Betts (2002) draw attention to this disadvantage in their Mid-Term Review of the Second Mental Health Plan for Australia, stating that people with mental illness face severe difficulties in accessing accommodation, education, social security, transport and employment. People with mental illness require appropriate inpatient treatment when in the acute stages of illness but recent Australian literature shows that they prefer to reside in the community, indicating that they value their personal autonomy highly (Newton et al. 2000). Successful community integration and a decrease in the stigma attached to those exhibiting signs of mental illness requires a concerted and comprehensive approach at the local and national levels, with clear and effective links between various social and health services.

In Australia and New Zealand today, psychiatric services are provided by public, private and non-government organisations. They are located in hospital and community settings and include: psychiatric emergency services and 24-hour crisis teams; continuing care and consultancy teams; mobile intensive community treatment teams (MITT); inpatient services comprising intensive care, sub-acute and asylum services either within psychiatric wards in general hospitals or psychiatric hospitals (Ash et al. 2001) (Ch 21 provides a full description of these settings and services).

THE CURRENT GLOBAL PERSPECTIVE

In 1991, the United Nations established the Principles for the Protection of Persons with Mental Illness and the Improvement of Mental Health Care, reflecting an international understanding and awareness of the individual and unique needs of those with mental illness and the responsibilities incumbent on the 'state and professional communities to respond adequately and ethically to these needs' (Singh 2001, p 43). An overarching statement of the fundamental human rights of those with mental illness guides the twenty-five principles (Box 4.1).

The World Health Organization (WHO 2001b) also recommends that all mental health policies be anchored by the four guiding principles of:
- access
- equity

- effectiveness
- efficiency.

A description of each of these principles is given in Box 4.2.

Box 4.1 Rights of the mentally ill

Rights of the mentally ill include:
- rights in regard to confidentiality of all information about the person with mental illness in regard to their care
- the right to live and work in the community (further reinforced by the document Mental Health around the World: Stop Exclusion: Dare to Care (WHO 2001a))
- protection of minors and others deemed not to be able to give informed consent
- the right to voluntary treatment, wherever possible by those specifically qualified to care for such individuals and in approved mental health facilities
- the right to receive appropriate medical treatment including medication, prescribed by mental health professionals, but never as punishment or for the convenience of others
- the right that no treatment shall be given without informed consent other than when held as an involuntary client
- the right that physical restraint or involuntary seclusion of a client shall not be used unless it is a last resort, used to prevent imminent harm to the client or others
- the right that involuntary admission will only occur if authorised by a qualified mental health practitioner, that the person is suffering from a mental illness, that treatment occurs in an approved mental health facility, that a second medical opinion is sought where possible and that appropriate treatment can only be given within a mental health facility
- the right to make a complaint.

Source: Singh B 2001, The global perspective in mental health. In: Meadows G & Singh B (eds), *Mental Health in Australia: Collaborative Community Practice*, Oxofrd University Press, London. pp 44–5.

Box 4.2 WHO principles for guiding mental health policy

- *Access*: the right to obtain treatment for mental health issues based on need not on ability to pay
- *Equity*: mental health resources should be fairly distributed across the population as indicated by need
- *Effectiveness*: mental health services should be aimed solely at improving health for individuals and collectivities
- *Efficiency*: resources should be distributed in such a way as to maximise gains for individuals and society as a whole.

Source: World Health Organization 2001, *Mental Health, New Understanding, New Hope*, WHO, Geneva. Online: http://www.who.int/whr2001/2001/main/en/

These WHO recommendations have been adopted in Australian and New Zealand mental health care law, and enshrined in the various State and Territory Mental Health Acts, which are described later.

AUSTRALIAN NATIONAL MENTAL HEALTH POLICY

The material in this section is drawn largely from national policy documents that describe the direction of federal governments in the ongoing reform of mental health services in Australia since the early 1990s. An understanding of policy direction is important in order to appreciate the current and future course of mental health care and its impact on the shape of mental health nursing in the future.

In 1992 Australian state health ministers gave full support to the National Mental Health Strategy (Australian Health Ministers 1998), which operationalised the National Mental Health Plan (Australian Health Ministers 1992a). The National Mental Health Strategy established twelve priority areas. These are listed in Box 4.3.

Box 4.3 Priorities of the National Mental Health Strategy

- consumer rights
- linking mental health with other sectors
- promotion and prevention
- carers and non-government organisations
- legislation
- standards
- monitoring and accountability
- service mix
- primary care services
- mental health workforce
- research and evaluation
- the relationship between mental health and general health services

Source: National Mental Health Strategy (Australian Health Ministers 1998)

The urgent need for reforms and additional funding for mental health services was recognised with the release of the findings of the Report of the National Inquiry into the Human Rights of People with Mental Illness (HREOC 1993). This damning report highlighted the often appalling experiences of consumers of mental health services in inpatient care, the perpetuation of stigma and the consequent isolation of people living with mental illness.

In 1997, the Evaluation of the National Mental Health Strategy (Australian Health Ministers 1998) concluded that considerable progress had been made in the areas of:
- carer and consumer rights and involvement
- reducing the focus on inpatient services and bringing mental health services within the structures of mainstream health services

- improving links between mental health and other sectors
- national initiatives on prevention and promotion.

The framework for the future directions outlined in the Evaluation established the basis for developing the Second National Mental Health Plan (Australian Health Ministers 1998). This plan built on the achievements of the First National Mental Health Plan (Australian Health Ministers 1992a) and identified the following priority areas:

- promotion/prevention
- development of partnerships in service reform
- the quality and effectiveness of service delivery.

In addition to the development of specific mental health policy and strategic frameworks, the inclusion of mental health, and particularly depression, as one of the seven National Health Priority Areas further encouraged State and Territory governments' focus on mental health.

The Second National Mental Health Plan
In terms of prevention and promotion, the Second National Mental Health Plan emphasised the use of a range of settings in which mental health promotion and community education could occur, and the groups of workers who should be targeted to undertake activities in this area. A key development in this area of the plan was a population health approach to mental health, with acknowledgment that different groups within the population required different types of services and interventions.

Although the First National Mental Health Plan enunciated the need to develop links and partnerships with a range of groups outside the specialist mental health sector, it was not until the Second National Mental Health Plan that the groups with whom partnerships should be established were specified (see Box 4.4).

Box 4.4 **Partnership groups**

- consumers, families and carers
- private psychiatrists and the private mental health sector
- the wider health sector
- non-government agencies
- the broader community
- general practitioners
- emergency services
- other government agencies
- community support services
- a range of priority partnerships for indigenous mental health

Source: Second National Mental Health Plan (Australian Health Ministers 1998)

The third area that the Second National Mental Health Plan (Australian Health Ministers 1998) focused on was improving the quality and effectiveness of mental health services, with emphasis on improving consumer outcomes across the lifespan. The plan emphasised the need for:

- further development and implementation of the national standards for mental health services
- the preparation and dissemination of clinical standards
- the establishment of benchmarks and best practice models using evidence-based practice
- the expansion of education and training to support both specialist mental health and primary health care staff to respond effectively to the changes envisaged within the Plan
- enhancing the quality and effectiveness of services provided.

National Action Plan for Prevention, Promotion and Early Intervention
While the Second National Mental Health Plan (Australian Health Ministers 1998) broadly identified prevention and promotion as key priorities for action, the National Action Plan for Promotion, Prevention and Early Intervention for Mental Health 2000 (Department of Health and Aged Care 2002a) clearly articulated the population health approach to mental health. Such an approach seeks to develop strategies which attend to the mental health status and mental health needs of whole populations. The Action Plan emphasised the continuum of care from universal prevention through to long-term, individual care and the overlap between prevention, early intervention and treatment (see Figure 4.1).

Central to the Action Plan is attention to improving family environments, building family-friendly workplaces, enhancing parenting skills, reduction of abuse and neglect, and increased attention to early identification and intervention.

CRITICAL THINKING CHALLENGE 4.1

- In your own words, define promotion and prevention in mental health.
- How can you assist clients and their families to consider their lifestyle behaviours (lack of exercise, long working hours, use of alcohol or other drugs) to minimise mental health problems, including depression?
- How do you minimise stress in your own life?

The National Action Plan for Depression
The National Action Plan for Depression (Department of Health and Aged Care 2002b) builds on the Second National Mental Health Plan (Australian Health Ministers 1998) by applying a population health approach to depression. Strategies are proposed to: enhance skills to manage adverse events (protective factors); introduce mental health programs into schools; support children of parents with depressive disorders; enhance skills of primary health care and specialist mental health providers in screening for and intervening in depression; and develop culturally appropriate approaches to depression in the Aboriginal and Torres Strait Islander community.

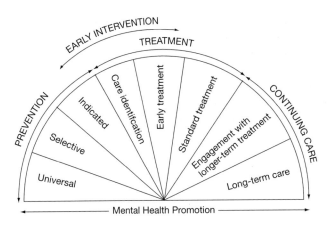

Figure 4.1 Spectrum of interventions for mental health problems (from Department of Health and Aged Care 2002, *National Action Plan for Promotion, Prevention and Early Intervention in Mental Health*, AGPS, Canberra)

The Second National Mental Health Plan mid-term evaluation

In 2001, Thornicroft & Betts (2002) reviewed the Second National Mental Health Plan and reported progress in a number of areas including consumer and carer participation, partnership development, and quality and effectiveness. They emphasised that consolidation was required and proposed options for future directions.

The negotiation of the Australian Health Care Agreement between the Commonwealth, States and Territories is a key component of the National Mental Health Strategies extension. The emphasis for the future is placed on:

- reaffirmation of the National Mental Health Policy for 2003–08
- continuity of care
- improving access to and the quality of effective primary and secondary interventions within the mental health system
- enhancing the capacity of services to meet the needs of under-served populations, such as indigenous people, older Australians and those living in rural and remote areas
- enhanced training of the mental health workforce
- development of links between service sectors.

Through these mechanisms a consistent approach has been adopted nationally.

NEW ZEALAND MENTAL HEALTH POLICY

Following major structural changes throughout the 1980s, the New Zealand Government set about constructing a national mental health strategy to address recurring issues within mental health services. Deinstitutionalisation had seen the closure of psychiatric hospitals and their replacement with mental health units located within general hospitals. At the same time specialist forensic services and drug and alcohol services developed separately. A set of five strategic directions was established by the Ministry of

Health (MOH) in 1994 as part of an overall strategy for mental health. Over the following ten years the National Mental Health Strategy has developed, along with a set of standards for mental health care and a number of initiatives in workforce and service development. The Mental Health Commission (MHC) was established in 1996 to oversee implementation of the National Mental Health Strategy. The principal document that guides the work of the Commission is the *Blueprint for Mental Health Services* (MHC 1998). Originally envisaged as having a time-limited role, the Commission planned to have completed its work by 2001. Such is the complexity of reform, and the scope of issues to be addressed, that the Commission still existed in 2003, with many aspects of the mental health strategy still to be achieved.

Chapter 5 refers to areas of mental health policy as part of a discussion of professional issues. This section reviews the recent development of mental health policy in New Zealand and discusses the role of the Mental Health Commission in monitoring policy implementation.

Treaty of Waitangi (1840)

The Treaty of Waitangi is regarded by many as New Zealand's founding constitutional document, and as the basis for development of economic, health and social policy (Durie 1994). Both the Ministry of Health and the Mental Health Commission accord the Treaty a central place in policy development and service provision and recognise the special health issues facing Maori, the indigenous people of New Zealand. Publications of both bodies make specific reference to Maori, Pacific and other cultural needs in the development of mental health policy and services.

The National Mental Health Strategy

The National Mental Health Strategy was launched in 1994 with the publication of *Looking Forward: Strategic Directions for the Mental Health Services* (Ministry of Health 1994). The closure of hospitals revealed gaps in community-based services that the new strategy was designed to rectify. *Looking Forward* stated that a new direction was needed in the post-institutional era of mental health care, and set two key goals for the National Mental Health Strategy. These were:

- to decrease the prevalence of mental illness and mental health problems within the community
- to increase the health status of and reduce the impact of mental disorders on consumers, their families, caregivers and the general community (Ministry of Health 1994).

Based on the Australian Tolkein report (Andrews 1994), *Looking Forward* set a national benchmark of three per cent for provision of mental health services for those most severely affected by mental illness. However, the National Mental Health Strategy was not concerned only with expanding the range of available services. In addition, the five strategic directions set for mental health reflected concern for consumer responsiveness, cultural responsiveness, quality of care and access to health care. The five strategic directions of *Looking Forward* are:

1 implementing community-based mental health services
2 encouraging Maori development in planning, developing and delivering mental health services
3 improving quality of care
4 balancing personal rights with protection of the public
5 developing a national alcohol and drugs policy.

By 1996 there was recognition that more specific policy and targeted funding were necessary in order to achieve the objectives of the National Mental Health Strategy. A 1996 report (the Mason Report) (Mason, Johnston & Crowe 1996) identified continuing problems with mental health services and made numerous recommendations for change. Among the recommendations was that of creating a national mental health monitoring body, subsequently established as the Mental Health Commission (see discussion below). A further policy document, *Moving Forward: The National Plan for More and Better Mental Health Services* (Ministry of Health 1997a) set more specific targets for service development. The benchmarks set in *Moving Forward* include the range of mild, moderate and severe mental disorders among the adult population, and are shown in Figure 4.2.

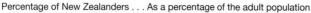

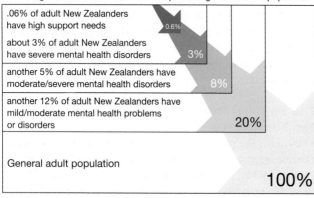

Figure 4.2 Estimated prevalence of mental health problems amongst adult New Zealanders (from New Zealand Ministry of Health 1997, *Moving Forward: The National Plan for More and Better Mental Health Services*, MOH, Wellington, p 11)

Moving Forward also established two further strategic directions: developing the mental health services infrastructure, and strengthening promotion and prevention. These new strategic directions expanded the scope of the mental health strategy to include workforce development and research, and to broaden the focus beyond that of treatment services. To provide services based on the benchmarks shown in Figure 4.2, the National Mental Health Strategy modelled service provision to include the mental health service sector as well as primary health care and public health services, and social service agencies. Mental health was seen as an issue not just for mental

health services, but across the range of mental health and social services. The model of service delivery is shown in Figure 4.3.

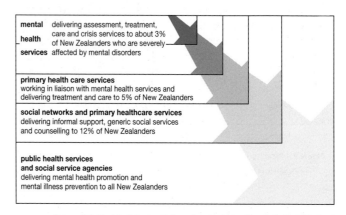

Figure 4.3 Model of service delivery for mental health care in New Zealand (from New Zealand Ministry of Health 1997, *Moving Forward: The National Plan for More and Better Mental Health Services*, MOH, Wellington, p 11)

Mental Health Commission

The Mental Health Commission was established in 1996 in response to a recommendation of the 1996 Mason inquiry. The Mason report stated that a process of independent monitoring of mental health policy and service delivery was necessary to address issues identified in mental health services. The role of the Commission is to monitor the implementation of the National Mental Health Strategy. The key functions of the Commission are to:

■ monitor and report to government on the performance of the Ministry of Health and the Health Funding Authority in the implementation of the government's National Mental Health Strategy
■ work with the sector to promote better understanding by the public of mental illness, and eliminate discrimination
■ strengthen the mental health workforce.

The work of the Commission is guided by its key document, the *Blueprint for Mental Health Services* (MHC 1998). The *Blueprint* describes services required to fully implement the National Mental Health Strategy, and is focused on the goal of decreasing the prevalence of mental illness and mental health problems in the community. The *Blueprint* is described by the Commission as:

a national mental health service development plan, setting out the Commission's view of the qualitative and quantitative changes needed . . . to realise the objectives of the Government's National Mental Health Strategy.

(MHC 1998, p 1)

As part of its role in facilitating the implementation of the National Mental Health Strategy, the Mental Health Commission conducts reviews of aspects of mental health services, and produces reports on issues of broad significance to mental health. The full range of publications is available from the Commission's website (http://www.mhc.govt.nz).

Recovery focus

The Mental Health Commission promotes recovery-focused care as part of its mandate to promote better mental health services (Ch 2 also discusses a recovery approach to mental health care). Recovery is a concept with a long history in mental health care (Clinton & Nelson 1999), but the Commission's work is linked to the consumer advocacy movement, rather than having a medically oriented meaning of recovery as cure of illness (MHC 1998). The Commission defines recovery as:

> liv[ing] well in the presence or absence of ... mental illness and the many losses that may come in its wake, such as isolation, poverty, unemployment and discrimination. Recovery does not always mean that people will return to full health or retrieve all their losses, but it does mean that people can live well in spite of them.
>
> (MHC 1998, p 1)

Recovery is not a model of care, but a philosophical orientation to mental health and mental health service. It is regarded as consistent with a range of models of mental illness and mental health care. Within the Mental Health Commission's approach, recovery is both subjectively defined by consumers and observable in the attitudes, skills and knowledge of mental health workers (MHC 2001). Central to recovery philosophy is the notion of *hope*. The traditional medical notion of recovery stresses cure from disease, with the result that without a cure there is no recovery. In contrast, the consumer advocacy model of recovery used by the Commission emphasises that recovery is always occurring, and can be assisted by mental health workers who have integrated recovery principles into their clinical practice. The idea that recovery is a continuous process rather than an end point which may or may not be achieved encourages both consumers and clinicians to maintain an attitude of hope. To promote a recovery focus in mental health services, the Commission has developed a set of ten competencies for employees of mental health services (MHC 2001). The competencies seek to define the 'attitudes, skills, knowledge and behaviour required of the mental health workforce' (MHC 2001, p 3) if it is to provide recovery-focused services. Although primarily intended as a resource for education providers, the recovery competencies are a useful reflective tool for practitioners in all disciplines. They provide a basis for discussion in clinical supervision, service audit, setting practice guidelines and reviewing services with consumers.

Consumer participation

Consumer participation is central to the work of the Mental Health Commission and is an inherent aspect of a recovery orientation. Recovery Competency Nine states:

> A competent mental health worker has knowledge of the service user movement and is able to support their participation in services.
>
> (MHC 2001, p 7)

Consumer involvement is built into the governance processes of the Commission, with consumers constituting one of the five reference groups that inform the Commission's work. Participation of consumers is considered necessary for the improvement of the quality and responsiveness of mental health services. In addition to the commitment to consumer participation by the Commission, Standard Nine of the National Mental Health Sector Standard (Standards New Zealand 2001a) states that consumers should be involved in every level of the mental health service. Most New Zealand mental health services now employ consumers in an advisory, educational or caregiving capacity. Expansion of the consumer workforce, provision of training opportunities and active recruitment policies are seen as necessary to extend the current level of consumer participation in mental health services.

CRITICAL THINKING CHALLENGE 4.2

- What skills do you consider consumers would bring to mental health services?
- What do you think nurses can learn from consumer participation in service delivery?
- What are some of the barriers to involving consumers in services?
- What opportunities does your service area or education program provide for collaboration with consumers?

Maori mental health

The issue of Maori mental health is recognised as a priority area for service development. Improvement in Maori mental health was the objective of Strategic Direction 2 of *Moving Forward* (MOH 1997a). This document referred to the past tendency of services to operate in a monocultural manner and their need to increase their responsiveness to Maori. The *Blueprint* (MHC 1998) identified improvement of services to Maori as crucial to the National Mental Health Strategy. Commitment to Maori mental health is also seen in Standard One of the National Mental Health Sector Standard (Standards New Zealand 2001a), which specifies the need to provide mental health services appropriate to Maori needs. Competency Seven of the Mental Health Commission's recovery competencies emphasises the need for mental health workers to demonstrate awareness of cultural safety and knowledge of Maori protocols and models of care (MHC 2001).

Mental health problems are considered to be the major health concern of Maori (Durie 1997) and to involve patterns of presentation that reflect problems experienced in accessing mainstream services. Compared to non-Maori, a significant proportion of Maori referrals come from law enforcement and welfare agencies (Te Puni Kokiri 1996). This pattern of referral and the importance of cultural identity in mental health care suggest a need for Maori cultural solutions to Maori mental health problems. This has implications for both Maori and mainstream services.

Te Puawaitanga (the Maori Mental Health Strategy), (MOH 2002a) is part of a wider strategy for Maori mental health, involving access to the institutions of Maori society such as te reo (language), land and marae (meeting places) (MOH 2002a, p 3). This reflects a cultural perspective of health as a product of social integration and access to social resources. The strategy sets specific service targets for Maori mental health, and aims to provide service providers with a nationally consistent framework for development of services to Maori (MOH 2002a).

To improve Maori mental health, Te Puawaitanga envisages that Maori consumers should have a choice between mainstream or Maori-specific (kaupapa Maori) mental health services. The strategy sets a three per cent benchmark for provision of service to Maori with high needs (MOH 2002a), and identifies Maori workforce development as essential to provision of these services.

National mental health standards

As part of the commitment to improved quality of services, the Ministry of Health developed an initial set of mental health standards in 1997 (Ministry of Health 1997b). These were the first specific standards written for mental health services and were designed to enable measurement of progress towards achievement of the National Mental Health Strategy. The standards were revised in 2001 and developed as a new document, the *National Mental Health Sector Standard* (Standards New Zealand 2001a). This document contains eighteen individual standards covering cultural issues, safety, privacy, assessment, consumer participation, management and reducing discrimination. The standards aim to achieve national consistency and continuous improvement in mental health services. An audit workbook has been developed to measure services provided against the standard (Standards New Zealand 2001b). Although standards do not capture the experience of consumers receiving care, and are not specific to nursing, they provide a definition of the broad quality of service consumers can expect. (Standards of practice for nursing are discussed in Ch 5.)

Primary Health Care Strategy

Mental health has evolved in isolation from the rest of the health sector, and as a result has developed its own services, facilities, service systems and workforce. While there are obvious advantages to the development of specialist skills, this separation carries the risk of creating barriers between different parts of the health system, with the result that the mental health needs of consumers in the wider health sector are not always met. The New Zealand Primary Health Care Strategy (MOH 2001) seeks greater integration of health services, especially at the level of primary care. The epidemiological model used to develop the National Mental Health Strategy suggests that three per cent of the New Zealand population experience severe mental health problems. Most of the care of this group of consumers is provided in the mental health sector, but a further seventeen per cent of the population have less severe mental health problems that can be treated in primary care (MOH 2002b). It is in the primary care sector that individuals first present with a range of mental health problems such as depression, anxiety, substance abuse, child and youth mental health problems and suicidality (MOH 2002b). The rate of treatable mental health problems in primary care is considered to be as high as fifty per cent, with depression considered to be a leading cause of mental health problems. The Primary Health Care Strategy is designed to achieve high rates of detection and more effective treatment for mental health problems presenting in primary care, and to contribute to the National Mental Health Strategy goals of reducing the prevalence and impact of mental health problems in the community.

The past ten years has been a period of intense policy development in mental health, beginning with the release of the first National Mental Health Strategy document, *Looking Forward*, in 1994. The closure of psychiatric hospitals together with greater recognition of the prevalence of mental health problems created a need for a range of new services as well as development of existing services to meet the diverse mental health needs of New Zealand society. The Mental Health Commission has provided a monitoring framework and continues to guide the development of new policy.

MENTAL HEALTH LAW

Legal provision to protect individuals from the consequences of behaviour resulting from mental illness, or to protect others from such behaviour, has a long tradition in Western societies (Rosenman 1994). Usually based on an ethical justification of paternalism, mental health law provides States with the right, known as *parens patriae*, to restrain the autonomy of individuals by physically removing them from society, or by placing conditions on their choices as members of society. In some cases the ethical justification for this form of legal coercion is that of justice; that is, some people with mental illness are legally coerced in order that the interests of others will be protected. Mental health legislation provides clinicians with a legal framework within which to provide involuntary treatment to individuals who meet the criteria of that

THE AUSTRALIAN AND NEW ZEALAND POLITICO-LEGAL CONTEXT 53

legislation. Individuals meeting these criteria are placed under involuntary status, or civil commitment, until such time as their clinical state no longer meets the criteria for involuntary treatment. A further purpose of mental health legislation is to define the rights of those placed under civil commitment, and to ensure their appropriate treatment.

The WHO document *Mental Health Care Law: Ten Basic Principles* (WHO 1996) distils the United Nations' (1991) principles, focusing particularly on the promotion of mental health, the prevention of mental disorder and the right of those with mental illness to be assisted in self-determination. Of particular interest to mental health nurses is the Principle of the Provision of the Least Restrictive Type of Mental Health Care (WHO 1996). This principle refers to the selection of the least-restrictive option when considering the individual's illness, the treatment available, the person's level of autonomy, the person's acceptance and cooperation, and the potential harm that could be caused to self and others. Further, the principle emphasises that individuals ought to be treated in the community in which they live, and if institution-based treatment is required, then the use of physical or chemical restraints must be a last resort and administered under the close scrutiny of the health-care provider (WHO 1996). The next section will consider mental health legislation in New Zealand and Australia, and the issues it raises for the practice of mental health nursing.

New Zealand mental health legislation

The *New Zealand Mental Health (Compulsory Assessment and Treatment) Act (1992)* and subsequent amendment (1999) were introduced towards the end of the period of deinstitutionalisation and reflect a shift from a therapeutic to a legal standard in decisions about involuntary treatment. The shift from a therapeutic to a legal standard in mental health care has been called 'the new legalism' (Verdun-Jones 1986; Vestegaard 1994) and has influenced mental health legislation in many Western countries. Clients have access to legal counsel, appeal processes and reviews of their status under legislation by courts of law. For nurses, the Act introduced changes in their responsibilities by creating a range of new roles, from providing advice to the public to the exercise of temporary holding powers.

An earlier part of this chapter discussed deinstitutionalisation, the closure of psychiatric hospitals and the reduced focus on custodial care in favour of care in the community. Deinstitutionalisation is based on the concept of the least-restrictive alternative, a concept that underpins mental health legislation in New Zealand (Bell & Brookbanks 1998). By this standard a decision to place a person under involuntary status does not mean that that person needs to be admitted to hospital. Treatment can occur in a hospital or in any other place deemed suitable by the treating clinician, including the person's home.

In practice, most individuals who are acutely disturbed within the meaning of the Mental Health Act are admitted to hospital. However, the intent and wording of the Act allows clinicians to explore less restrictive alternatives such as care in a community respite facility or care at home.

Criteria for invoking mental health legislation involve two components: 'abnormal state of mind'; and serious danger to self or others (Bell & Brookbanks 1998). Mental disorder is defined (Section 2) as:

an abnormal state of mind (whether of a continuous or intermittent nature), characterised by delusions, or by disorders of mood or perception or volition or cognition, of such a degree that it:

(a) Poses a serious danger to the health or safety of that person or of others; or

(b) Seriously diminishes the capacity of that person to take care of himself or herself

As with the Victorian legislation cited later in this chapter, there are certain exclusions to the application of the New Zealand legislation. Section 4 of the Act specifies that the Act cannot be invoked solely by reasons of the person's

- political, religious or personal beliefs
- sexual preferences
- criminal or delinquent behaviour
- substance abuse, or
- intellectual disability (MHA 1992).

In keeping with recognition of the Treaty of Waitangi, Section 5 of the New Zealand Mental Health Act requires that powers be exercised under the Act with respect for the cultural identity of consumers.

For an individual to be placed under mental health legislation there first needs to be an application by a member of the public and an accompanying medical certificate. Following an initial assessment examination, the person may be required to undergo further periods of assessment and treatment, coordinated by a 'responsible clinician' appointed under the Act. During this time the individual can apply under Section 16 of the Act for a review of their condition by a judge. At the conclusion of the assessment, if the person is thought to meet the criteria for compulsory treatment, the responsible clinician applies to the court for a Compulsory Treatment Order (CTO). Compulsory Treatment Orders can be either inpatient orders or community treatment orders, and are for an initial period of six months. Other provisions of the Act apply to clients following the issue of a CTO. These include Special and Restricted client status, Review Tribunals, and rights under the Act. A detailed outline of the process of compulsory assessment and treatment, including definitions of key concepts, is available in the Ministry of Health guidelines (MOH 2000).

Nurses are involved through a number of statutory roles in facilitating assessment and treatment under the Mental Health Act. The role of Duly Authorised Officer (DAO) involves providing assistance to members of the public who may be concerned that a person is mentally disordered and in need of treatment under the Act. Although the legislation does not specify the professional background of individuals acting as DAOs, in the majority of cases this role has been assumed by nurses. Concerns have been expressed that nurses acting as DAO, especially with consumers for whom they may be also acting in a case management role, may, by acting in the DAO role, jeopardise the therapeutic relationship they have with those consumers (Street & Walsh 1994). The role involves considerable skills in mental status and mental health assessment (Street & Walsh 1998), and was developed in recognition of the fact that nurses constitute a large and accessible group of mental health professionals with those skills. Despite this concern, Foster (1998) has argued that the DAO role provides an opportunity for consumer advocacy, particularly in situations where the DAO assessment might show that there is no need to invoke the Act.

As discussed above, clients under involuntary status may appeal under Section 16 of the Act for a review of their condition by a District Court Judge. In most cases the second health professional providing an opinion to the court is a nurse. The role of second health professional is one for which few nurses have specific preparation, and about which they feel a sense of conflict between a legally custodial and a therapeutic role (Fishwick, Tait & O'Brien 2001).

The Mental Health Act applies only to individuals placed under involuntary treatment orders. An issue that arises for nurses in inpatient settings is that someone who is a voluntary client may experience a deterioration of their mental state to the point where a nurse considers that to allow that person to leave the inpatient facility would be a dereliction of their duty of care. In these circumstances nurses are empowered under Section 111 to detain the person for a period of up to six hours, subject to the condition that a medical review of the person's mental state is arranged. The Section 111 holding power recognises the assessment skills of the nurse and potential for crises to occur that require an immediate response.

Australian mental health legislation

Each Australian State and Territory has mental health legislation (Mental Health Acts) designed to achieve the following objectives: to protect individuals with mental illness from inappropriate treatment; to direct the provision of mental health care and the facilities in which it is provided; and to instruct the practice of mental health professionals in principles of treatment and care. Australian Mental Health Acts without exception detail the prescribed actions around the use of physical treatments such as electroconvulsive therapy and psychosurgery as well as medical interventions. Seclusion practices are prescribed in most, but not all, Mental Health Acts in Australia. While Mental Health Acts vary in regard to the requirements of psychiatrists and mental health nurses, core issues such as a definition of mental illness, basic criteria for the admission and detention of voluntary and involuntary clients reflect the United Nations' human rights principles and are present in all state and territory Acts. Mental illness is generally defined as a medical condition characterised by a significant disturbance of thought, mood, perception or memory (*Victorian Mental Health Act 1986*, amended 2003). In the past, people with beliefs or behaviours judged by society in general, or the State, to be abnormal, deviant or immoral, were labelled as mentally ill. A number of Mental Health Acts go so far as to identify behaviours and personal characteristics that are *not* indicative of mental illness:

- particular political views or activities
- particular religious views or activities
- particular philosophy
- particular sexual preference or sexual orientation
- particular illegal conduct or use of drugs and/or alcohol
- having an antisocial personality
- being intellectually disabled (*Victorian Mental Health Act 1986*, amended 2003).

Most Australian Mental Health Acts involve the care and treatment of both voluntary and involuntary clients. Care has been taken in amendments made to Acts in recent years to embrace the client's perspective and to provide appropriate and timely response to complaints about care that has been received during treatment (in the hospital and the community). Detained clients are more likely than ever before to receive care in the community, and Australian Mental Health Acts provide for this context of care using community-based treatment orders. In some circumstances (such as refusal of depot medication), clients may be forcibly removed to hospital for treatment. Geography and isolation factors also affect differences in legislation. In the Northern Territory, for example, ambulance officers may detain clients (for a maximum of six hours) who are deemed to be mentally ill and requiring immediate treatment.

Community visitors (for example, *Tasmanian Mental Health and Related Services Act 1996*), or Official Visitor Programs are external, independent mechanisms introduced to advocate for people with mental health problems having treatment.

Voluntary and involuntary admission of psychiatric clients

Two criteria common to Australian Mental Health Acts regarding the voluntary (i.e. with their full permission) admission of individuals are that: the severity of the mental illness requires treatment in an approved mental health facility; and the individual is suffering from an acute episode of a mental illness. Mental Health Acts generally include statements about the need to involve clients in all appropriate aspects of their care and treatment regardless of their status (voluntary or detained). Circumstances occur where a person may have been admitted voluntarily and then requests to leave but may be deemed too unwell to do so and is then detained against their will. For a person to be detained, the following criteria must *all* apply:

■ The person appears to be mentally ill.

■ Immediate treatment is required and can be obtained in an approved mental health facility.

■ Due to the illness the person needs to be detained for treatment as an involuntary client for the person's own safety (physical or mental) or for protection of members of the public (*Queensland Mental Health Act 2000*; *Victorian Mental Health Act 1986*, amended 2003).

Compulsory or involuntary admission (detention to an approved psychiatric institution) is controversial as it involves the removal of, by the State or Territory under the auspices of the Mental Health Act, an individual's freedom and autonomy, raising complex legal and ethical issues about the role of the State in controlling individuals deemed to be mentally ill. Mental Health Acts vary in the periods of time for which they specify that people can be detained involuntarily when first admitted to a mental health unit. Generally speaking, a person may be detained against their will for an initial period of twenty-four hours by a medical practitioner, but then must be reviewed by a psychiatrist as soon as is practicable. The person may then be further detained for a period of twenty-one days, or the detention may be revoked and the person assume voluntary status. In the latter case clients then have the right to appeal through the Guardianship Board to review their voluntary status (*South Australian Mental Health Act 1993*, Section 12; *Queensland Mental Health Act 2000*). In certain circumstances treatment orders and orders for forced treatment in mental health facilities and the community can be placed on individuals who refuse, or fail to undergo, treatment. The principle here is that the treatment is in the best interests of the client and that treatment will alleviate their symptoms of mental illness. Under any of the continuing detention orders, clients have a right of appeal, which is heard through a sitting of the state or territory Guardianship Board. For consumers there is an uneasy tension between self-determination and the determinations made by mental health authorities, 'in their best interests' (in this case, the Guardianship Board).

Three confounding issues are: the different words used for 'compulsory detention' in the various state and territory Mental Health Acts (for example, 'section' is used in one State, 'schedule' or 'order' in another); the length of time for which a person may be detained; and the varying conditions surrounding the use of seclusion and restraint. Although all Australian Mental Health Acts have adopted tenets of least-restrictive and consumer-focused practice in relation to the law, the continuing differences remain confusing and potentially unhelpful for those who may require admission in more than one State or Territory over time.

The use of control measures in mental health nursing practice must also be understood in the social context of mental health legislation and increasing focus on 'risk management' of individuals in society (mentally ill or otherwise) deemed to pose a risk to the general public, including health professionals. The next section briefly explores the notion of dangerousness and risk management as recent concepts in the care and treatment of people in health settings and, in particular, mental health service delivery.

Risk management and the concept of dangerousness

The growth of the concept of risk in health care can be seen to be reflected by the perception of the general public that people with mental illness have an increased capacity for violence and being a danger to others (Morgan 1998). Although there are indications that client violence is increasing in the inpatient setting (Whittington & Wykes 1994) and the community (Fry et al. 2002), it is not known whether this is due to a real increase, previous under-reporting, a worsening level of risk in the workplace, or an increased awareness of the subject of violence in society in general (Morgan 1998).

The impact of the media in raising alarm about people with mental illness being violent in the community is also a factor in negative perceptions about people with mental illness. However, statistics concerning the rate of violence among people with mental illness in the community do not confirm the attention given by the media. More balanced debates about this emotive subject remind us that people living with mental illness also have to bear the stigma and 'presumed guilty' label without a voice to present their view when fatalities in the community occur (Sayce 1995). Some basic truths remain: the diagnosis of mental illness is not a predictor of violence; incidents are more likely to be linked to the situational context; and alcohol or other drugs are often also involved in the incident (Morgan 1998, p 266).

The concept of dangerousness has become commonly used to assess the behaviour of the client in a health-care setting, though historically it was used to describe the likelihood of a forensic client re-offending when released into the community (Mason & Chandley 1999). The term 'forensic client' can be defined as a person who has committed a crime while mentally ill and is remanded in custody in an approved mental health service, within a prison, remand centre or forensic psychiatric hospital. Mental health nurses working on forensic psychiatric wards face unique challenges when working with vulnerable people in an extreme environment (Mason & Mercer 1998, p 84). Mason & Mercer (1998) state that this group of nurses, like all nurses working in prisons, have contradictory responsibilities, namely that they have to exert control over clients while maintaining ethical professional practice and protecting the public. 'Nursing practice in corrections is concerned with issues such as: mental illness, criminal acts, morality, treatment, containment and punishment' (Mason & Mercer 1998, p 85, drawing on Burnard 1992). In short, forensic mental health nurses must provide nursing care and obey the correctional codes of the institution. Given the nature of some of the crimes committed by this group of clients, risk assessment is a core and vital component of their role.

State and Territory governments around Australia have responded to concerns about the occupational health and safety of health professionals in the healthcare setting by implementing policies to guide practice in the management of aggression and violence in the workplace, citing the increase in risk and violence as the driving force. However, in some States, the adoption of strategies such as refusing service to clients who exhibit agitated or aggressive behaviour suggests a draconian, zero-tolerance approach. This approach does not take into account the need for treatment for individuals who exhibit behaviours such as agitation, anxiety or extreme fear that is a symptom of their illness. While the assessment of risk is imprecise—one paper indicates that health professionals may get it wrong up to half the time (Monahan 1984)—mental health nurses are required to be prepared with the skills and knowledge associated with this aspect of nursing care.

CRITICAL THINKING CHALLENGE 4.3

- Have you ever felt at risk in the nursing setting?
- What risk assessment policies and procedures are you aware of in nursing settings?
- How would you respond to statements from people you know about all 'mad' people being dangerous?

Duty of care and right to self-determination

That nurses owe a duty of care to clients and their fellow employees at work is a well-accepted premise. Duty of care involves both *acts* and *omissions*, meaning that liability can arise as much by a failure to perform a particular act as it can by doing it and doing it badly (Staunton & Whyburn 2002).

Alexander (1998, p 38) cites duty of care as deriving from the 'neighbour principle'. The essence of this principle is that 'you must take reasonable care to avoid acts or omissions which you can reasonably foresee would be likely to injure your neighbour'. At law, this can be any person who is likely to be affected by your acts or omissions. The justification for medical treatment against the will of the client is the common law duty of clinicians to provide whatever care is needed in an emergency to preserve life. Treatment against the client's wishes in an emergency is justified using the concept of urgent necessity (Hatcher & Samuels 1998).

CASE STUDY: Melissa—an incident of self-harm

Melissa is a 19-year-old woman brought into the department via ambulance following deliberate self-harming behaviour. Melissa has had a fight with her boyfriend, Brett, who wants to end their two-year relationship. Melissa has made a laceration to her left wrist with a knife that requires suturing. The mental health nurse talks to Melissa when she first arrives in the department. Melissa is reasonably calm on presentation, albeit abrupt, and agrees to have her wrist attended to. She is vague about the intent attached to this gesture and admits to having cut her wrist twice in the past under similar circumstances. She has had a recent admission to the mental health unit but is adamant about not wanting to return there. Instead she emphasises that she simply wants to be treated and to go home.

During the admission procedure Melissa has a disagreement with a nurse who insists that she change into a gown. Melissa quickly becomes distressed, loud and angry, her speech abusive. Melissa allows an emergency registrar to assess the laceration though she continues to vent her anger. She has limited sensation and movement in two fingers, indicative of nerve and tendon damage. The registrar decides that a plastic surgery consultation is necessary. The wound is cleaned and dressed.

The plastic surgery registrar arrives in the department and is met with Melissa's distress and hostility. He wants Melissa to have a repair of her laceration but she seems intent only on arguing. She refuses to sign the consent form for the operation even though it is explained to her that she will suffer some permanent impairment in function if she does not have the procedure.

Discussion

Mental health legislation has no bearing on involuntary medical or surgical treatment and does not allow for procedures or treatment to be performed or administered against the client's will (Hodgkinson et al. 1995). Mental health legislation is therefore of little assistance in the initial management of Melissa. Her presentation appears to arise as a consequence of a mental disorder, but medical attention is the priority rather than treatment of any mental illness or disorder (Hull & Haut 1999). Melissa has injured herself and requires medical treatment, although her injury is not life-threatening. At issue is her competence to refuse the surgical procedure that is required and the medical necessity attached to the procedure. Her capacity to consent to treatment is questionable given her extreme state of distress.

CASE STUDY: Ron—an aggressive and distressed client

Ron is a 21-year-old man who presents one evening with his mother. He has smoked cannabis on a regular basis (with occasional amphetamine use) for several years but decided to stop one week ago. Ron has always had a problem with aggression but since he has stopped smoking cannabis it has become worse. Several friends have distanced themselves from him recently because he has started fights with strangers. Ron has also been aggressive toward his brother, who he lives with, and last night broke some furniture in their flat during an argument. He punched a wall during the argument and injured his hand, which is now swollen and very painful.

Ron is calm at triage and tells the nurse that along with his painful hand he has an anger problem and wants assistance. He says that the cannabis controlled his aggressiveness to a degree but now, without it, he is much worse. He feels constantly agitated and restless. The department is busy this particular evening and Ron and his mother are left in the waiting area for almost two hours. Ron becomes increasingly angry about having to wait and tries to leave on several occasions but his mother is able to persuade him to stay.

The medical officer who comes to see Ron in view of his aggressive behaviour calls for security, writes a schedule and tells the nursing staff that Ron cannot leave the department until he has seen a psychiatric registrar. The psychiatric registrar soon arrives to speak to Ron. By now it is late in the evening. She finds him outside in a highly distressed state, circled by security guards and ED staff who are trying to reason with him. His voice is loud and he is gesticulating wildly. He repeatedly states that he just wants to go home. His mother is tearful and upset, standing to the side of the commotion with a nurse from the department.

Discussion

Ron is highly distressed and potentially violent. His reaction to the long wait highlights his difficulty with anger management. Violence or aggressiveness alone, however, is not sufficient for detention under the Mental Health Act. Ron is a risk to others and probably himself, but whether this is due to mental illness has not been established. He exhibits the most common risk factors associated with violent clients—male gender, a history of violence, drug or alcohol abuse and personality disorder (Kao & Moore 1999). His hand requires attention and his pain contributes to his risk of aggression but his injury would not be considered medically urgent.

Health-care professionals must balance the necessity of emergency medical treatment and their duty of care against the client's autonomy based on his or her capacity. A competent client has the right to withhold consent to examination, investigation or treatment even if such a decision is likely to result in death. This right to self-determination takes priority in law over the duty of care that health-care professionals feel obliged to practise (Bieger & Stewart 2001).

To achieve competence, three factors must be assessed and met:

- The client understands information on the proposed treatment, is able to retain it, and understands the consequences of non-treatment.
- The client believes the information.
- The client is able to weigh up that information and arrive at a choice.

The decision regarding capacity to refuse treatment must have been made with a senior doctor and must take into account the effect of physical and mental illness, alcohol and any drugs that may have been taken. Whether drugs that have been taken impede capacity should be considered urgently (Hassan et al. 1999).

Temporary mental incapacity also occurs as a result of intoxication and in states of high emotional arousal. These factors are most often operating in uncooperative clients who deliberately harm themselves (Feldman 1999). In the case studies above, Melissa's and Ron's distress has clouded their judgment, but this is temporary, and both of them may only require a little time to regain composure. It could be argued that both Melissa and Ron lack capacity due to extreme emotional arousal but detaining them forcibly would seem an excessive measure. Neither has a life-threatening medical condition, and if either Melissa or Ron were to leave the department it is unlikely that anything serious would eventuate.

Managing behavioural emergencies

The first priority with behavioural emergencies is to reason with the client and then try to persuade him or her to accept treatment voluntarily (Hodgkinson et al. 1995). It is beneficial for all emergency department staff to be trained in communication and negotiation. Attempts to force treatment on clients often leads to further resistance, but giving them the chance to vent their feelings and thereby establishing rapport often alleviates these difficult situations (Plummer 1999).

Emergency departments are especially susceptible to aggressive situations as the environment is filled with emotional stress and clients may endure prolonged waiting times, confusion, and gaps in communication. Violence rarely erupts suddenly. Frequently, aggression follows a period of mounting tension. In a typical scenario, the client first becomes angry, then resists authority, and finally becomes confrontational and overtly violent. Although it is necessary to deal with violence, it is better to recognise signs of impending violence and prevent it before it happens (Kao & Moore 1999).

The *Code of Ethics for Nurses in Australia* (ANC 2002) reinforces the respect that nurses have for individual needs, values and culture in the provision of health care which 'includes the development of confidence and trust in the relationship between nurses and the people for whom they care' (ANC 2002, p 3). It is essential that clinicians work at establishing trust and developing rapport from the moment a client enters the emergency department. Support, reassurance and gaining trust are especially important with people who are reluctant to accept treatment. Wherever possible there should be an avenue for compromise in the management of challenging behaviour.

Clinicians must be cognisant of circumstances where a potential for conflict exists. To decrease the likelihood of a situation escalating means recognising this possibility in its infancy, not its adolescence. Negotiating for cooperation from a client greatly diminishes the potential for further difficulties. The risk of a personal battle, the 'dominance reciprocal', between the clinician and client is particularly high with resistive clients and must be consciously avoided (Shea 1998). It is also important for clinicians to be attentive listeners and to respond verbally in a calm and soothing tone of voice. Nurses need to be particularly mindful of their own non-verbal communication, avoiding vocal qualities that may convey sarcasm, frustration, anger or an overly authoritarian demeanour. A conciliatory manner and supportive statements are required, rather than condescension (Rallis-Peterson 2001).

Expert consensus guidelines on the treatment of behavioural emergencies developed by Allen et al. (2001) recommend beginning with the least paternalistic or aggressive approaches—verbal intervention, offering food, beverage or other assistance, or voluntary medication—before moving to more intrusive strategies. Rallis-Peterson (2001) recommends that the emergency department have 'greeters' to direct clients and family members and to keep clients informed about delays. She also suggests that a coordinated response team be formed to manage clients who are out of control or threatening towards staff.

The main difficulty with a behavioural emergency is that an intervention is required but there is often a stand-off between the individual at the centre of the incident and those responsible for managing it (Allen et al. 2001). Physical restraint is a final response to imminent, dangerous behaviour when less restrictive measures fail or are not appropriate (Karas 2002). Many violent individuals will back down to a team response. A 'show of force' also protects the person's ego as it allows them to rationalise that they would have fought back if the odds had not been so overwhelming (Kao & Moore 1999).

Clinicians may not appreciate the detrimental, physical and psychological effects of restraining a client. Offering choices to the client should be factored into the decision-making process with an awareness of the adverse impact of heavy-handed or injudicious reliance on forced medications.

Managing clients who threaten to leave

The promotion of the health, safety and welfare of people at work is enshrined in legislation and overrides all other legal statutes and regulations. Both Melissa and Ron are a concern if they leave the department, and strategies should be employed to reduce the possibility of them leaving until their disposition is arranged. However, staff also need to consider their own safety as a priority and not place themselves at risk of becoming a casualty (NSW Health Department 2002).

No clinician should feel they have to pursue and physically restrain an 'at-risk' client who leaves the department prior to the completion of their treatment, especially in the absence of a coordinated response team. Restraining a client without a prearranged response is ill-advised as it places in jeopardy the safety of the client and staff members. A description of the events surrounding the client leaving the department and the individuals and organisations that have been notified (such as the police, relatives and friends, general practitioner or community mental health team) should be documented in the client's file. Clear, accurate documentation is essential and is the best defence against litigation (Kao & Moore 1999). While this may not be a satisfactory clinical outcome, duty of care is being extended to the client to as reasonable a degree as can be expected in the situation.

Management of deliberate self-harm and aggression is often unclear and confusing in the emergency department setting. Due to such uncertainty and in an attempt to feel less legally vulnerable in these situations, the decision is often made to place such presentations under the Mental Health Act. While such a decision is understandable it is usually an inappropriate use of statutory law and provides clinicians with no greater protection than treating someone under duty of care.

Nurses must be familiar with the ethical and legal considerations relevant to clients who present to the emergency department with self-harm and aggressiveness and follow a logical approach between the duty of care nurses are beholden to extend to a client and the client's right to self-determination. Working effectively with difficult clients requires the establishment of rapport. This is especially true in cases where a potential for disruption exists. Managing resistive clients requires flexibility, adept use of interpersonal skills and conscious control over the non-verbal qualities that can be conveyed in human interaction.

The final section of this chapter deals with the current shortage of nurses and mental health nurses locally and globally, outlining reasons for this situation and implications for the discipline of mental health nursing.

THE PROFESSION IN CRISIS

There is an acute shortage of mental health nurses in Australia today. In rural and regional areas the problem is exacerbated, with anecdotal reports suggesting that as many as forty per cent of mental health professional positions in Central Australia remain unfilled (Riley S, Healthcare Management Advisers, personal communication 2002). Where there are inadequate numbers of staff, turnover is high, affecting morale and the quality of care being delivered. The population of mental health nurses is also ageing; for example, in South Australia well over fifty per cent of nurses are over forty-five years of age. The shortage of mental health nurses mirrors the increasing shortage of general nurses worldwide. While explanations for why up to thirty per cent of the newly graduated workforce leave nursing within the first three years of their practice are complex, they clearly include increasingly difficult working conditions, burnout, low pay, and family non-friendly working hours. Australia is not alone in regard to the problems of the mental health nursing workforce. Burnout, a lack of organisational belonging and a sense of powerlessness and lack of control over one's work have been reported in the international literature (Melchior et al. 1997).

Because of concerns about the future of the Australian mental health nursing workforce, a scoping study was commissioned to the Australian and New Zealand College of Mental Health Nurses Inc by the Mental Health Branch of the Department of Health and Aged Care in 1999. The findings revealed problems with the education, recruitment, retention and employment of mental health nurses. Relatively few undergraduate nurses consider a career in mental health nursing, imposing the same stigma on the mentally ill as the general public. Undergraduate programs do not contain adequate educational preparation to remove this stigma; many academics argue that there is 'just not room' in the three-year educational preparation of general nurses for predominantly acute physical care, to include psychiatric nursing theory and practice. Mental health services often disempower clients and mental health nurses alike in the perpetuation of anachronistic and paternalistic management practices (Clinton & Hazelton 2002). These authors go on to argue that arrangements for the preparation of highly experienced mental health nurses to become nurse practitioners and to work in autonomous nursing positions are relatively non-existent, halting career paths for committed and motivated clinicians.

Further, given that in many States and Territories of Australia general nurses may work in mental health settings without formal qualifications, there is little direct incentive for nurses to gain formal qualifications in mental health. Thus, the suggestion that there may be a demise of the mental health nurse as we know it is not alarmist and is supported by many commentators in Australia (Happell 1997; Holmes 2001). Workforce planning around Australia has given little thought to the changing nature of nursing graduates and whether university-educated students see the attraction of the current scope of mental health nursing practice. So which way forward? Clinton & Hazelton (2002) suggest that there is little point in waiting for the State or Territory or Australian Commonwealth Government to make change. Mental health nurses must 'do it for themselves', must take responsibility for leading reforms, just as consumers took the initiative during the 1990s, and voice their vision of the raison d'etre of the profession. In doing this, mental health nurses must be careful to work in partnership with those for whom they care—in the end we are all consumers of mental health services in one form or another.

CRITICAL THINKING CHALLENGE 4.4

- What would you change about your workplace to improve your daily working life?
- What mental health nursing practices do you strongly agree/disagree with? What evidence do you base this on?
- Do you feel disempowered in the workplace? If so, by what or whom?
- How would you describe the work of a mental health nurse to someone who was interested in entering the field?
- How can mental health nurses become more active as agents of change?

CONCLUSION

This chapter has explored a number of contemporary legal and political issues associated with mental health nursing practice in Australia and New Zealand. There are many challenges facing mental health nurses, including changes to the role of the mental health nurse, ongoing policy developments in the provision of mental health services and the need to balance the caring and controlling functions of mental health nursing practice. Such challenges serve to facilitate opportunities for reform, practice developments and the development of new partnerships with those for whom we care.

EXERCISES FOR CLASS ENGAGEMENT

■ Discuss contemporary developments in mental health services globally and in Australia and New Zealand, and their impact on how people with mental illness are cared for in the community.

■ Examine the role of the mental health nurse in contemporary practice. Discuss the tension between caring and controlling functions of the role of the mental health nurse, using examples from practice.

■ Discuss the concept of dangerousness in relation to nursing practice in mental health settings.

■ Think about some recent clinical experiences you have had with clients with mental health problems, and discuss your responses to the following questions with your group or class members.

● Identify some caring and controlling functions you have observed or been involved with.

● How did you feel about being involved in controlling interventions with clients?

● Were there alternatives that could have been less restrictive?

● What are your own beliefs about how and where people with mental illness should be cared for?

● Should State and Territory legislation have the power to contain or control people with a mental illness to protect them from themselves and/or other people?

REFERENCES

Alexander L 1998, Duty of care: legal issues for nurses, *Lamp*, 5(5), p 38.

Allen MH, Currier GW, Hughes DH, Reyes-Harde M & Docherty JP 2001, The expert consensus guidelines series: Treatment of behavioural emergencies, *Post Graduate Medicine*, Supplement May 1-88.

Andrews G 1994, The Tolkein Report—1994. A Model for Matching the Available Workforce to the Demand for Services, unpublished paper.

Ash D, Burvill P, Davies J, Hughson B, Meadows G, Nagle T et al. 2001, Mental health services in the Australian States and Territories. In: Meadows G & Singh B (eds), *Mental Health in Australia Collaborative Community Practice*, Oxford University Press, Melbourne.

Australian Health Ministers 1992a, *The National Mental Health Plan*, Australian Health Ministers' Conference 1992, AGPS, Canberra.

Australian Health Ministers 1992b, *National Mental Health Policy*, Australian Health Ministers' Conference 1992, AGPS, Canberra.

Australian Health Ministers 1998, *Second National Mental Health Plan*, Mental Health Branch, Commonwealth Department of Health and Family Services, AGPS, Canberra.

Australian Nursing Council 2002, *Code of Ethics for Nurses in Australia*, ANC, Canberra.

Bell S & Brookbanks W 1998, *Mental Health Law in New Zealand*, Brooker's, Wellington.

Biegler P & Stewart C 2001, Assessing competence to refuse medical treatment, *Medical Journal of Australia*, 174(10), pp 522–5.

Clinton M & Hazelton M 2002, Towards a Foucauldian reading of the Australian mental health nursing workforce, *International Journal of Mental Health Nursing*, 2(1), pp 18–23.

Clinton M & Nelson S 1999, Recovery, mental illness and mental health nursing. In: Clinton M & Nelson S (eds), *Advanced Practice in Mental Health Nursing*, Blackwell Science, Oxford.

Department of Health and Aged Care 2002a, *National Action Plan for Promotion Prevention and Early Intervention in Mental Health*, Department of Health and Aged Care, AGPS, Canberra.

Department of Health and Aged Care 2002b, *National Action Plan for Depression*, Department of Health and Aged Care, AGPS, Canberra.

Durie M 1994, *Whaiora. Maori Health Development*, Oxford University Press, Auckland.

Durie M 1997, Puahou: A Five Point Plan for Improving Maori Mental Health, unpublished paper, Maori Mental Health Summit.

Feldman E 1999, No case law supports sectioning under the Mental Health Act in these circumstances, *British Medical Journal*, 319(7214), p 916.

Fishwick M, Tait B & O'Brien AJ 2001, Unearthing the conflicts between carer and custodian. Implications for mental health nurses in Section 16 hearings under the Mental Health (Compulsory Assessment and Treatment) Act (1992), *Australian and New Zealand Journal of Mental Health Nursing*, 10, pp 187–94.

Foster B 1998, Ethical practice and legal responsibility for duly authorized officers: achieving a balance, *Australian and New Zealand Journal of Mental Health Nursing*, 7(1), pp 41–5.

Fry AJ, O'Riordan D, Turner M & Mills K 2002, Survey of aggressive incidents experienced by community mental health staff, *International Journal of Mental Health Nursing*, 11, pp 112–20.

Happell B 1997, Psychiatric nursing in Victoria: a profession in crisis, *Journal of Psychiatric and Mental Health Nursing*, 4(6), pp 417–22.

Hassan TB, MacNamara AF, Davy A, Bing A & Bodiwala GG 1999, Lesson of the week: managing patients with deliberate self-harm who refuse treatment in the accident and emergency department, *British Medical Journal*, 319(7202), pp 107–9.

Hatcher S & Samuels A 1998, Medicolegal aspects of managing self-harm in the emergency department, *New Zealand Medical Journal*, 111(1069), pp 255–8.

Hodgkinson DW, Gray AJ, Dalal B, Wilson P, Szawarski Z, Sensky T, Gillett G & Yates DW 1995, Ethical debate: doctors' legal position in treating temporarily incompetent patients, *British Medical Journal*, 311(6997), pp 115–18.

Holmes C 2001, Postdisciplinarity in mental health-care: an Australian viewpoint, *Nursing Inquiry*, 8(4), pp 230–9.

Hull A & Haut F 1999, Managing patients with deliberate self-harm who refuse treatment in the accident and emergency department. Advice and procedure require correction, *British Medical Journal*, 319(7214), p 916.

Human Rights and Equal Opportunity Commission 1993, *Human Rights and Mental Illness: Report of The National Inquiry Into the Human Rights of People with Mental Illness*, AGPS, Canberra.

Kao LW & Moore GP 1999, The violent patient: Clinical management, use of physical and chemical restraints, and medicolegal concerns, *Emergency Medicine Practice*, 1(6), pp 1–24.

Karas S 2002, Behavioural emergencies: differentiating medical from psychiatric disease, *Emergency Medicine Practice*, 4(3), pp 1–20.

Mason K, Johnston J & Crowe J 1996, *Inquiry Under Section 47 of the Health and Disability Services Act 1993 in Respect of Certain Mental Health Services. Report of the Ministerial Inquiry to the Minister of Health, Hon Jenny Shipley*, Ministerial Inquiry to the Minister of Health, Wellington.

Mason T & Chandley M 1999, *Managing Violence and Aggression: A Manual for Nurses and Health Care Workers*, Churchill Livingstone, Edinburgh.

Mason T & Mercer D 1998, *Critical Perspectives in Forensic Care: Inside Out*, Macmillan, London.

Maude P 2001, From Lunatic to Client: A History/nursing Oral History of the Treatment of Western Australians who Experienced a Mental Illness, unpublished doctoral thesis, University of Melbourne, Melbourne.

Melchior MEW, Bours JJW, Schmitz P & Wittich Y 1997, Burnout in psychiatric nursing: a meta analysis of related variables, *Journal of Psychiatric and Mental Health Nursing*, 4, pp 193–201.

Mental Health Commission 1998, *Blueprint for Mental Health Services. How Things Need to Be*, Mental Health Commission, Wellington.

Mental Health Commission 2001, *Recovery Competencies for New Zealand Mental Health Workers*, Mental Health Commission, Wellington.

Mental Health (Compulsory Assessment and Treatment) Act (1992) (and amendments), Government Printer, Wellington.

Ministry of Health 1994, *Looking Forward: Strategic Directions for the Mental Health Services*, Ministry of Health, Wellington.

Ministry of Health 1997a, *Moving Forward: The National Plan for More and Better Mental Health Services*, Ministry of Health, Wellington.

Ministry of Health 1997b, *National Mental Health Standards*, Ministry of Health, Wellington.

Ministry of Health 2000, *Guidelines to the Mental Health (Compulsory Assessment and Treatment) Act (1992)*, Ministry of Health, Wellington.

Ministry of Health 2001, *Primary Mental Health Care Strategy*, Ministry of Health, Wellington.

Ministry of Health 2002a, *Te Puawaitanga. Maori Mental Health National Strategic Framework*, Ministry of Health, Wellington.

Ministry of Health 2002b, *Primary Mental Health: A Review of the Opportunities*, Ministry of Health, Wellington.

Monahan J 1984, The prediction of violent behaviour: toward a second generation of theory and policy, *American Journal of Psychiatry*, 141(1), pp 10–15.

Morgan S 1998, The assessment and management of risk. In: Brooker C & Repper J (eds), *Serious Mental Health Problems in the Community: Policy, Practice and Research*, Balliere Tindall, London.

New South Wales Health Department circular 2002/19 2002, Effective Incident Response: A Framework for Prevention and Management in the Health Workplace, Sydney.

New South Wales Mental Health Act, 1990, New South Wales Government.

Newton L, Rosen A, Tennant C, Hobbs C, Lapsley HM & Tribe K 2000, Deinstitutionalisation for long term mental illness: an ethnographic study, *Australian and New Zealand Journal of Psychiatry*, 34(3), pp 484–90.

Plummer WP 1999, The Mental Health Act and consent to treatment. *eBMJ*. Online: Rapid responses for Hassaan et al., http://bmj.bmjjournals.com/cgi/eletters/319/7202/107#3833, accessed 22 March 2004.

Rallis-Peterson D 2001, When a patient turns violent, *RN*, 64(5), pp 32–5.

Rosenman S 1994, Mental health law: an idea whose time has passed, *Australian & New Zealand Journal of Psychiatry*, 28(4), pp 560–5.

Sayce L 1995, Response to violence: a framework for fair treatment. In: Crichton J (ed.), *Psychiatric Patient Violence: Risk and Response*, Duckworth, London.

Shea S 1998, *Psychiatric Interviewing. The Art of Understanding*, WB Saunders, Philadelphia.

Singh B 2001, The global perspective in mental health. In: Meadows G & Singh B (eds), *Mental Health in Australia: Collaborative Community Practice*, Oxford University Press, London.

South Australian Mental Health Act 1993. Online: http://www.austlii.edu.au/au/legis/sa/consol-act/mha1993128/s12html.

Standards New Zealand 2001a, *National Mental Health Sector Standards*, Standards New Zealand, Wellington.

Standards New Zealand 2001b, *National Mental Health Sector Standard: Audit Workbook*, Standards New Zealand, Wellington.

Staunton P & Whyburn B 2002, *Nursing and the Law* (4th edn), Churchill Livingstone, Sydney.

Street AF & Walsh C 1994, The legislation of the therapeutic role: implications for the practice of community mental health nurses using the New Zealand Mental Health (Compulsory Assessment and Treatment) Act of 1992, *Australian and New Zealand Journal of Mental Health Nursing*, 3, pp 39–44.

Street AF & Walsh C 1998, Nursing assessments in mental health New Zealand, *Journal of Advanced Nursing*, 27(3), pp 553–9.

Te Puni Kokiri 1996, *Nga ia o te oranga hingearo Maori. Trends in Maori mental health 1984–1993*, Te Puni Kokiri, Wellington.

Thornicroft G & Betts V 2002, *International Mid-term Review of the Second National Mental Health Plan for Australia*, Mental Health and Special Programs Branch, Department of Health and Ageing, Canberra.

United Nations Declaration 1991, Principles for the Protection of Persons with Mental Illness and for the Improvement of Mental Health Care as set out by the United Nations Human Rights Commission, Geneva.

Verdun-Jones SN 1986, The dawn of a 'new legalism' in Australia? The New South Wales Mental Health Act, 1983 and related legislation, *International Journal of Law and Psychiatry*, 8(1), pp 95–118.

Vestegaard J 1994, The Danish Mental Health Act of 1989: psychiatric discretion and the new legalism, *International Journal of Law and Psychiatry*, 17(2), pp 191–210.

Victorian Mental Health Act 1986, amended 2003, AGPS, Melbourne.

Whittington R & Wykes T 1994, The prediction of violence in a health care setting. In: Wykes T (ed.), *Violence and Health Care Professionals*, Chapman Hall, London.

World Health Organization (WHO) 1996, *Mental Health Care Law: Ten Basic Principles*, WHO, Geneva.

World Health Organization (WHO) 2001a, *Mental Health around the World: Stop Exclusion: Dare to Care*, brochure, WHO, Geneva.

World Health Organization (WHO) 2001b, *Mental Health, New Understanding, New Hope*, WHO, Geneva. Online: http://www.who.int/whr2001/2001/main/en/chapter4/Box 5.1. Rights of the Mentally Ill.

PART

2

Mental Health
and Wellness

INTRODUCTION

This chapter discusses key issues related to the professional practice of mental health nursing. The past twenty years have seen the final devolution of mental health care from predominantly hospital-based services to integrated hospital and community care, together with the development of a wide range of clinical specialisations within mental health nursing. In parallel with that process of change has been the move within nursing education to degree-based generic preparation for practice and, in some centres, the development of mental health nursing as a postgraduate specialty. Mental health nursing has responded to these challenges by developing standards for practice, practice competencies and models of advanced practice. The scope of practice has been extended to include the nurse practitioner role and prescribing. At the same time that the profession has been developing its own structures and processes, it has developed responses to the complex ethical issues that the changing mental health context demands. This chapter explores the professional context of practice, including the roles of professional and industrial nursing organisations, mechanisms of professional self-regulation and development of advanced practice and nurse practitioner roles. It also outlines the principles of ethical conduct and discusses some ethical issues commonly encountered in mental health nursing.

REGULATION OF PROFESSIONAL PRACTICE

Regulation of nursing is managed by statutory authorities in each Australian State or Territory and in New Zealand. Their primary purpose is to ensure public safety through maintaining professional standards. Regulatory authorities set and monitor standards in the interests of the public and the professions, and maintain registers of individuals licensed to practise nursing. In addition, they accredit educational institutions and nursing programs, provide complaints and disciplinary processes, and produce publications on key areas of policy. Individual nurses are granted a licence in the form of a practising certificate, entitling them to practise, subject to meeting criteria for registration. In both Australia and New Zealand there are two levels of nurse: enrolled and registered. In both countries, enrolled nurses, while accountable for their practice within the relevant framework of competencies, work under the direction and supervision of registered nurses.

Changes in educational preparation for practice have meant that qualifications for practice and categories of registration vary from one authority to another. There are even problems with the terms 'mental health nurse' or 'psychiatric nurse' because there is no accepted credentialling process that regulates the use of either term. For example, while a nurse gaining comprehensive registration in New Zealand is licensed to practise in any nursing specialty within New Zealand (excluding midwifery, which has a separate process of registration), the same nurse may have to undertake additional educational preparation to practise in some Australian States or Territories. Similarly, the individual States and Territories set their own registration criteria, creating a plethora of regulatory regimens throughout Australia and New Zealand.

Mutual Recognition Acts in the States and Territories provide mechanisms for nurses to have their registrations recognised from one State or Territory to another. The New Zealand Trans-Tasman Mutual Recognition Act (TTMRA), which came into effect in 1997 (ACT Parliamentary Council), allows applicants with nursing and midwifery registration in the Australian Capital Territory, New South Wales, Victoria, Tasmania, South Australia and the Northern Territory to apply to the Nursing Council of New Zealand under TTMRA for recognition of their registration. Contact details for the various Australian and New Zealand registering authorities are provided in Box 5.1.

Although States and Territories manage the process of regulating nursing, the Australian Nursing Council (ANC) provides a coordinating national role on regulatory issues affecting Australian nurses. The ANC is a representative body comprising members from each of the States and Territories, and two members of the public. The ANC maintains a national set of competency standards for nursing, guidelines for accreditation of nursing courses, and frameworks for dealing with ethical, professional and disciplinary matters.

Because of the move towards comprehensive education and the closer collaboration between the States established by the ANC, all States have reviewed their registers, and nurses are placed largely on a single register, with the employing authority making the decision as to whether or not they are competent to practise. This has, in effect, deregulated the market for nursing, but has largely disregarded the need for specialty preparation in mental health. Western Australia and South Australia have maintained separate registers of mental health nurses, while others such as Victoria and Queensland have made provision for endorsement of a mental health specialty qualification. New South Wales and New Zealand each maintain single registers with no endorsement or recognition for specialty mental health qualifications. In most Australian States, nurses who hold current registration, even without a mental health qualification, can work in mental health. However, in most States restrictions exist for nurses who hold only mental health qualifications and wish to work in general health settings.

In New Zealand, nurses with a comprehensive registration can work in any health setting, although some services will only employ new graduates who are enrolled

in a specialty mental health nursing program. However, there is no restriction on employment of comprehensive nurses, and those without postgraduate preparation in the specialty are not prevented from practising in mental health. Under the *New Zealand Nurses' Act (1977)*, nurses must practise within their scope of practice, meaning that those prepared in the previous hospital-based general programs cannot practise in mental health. The Nurses' Act is due to be replaced by a *Health Practitioners' Competency Assurance Act (2003)* which will establish a single regulatory body for all New Zealand health professionals (Ministry of Health 2001).

As mental health nursing develops, regulatory bodies need to develop regimens to credential those with specialist education in mental health, and to support new roles such as nurse practitioner. This includes specifying competencies and educational requirements, providing processes of accreditation and monitoring, and systems of accountability. However, it should be noted that nurse practitioners are professionals who practise with a high degree of autonomy, and so are expected, in addition to the regulatory controls of registration bodies, to maintain their own systems of professional monitoring and review.

The regulation of nursing practice is a political and professional issue. Definition of the mental health scope of practice and protection of consumers through employing only practitioners prepared within that scope are issues that require an assertive approach on the part of professional nursing bodies. What is at stake is the specialist nature of mental health care, recognition of the skills of mental health nurses, and acceptance that mental health consumers have needs that cannot adequately be met by generalist nurses without specialty preparation. The Australian and New Zealand College of Mental Health Nurses has proposed a credentialling process for mental health nurses. The proposed process requires specialist postgraduate mental health nursing education, current practice in mental health, and an auditable record of professional development (Chesterson 2002). Such a process, if adopted throughout Australia and New Zealand, would recognise the specialist nature of mental health nursing, and would provide protection for consumers in the form of uniform minimum professional standards.

Box 5.1 **Australian and New Zealand regulatory bodies**

AUSTRALIA

Australian Nursing Council
First Floor, 20 Challis Street, Dickson, ACT 2602
PO Box 873, Dickson, ACT 2602
ph: +61 2 6257 7960, fax: +61 2 6257 7955
general enquiries email: anc@anc.org.au
http://www.anci.org.au/

Australian Capital Territory Nurses Board
PO Box 1309, Tuggeranong, ACT 2901
ph: +61 2 6205 1599, fax: +61 2 6205 1602
www.healthregboards.act.gov.au

New South Wales Health Professionals Registration Board
PO Box K599, Haymarket, NSW 2000
ph: +61 2 9219 0222 or 1800 241 220,
fax: + 61 2 9212 7126
http://www.nursesreg.nsw.gov.au

Nurses Board of Victoria
GPO Box 4932, Melbourne, Vic 3001
ph: +61 3 9613 0333, fax: +61 3 9629 2409
www.nbv.org.au

Nursing Board of Tasmania
PO Box 847, Sandy Bay, Tas 7006
ph: +61 3 6224 3991, fax: +61 3 6224 3995
www.nursingboardtas.org.au

Health Professionals Licensing Authority
GPO Box 4221, Darwin, NT 0801
ph: +61 8 8999 4157, fax: +61 8 8999 4196
www.nt.gov.au/health/org_supp/prof_boards/

Nurses Board of South Australia
PO Box 7106, Adelaide, SA 5000
ph: +61 8 8223 9700, fax: +61 8 8223 9707
www.nursesboard.sa.gov.au

Nurses Board of Western Australia
Locked Bag 6, East Perth, WA 6892
ph: +61 8 9421 1100, fax: +61 8 9421 1022
www.nbwa.org.au

Queensland Nurses Council
GPO Box 2928, Brisbane, Qld 4001
ph: +61 7 3223 5111, fax: + 61 7 3223 5115
http://www.qnc.qld.gov.au

NEW ZEALAND

Nursing Council of New Zealand
Level 12, Mid City Tower, 139–143 Willis Street, Wellington, New Zealand
PO Box 9644, Wellington, New Zealand
ph: +64 4 802 0247, fax: +64 4 801 8502
general enquiries email: admin@nursingcouncil.org.nz
http://www.nursingcouncil.org.nz

PROFESSIONAL AND INDUSTRIAL BODIES

Mental health nurses practise in a complex professional environment that requires a clear sense of professional identity and clear frameworks for practice. While broad frameworks for professional practice are provided by legislation and by nursing regulatory bodies, a wide range of professional issues are regulated through professional nursing bodies. In addition, the profession has a role in monitoring the social context of practice through involvement in the development of legislation, policy and local services. A related issue is the maintenance and improvement of nurses' employment conditions. Much of this work is carried out by nurses within the various professional and industrial bodies.

The range of professional and industrial nursing bodies can be divided into those whose primary focus is professional issues, such as the colleges of nursing, and those whose primary focus is providing workplace representation and bargaining over salary and conditions of employment. However, this distinction disguises the overlap between these bodies, as conditions of employment have a direct effect on ability to meet professional standards, and the realisation of the expectations of professional bodies can affect conditions of employment. The issues of numbers of beds provided by a mental health service, and the number of staff allocated to different sections of the service demonstrate the overlapping functions of professional and industrial organisations. While these may be primarily industrial issues in terms of their immediate impact on nurses' conditions of employment, they also have the potential to affect standards of clinical practice. Both professional and industrial bodies have an interest in quality-of-service issues. Many nurses belong to more than one nursing body, as the functions of those bodies meet differing needs.

There are many organisations representing the professional and industrial interests of mental health nurses. As employees and as a professional group, nurses have a wide range of interests that require professional advocacy and articulation. While membership of professional bodies or industrial bodies is not compulsory in Australia or New Zealand, individual nurses need to reflect carefully on the advantages of membership and their responsibilities as health professionals to support the representative bodies that maintain their conditions of employment and advocate on professional issues. Professional and industrial bodies negotiate with employers and policy makers on employment and professional issues, and have an important role in informing members on current issues in health care. They may also play an advocacy role in the case of disputes or inquiries, and provide legal advice to nurses facing complaints or disciplinary proceedings. Some organisations provide indemnity insurance, which can be a valuable protection against the costs of legal advice. Some of the key professional and industrial bodies in Australia and New Zealand are listed in Box 5.2.

In both Australia and New Zealand, changes to employment law throughout the 1990s saw a reduction in the power of industrial unions, and a loss of national award structures. Employers argued for greater flexibility in industrial matters, negotiating with individual worksites rather than unions covering a range of sites, or with national unions. The changed industrial environment coincided with recruitment and retention problems in mental health nursing, and affected the ability of services to provide an appropriately skilled workforce (Clinton & Hazelton 2000a; Mental Health Commission 1998; Ministry of Health 1996).

A related issue is the development of a 'casual' nursing workforce, especially in inpatient settings. Nurses employed on a casual basis may not have the familiarity with consumers that is gained by regular employment in mental health services, and are frequently not union members, thus diminishing the resources available to unions to advocate on industrial and professional issues.

NURSING EDUCATION

The first training programs for psychiatric nurses commenced in Sydney in 1887 and in Auckland in 1907. Registration for psychiatric nurses began in New Zealand in 1907 (Psychiatric nursing training 1945) and in Australia in 1911 (Maude 2001). The early programs of education in psychiatric nursing were based in psychiatric institutions and were apprentice-style programs with students spending the greater proportion of their time meeting the service needs of the institutions. While this had the benefit of providing nursing students with a great deal of exposure to the clinical practice of nursing, it provided limited opportunities to develop academic and theoretical skills.

Educational preparation for practice in mental health nursing underwent a tremendous period of change in the latter half of the last century. From a specialist, service-based training based in psychiatric hospitals, mental health nursing came to be included in generic (comprehensive) nursing degree programs within the tertiary education sector. This process began in New Zealand in 1973 (Department of Health 1986) and in Australia in 1984 (National Education Review Secretariat 2002). The last hospital-based programs ceased in New Zealand in 1987 and in Australia in 1994. Although there are distinct advantages in separating education from employment, the change in the educational preparation of nurses for practice in the mental health specialty has not been without problems. Reviews of nursing education have stressed the importance of mental health within undergraduate education, citing the need to maintain an effective and skilled workforce (KPMG Consulting 2001; National Education Review Secretariat 2002). However, some pressing problems that remain are the loss of specialty focus in undergraduate programs, recruitment into the mental health specialty, and access to postgraduate education.

Box 5.2 Professional and industrial bodies in mental health nursing

Australian and New Zealand College of Mental Health Nurses

The Australian and New Zealand College of Mental Health Nurses (ANZCMHN) was established in 1974, and is a nursing body which represents the professional interests of mental health nurses in Australia and New Zealand. Members of the College work in a variety of settings throughout the public and private health-care and education sectors. The majority of members work in clinical practice in hospital or community services. There are 1600 College members in branches in each state of Australia and in New Zealand. The College produces the quarterly *International Journal of Mental Health Nursing* (http://www.anzcmhn.org).

Australian Nursing Federation

The Australian Nursing Federation (ANF) was established in 1924 and is the largest nursing organisation in Australia. The ANF is Australia's only national nursing union. The ANF's core business is the industrial and professional representation of nurses through the activities of a national office and branches in every State and Territory. The ANF has 120,000 members and produces the *Australian Nursing Journal* and *The Australian Journal of Advanced Nursing* (http:/www.anf.org.au).

Health Services Union of Australia

The Health Services Union of Australia was established in Victoria in 1911 as the Hospital and Asylum Attendants and Employees' Union and has branches in most Australian States. Branches represent nurses employed in psychiatric, intellectual disability and alcohol and drug services. The principal function of branches is to provide an association of members for the purposes of bargaining for reasonable wages, conditions of employment and career standards (http://www.hsua.asn.au/).

New Zealand Nurses' Organisation (NZNO)

The New Zealand Nurses' Organisation was established in 1909 and is New Zealand's largest nursing organisation, with 24,000 members. NZNO has branches throughout New Zealand, and represents members in the promotion of nursing and midwifery and participation in health and social policy development. NZNO produces the monthly *Kai Tiaki: Nursing New Zealand* (http://www.nzno.org.nz).

Public Service Association (PSA)

The Public Service Association (PSA) is New Zealand's largest state sector union and has 40,000 members in public services, health services and local government. The PSA represents nurses in many mental health services and participates in negotiation over salary and conditions of employment, as well as providing an advocacy role on mental health issues (http://www.psa.org.nz).

Royal College of Nursing Australia (RCNA)

The Royal College of Nursing Australia (RCNA) is a professional organisation representing nurses from all practice areas throughout Australia. The RCNA represents Australian nurses on policy-making bodies and committees and by promoting the professional development of nurses. The RCNA is the Australian member of the International Council of Nurses (ICN), representing Australian nursing to the world. It produces a monthly newspaper, *Nursing Review*, and a quarterly journal, *Collegian* (http://www.rcna.org.au).

STANDARDS OF PRACTICE

The professionalisation of mental health nursing is reflected in the development of standards of practice for both Australia and New Zealand (ANZCMHN 1995a,b). The growing emphasis on accountability in mental health care means that development of standards has assumed increasing significance (Rodgers 2000). The standards cover the broad scope of professional practice and include a rationale for each standard, attributes related to each standard, and performance criteria. A comparison of the Australian and New Zealand standards of practice is shown in Table 5.1.

The standards represent the commitment of mental health nurses to accountability in the professional practice of nursing. They have been recognised as a benchmark in examining the quality of mental health nursing care (Health and Disability Commissioner 2002; O'Brien 2002/2003). As broad statements of expected quality of care the standards are not directly measurable. However, clinical indicators have been developed to measure their achievement in practice (O'Brien et al. 2002; Skews et al. 1998, 2000). Clinical indicators are objective statements of specific outcomes or processes of care, which enable quantitative measurement of the quality of care (Idvall, Rooke & Hamrin 1997). They are an accepted means of measuring the achievement of practice standards. The Australian and New Zealand clinical indicator studies found high levels of achievement of some standards of practice, but also a significant number of areas of possible improvement, a finding similar to that of the Australian scoping study (Clinton & Hazelton 2000b). Continued monitoring of achievement of standards of practice is essential for any group claiming professional status, as self-regulation is recognised as a defining characteristic of professions.

Mental health nursing standards of practice describe the expected performance of nurses providing mental health care, but nurses in both countries also work within national systems of service standards that govern the practice of all mental health professionals (Commonwealth of Australia 1998; Standards New Zealand 2001). The coexistence of nursing professional standards and

Table 5.1 Standards of practice for mental health nursing in Australia and New Zealand

Australia[1]	New Zealand[2]
The mental health nurse:	The mental health nurse:
1 Ensures his or her practice is culturally safe through the sensitive and supportive identification of cultural issues	1 Ensures her or his practice is culturally safe
2 Establishes partnerships as the working basis for therapeutic relationships	2 Establishes partnerships as the basis for therapeutic relationships with consumers
3 Provides systematic nursing care that reflects contemporary nursing practice and the client's health-care/treatment plan	3 Provides nursing care that reflects contemporary nursing practice and is consistent with the therapeutic plan
4 Promotes health and wellness of individuals, families and communities	4 Promotes health and wellness in the context of their practice
5 Commits to ongoing education and professional growth and develops the practice of mental health nursing through the use of appropriate research findings	5 Is committed to ongoing education and contributes to the continuing development of theory and practice in mental health nursing
6 Practises ethically, incorporating the concepts of professional identity, independence, interdependence, authority and partnership	6 Is a health professional who demonstrates the qualities of identity, independence, authority and partnership

1 Source: Australian and New Zealand College of Mental Health Nurses (ANZCMHN) 1995a, Standards of practice for mental health nursing in Australia, ANZCMHN, Greenacres, SA.

2 Source: Australian and New Zealand College of Mental Health Nurses (ANZCMHN) 1995b. Standards of practice for mental health nursing in New Zealand, ANZCMHN, Greenacres, SA.

national service standards reflects the interdisciplinary nature of mental health care (Holmes 2001) and the demand for nurses to meet standards of their own profession as well as those of the service sector.

COMPETENCIES

In order to ensure a framework of safety that will protect the public, professions specify sets of competencies that describe the expected skills of all practitioners within a particular discipline. In nursing, competencies are set by regulatory bodies and by professional nursing organisations. The Australian Nursing Council (ANC) and the Nursing Council of New Zealand (NCNZ) provide competencies for enrolled and registered nurses, and in addition state and national bodies provide competencies for nurse practitioners and nurse prescribers. Where renewal of the annual practising certificate was formerly a procedural matter involving documentation and payment of a fee, nurses in future will have to demonstrate continuing competency in order to retain their registration. Competence-based practising certificates are due to be introduced in New Zealand in the near future (NCNZ 2001). Nurses in Australia must declare continuing competence in order to renew their annual practising certificate. State regulatory authorities conduct audits of competence in which nurses are expected to produce documentary evidence of continuing competence.

In addition to competencies specified by the profession, competencies set outside the profession also have the potential to affect practice. The New Zealand Mental Health Commission (MHC) has developed a set of recovery competencies that apply to all mental health workers in New Zealand (MHC 2001a). The competencies are shown in Box 5.3. The recovery competencies focus on attitudes of

mental health workers and choices offered to consumers. They are additional to the competencies expected of health professionals, for example in providing skilled assessment and intervention and the safe administration of medication.

> **Box 5.3 Recovery competencies for New Zealand mental health workers**
>
> A competent mental health worker:
> 1 understands recovery principles and experiences in the Aotearoa/NZ and international contexts
> 2 recognises and supports the personal resourcefulness of people with mental illness
> 3 understands and accommodates the diverse views on mental illness, treatments, services and recovery
> 4 has the self-awareness and skills to communicate respectfully and develop good relationships with service users
> 5 understands and actively protects service users' rights
> 6 understands discrimination and social exclusion, its impact on service users and how to reduce it
> 7 acknowledges the different cultures of Aotearoa/NZ and knows how to provide a service in partnership with them
> 8 has comprehensive knowledge of community services and resources and actively supports service users to use them
> 9 has knowledge of the service user movement and is able to support their participation in services
> 10 has knowledge of family/whanau perspectives and is able to support their participation in services.
>
> Source: Mental Health Commission 2001b, Recovery competencies for New Zealand mental health workers, Mental Health Commission, Wellington.

CAREER PATHWAYS

While mental health nursing was located primarily in psychiatric hospitals, the hierarchical nature of those institutions provided some structure to the careers of nurses. With the devolution of care to community settings and acute units attached to general hospitals, mental health nurses lost the opportunities for career advancement provided by large hospitals. Nurses wishing to gain career advancement sought academic or managerial, rather than clinical, appointments. This has challenged the profession to develop and lobby for career progression based on experience and clinical expertise.

Career pathways for nurses need to consider the diversity of nursing, and encourage nurses to pursue careers in clinical practice, education, management and research. All these choices require a sound foundation in clinical practice that is further enhanced by education and professional development.

The nurse practitioner development (discussed below) represents a career pathway for nurses that recognises their clinical expertise and its contribution to health outcomes, and encourages their retention in the nursing workforce. Thus nurse practitioners can be said to work on two levels, maximising health gains to consumers, and providing a career structure that will encourage the retention of the most experienced and skilled practitioners in the nursing workforce.

ADVANCED PRACTICE

In recent years, nurses in Australia and New Zealand have developed advanced practice roles. In some cases advanced practitioners extend that role to that of *nurse practitioner*, a title that requires licensing by a nursing regulatory body. The growth of advanced practice roles is part of a global development in nursing aimed at maximising the nursing contribution to health care, and improving health outcomes. The concept of advanced practice recognises that nurses seeking career progression do not always wish to follow careers in management or education, but may wish to retain their clinical focus while incorporating aspects of research, education and service leadership into their roles. Advanced practice roles recognise the contribution that experienced clinicians make to consumer outcomes, and their importance to the development of the nursing workforce.

Advanced roles have existed in the United States since the 1940s, where Hildegard Peplau was involved in the education of nurses with skills in psychotherapy, and with the development of the clinical nurse specialist role (Rice 2000). The terms 'advanced practitioner' and 'nurse practitioner' are often discussed synonymously in US literature, where both are used to refer to a nurse who has been authorised by a registering body to practise at an advanced level. There are currently a number of credentialled, advanced practice roles in the United States, where there have been calls for the multiplicity of roles to be replaced with a single 'blended' advanced practice role (Moller & Haber 1996).

The International Council of Nurses (ICN) applies a single definition to advanced practice nurse and nurse practitioner if those roles have been subject to credentialling in the context within which the nurse practises (ICN 2003). However, in Australia and New Zealand, 'nurse practitioner' is the title applied to nurses who are licensed in advanced practice roles.

Advanced practice is a level of nursing that involves specialisation within a scope of practice, increased clinical expertise, ability to provide nursing leadership, application of research to practice, teaching and consultancy (UKCC 1994). Advanced practitioners have usually received postgraduate education within their specialty, and possess a range of clinical skills within that specialty (Fulbrook 1998). Another definition of advanced practice in mental health stresses the development of skills of critical reflection on practice and on the social conditions of nursing practice and mental health (Crowe 1998). Such a definition emphasises the contextual nature of mental health and clinical practice rather than describing skills and attributes in isolation.

It is clear that mental health nursing involves a range of skills that extends far beyond the traditional skills of observation and engagement that characterised nursing in the era of hospital care. However, the skills of interpersonal engagement continue to provide a core around which advanced practice roles are developing. Competencies for advanced practice developed in New Zealand (ANZCMHN 2002) emphasise the central role of relationships in advanced practice mental health nursing. As advanced practice roles develop, mental health nurses will continue to build on the core concept of the interpersonal relationship, with skills specific to the diverse needs of consumers in specialist mental health services.

NURSE PRACTITIONERS

While advanced practitioners are nurses with advanced clinical expertise who provide clinical nursing leadership, they hold the same registration status as other nurses, and are not necessarily licensed to practise in extended roles. Nurse practitioners are those advanced practitioners who have extended education within a defined scope of practice, and who are licensed to practise within an extended role. Nurse practitioners represent a shift from health services based mainly on treating problems when individuals present with symptoms to those based on population health needs and primary health care. The role of nurse practitioner has been established in New Zealand (Ministry of Health 2002), New South Wales (Appel & Malcom 2002), Victoria, South Australia and the Australian Capital Territory.

In the United States, where nurse practitioners (or licensed advanced nurse practitioners) have been involved in health care for a number of decades, one of the major influences on the development of the role was the recognition that significant populations do not receive adequate health

services. For this reason nurse practitioners define the population of patients to whom they will provide a service, and specify how their skills will benefit that population. To achieve this, nurse practitioners need a sound understanding of the principles and practice of evidence-based care, and of measuring achievement of outcomes of care.

Mental health consumers represent a population that has traditionally been under-served by primary health care, whose physical health problems have been under-detected and under-treated, and who do not readily access health services due to barriers of transport, cost and issues of trust (Dickey et al. 2001). In addition, there is the potential for development of nurse practitioner roles within scopes of practice that involve early intervention, care of indigenous populations, misuse of substances, eating disorders, forensic services, primary care and a wide range of other specialties within mental health.

Because the nurse practitioner focuses on meeting the needs of under-served populations, rural communities are considered one of the population groups that could benefit from the nurse practitioner role (Ministry of Health 2002; NRB 1999). Traditionally, general medical practitioners have been hard to recruit to rural settings (Gill et al. 2001; Hays et al. 1997), creating an area of health need that could be met by nurse practitioners. Nurses have practised in extended roles in rural areas for some time (Appel & Malcom 2002), where they have frequently functioned as the only health professional providing direct contact. For these nurses, the nurse practitioner role recognises and formalises their existing practice. Similarly, in mental health, there is difficulty in providing sufficient psychiatrists to meet consumer needs (Andrews 1995), especially in rural and remote areas.

The current process of licensing nurse practitioners allows for experienced nurses with postgraduate certificates or diplomas to apply for nurse practitioner status. Most nursing authorities have signalled that, in the near future, Masters preparation and an appropriate level of experience will be the minimum criteria for application for accreditation as a nurse practitioner (Appel & Malcom 2002; Ministry of Health 2002).

Development of the nurse practitioner role has not come without resistance and opposition from those who see this expanded role encroaching on their professional domain (Loff & Cordner 1998). One of the potential sources of conflict as the nurse practitioner role develops is in the area of boundaries between different health-care providers. The nurse practitioner is envisaged as a collaborative health professional who develops collegial relationships with health colleagues and negotiates decision-making with them.

Research into the effectiveness of nurse practitioners has focused on two areas of outcome: cost effectiveness and clinical effectiveness. Nurse practitioners are most often compared to medical practitioners in evaluation studies, and despite the limitations of this approach, studies have so far demonstrated the greater or equal cost and clinical effectiveness of nurse practitioners (Horrocks, Anderson & Salisbury 2002; McManus et al. 2002; Mundinger et al. 2000; Venning et al. 2000).

As more nurse practitioners gain accreditation they will face challenges in defining models of practice that may be quite different from the models of clinical service delivery currently used. Suggested models include integrated nursing teams, consultancy, independent practice and provision of specialty services (Ministry of Health 2002). Development of new models of service delivery suggests that outcome studies will need to be developed that take account of the design and aims of services, and which measure the specific outcomes that have been planned. In addition, development of the nurse practitioner role will require careful attention to the legal and policy context to support the nurse practitioner development (Offredy 2000).

PRESCRIBING

Nurses have long influenced the pattern of medications prescribed to consumers by suggesting to doctors specific medications and medication regimens, based on their knowledge of consumers' preferences and responses, assessment of consumers' clinical state, and knowledge of the actions and interactions of psychotropic medications (Bailey 1999). In many areas, nurses practising as nurse practitioners are seeking to formalise this practice in the form of independent prescribing. Advanced practice nurses in the United States have been licensed to prescribe since 1977 (Fennell 1991), and currently forty-eight of the States extend prescribing authority to nurses (Pearson 1998). As with the nurse practitioner role, the intention of extending prescriptive authority to nurses is to fully utilise the capacity of nurses to provide health care (Bailey 1999), and to make health care more accessible to consumers.

In several Australian States and in New Zealand, legislation has allowed nurses who meet defined educational criteria to gain prescribing authority. Like the nurse practitioner development, this has not occurred without controversy. Medical practitioners have not always supported extension of prescribing authority to nurses (Clinton & Hazelton 2000b), arguing that nurses do not have adequate educational preparation for this role (Maling 2000), and there are questions within the profession about whether prescribing is a legitimate aspect of mental health nursing (Hemingway 2003). There is qualified support for prescribing by mental health nurses in Australia (McCann & Baker 2002). However, there are also complex legal, professional and clinical issues that need to be addressed. As more nurses are credentialled as nurse practitioners it seems likely that there will be growth in the number of nurses applying for prescriptive authority.

Prescribing does not stand alone as a clinical skill, but is embedded in a body of skills in assessment, diagnosis

and treatment. For a nurse or any health practitioner to prescribe safely and competently, they are required to demonstrate theoretical understanding and practical skills in health assessment, pharmacodynamics and pharmacokinetics. Regulatory bodies provide frameworks of competencies for prescribing and approve educational programs for nurse prescribers. Development of prescribing authority for nurses requires close collaboration with existing prescribers as nurses undertake the necessary clinical programs in prescribing. There is some evidence that nurses' prescribing patterns are different from those of doctors, with nurses prescribing medication less readily and in lower doses (Avron 1991; Safriet 1992). Negotiation with consumers about preferences in relation to medication will be an important aspect of nurse prescribing, as nurses seek to develop collaborative, consumer-focused models of prescribing.

ETHICS AND PROFESSIONAL PRACTICE

Eliot Freidson, a medical sociologist, defined a profession as 'an occupational group that reserves to itself the authority to judge the quality of its work' (Freidson 1989, p 9). This asserts that an occupation earns the right to call itself a profession partly through the credibility and trust that is built with the people to whom they provide a service. For nursing to assert itself as a profession, ethics and identity are inseparable. This is because the identity of nursing, and the self-regulatory processes that ensure continued trust within the community, are inextricably interwoven. In other words, nursing and nursing practice are guided by the law, ethical principles and the public image of the nurse as an ethical practitioner. The nurse must practise in accordance with the law and adhere to a code of ethical conduct.

Within the health professions there is a long history of debate concerning the professional codes of conduct and ethics required to guide practice and research with humans. Many professional groups have developed their own codes of ethics, which provide guidance to their members as to the nature of proper conduct and their obligations to the public. Most of these professional ethical codes consider three principal areas:

- standards of professional competence
- standards of professional integrity
- standards of professional etiquette.

These guiding ethical codes originate from ancient Greek (fifth century BC) thinking concerning ethics and have continued to influence ethical decision-making and thinking to the present day. The post World War II Nuremberg Code of 1949 inspired the formation of a medical code of ethical conduct—the Declaration of Geneva. In 1964 the Declaration of Helsinki (extended in 1975) guided the development of codes of ethical conduct for health research (Plueckhahn, Breen & Cordner 1994). Three contemporary developments worth noting are:

1 the Australian National Health and Medical Research Council *National Statement on Ethical Conduct in Research Involving Humans* (2001)
2 the *Code of Ethics for Nursing in Australia* (Australian Nursing Council 2000), which was first developed in 1993 and arose from the ANRAC Nursing Competencies Assessment project. The findings arising from this project indicated a need for nurses to have a code to guide ethical and cultural practice.
3 the New Zealand Nurses Organisation (1995) *Code of Ethics*.

The four principles guiding ethical conduct are listed in Box 5.4.

Box 5.4 **Principles of ethical conduct**

Autonomy—The person should have the right to make their own decisions, provided these decisions do not violate other people's autonomy. For people to be able to make autonomous decisions they must be free of the control of others and be informed of their options.
Beneficence—Beneficence in regard to nursing research or clinical care implies that what is conducted is good for the wellbeing of the person. Beneficence is the deliberate bringing about of positive action or intervention.
Non-maleficence—This means above all to do 'no harm' and implies both the duty of care to avoid actual harm as well as to consider the risks of any potential harm.
Justice—Justice refers to what society's expectations are of what is fair and right. The characteristics of justice imply that equality, access and no evidence of subordination exist (Hawley 1997).

Although the Australian and New Zealand College of Mental Health Nurses has developed standards of practice for Australia and New Zealand (ANZCMHN 1995a,b) and competencies for advanced practice (ANZCMHN 2002), the College has not yet developed a separate code of ethics for mental health nurses.

Internationally, professional nursing organisations have identified the need for a code of ethics to guide practice. All members of the American Psychiatric Nurses Association are expected to adhere to a code of ethics established by the Association. A website providing useful information about how other organisations have approached ethical codes of practice, as well as general information about professional ethics is at: http://hometown.aol.com/egeratylsw/ethics.html.

Ethical issues in mental health practice

People experiencing mental illness are, by the very nature of their disorder, possibly the most politically powerless and vulnerable group within society (Human Rights Commission, Australia 1993). The manifestations of

mental illness often include low self-esteem, withdrawal, self-doubt and distortions in thinking. Consequently, this is a population of people who find autonomy difficult to achieve and have difficulty advocating for themselves. Ethical issues abound in mental health and nurses practising in this area are confronted daily with the need for ethical decision-making. This section considers the following areas of mental health nursing practice, taking into consideration the need for ethical decision-making:

- psychiatric diagnosis
- psychiatric treatment
- suicidal behaviour
- involuntary commitment
- deinstitutionalisation
- therapy.

Psychiatric diagnosis

Psychiatric diagnosis should be the most fundamental aspect of mental health care delivery under ethical examination. The effects of diagnosis on an individual may include loss of personal freedom, imposed treatment regimens and the possibility of being labelled for life as mentally ill. Diagnostic labelling and hospitalisation of people with mental illnesses often marginalise them from their community and thus jeopardise their chances of achieving or regaining social integration. Consider a consumer who leaves the ward, steals a gardener's car and later returns to the hospital safely with the car and a carton of beer. When asked why he did such a thing, he advises that it was not something he would normally do, but since he was classified as insane he might as well act that way. This story demonstrates how labels can attract behaviour. The scenario may be explained as merely an impulsive act, but a person who feels they have been labelled may demonstrate that very behaviour, to challenge the assumption.

Diagnosis is a powerful tool. It has the capacity to describe behaviour that is odd or objectionable, and also has been used to explain behaviour that is unlawful, such as acts of theft or violence. In the latter case, the law recognises that mental illness compromises a person's free will and can classify them as not legally responsible for their actions. Therefore, a diagnosis of mental illness can, in some cases, benefit a person. However, the process of psychiatric diagnosis has been reported as being of poor or questionable reliability (Reich 1991). In mental health, objective signs of mental distress are not always evident, so diagnosis may be a difficult procedure. Consumers may not always have sufficient trust in professionals to tell the full story, and some aspects of their history may be too painful to recount in full. Also, consumers, like others, are influenced by processes such as denial and fantasy in describing their lives. A diagnosis is often made on subjective data and has been found to vary according to the psychiatrist's own bias (Reich 1991), or the impression the consumer gives to the psychiatrist. Diagnosis plays a powerful role within some people's lives, but it has its limits. People can be left

with a lifelong label and care must be taken not to identify cultural differences as signs of mental illness.

A diagnosis of mental illness may label the consumer as deviant from the normal population and result in pre-determined clinical and social behaviours, in both the person diagnosed and those health-care professionals caring for the consumer. Illich (1977) suggests that people are transformed into consumers by labelling and the disabling dependence that requires self-care, while individuals are transformed into clinicians by enculturation that attributes to them the power to diagnose and heal all ills. If a consumer is described to you as 'Mr Brown, the man who has been hearing voices and is afraid that others are talking about him', you will have certain expectations based on this description. However, if Mr Brown is described as 'the schizophrenic in room 4', how might your initial perceptions differ? There are strong messages in the words we use, especially when they become labels.

Some of the questions that need to be considered are: who has the right to decide what types of behaviours are considered to be mental illness rather than moral deviance?, how do we classify people who become verbally abusive when drunk, who are addicted to psychoactive substances, antisocial, have sexual preferences different to our own, hold unusual religious beliefs or who gamble excessively? Some of these you may see as mental illness, but other people would disagree with you. We do have systems of classification that differentiate normal from abnormal behaviour—for example, the *Diagnostic and Statistical Manual of Mental Disorders* (DSM-IV-TR) (American Psychiatric Association 2000) and the *International Classification of Diseases* (ICD), but these reflect contemporary beliefs about behaviour rather than objective standards (Moorey 1998). The cultural sensitivity of these diagnostic criteria and the disempowerment that the consumer feels from the confusing terminology used have also been questioned.

Psychiatric treatments

There is an increasing body of literature documenting patients' experiences of psychiatric treatment. Quirk & Lelliot (2001) usefully summarise research from the United Kingdom which indicates that nurse–patient relationships are considered to be a core component of inpatient care by patients as well as nurses, but this contact is often perceived to be limited. Furthermore, patients appreciate 'humane' qualities in nurses (Quirk & Lelliot 2001, p 1568). Patients are critical of the use of coercive practices such as restraint and seclusion, and perceive their use by nurses as punishment (Rogers & Pilgrim 1994). Worldwide, patient length of stay has decreased, while admission rates have increased, resulting in changes to the overall milieu of the ward, where acute interventions and containment are the predominant care provided, and less attention is paid to rehabilitation and comprehensive discharge planning. Within this climate, patients report that being in hospital is often boring and that they do not always feel safe (Quirk & Lelliot 2001).

Given that the Australian and New Zealand policy frameworks support increased consumer and carer involvement in aspects of treatment such as medication management and discharge planning, more research is indicated to explore the experiences of patients and their expectations of care. As an example of attempts to explore these issues further, a study by Johannsson & Lundman (2002) describes patients' experiences of involuntary care. Their findings revealed that patients perceive both supportive and controlling interventions which provide both 'good opportunities for care as well as great losses' (Johansson & Lundman 2002, p 639). Controlling interventions resulted in patients feeling that their autonomy was restricted, that they had been violated by an intrusion on their physical integrity and not receiving information about their care or not being involved in care. Conversely, caring interventions included being consulted about their care planning, being given freedom to go outside and nurses' flexibility about care. This resulted in patients feeling respected as individuals and being protected (Johansson & Lundman 2002, p 642). Similar findings also emerged in an ethnographic study exploring the process of constant observation of patients deemed to be at risk of suicide (Fletcher 1999). In this study, both nurses and patients identified therapeutic and controlling categories of nursing interventions. Some differences in perceptions related to patients not recognising nursing actions such as assessment, and nurses' explanations of nursing care suggest that nurses need to reflect carefully on the care they are providing and on how what they are doing is understood by patients.

Other authors have written about similar patient experiences of care and control in relation to the compulsory administration of medication, a necessary function of mental health nurses in both the inpatient setting and the community. Patients who experience forced medication report negative responses to that experience (Haglund, von Knorring & von Essen 2003). While a minority of patients gave retrospective approval for the forced administration, this was in fact a smaller number than expected by nurses. All patients spoke of the need to be offered alternatives, for nurses to take more time in discussing the need to take the medication, and to have the medication in a form other than injection.

CRITICAL THINKING CHALLENGE 5.1

Using the four principles of ethical conduct, consider when and if it is appropriate to administer an intramuscular injection of medication against a consumer's will.

Psychopharmacology—Until the 1950s there were few treatments for mental illness. The drugs prescribed for mental illness are potent agents, often causing major side-effects, creating problems with toxicity and, in the case of tranquillisers such as the benzodiazepines, causing

dependence. Psychotropic medications can also interact with other therapeutic agents, and so need to be monitored closely. These effects counter the argument that these drugs have been the single most important development in the treatment of mental illness (Krauss & Slavinsky 1982).

With respect to drug treatment, a question that needs to be considered is: What are a person's rights when placed on psychopharmacological agents? These rights should include access to effective professional treatment, information concerning the drug prescribed (desired effects, side-effects, contraindications, complications), and the freedom to accept or refuse treatment. These rights may be limited if the person is an involuntary patient under mental health legislation. However, all consumers should have some voice and choice in the selection of drugs. If the side-effects of a particular drug are difficult to live with, the person should be able to ask for a review and change of treatment.

Muir-Cochrane (2000, 2001) established that community mental health nurses found the task of forcible administration of medication in the community setting (i.e. in the patient's home) a less controlling encounter as the nurse attempted to convey respect for the context of the encounter. Nevertheless, forced administration of medication was recognised as a controlling task, one that nurses felt was a medical function, a difficult and uncomfortable, but inevitable, component of their responsibilities. To approach patients in their own home respectfully, without confrontation and with attempts to minimise antagonism were appropriate and inherent strategies used by community mental health nurses (Muir-Cochrane 2000).

Electroconvulsive therapy—Electroconvulsive therapy (ECT) is used mainly for major depression. A major ethical problem occurs when a psychiatrist prescribes ECT in order to reduce the risk of self-harm or harm through neglect, but the person does not give consent. The thought of having ECT can be traumatic to consumers due to negative perceptions about this form of treatment. All treatments need to be carefully negotiated with the consumer. In the case of the depressed person, their lowered mood and pessimistic outlook may mean that they are unable to see any solution to their depression. Some consumers may say that they do not deserve help. In the case of refusal of consent, doctors in some Australian States and in New Zealand require a second opinion and have the power under mental health legislation to administer ECT without the consumer's consent. Nurses need to ensure that these consumers and their families have been informed of the nature of the procedure and of why consent has been provided by another source.

Seclusion—Seclusion is generally defined as the removal of a person to a locked room, from which they may not leave, in order that the person may regain control and return to the ward environment. The wording in Mental

Health Acts suggests that seclusion is not deemed in law to be a treatment *per se* but rather a management tool enabling other treatments such as medication or counselling to be given (Muir-Cochrane, Holmes & Walton 2002).

Seclusion has also been identified as constituting a unique form of restraint, which 'effectively removes all social contact' (Alty & Mason 1994, p 4). This has been confirmed by Wallace (1997) in the context of Australian literature on the legal implications of restraint, indicating that clinicians should exercise special caution, particularly in relation to aspects of care that impinge upon personal freedom and rights (Holmes 1998). In Australia, in 1993, the Human Rights and Equal Opportunity Commissioner expressed concern about consumer reports that they experienced a loss of dignity when secluded, and that seclusion constituted a 'humiliating breach of their human rights' (HREOC 1993, p 271). Such a comment must be viewed in light of Farrell & Dares' (1996, p 179) subsequent warning that 'in an era of increasing focus on human rights' there will be demands for 'treatment which is more curative and supportive rather than disempowering and punitive'. The current focus on human rights paves the way for patients and their advocates to increasingly seek redress in litigation (Muir-Cochrane, Holmes & Walton 2002, p 502).

Seclusion is generally deemed lawful when: it is used for patients receiving treatment for mental illness; it is necessary to protect the person or any other person from an immediate or imminent risk to his or her health or safety or to prevent the person from absconding; or it has been approved by an authorised psychiatrist or senior psychiatric nurse on duty. Most Mental Health Acts state that a patient in seclusion must be subject to regular review (varying from continuous observation to five to fifteen minutes) by a registered nurse and between four and eight hours by a registered medical practitioner. Patients must be given appropriate bedding, food and drink, and have access to toilet and hygiene facilities. These provisions are mentioned in some, but not all, Mental Health Acts. In New Zealand, guidelines for seclusion are provided in the *Restraint minimisation and safe practice* standard (Standards New Zealand 2001), which aims to limit the use of restraint and seclusion, and to provide for safe practice where seclusion is used. Some settings monitor patients from video screens in the nurses' station, while others post nurses outside the seclusion room door for the duration of the seclusion episode. Thus, variation occurs across Australia in the policies within psychiatric units prescribing the monitoring, review and observation practices for the duration of seclusion episodes (Muir-Cochrane, Holmes & Walton 2002).

The differences in relation to the prescription and practice of seclusion reflects the tension between the protection of patients when acutely unwell and the need to provide care within the least-restrictive environment.

While World Health Organization (WHO 1996) documents suggest that authorities should pursue the elimination of isolation rooms and the prohibition of the provision of new ones, such recommendations have not yet been fully addressed in Australian or New Zealand legislation. It is recognised therefore that the legal requirements for the definition and management of seclusion attempt to protect the individual concerned and provide practical approaches to difficult situations. However, the differences in Mental Health Acts concerning seclusion point to the lack of consensus about what constitutes seclusion and under what circumstances it can be applied. Such differences in mental health legislation are likely to be a source of confusion to consumers and carers who move between States and Territories and raise questions about why such variations exist. The challenge for mental health nurses is to be aware of patients' previous experiences of hospitalisation.

Suicidal behaviour

Care of the suicidal consumer is possibly the most challenging clinical situation a mental health professional must face. The problem of suicide within the Australian population is well documented but few realise that the number of unsuccessful attempts at suicide is eight to ten times the figure for actual suicide (Cantor & Neulinger 2000). This widespread incidence of suicide renders it hard to ignore, and so it remains a confronting issue. The prospect of members of our community considering whether they wish to live at all destroys the image of life as cherished and worthwhile and makes us face the reality of our own mortality. The ethical debate about suicide largely centres on the justification for intervening in a person's choice to live or die. Health-care workers have a duty to intervene by preventing the suicidal act or treating the person who has made an attempt on their own life. This duty arises from our need to abide by the law but also our moral need to do no harm.

Involuntary treatment

Guidelines for ethical conduct are particularly relevant to mental health nurses because involuntary status under mental health legislation places restrictions on the therapeutic nurse–consumer relationship. Consumers who feel that they have few rights and are restricted by legislation may be less likely to engage in a working relationship with a mental health nurse. In this situation, where the consumer's actions are subject to mental health legislation, the nurse exercises social control over the consumer. If the consumer is hospitalised, the nurse can initiate PRN medication and restrain and seclude the consumer under medical authority. Mental health is not an area where the nurse can always refer the consumer to doctors for the answers, because the nurse is often the person delivering care, and it is often the nurse's actions that the consumer is questioning.

While the relationships that mental health nurses form with patients are recognised as central to the provision of care (Forchuk 1995; Peplau 1994), inevitable dynamics within this relationship are power and control. Issues of power and control were first brought into the psychiatric literature with the work of Goffman (1961) in the famous text *Asylum*, which described the relationship between patients and nurses as being controlled by the organisational rules and rigid hierarchical structure of the psychiatric hospital. Mental health nurses are in a unique position through the types and duration of therapeutic relationships that they can establish with patients. However, it is important to recognise the dichotomy between the caring and controlling functions mental health nurses must undertake as part of their professional practice. This often places nurses in difficult situations, ones that are not common to other health professionals (Muir-Cochrane 1998, 2000). The use of coercion is an uncomfortable component of nursing practice. It may be subtle ('encouraging', 'deciding for', 'trading off', 'persuading') and be seen as a weak form of paternalism justified by the goal of benefiting or avoiding harm to the person whose will is overridden (Morrall & Muir-Cochrane 2002, p 8).

When a person is committed to a mental health facility, the major ethical debate centres around legal rights versus moral rights. When should a person be admitted involuntarily under mental health legislation? This question is usually answered by saying: 'When the person is a danger to themselves or others'. However, consider whether you would feel comfortable committing this person to a mental health facility if the person was a member of your family or a close friend.

A consumer voluntarily seeking treatment for a mental illness should be treated as fully competent and retains the right to give or withhold consent to treatment (Wallace 1995). An involuntary consumer is admitted to hospital under mental health legislation and has limited legal capacity to refuse or consent to treatment (Stagno & Agich 1997). The ethical principles guiding treatment of the involuntary consumer are beneficence and non-maleficence. These require that the committed person be kept from harm and experience benefits as a result of their committal. But are such paternalistic actions ethically justifiable? Utilitarianism asserts that paternalistic actions are justified when the person is being protected from harm and does not have the capacity to make decisions by themselves (Mappes & Zembaty 1991). Consent to treatment is required from every competent person. In the case of an emergency, consent is often implied because of the nature of the condition (for example, when an unconscious individual arrives at an emergency department). A determination of incompetency which is assessed by a psychiatrist requires that the person has a mental disorder that impairs their judgment and ability to make sound decisions.

We can be advocates for a consumer but we must ensure that we advocate in collaboration with them, or else we risk being paternalistic. Paternalism is when the nurse believes that they know what is best for the client, that they are most qualified to speak on the patient's behalf, and that the patient is not sufficiently capable of doing so. Although the intention is good, client autonomy is at risk. All consumers should be treated with the same degree of respect that you would require and, whenever practicable, the person's autonomy should be maintained. This would ensure that the person maintains their integrity and does not feel so vulnerable and powerless.

Deinstitutionalisation

Deinstitutionalisation of the mentally ill has occurred since the early 1950s. The history of the movement and the reasons for it occurring raise a number of ethical issues. While many people were discharged from mental health hospitals to supportive settings, and a few others required no follow-up, thousands of consumers have been discharged to inadequate housing or even to the streets (Trow 1999). The reasons for deinstitutionalisation were many: overcrowding, high costs, greater community awareness of the needs of the mentally ill, the availability of pharmacological treatments, and sociopolitical movements such as the mental hygiene movement (Maude 2001). In addition, consumers have campaigned for less restrictive mental health care than that provided in institutional settings (Curtis & Diamond 1997).

People experiencing the often debilitating nature of mental illness face the same economic challenges as all other citizens, but they have the added burden of stigma and the personal cost of their illness. Issues such as equity of access to health care, affordable accommodation, adequate income and meaningful work are all made much harder with the complication of mental illness.

Therapy

The consumer places their trust in the therapist, expecting that the therapist will not exploit it. The relationship between therapist and consumer is therapy's strength and weakness. The therapist gains recognition as a health professional, and also power within the relationship. The ethical issue is how to use this power. Does the power remain egalitarian or become authoritarian? And to what extent does transference within the relationship hinder the therapeutic process? The therapist may become the most important person in the consumer's life and runs the risk of assuming priority over all other people in the consumer's life.

In general, the ethical guidelines for one-on-one therapy and group work are threefold. First, to protect the consumer from exploitation, incompetence and pressure to perform; second, to uphold the right of the consumer to be provided with information and make informed decisions concerning their life; and third, to foster personal growth and wellness (Bancroft 1995). The first two goals protect the consumer and promote the consumer's rights.

The third goal outlines the true goal of therapy. It is often taken for granted that therapy is always beneficial to the consumer. After all, to look at oneself or share beliefs during group or individual therapy should help us to grow and understand why our lives have evolved as they have. This aim is compromised when the therapy is focused on the needs of the therapist or institution, rather than on those of the consumer. In extreme cases this can lead to unprofessional conduct, including sexual exploitation of the consumer (Horsfall & Stuhlmiller 2000).

Professional boundaries—The therapeutic relationship is a privileged relationship for both the consumer and the clinician. However, responsibility for maintaining the required professional standards rests with clinicians, who need to have safeguards in place that will enable issues involving professional standards to be identified and appropriately managed. These include reflective practice, especially use of a co-therapist or supervisor to discuss consumer care confidentially. You may notice at times when you are working closely with a consumer, feelings of impending friendship, wanting to save the consumer from reckless behaviour, boredom with their lack of progress, or a sense of knowing better than the consumer what their needs are. These are all signs of potential counter-transference. The clinician needs to be aware of the boundaries needed to keep the therapy sessions therapeutic and consumer-centred. When a nurse moves outside the therapeutic relationship and establishes a friendship or social relationship with a consumer, the professional boundaries between the nurse as therapist and the consumer become confused. When professional boundaries are blurred, the relationship can become non-therapeutic and potentially harmful to both the consumer and the nurse. Ethical decision-making principles are especially important to ensure that professional boundaries are not transgressed. Horsfall, Cleary & Jordon (1999, p 7) have identified examples of professional boundary transgression from the available literature (see Box 5.5).

Behaviour modification—The major ethical issues when considering behaviour modification are misuse of power, control and the potential dehumanisation of the consumer. Behaviour therapy is often questioned because, unlike psychotherapy, it does not expand the consumer's awareness. For many, it fosters a machine model of human beings and portrays the therapist as a technician who manipulates the consumer (Bancroft 1995). Behaviour modification is often conducted against the person's will and, in the case of the involuntary consumer, behaviour modification methods have often been applied without consent.

Behavioural controls manifest in the form of positive reinforcement by rewarding desirable behaviour, and negative reinforcement by punishing undesirable behaviour. These forms of behavioural manipulation have in the past taken the form of token economies within mental health/psychiatric units. The nurse holds the cigarettes and the consumer may have one on the half hour but only if there has been no disturbing behaviour. However, signs of the token economy persist when privileges are withheld because the consumer fails to comply with ward rules.

> When considering behaviour modification, the questions that should be asked are:
> - Who sets the standard of behaviour?
> - How will reward and negative reinforcement be carried out?
> - Has this decision been made with consideration of the consumer's needs and benefit?

Confidentiality—Consumers often tell us stories and ask that we keep them a secret. Confidentiality is a primary principle of the therapeutic relationship, but how can it be upheld if the consumer reveals information that must be shared with the rest of the team? Nurses working in groups should never promise to keep a secret. These are appropriate within a friendship, but never within a therapeutic relationship. It is paramount

Box 5.5 Examples of professional boundary transgression

- Sharing confidential consumer information with others outside the treatment team
- Taking consumers to social events outside work hours
- Inviting a consumer home
- Having a sexual relationship with a consumer during or following treatment
- Conducting inappropriate or unnecessary examinations or interviews
- Physical, sexual or verbal abuse
- Entering into a business transaction with a consumer
- Allowing personal matters to intrude on clinical work
- Inappropriately exempting consumers from responsibilities
- Giving or receiving inappropriate gifts
- Disclosing personal feelings without therapeutic justification
- Making seductive comments about a consumer's appearance or being flirtatious
- Having an ongoing social relationship
- Entering into a financial relationship with a consumer
- Not disclosing relevant change within a relationship to other team members
- Using nursing procedure to engage in inappropriate contact or prolonging contact

Source: Horsfall J, Cleary M & Jordon R 1999, *Toward Ethical Mental Health Nursing Practices*, Australian and New Zealand College of Mental Health Nurses Inc, Greenacres, SA.

that the consumer is made aware that all necessary information will be shared with the team and that this information will remain within the team. So, too, when commencing a discussion during group therapy it is always important to remind people that what they share with the group is for the group alone and not to be taken out of the room.

CONCLUSION

The future of mental health nursing seems likely to become more rather than less complex. Current issues of regulation of practice, credentialling of mental health nurses and education look set to continue to occupy the profession in the foreseeable future. At the same time the development of advanced practice and nurse practitioner roles represent a future in which mental health nurses will play an increasing role in the provision and development of clinical services. The increasing role of generic mental health workers and the growing diversity of services challenge nurses to articulate their contribution to mental health care and consumer outcomes. So, too, the complexities of the ethical and legal issues concerning the care of vulnerable populations, such as the mentally ill, requires constant scrutiny. Mental health nursing is fraught with ethical issues arising from classification of mental illness, diagnosis, treatment and working within the constraints of mental health legislation. While there are existing codes of ethics for nurses, a code of ethical conduct specific to mental health nursing is required to guide practice in the complex challenges of mental health care.

Mental health nursing will need a strong professional voice and organisation to support practitioners in the services of the future. The profession has already responded to the challenge of deinstitutionalisation by re-focusing on community-based roles while still retaining an essential role in inpatient services. Growing recognition of the prevalence and burden of mental illness, together with increasing specialisation within mental health, will require similar resourcefulness and adaptability as mental health nurses work to maintain a profession that is both rewarding to practitioners and valued by consumers.

EXERCISES FOR CLASS ENGAGEMENT

ETHICAL DILEMMAS

You could split into discussion groups or individually consider the following case studies. Read the four case studies and consider appropriate responses to the questions that follow.

Case study 1
A 33-year-old woman reports that she wants to die as she cannot get over the death of her husband and six-year-old son in a motor vehicle accident eleven months ago. She has no family and has lost her home because she is on an unemployment benefit and is unable to pay the mortgage. She feels the pain is too great and just wants it to end.

Case study 2
A 59-year-old male widower, who has been diagnosed with liver and bowel cancer, presents with considerable pain and distress. He advises the nurse that he has always believed in euthanasia and has decided that his time is now up. He does not want to be a burden on his daughter and wishes to die with dignity. He is open about his wish to die and has planned his suicide. All his affairs are in order. He believes that he will carry this out sooner rather than later, as the pain is now too great and he just wants it to end.

Case study 3
A 15-year-old girl arrives at the emergency room after ingesting twenty-four Panadol tablets. She has been struggling with anorexia nervosa since she was eleven and now feels that her life is heading nowhere. She is transferred as an involuntary consumer to the local mental health hospital and prescribed a course of electroconvulsive therapy, which is given without her consent. Three weeks later she remains suicidal and is now being tube fed. She wants to be left alone as she can't face the pain of life anymore.

Case study 4
An 84-year-old famous actor has refused food and fluid for six days as she does not want to live anymore. She has right-sided paralysis following a cerebrovascular accident. She wants to be remembered as young and beautiful. She feels that her life has been full and now wants it to end, as she feels that her future prospects are hopeless.

Questions
- In the above four studies, who is making a rational choice to die?
- What are our responsibilities in each case as health professionals?
- Do health professionals have the right to stop people when they wish to die?

LOCAL SERVICES
Contact your local city council and look at the web page for your national/state health department and find out what services are available to people with mental illness in your area. Are these local services adequate?

REFERENCES

Alty A & Mason T 1994, *Seclusion and Mental Health: A Break with the Past*, Chapman and Hall, London.

American Psychiatric Assocation (APA) 2000, *Diagnostic and Procedural Manual of Mental Disorders* (4th edn, text rev.), APA, Washington.

Andrews G 1995, Workforce deployment: reconciling demands and resources, *Australian and New Zealand Journal of Psychiatry*, 29(3), pp 394–402.

Appel AL & Malcom P 2002, The triumph and continuing struggle of nurse practitioners in New South Wales, Australia, *Clinical Nurse Specialist*, 16(4), pp 203–10.

Australian and New Zealand College of Mental Health Nurses (ANZCMHN) 1995a, *Standards of Practice for Mental Health Nursing in Australia*, ANZCMHN, Greenacres, SA.

Australian and New Zealand College of Mental Health Nurses (ANZCMHN) 1995b, *Standards of Practice for Mental Health Nursing in New Zealand*, ANZCMHN, Greenacres, SA.

Australian and New Zealand College of Mental Health Nurses (ANZCMHN) 2002, *Competencies for Advanced Practice in Psychiatric Mental Health Nursing in New Zealand*, New Zealand Branch, ANZCMHN, Auckland.

Australian National Health and Medical Research Council 2001, *National Statement on Ethical Conduct in Research Involving Humans*, ANHMRC, Canberra.

Australian Nursing Council 2000, *Code of Ethics for Nursing in Australia*, ANC, Canberra.

Avron J 1991, The neglected medical history and therapeutic choices for abdominal pain: a nationwide study of 799 physicians and nurses, *Archives of Internal Medicine*, 151, pp 694–8.

Bailey K 1999, Framework for prescriptive practice. In: Shea CA, Pelletier LR, Poster EG, Stuary GW & Verley MP (eds), *Advanced Practice in Psychiatric and Mental Health Nursing*, Mosby, St Louis, pp 297–313.

Bancroft J 1995, Ethical aspects of sexuality and sex therapy. In: Bloch S & Chodoff P (eds), *Psychiatric Ethics* (2nd edn), Oxford University Press, Oxford, pp 215–42.

Cantor C & Neulinger K 2000, The epidemiology of suicide and attempted suicide among young Australians, *Australian & New Zealand Journal of Psychiatry*, 34(3), pp 370–87.

Chesterson J 2002, Setting the Standard: Credentialling and Mental Health Nursing Practice, paper presented at the 28th International Conference of the Australian and New Zealand College of Mental Health Nurses, Sydney, Australia, October 2002.

Clinton M & Hazelton M 2000a, Scoping mental health nursing education, *Australian and New Zealand Journal of Mental Health Nursing*, 9(1), pp 2–10.

Clinton M & Hazelton M 2000b, Scoping practice issues in the Australian mental health workforce, *Australian and New Zealand Journal of Mental Health Nursing*, 9(3), pp 100–9.

Commonwealth of Australia 1998, *National Standards for Mental Health*, AGPS, Canberra.

Crowe M 1998, Developing advanced mental health nursing practice: a process of change, *Australian and New Zealand Journal of Mental Health Nursing*, 7(2), pp 86–94.

Curtis LC & Diamond R 1997, Power and coercion in mental health practice. In: Blackwell B (ed.), *Treatment Compliance and the Therapeutic Alliance*, Harwood Academic, Australia, pp 97–122.

Department of Health 1986, *Review of the Preparation and Initial Employment of Nurses*. Report to the Director-General of Health, Department of Health, Wellington.

Dickey B, Normand S-LT, Weiss RD, Drake RE & Azeni H 2001, Medical morbidity, mental illness and substance use disorders, *Psychiatric Services*, 53(7), pp 861–7.

Farrell GA & Dares G 1996, Seclusion or solitary confinement: Therapeutic or punitive treatment?, *Australian and New Zealand Journal of Mental Health Nursing*, 5(4), pp 171–9.

Fennell KS 1991, Prescriptive authority for nurse-midwives: a historical review, *Nursing Clinics of North America*, 26(2), pp 511–22.

Fletcher RF 1999, The process of constant observation: perspectives of staff and suicidal patients, *Journal of Psychiatric and Mental Health Nursing*, 6(1), pp 9–14.

Forchuk C 1995, Uniqueness within the nurse–patient relationship, *Archives of Psychiatric Nursing*, 9(1), pp 34–9.

Freidson E (ed) 1989, *Medical Work in America: Essays on Health Care*. Yale University Press, New Haven.

Fulbrook P 1998, Advanced practice. The 'advanced practitioner' perspective. In: Rolffe G & Fulbrook P (eds), *Advanced Nursing Practice*, Butterworth Heinemann, Oxford, pp 87–102.

Gill D, Palmer C, Mulder R & Wilkinson T 2001, Medical student career intentions at the Christchurch School of Medicine. The New Zealand Wellbeing, Intentions, Debt and Experiences (WIDE) survey of medical students pilot study. Results part II, *New Zealand Medical Journal*, 114(2), pp 465–7.

Goffman I 1961, *Asylum: Essays on the Social Situation of Mental Patients and Other Inmates*, Penguin, London.

Haglund K, von Knorring L & von Essen L 2003, Forced medication in psychiatric care: patient experiences and nurses perceptions, *Journal of Psychiatric and Mental Health Nursing*, 10(1), pp 65–72.

Hawley G 1997, *Ethics Workbook for Nurses: Issues, Problems and Resolutions*, Social Science Press, Wentworth Falls, NSW.

Hays RB, Veitch PC, Cheers B & Crossland L 1997, Why doctors leave rural practice, *Australian Journal of Rural Health*, 5(4), pp 198–203.

Health and Disability Commissioner 2002, Southland District Health Board Mental Health Services February–March 2001. A report by the Health and Disability Commissioner, Health and Disability Commissioner, Auckland.

Health Workforce Advisory Committee 2002, *The New Zealand Health Workforce: A Stocktake of Issues and Capacity 2001*, HWAC, Wellington.

Hemingway S 2003, Nurse prescribing for mental health nurses: scripting the issues, *Journal of Psychiatric and Mental Health Nursing*, 10, pp 239–45.

Holmes C 1998, *The Policies and Practices of Seclusion: An Advisory Report for the Western Sydney Area Mental Health Service*, Western Sydney Area Mental Health Service, Parramatta, NSW.

Holmes CA 2001, Postdisciplinarity in mental health-care: an Australian viewpoint, *Nursing Inquiry*, 8(4), pp 230–9.

Horrocks S, Anderson E & Salisbury C 2002, Systematic review of whether nurse practitioners working in primary care can provide equivalent care to doctors, *British Medical Journal*, 324(7341), pp 819–23.

Horsfall J & Stuhlmiller C 2000, *Interpersonal Nursing for Mental Health*, McLennan & Petty, Sydney.

Horsfall J, Cleary M & Jordon R 1999, *Toward Ethical Mental Health Nursing Practice*, Australian and New Zealand College of Mental Health Nurses, Inc., Greenacre, SA.

Human Rights Commission, Australia 1993, *National Inquiry Into the Rights of People with Mental Illness: The Burdekin Report* (vols 1 & 2), AGPS, Canberra.

Human Rights and Equal Opportunity Commission (HREOC) 1993, *Human Rights and Mental Illness: Report of the National Inquiry into the Human Rights of People with Mental Illness*, AGPS, Canberra.

International Council of Nurses (ICN) 2003, Definition and characteristics for nurse practitioner/advanced practice nursing roles. Online: http://www.icn.ch/networks_ap.htm#definition, accessed 19 February 2003.

Idvall E, Rooke L & Hamrin E 1997, Quality indicators in nursing: a review of the literature, *Journal of Advanced Nursing*, 25(1), pp 6–17.

Illich I 1977, *Limits to Medicine*, Penguin, London.

Johannsson IM & Lundman B 2002, Patients' experiences of involuntary psychiatric care: good opportunities and great losses, *Journal of Psychiatric and Mental Health Nursing*, 9(6), pp 639–47.

KPMG Consulting 2001, *KPMG Strategic Review of Undergraduate Education. Report to the Nursing Council*, KPMG Consulting, Auckland.

Krauss J & Slavinsky A 1982, *The Chronically Ill Psychiatric Patient and the Community*, Blackwell, Boston.

Loff B & Cordner S 1998, Nurses in New South Wales get greater powers, *Lancet*, 3(52), p 797.

Maling T 2000, Extended prescribing rights—a statutory right or hard earned privilege?, *New Zealand Medical Journal*, 113(1119), pp 410–11.

Mappes T & Zembaty J 1991, *Biomedical Ethics* (3rd edn), McGraw-Hill, New York.

Maude P 2001, From Lunatic to Client: A History/Nursing Oral History of the Treatment of Western Australians who Experienced a Mental Illness, unpublished doctoral thesis, University of Melbourne, Melbourne.

McCann TV & Baker H 2002, Community mental health nurses and authority to prescribe medications: the way forward?, *Journal of Psychiatric and Mental Health Nursing*, 9(2), pp 175–82.

McManus RJ, Mant J, Meulendijks CFM, Salter RA, Pattison HM, Roalfe AK et al. 2002, Comparison of estimates and calculations of risk of coronary heart disease by doctors and nurses using different calcuation tools in general practice: cross sectional study, *British Medical Journal*, 324(7335), pp 459–64.

Mental Health Commission (MHC) 1998, *Blueprint for Mental Health Services in New Zealand. How Things Need To Be*, Mental Health Commission, Wellington.

Mental Health Commission (MHC) 2001a, *A Competency Framework for the Mental Health Workforce. A Report of the National Mental Health Workforce Development Co-ordinating Committee*, Mental Health Commission, Wellington.

Mental Health Commission (MHC) 2001b, *Recovery Competencies for New Zealand Mental Health Workers*, Mental Health Commission, Wellington.

Ministry of Health 1996, *Report on the National Working Party on Mental Health Workforce Development*, Ministry of Health, Wellington.

Ministry of Health 2001, *Summary of Submissions on the Health Professionals' Competency Assurance Bill Discussion Paper*, Ministry of Health, Wellington.

Ministry of Health 2002, *Nurse Practitioners in New Zealand*, Ministry of Health, Wellington.

Moller MD & Haber J 1996, Advanced practice psychiatric nursing: the need for a blended role, *Online Journal of Issues of Nursing*. Online: http://www.nursingworld.org/ojin/tpc1/tpc1_7.htm, accessed 26 January 2003.

Moorey J 1998, The ethics of professional care. In: Barker P & Davidson B (eds), *Psychiatric Nursing: Ethical Strife*, Arnold, London, pp 39–56.

Morrall P & Muir-Cochrane E 2002, Naked social control: seclusion and psychiatric nursing in post-liberal society, *Australian ejournal for the Advancement of Mental Health*, 1(2), online: http://ausienet.flinders. eduau/journal/.

Muir-Cochrane E 1998, The role of the community mental health nurse in the administration of depot neuroleptic medication: 'Not just the needle nurse', *International Journal of Nursing Practice*, 4(4), pp 254–60.

Muir-Cochrane E 2000, The context of care: issues of power and control in community mental health nursing, *International Journal of Nursing Practice*, 6(6), pp 292–9.

Muir-Cochrane E 2001, The case management practices of community mental health nurses: doing the best we can!, *Australian and New Zealand Journal of Mental Health Nursing*, 10(4), pp 210–20.

Muir-Cochrane E, Holmes C & Walton J 2002, Law and policy in relation to the use of seclusion in psychiatric hospitals in Australia and New Zealand, *Contemporary Nurse*, 13(2/3), pp 105–292.

Mundinger MO, Kane RL, Lenz ER, Totten AM, Tsai WY & Cleary PD 2000, Primary care outcomes in patients treated by nurse practitioners or physicians: a randomized trial, *Journal of the American Medical Association*, 283, pp 59–68.

National Education Review Secretariat 2002, *National Review of Nursing Education*, Commonwealth of Australia, Canberra.

New Zealand Nurses Organisation 1995, *Code of Ethics*, NZNO, Auckland.

Nurses Registration Board (NRB), New South Wales 1999, Professional and educational matters, *NRB Board Works. Newsletter of the Nurses Registration Board, New South Wales*, November, p. 2.

Nursing Council of New Zealand (NCNZ) 2001, *Guidelines for Competence-Based Practising Certificates for Registered Nurses*, Ministry of Health, Wellington.

O'Brien AJ 2002/2003, Judging care against standards in mental health, *Kai Tiaki Nursing New Zealand*, 8(11), pp 22–3.

O'Brien AP, O'Brien AJ, McNulty N, Morrison-Ngatai E, Skews G, Ryan T et al. 2002, *Clinical Indicators for Mental Health Nursing Standards of Practice in Aotearoa/New Zealand*, Massey University, Palmerston North.

Offredy M 2000, Advanced nursing practice: the case of nurse practitioners in three Australian states, *Journal of Advanced Nursing*, 31(2), pp 274–81.

Pearson L 1998, Annual update of how each state stands on legislative issues affecting advanced nursing practice, *Nurse Practitioner*, 23(1), pp 14–66.

Peplau H 1994, Psychiatric mental health nursing: challenge and change, *Journal of Psychiatric and Mental Health Nursing*, 1, pp 3–7.

Plueckhahn V, Breen K & Cordner S 1994, *Law and Ethics in Medicine for Doctors in Victoria*, Henry Thacker Print, Geelong.

Psychiatric nursing training 1907, *Kai Tiaki*, 38(1), pp 3–4.

Quirk A & Lelliott P 2001, What do we know about life on acute psychiatric wards in the UK: a review of the research evidence, *Social Science and Medicine*, 53, pp 1565–74.

Reich W 1991, Psychiatric diagnosis as an ethical problem. In: Bloch S & Chodoff P (eds), *Psychiatric Ethics* (2nd edn), Oxford University Press, Oxford, pp 101–34.

Rice MJ 2000, Certification standards for advanced practice psychiatric nursing, *Perspectives in Psychiatric Care*, 36(1), pp 33–4.

Rogers A & Pilgrim D 1994, Service users of psychiatric nurses, *British Journal of Nursing*, 3(1), pp 16–18.

Rodgers SJ 2000, The role of nursing theory in standards of practice: A Canadian perspective, *Nursing Science Quarterly*, 13(3), pp 260–1.

Safriet B 1992, Health care dollars and regulatory sense: The role of advanced practice nursing. *The Yale Journal on Regulation*, 9(2), 417–87.

Skews G, Armitage P, Hoot S, Hunt G & Armitage P 1998, *Clinical indicators for standards of practice: development and validation*. South Australia, ANZCMHN.

Skews G, Armitage P, Hoot S, Hunt G & Armitage P 2000, Development and validation of clinical indicators for mental health nursing standards of practice, *Australian and New Zealand Journal of Mental Health Nursing*, 9(1), pp 11–18.

Stagno S & Agich G 1997, Consent in patients with mental illness, *Current Opinion in Psychiatry*, 10(5), pp 423–6.

Standards New Zealand 2001, *Mental Health Sector Standards*, SNZ, Wellington.

Trow C 1999, Revolving door syndrome: the deinstitutionalisation of mental health services in New Zealand, *Whitireia Nursing Journal*, 6, pp 33–42.

United Kingdom Central Council for Nursing, Midwifery and Health Visiting 1994, *The Future of Professional Practice. The Council's Standards for Education and Practice Following Registration*, UKCC, London.

Venning P, Durie A, Roland M, Roberts C & Leese B 2000, Randomised controlled trial comparing cost effectiveness of general practitioners and nurse practitioners in primary care, *British Medical Journal*, 320(7241), pp 1048–53.

Wallace M 1995, *Health Care and the Law* (2nd edn), The Law Book Company, Sydney.

Wallace M 1997, Restraint: some legal implications, *Collegian*, 4(2), pp 15–19.

World Health Organization (WHO) 1996, *Mental Health Care Law: Ten Basic Principles*, WHO, Geneva.

5

Professional and Industrial Issues

Anthony O'Brien, Phillip Maude and Eimear Muir-Cochrane

KEY POINTS

- Nurses licensed to practise by state regulatory authorities are known as registered and enrolled nurses.
- The regulation of nursing occurs through a variety of legislative, professional and industrial bodies.
- There is no universally accepted credential for mental health nurses.
- Mental health nurses are now educationally prepared for practice in generic, rather than specialist, nursing programs.
- Accountability in nursing is achieved through adherence to standards of practice.
- Authority to continue to practise is increasingly being determined by declared competence.
- Mental health nurses have developed advanced and extended roles, in some cases including nurse practitioner roles and prescriptive authority.
- As the largest single group within the mental health workforce, mental health nurses play an important role in the development of mental health services that protect the rights of consumers and their carers and in ensuring that their needs are met.
- The claim to professional status requires nurses to practise within a code of ethics.
- Mental health care involves reflection on ethical issues and the use of principles of ethical reasoning.
- Codes of ethics guide members of the professions as to the nature of proper conduct and their obligations to the public.
- Mental health nurses are confronted with ethical issues on a daily basis.
- Diagnosing a person with a mental illness has powerful and potentially detrimental consequences for that person.
- Nurses need to consider the ethical issues arising from their choice of intervention and from many of the treatments prescribed in psychiatry.

KEY TERMS

- advanced practice
- code of ethics
- competency
- confidentiality
- deinstitutionalisation
- ethics
- mental health nursing
- nurse practitioner
- nursing education
- nursing organisations
- profession
- psychiatric nursing
- regulation
- standards of practice

LEARNING OUTCOMES

The material in this chapter will assist you to:
- outline the roles of professional and industrial organisations in mental health nursing
- discuss the influence of education on preparation for practice in mental health nursing
- discuss the roles of advanced practitioner and nurse practitioner in mental health nursing
- identify common ethical issues in mental health nursing
- apply ethical principles to the analysis of ethical issues in mental health nursing.

6

Mental Health in Australia and New Zealand

Pamela Wood, Pat Bradley and Ruth De Souza

KEY POINTS

- An appreciation of the prevalence of mental disorders will help the mental health nurse to understand the impact that mental disorders have on the health-care system, the health outcomes of individuals and demands for community services.
- The extent of disability associated with mental health disorders can have significant influence on an individual's ability to function in all aspects of their life, including the individual, significant others, work colleagues and social contacts.
- The outcomes associated with many mental disorders may be influenced by gender differences.
- Culture consists of a body of learned behaviours, passed on by role modelling, learning and lore, which is used by the individual to interpret experience and to generate social behaviour.
- An awareness of cultural factors can enhance the mental health nurse's ability to offer individualised, holistic care within a therapeutic relationship, and to value the contribution that cultural interventions can make to the therapeutic environment.
- Openness to diversity in cultures offers the mental health nurse the opportunity to reflect on his or her own beliefs and values about health, what it means to be healthy, and what he or she recognises as mental wellbeing.
- The culturally competent mental health nurse will aim to 'enter' the client's experience, while maintaining a strongly rooted sense of his or her own lived experience and developmental learning.
- The culturally safe mental health nurse will aim to provide care that is deemed culturally safe by the client.

KEY TERMS

- consumer
- cultural awareness
- cultural competence
- cultural safety
- cultural sensitivity
- culture
- disability
- ethnocentrism
- gender
- incidence
- mental health
- mental health disorders
- morbidity
- mortality
- prevalence
- stigma

LEARNING OUTCOMES

The material in this chapter will assist you to:
- develop an awareness of the prevalence of mental health disorders and the impact this has on the community and society
- understand the concept of disability in relation to mental illness and how the levels of disability are determined
- appreciate the negative influences of misconceptions and discrimination experienced by people with a mental health disorder
- understand how individuals can positively influence mental health outcomes for consumers, carers and communities
- describe the relevance of culture and gender issues to mental health outcomes for the individual and their family, friends and carers
- understand the importance of cultural diversity in negotiating health-care strategies that achieve outcomes endorsed by the client
- use resources available for research, continuing education and professional development.

INTRODUCTION

This chapter explores two interrelated facets of mental illness. The first section discusses the prevalence of mental illness in Australia and New Zealand and its impact on the individual, family, carers and health systems. Other factors such as misconceptions, gender issues and perceptions of mental illness will be shown to have the potential to contribute to the degree of disability experienced by a person who is ill or recovering from illness. The role of the media in shaping opinions and ideas is also examined. The second section of this chapter deals with the impact of culture, including gender and ethnicity, on the way in which mental disorders are perceived and managed by individuals and communities. Issues of stigma and stereotyping are explored, models of cultural competence and cultural safety are introduced, and the importance of self-reflection in mental health nursing practice is emphasised.

INCIDENCE AND PREVALENCE OF MENTAL HEALTH DISORDERS

The worldwide burden of mental health problems and disorders is high and is expected to increase—for example, depression is expected to become one of the greatest health problems in the world by the year 2020 (Murray & Lopez 1996). Mental disorders cause considerable personal, social and financial distress to individuals, and have a huge impact on health-care funding, implementation of service provision and community resources. In order to gauge the full extent of the problem, many countries have conducted research into the prevalence and consequent impact of mental disorders on the individual, society and health-care funds. Both the Australian and New Zealand governments have conducted extensive research to determine the extent of mental disorders in the community and the impact this has had on the individual, community and government spending. A brief overview of the findings is presented below.

Australian National Survey of Mental Health

Studies undertaken by the Australian National Survey of Mental Health include three studies on adult Australians, psychosis, and children and adolescents. Information on these can be found at the following websites:

- http://www.mentalhealth.gov.au/resources/reports/pdf/psychot.pdf ('People Living with Psychotic Illness: An Australian Study')
- http://www.mentalhealth.gov.au/resources/young/pdf/young/pdf ('Child and Adolescent Component of the National Survey of Mental Health and Wellbeing').

The National Survey of Adult Australians (aged 18 to 99 years) conducted by the Australian Bureau of Statistics in 1997 examined mental illness, anxiety disorders, affective disorders and substance abuse disorders. This survey revealed that 9.7 per cent of all people (*n* = 10,000) who participated in the study suffered from an anxiety disorder

(7.1 per cent of men and 12 per cent of women); 5.8 per cent of all people surveyed suffered from an affective disorder (4.2 per cent of men and 7.4 per cent of women); and 7.7 per cent of people surveyed suffered from a substance abuse disorder (11.1 per cent of men and 4.5 per cent of women) (Andrews et al. 1999).

The overall results showed that over a twelve-month period an estimated 18 per cent of Australians are affected by one or more mental disorders. From this it is anticipated that one in five people in Australia will be affected by a mental health problem at some stage in their lives (Commonwealth Department of Health and Aged Care (CDHAC) & Australian Institute of Health and Welfare 1999). Results from the Child and Adolescent component of the National Survey of Mental Health and Wellbeing were published in October 2000. The survey included 4500 children between the ages of four and seventeen, with the results indicating that 14–20 per cent of children had mental health problems (Zubrick et al. 1995; Sawyer et al. 2000). Interestingly, the prevalence of mental disorders drops to 6 per cent among Australians aged 65 years and over. Dementia is strongly related to age, affecting 1.6 per cent of those aged 65–70 years and 39 per cent of those aged 90–94 years (Henderson & Jorm 1998).

Survey results for people living with a psychotic illness, undertaken in 1997–98, revealed that illnesses included schizophrenia, bipolar affective disorders and delusional disorders. The survey covered 3800 Australians aged 18 to 64 years who attended mental health services in four States of Australia (Jablensky et al. 1999). The results of the survey revealed that approximately four to seven per 1000 adults living in the urban area suffered from a psychotic illness—that is, 0.3–0.5 per cent of the population (Jablensky et al. 1999). A further breakdown of these results indicates that 62.4 per cent (approximately 34,000 people, or 0.25 per cent of the population) had schizophrenia or a closely related disorder: 11.4 per cent (approximately 6200 or 0.05 per cent of the population) had bipolar disorder and 8.1 per cent (approximately 4400 people or 0. 03 per cent of the population) had a depressive psychosis (Meadows & Singh 2001).

New Zealand National Survey of Mental Health

The New Zealand Mental Health Commission was established as a Ministerial Committee in 1993 and began operating in 1996. The committee was established following the release of recommendations from the 1996 Mason inquiry into Mental Health Services. The *Mental Health Commission Act 1998* was established to:

- monitor and report to government on the performance of the Ministry of Health and Health Funding Authority in the implementation of the National Mental Health Strategy
- work to promote a better understanding by the public of mental illness and to eliminate discrimination

■ strengthen the mental health workforce (Mental Health Commission 2003).

Following research into the prevalence of mental health problems, a report to the New Zealand Minister of Health in August 2002 claimed that approximately 20 per cent of the adult population will have a diagnosable mental illness (including drug and alcohol disorders) at some time in their life. Rather than discuss the incidence surrounding each individual illness, the Mason inquiry discusses the prevalence of mental disorders in relation to the severity of the disorder. For example, it is reported that 0.06 per cent of adult New Zealanders have high support needs, approximately 3 per cent have severe mental health disorders, 5 per cent have moderate/severe mental disorders and a further 12 per cent have mild/moderate mental health problems or disorders (Powell 2002). From this it is anticipated that, as with the Australian statistics, one in five people in New Zealand will have a mental disorder at some stage of their life.

Co-morbidity (the presence of more than one mental health disorder) is common at all ages. Research has found that the development of one mental disorder increases the likelihood of developing a range of other mental health problems. For example, the results of the Australian 1997 Survey of Mental Health and Wellbeing highlight this fact, with the findings that almost one in four people with an anxiety, affective or substance use disorder also had at least one other mental disorder (Andrews et al. 1999). It was also found that 23 per cent of children with a mental disorder exhibited symptoms that met the criteria for another disorder (Sawyer et al. 2000). Around 15 per cent of the general population has a substance use disorder; and approximately 50 per cent of all people with a psychotic disorder may also use alcohol or other illicit drugs. Likewise, there is also a high incidence of substance use among people with bipolar disorders and mood disorders (Regier et al. 1990).

GENDER DIFFERENCES

There are unmistakable gender differences in the prevalence of mental disorders. The results of recent studies indicate that females are twice as likely as males to develop anxiety-related disorders and have a substantially higher incidence of reported affective disorders. Females report higher rates of depression across all age groups, the highest being those aged 18–24 years. Males, on the other hand, have a much higher occurrence of substance-abuse disorders. Both genders have the same reported incidence of psychotic disorders; although males generally experience an earlier onset and have a poorer outcome, females tend to have more affective symptoms and generally have more periods of remission than males (Jablensky et al. 1999). It is unclear whether the differences are a result of schizophrenia or the normal differences in brain structure and function between males and females (Meadows & Singh 2001).

The prevalence of depressive and anxiety disorders in children and adolescents (those aged 13–17 years) does not match the pattern for adults, in that both genders in this group have similar prevalence for depressive and anxiety-related disorders. However, males have a higher prevalence of attention deficit hyperactivity disorder and conduct disorder than females in all age groups (Sawyer et al. 2000). This tends to lead to problems associated with the legal system and a higher use of mental health facilities for male children and adolescents. The above figures are not restricted to the Australian population; similar results have been found in studies conducted in many other countries.

The discussion of gender differences in mental health cannot be limited to the statistics alone; there are many factors involved, such as the acceptance of treatment and the amount of disability suffered by individuals. As already discussed, females are more likely to report recent episodes of depression and anxiety disorders, and to seek treatment for mental health problems, whereas men tend to be more reluctant to seek professional help. This delay in seeking assistance may be attributed to a number of things, such as the stigma associated with mental health services, the belief that seeking help is a sign of weakness and therefore a threat to an individual's manhood; or, if in full-time work, it may be difficult to attend clinics. This delay results in poor access to early intervention and prevention services, which may lead to increased disability caused by the disorder. In general, men have a stronger tendency to turn to alcohol and other drugs as a means of dealing with their emotional problems, which does little more than exacerbate the problem in the long term (Nielsen, Katrakis & Raphael 2001).

Although women access services, they may have concerns about taking medications for their illness if they are pregnant, likely to become pregnant or are breastfeeding, for fear of the effects the medications may have on the baby. A pregnant women or nursing mother may well be limited in the medications she is able to take, leaving her susceptible to relapse due to inadequate treatment. Women are more likely than men to discontinue successful treatment because of medication-related weight gain and adverse side-effects. Women with severe mental illnesses such as bipolar disorder and major depression are at increased risk for an episode after childbirth, with some women experiencing their first episode at this time (Fullagar & Gattuso 2002; Meadows & Singh 2001).

Because of the later onset of some severe mental illnesses many women may already be married and be mothers before the initial onset of their illness. This may indicate that although the woman has support and security, ongoing severe mental illness may have a detrimental effect on her relationships with her husband and children, leading to family breakdown and long-term hardship (National Institute of Mental Health, http://www.nimh.nih.gov/wmhc/research.cfm).

Men with severe mental illness such as schizophrenia generally have worse outcomes than females, as measured by early onset, cognitive disabilities and social impairments. The earlier onset usually prevents males from developing personal relationships, which leads to most remaining single, childless and with reduced employment prospects. Women with schizophrenia seem to have an increased risk of relapse at times of rapid changes in their levels of oestrogen, such as at menopause or before the onset of menstruation (Fontaine 2003; Fullagar & Gattuso 2002).

CRITICAL THINKING CHALLENGE 6.1

■ Investigate some possible reasons why females have a higher incidence of anxiety and affective disorders. You should consider biological, psychological and cultural influences.

■ Why do you think men have a much higher incidence of substance abuse? It will help to make a list of your thoughts.

■ Do you think the figures as stated in this chapter are a true indication of the prevalence of mental health disorders between the sexes? Give at least five reasons to support your answer.

THE COST OF MENTAL DISORDERS

The direct monetary cost of mental illness is high. In 1997 the Australian Commonwealth Government spent $659 million on mental health; the States and Territories spent $1267 million; and $156 million was spent in private hospitals (Meadows & Singh 2001). The New Zealand Government increased its budget for both secondary and tertiary mental health services to $687 million in the year 2001 (Powell 2002).

These figures have not taken the hidden (indirect) cost of mental health into consideration—that is, the health costs and loss of earnings for families and carers, the community and welfare costs, charity agencies and the coronial work in the case of suicide. In addition, it has been estimated that only 38 per cent of adult Australians with a mental disorder actually receive help for their problem (McLennan 1998) and only 29 per cent of children and adolescents with a mental health problem had been in contact with a professional service (Sawyer et al. 2000). These findings are consistent with studies conducted in other countries. The actual cost of mental health problems is unknown and potentially underestimated.

DISABILITY AND MENTAL HEALTH

Disability in mental health refers to an individual's impairment in one or more important areas of functioning. Mental health disorders are a leading cause of disability

and account for 11 per cent of all disease burden worldwide (Murray & Lopez 1996). In 1990, five of the ten leading causes of disability worldwide were mental disorders: unipolar depression, alcohol abuse, bipolar affective disorder, schizophrenia and obsessive-compulsive disorder (Ministry of Health 1997). Among these disorders depression was ranked fourth, but the World Health Organization (WHO) has predicted that depression will be the second leading cause of disability in the world by 2020 (WHO 1996).

Although mortality rates from mental disorders are not considered to be high, the impact of chronic disability on an individual's life can be measured in days out of their normal role. The severity of an individual's disorder can be measured using the Disability Adjusted Life Year (DALY) tool developed by the WHO Harvard School of Public Health and the World Bank (Meadows & Singh 2001; Murray & Lopez 1996). This tool measures lost productivity associated with disability due to an individual's altered health status and is based on the years of life lost through living with disease, impairment and disability (Meadows & Singh 2001). The results from the Australian National Survey of Mental Health and Wellbeing indicate that chronic disability from a mental disorder accounts for 27 per cent of years lost to disability (Andrews et al. 1999).

Mental health problems cause considerable distress for individuals, families and friends as well as contributing to absenteeism from work or school and to the extensive use of community support services such as crisis lines and welfare groups. Mental disorders are more prevalent in the young, and therefore these people may become significantly disabled at a stage of their lives when they are completing education and establishing relationships and independence.

The type and length of illness (as measured by DALY) is a major factor when determining the effects of a particular illness on an individual's life. For example, people with a psychotic disorder may be socially isolated, unemployed and suffer considerable psychological and physical distress. Likewise, anxiety disorders have a profound effect on a person's work, social and family life. The Anxiety Disorders Foundation of Australia NSW Branch Inc. (1998) states that one in twelve Australians (1,360,000 people) suffer from an anxiety disorder and that people suffering from an anxiety disorder have a higher risk of suicide, drug and alcohol abuse, causing considerable disability to sufferers.

People with some mental disorders such as psychotic disorders or severe depression may well be unable to attend adequately to their hygiene needs, or shop and/or prepare meals, or to make sure their environment is clean and safe, thus placing their physical wellbeing in jeopardy. Poor physical health places a huge burden on the sufferer, their family, the community and the health-care system. A significant number of people with mental health problems are living below the poverty line, requiring assistance from welfare groups (government and non-government). Even with assistance a number of people may not have the means to provide adequate nutritious food, heating, clothing, housing, electricity, telephone or furniture for themselves and their families. Some housing and accommodation is available through a number of agencies, but the demand is greater than the resources available (Pinches 2002). A relatively small number have turbulent illnesses and often find that they are turned out of accommodation because of disruptive behaviour (Robinson 2003). Many welfare agencies run homeless shelters but have limited resources to deal with the complex needs of those with mental disorders.

CRITICAL THINKING CHALLENGE 6.2

■ Write a short list (dot points) of what you think about people suffering from:
  ● diabetes
  ● schizophrenia.
■ How do you think these illnesses would affect peoples' lifestyles?
■ What would you expect to see if you walked into a psychiatric ward today? For example:
  ● What would the patients be doing?
  ● What would the nurses be doing?
■ What influences your perceptions of people with mental illness?
■ How could you test your perceptions against reality?

MISCONCEPTIONS ABOUT MENTAL HEALTH

Mental disorders cause considerable distress to individuals, their significant others and the community. Being diagnosed with any chronic health problem is distressing. When stigma, negative misconceptions and discrimination are all attached to the diagnosis, the illness can seem insurmountable to those concerned.

Misconceptions regarding mental health disorders have a negative impact on the perception of mental health issues. Some commonly held misconceptions are as follows:

■ All people with mental health disorders are violent and dangerous.
■ People who are mentally ill have an intellectual disability or brain damage.
■ People with a mental illness will never recover.
■ People with a mental illness should be locked up and kept away from society.
■ People who have schizophrenia have a split personality.

Unfortunately, misconceptions have influenced the general perception and treatment of mental health problems for centuries. In line with recent studies undertaken in conjunction with the Australian National Mental Health Strategy, research was conducted in 1993 to determine the community's attitudes, knowledge and beliefs regarding mental health issues at the time. The results confirmed that extensive ignorance and fear remain prevalent in the community, reinforcing the need for extensive education as a means of increasing public awareness of mental health issues (Commonwealth Department of Health and Aged Care 2000).

The high level of misunderstanding concerning mental health problems and mental illness in the community may well contribute to the low numbers of people seeking help or those who wait until they are in crisis before seeking help. Poverty and the resulting inability to access health care in some instances, the inability to travel to services, poor social skills or lack of support all contribute to delay in seeking help.

People who develop mental health disorders may have had their own preconceived ideas and prejudices in regard to mental health issues, before becoming ill. Many people believe it is the end of their life and will grieve for the life they had and for the aspirations they held for their future. While people are unwell, work or study can be interrupted. Unemployment often leads to financial hardship, forcing people to live below the poverty line, thus exacerbating the feelings of frustration, low self-esteem and entrapment. The potential for suicidal thoughts and behaviour is particularly high in this group of people (Fryer 1995; Mathers & Schofield 1998).

Parents and siblings will also have their own misconceptions and prejudices against the mentally ill. Parents may blame themselves for their child's illness, may be ashamed or embarrassed and try to hide the illness from extended family members, neighbours, friends and work colleagues. Siblings may also feel embarrassed and stop bringing friends home. They may be fearful that they too will develop a mental illness and may become afraid of their brother or sister. The acute phase of many mental health disorders, especially psychotic disorders, will cause major disruption to family life (Fontaine 2003). Parents may need to take time out from work, which will have financial implications for the family, and siblings may find it difficult to function at school or in the workforce. Both parents and siblings may well go through the grieving process as a result of the changes in their lives. Children who grow up with a parent who has a mental disorder are at higher risk of developing a mental illness, such as depression, through either genetic susceptibility or gaps in parenting (CDHAC & AIHW 1999; Davies 2002; Dean & Macmillan 2002).

As well as the stigma attached to mental illness, immigrants bear the added burden of their cultural difference and potential racial stigma. Language difficulties and culturally specific ways of expressing distress increase alienation from mainstream community groups and place this group of people at an increased risk of being misdiagnosed or receiving inadequate care and support.

NURSE'S STORY

When I was a young girl growing up in the 1960s I lived with my parents and siblings in a suburb next to a large mental health hospital in an Australian capital city. The hospital consisted of many buildings, some double storey and some single, spread out on a vast expanse of land. I remember big fences at the front of the hospital and the surrounding area being very dark due to the vacant land that surrounded the hospital.

People in the neighbourhood usually referred to the hospital as the 'nut factory' and the people in the hospital as 'nuts'. Sometimes the 'nuts' escaped and people were scared that their families wouldn't be safe. I remember my mother being afraid when my father wasn't home, for that very reason. Driving past the hospital at night was particularly scary, but at the same time you had to look so that you could tell the kids next door if you saw anything worth reporting. I too grew up afraid of 'those people' and didn't like walking near the hospital, even during the day.

Years later I was working as an enrolled nurse when I met and worked with a registered nurse who was also a mental health nurse. She used to talk to me about her experiences and to my surprise I became interested. I decided I would like to become a psychiatric nurse, so I rang the very same hospital near where I grew up, and arranged an interview!

I was successful in my application and so began my psychiatric nurse training in the mid-1970s. By this time the bars were off the windows and the high fences had been pulled down, but the stigma surrounding mental illness was rampant.

Can you imagine my family's response when I announced I was going to work in the 'nut factory'? I took along all of my preconceived stereotypical ideas, fears and misconceptions. On the first day, I remember being scared, but began to relax as I walked around the beautiful grounds, with its beautifully maintained lawns, garden beds, vegetable gardens and bird aviary, unharmed and intact. To my added surprise the patients (as they were referred to then) didn't look anything like what I expected—rather, they were all ordinary people who had an illness that needed to be treated.

I worked at that hospital for fifteen years and I often look back and smile as I remember all the interesting experiences I had there. Most of the hospital has now been demolished to make way for a housing estate, but I will always remember the people I met while working there, as they taught me not to be afraid and to recognise that mental illness is an illness just like chronic physical illnesses, and that the sufferers are mere mortals, just like you and me.

Even working in the 'general' medical/surgical arena, the skills learned as a mental health nurse are used every day. I currently teach mental health to undergraduate nurses, and with the assistance of my colleagues, strive to demystify all aspects of mental illness and provide students with a positive and fulfilling experience.

The media and misconceptions about mental illness

The media are very powerful in conveying information and influencing the community's attitudes and perceptions of social norms. Therefore it follows that media coverage and reporting, be it through films, television, newspapers, magazines, posters or pamphlets, are critical when attempting to form and influence community attitudes to mental health and mental illness and the people affected by it. Unfortunately, media coverage often reflects the widespread misunderstanding of mental health problems and mental disorders. This is particularly so in movies that have been released throughout the history of film. For example, the 1970s film *One Flew Over the Cuckoo's Nest* depicted patients in a psychiatric hospital as having few rights and being manipulated by the mental health nurses. Patients who were deemed 'difficult' were subjected to medical procedures in order to make their behaviour manageable. The 1990s film *Me, Myself and Irene* blatantly misconstrued the illness of schizophrenia. The illness was portrayed as a 'split personality' (a very common misconception) and violent, with terminology such as 'schizo' and 'psycho' being used frequently throughout the movie. Both films were very damaging to the image of mental illness and offensive to people who suffer from mental illnesses.

To highlight the inaccurate portrayal of mental illness in television and the media a one-year analysis of television drama programs (serials, plays and films) was conducted in the United States and found that:

73 per cent of people with a mental illness were depicted as violent, while 23 per cent of people were portrayed as homicidal maniacs. When the same study analysed media reports about mental illness on television and in newspapers, it found that nearly 90 per cent of stories depicted people with mental illness as violent and usually homicidal. This is grossly inaccurate.

(SANE Australia 2000)

Research into the reporting and portrayal of mental illness in the Australian and New Zealand media reveals similar attitudes and sensationalism. Newspaper reporting has a tendency to sensationalise issues related to mental disorders at times, thereby perpetuating negative stereotypes and unnecessary fears in the community (Blood 2002; Lindberg 2001; Mitchell 2003).

Just as the media can have a negative impact, it can also be used as a tool to educate and change public opinion by ensuring that accurate information is reported in a rational and sensitive manner. In order to achieve this, scriptwriters, journalists and newspaper editors need to be educated on mental health issues (Martin 1998). As a beliefs that may vary geographically or by age or status within the given community.

An attempt to define a person's culture only in terms of race or geography gives rise to stereotyping, generalisation and potential inaccuracies. It is strongly recommended that mental health nurses develop relationships with cultural intermediaries and ethnic support workers, because it is not possible to learn everything about all the cultures you will work with in your professional life (Fuller 1995). You might also want to enhance your knowledge by accessing reputable websites and publications to gain a deeper understanding of cultural diversity and the individual nurse's responsibility to respect diversity. Some useful printed and electronic resources are listed at the end of this chapter.

CRITICAL THINKING CHALLENGE 6.4

- What is meant by 'Western' culture?
- How helpful is this shorthand in explaining general population health beliefs in Australia and New Zealand?
- What do the advertising pages of popular magazines offer as an indication of popular 'Western' beliefs about health and wellbeing?

Indigenous health beliefs

Generally throughout Australia, traditional Aboriginal health models are determined by the Law generated by Dreaming beings, which provides a model for ideal relationships between human beings in society, between humans and the land, and between humans and other elements of creation. Traditional Aboriginal health beliefs embody a sense of holism. All elements of life—physical, spiritual, moral, social and environmental—must balance and interact in producing health. Illness, both physical and mental, may be brought about by transgression of any aspect of the Law, whether by commission or omission. Every action has repercussions on individual balance, by its effect on the balance of the whole (Rose 2000).

Not all aspects of traditional Aboriginal belief are open even to members of the Aboriginal community. Initiation to various levels of understanding is still very important in some areas, and not all are able to achieve full initiation. Some people are believed to have the power to curse—that is, to bring illness or death by supernatural means. Similarly, there are those who have the ability to restore health, by means of their strength in the Law. On a more everyday level, bush medicine is used by women for general health, for reproductive conditions and for the ailments of childhood, both curatively and preventively. Men's business and women's business are strictly delineated by the Law, and this must be respected in everyday talk and action as well as in health, illness and healing.

Maori understandings of health are also holistic in approach. Environmental health is important, as the health and wellbeing of the people reflect the effect of pollutants, neglect and damage on Papatuanuku (mother earth), Ranginui (sky father) and the realm of Tangaroa (the seas). Maori health models include *whare tapa wha*: where the four cornerstones of Maori health are whānau (family health), tinana (physical health), hinengaro (mental health) and wairua (spiritual health) (Durie 2001).

Traditional healing includes mirimiri (massage), rongoa (herbal treatments) and karakia (spiritual prayer). Traditional healers incorporate the spiritual dimension in assessment and therapy, and do so in a culturally relevant way. Standards for traditional Maori healing have been published and are available via the New Zealand Ministry of Health website (www.moh.govt.nz).

Other culturally and linguistically diverse (CALD) groups

Apart from the major indigenous cultural groups, mental health nurses in Australia and New Zealand will encounter many people from other cultural backgrounds who will provide challenges to their own beliefs regarding mental health. The cultural variety of migrant and refugee groups is broad and it is not the intention of this chapter to describe them. Many people from different cultures have experienced the stress that accompanies separation from country, families and communities, and also the trauma associated with forced removal or refugee status, torture and incarceration (WHO 2001).

Some factors suggested by Ferguson & Browne (1991) as affecting migrant health are listed in Box 6.2.

Box 6.2 Factors affecting migrant mental health

- previous personality, emotional health and coping mechanisms
- the stress of migration
- bereavement aspects of the migration process
- reception and ease of settlement into the host country
- support measures available and the size of the ethnic community
- cultural differences between the country of origin and the adopted country
- acceptability and availability of the adopted country's services
- social class, including under-employment and unemployment
- discrimination and racism

Source: Ferguson B & Browne E 1991 (eds), *Health Care and Immigrants: a Guide for Health Professionals*, McLennan & Petty, Sydney.

Some cultures predicate spiritual origins for mental disorder, including demonic possession, or punishment for sin. Others place great importance on 'cursing', 'ill wishing' or 'the evil eye'. Some believe that current ill health is a result of bad karma in previous lives, or of bad deeds by ancestors. Other cultures may be predisposed to presentation with somaticising complaints (see Ch 20).

The words and behaviours used to describe mental distress vary among cultures. It is important that the mental health nurse respects the value of other people's beliefs, and understands that these beliefs shape behaviour in response to illness or disease.

Cultural values and beliefs also shape the ways in which people make the decision to access services, and who is deemed an appropriate channel of communication between consumer and health service. Some cultures find mental illness so shameful that they will resist seeking any sort of help outside the family unit. In patriarchal cultures the senior male family member may make the decision as to who is to seek attention and under what circumstances. In some Aboriginal cultures a senior female family member will accompany a young client, rather than a parent or sibling; or a group of 'aunties' may take responsibility for a baby, rather than the blood-mother alone.

A central tenet of cultural safety is the ability to examine one's own beliefs and values, and therefore the mental health nurse needs to be aware of his or her own cultural bias when seeking histories and making assessments of presenting behaviours. Flexibility in approach will ensure that due respect is accorded the opinions and explanations of those bearing cultural authority.

Involving families can make care more effective, because the knowledge and expertise of family members (Mental Health Commission 1998) can be drawn upon. In New Zealand, guidelines have been developed to assist mental health staff to work effectively with families, and to assist families to establish and maintain working relationships with mental health services and staff (Ministry of Health 2000).

CRITICAL THINKING CHALLENGE 6.5

Consider your family unit.
- What health beliefs do members share?
- Do any members hold different health beliefs? If so, what has influenced their thinking?
- What health-care actions are taken within the family?
- Who makes decisions about when and how to seek health care outside the family?
- Are these decisions made individually or by group negotiation?
- How does your family's health culture influence your response to people with different health beliefs and values?

Culture and communication style

The essence of mental health nursing is the ability to communicate—to engage in meaningful interaction with others, aimed at therapeutic results. This means having an awareness of our own communication style, as well as that of our clients. A clear example is provided in the comparison of communication styles of Anglo-Celtic and Aboriginal Australian groups.

The Anglo-Celtic communication style is described as direct, dyadic and contained. The medical, and perhaps most notably the psychiatric, interview shows this style refined to a degree that is intrusive and threatening, even within mainstream culture (Carroll 1995; Dudgeon 2000). Aboriginal style is communal and continuous, indirect, allusive and group focused. This style is shown to be a cultural constant not only among Aboriginal language speakers, but also among Aboriginal people who speak English, or Aboriginal English, as a first language (Eades 1998).

To an Aboriginal client, the contained, direct, individually focused psychiatric interview is not conducive to information sharing, and may be interpreted as a show of hostility ('strong talk'). Aboriginal people may resort to silence or evasion to avoid direct questioning. Direct eye contact reinforces the effect of hostility. Time may be needed for family consultation, or direction from elders. All this may be seen by health professionals as prevarication or as evidence of ignorance or non-compliance (Harris 1995). Non-verbal expression and behaviours that appear self-injurious, aggressive or extreme to Anglo-Celtic health workers may carry a very different meaning for the individual concerned.

Culture and self-reflection

For the mental health nurse, culture is a vital element of therapeutic alliance. If we accept, as the basis of our human interaction, that all behaviour has meaning, then it is essential that we understand the cultural templates that shape behavioural and emotional responses. It is essential to reflect on our own beliefs and values about health, about what it means to be healthy, and what we recognise as mental wellbeing.

As mental health nurses, we must also reflect on the assumptions of our adopted culture of health-care professional. Health education, training and practice rely strongly on an assumption that all involved in health service delivery subscribe to 'Western' values concerning the application of scientific methods to everyday life and health behaviour.

The scientific or biomedical model of health care also assumes a power differential between professional and client, assigning the evaluation of health-care services and outcomes to the professional. Mental health nurses must be aware of power differentials inherent in social structures and service delivery models that marginalise or devalue the client's identity, beliefs and wellbeing, and prefer direct, practical and immediate assistance from the Western care system rather than long-term strategies (Fuller 1995).

Alternative models of care delivery

The biomedical model has failed to legitimise the traditional healers and networks of many communities, labelling them as supernatural and unscientific (Sue & Sue 1990). CALD clients often prefer support from their own community (Gauntlett et al. 1995), whether these are informal support networks or trusted folk healers, who share their beliefs about the role of religion or the supernatural, the role of the family in treatment and the context and process of treatment (Flaskerud 1984). Mental health workers need to develop some openness to compromise between conventional psychiatry and people's cultural beliefs (Wright 1991), particularly where cultural practices are preferred, such as massage or consultation with folk healers. There needs to be a broadening of our attitudes as to what constitutes legitimate mental health practice. Research into this could provide us with alternative frames of reference to Western definitions of mental health (Sue & Sue 1990).

Definition of the problem and diagnosis

Stern & Kruckman (1983) point out that the defining criteria for depression may vary greatly across cultures and so cannot necessarily be resolved by applying a Western concept of depression to them. Thus, the diagnosis and treatment of clients from CALD cultures may be inaccurate, even discriminatory and punitive (Flaskerud 1990). Referring to distress as depression can cause harm in cultures where discussion of mental health problems is stigmatised or taboo. However, Barnett, Matthey & Boyce (1999) argue that having a diagnosis means appropriate treatment and social and psychological support can be obtained. Fitzgerald et al. (1998) state, however, that the real debate is not whether distress exists, but rather how it is expressed and categorised and, secondly, whether a particular explanatory model should be predominant and common human experiences and responses pathologised. According to Fitzgerald et al. (1998, p 21), the key issue is: 'How can we best understand and respond to culturally influenced and contextualised experiences in meaningful and useful ways?'.

Structural barriers

Health-care practices by professionals continue to be predominantly monocultural despite recognition of the need to be responsive to culturally diverse populations. Durvasula & Mylvaganam (1994) suggest that a lack of awareness or knowledge of services, where they are located, and a scarcity of ethnically similar counsellors or counsellors who are bilingual, provide barriers to CALD consumers using mental health services. The Ministry of Health (1997) recommends that mental health promotion and prevention for Maori and Pacific Islanders be strengthened. It is recommended that traditional Pacific and Maori structures be used to promote mental health, including circulating Pacific-language descriptions of key Western mental illnesses.

Matching of client and provider

Research suggests that cultural similarity facilitates self-disclosure, a highly valued aspect of counselling (Jourard 1964, cited in Belkin 1988). Shared experiences are also thought to facilitate or enhance rapport (Belkin 1988). Furthermore, it is suggested that culture matching will increase the ability to understand language, nuance, communication styles and body language. In New Zealand, parallel services have been developed that are 'for Maori by Maori' and 'for Pacific by Pacific'. A review has shown that there is a paucity of culturally safe services for Maori and Pacific people (Ministry of Health 1997). Furthermore, the provision of resources and devolution of resources have not supported other views of mental illness (Mental Health Commission 1998). The *Moving Forward* national objectives state that more trained mental health workers are needed before culturally appropriate services can be provided by mainstream and kaupapa Maori mental health services (Ministry of Health 1997). Since then more parallel services have been established.

A better partnership is needed between education and health sectors so that training can be specifically targeted to Maori. The Pacific Island objective also recommends that work be done so that mental health services become more responsive to the diverse needs of Pacific peoples. The national objectives recommend educating consumers to participate in care provision as providers, community support workers and Maori and Pacific Island workers. A disadvantage of this is that mainstream services could fail to develop culturally responsive services. In addition, the Report of the National Working Party on Mental Health Workforce Development (Ministry of Health 1996), suggested that Maori consumers become integrated into the provider culture of mental health services, so that these services reflect the wealth of Maori consumer experience. This is in line with the request by Maori consumers to have more Maori community support workers, patient advocates and crisis teams.

Gender-appropriate service

Full attention must be given to the importance in many cultures of providing access to gender-appropriate health-care professionals. Many groups have strong rules about what is and is not appropriate in terms of male–female interaction. In some cultures males may not be given any information about issues to do with sexuality, pregnancy or childbirth. In others, males may only speak to other males of comparable rank in discussing some issues of behaviour associated with spirituality.

Interview style should also be flexible enough to allow the patient and family to contribute fully to negotiation of

---

Box 6.3 Strategies in the provision of cultural care

- Become aware of your own ethnocentrism—that is, the belief that your own group is superior to others (Henderson & Primeaux 1981). It has been well documented that counsellors are more likely to have good relationships with clients who fit the YAVIS client-model, namely, 'Young, Attractive, Verbal, Intelligent and Successful' (Schofield 1964, cited in Sue & Sue 1990). Clients from other cultures are often seen as having less of these qualities (D'Ardenne & Mahtani 1989). Your ethnocentrism may be reflected back to the client, causing them to withdraw or be seen as noncompliant and resistive (D'Ardenne & Mahtani 1989).
- Recognise that it is counterproductive to treat all people alike. There are characteristics that all people share, such as need for food and shelter, characteristics that some people share, such as language, and some that are unique to a group; these include racial or ethnic historical conditions such as slavery (Henderson & Primeaux 1981).
- Avoid creating stereotypes and generalisations.
- Recognise the limitations of your own expertise and enlist

the help of culturally appropriate practitioners as requested or required.

- Allow clients to define themselves rather than attempting to erase the clients' lived experiences with categories, notions of dysfunction or simplistic theories (MacKinnon 1993).
- Assist clients to optimally use the services available.
- Acknowledge with the client that there is a difference of cultures and encourage the client to be your teacher of what is culturally sensitive. Use photographs, books and articles of significance. Also try using other ways of communicating, such as music, drawing or painting.
- Sharing of cultural practices is by invitation. When you experience this, acknowledge it.
- Become knowledgeable, sensitive and aware of clients in their cultural setting (Wright 1991).
- Recognise that there is diversity within groups as well as between groups (Charonko 1992).
- Advocate for clients from ethnic minorities, particularly in regard to the way in which decisions are made in hospitals and the community (Wright 1991).

---

management/treatment options. With the presence of cultural intermediaries, support workers and linguistic interpreters as needed, and the provision of an appropriate area, it is possible to make space and time for full discussion. This may involve providing a large area, often an outside area, where adults and children can move about freely, and where discussion will not be intruded on by outsiders—a possible source of family 'shame' in Asian cultures.

It is important to ensure that all stakeholders are consulted or appropriately represented, especially the group's key opinion formers. If necessary, and if acceptable to the client, provision of conference phones or videoconferencing can enable extended family and other community stakeholders to become involved in discussion.

CRITICAL THINKING CHALLENGE 6.7

You are the assigned nurse for Guy, in the case described on the next page. You have been asked to develop a care plan.
- How might you go about rebuilding a therapeutic relationship with Guy and his family?
- Who should you involve in care-planning negotiations?
- What cultural factors may be significant?
- What social factors may apply?
- What interventions may be of use in ensuring that Guy receives the level of service that is his right?
- What treatment and management alternatives may be considered?
- How will treatment outcomes be evaluated, and by whom?

INCORPORATING CULTURALLY SAFE PRACTICE

Mental health nursing is about people—people of all cultures, socioeconomic groups and walks of life. So it follows that to provide quality care we must acknowledge the lived experiences of our clients, how these shape their beliefs and the acceptability of treatments. To provide quality care we must acknowledge cultural diversity. A system that does not consider race, culture, gender or social values does not serve the people it purports to (Speight et al. 1991). As professionals we need to be able to work with everyone (Kareem & Littlewood 1992).

Services must be accessible to all regardless of their culture and colour. However, we should not underestimate the effort involved in achieving this. For example, psychiatric nurses can be viewed by some as agents of social control (Wright 1991). We need to develop practical and realistic ways of supporting those whose cultural roots are different from our own and avoid projecting our own cultural expectations of what is therapeutic onto our clients.

In this section, the issues raised in the case study on the next page are examined in light of the authors' experience in working with consumers from traditional Aboriginal communities. Not all the issues are transferable to other cultural scenarios, but examples are given to show how mental health nurses can use support services to enhance patient outcomes, and how cultural awareness can be incorporated into flexible nursing service delivery.

As a first step in forging a therapeutic alliance, the mental health nurse must acknowledge the primacy of

CASE STUDY: Guy

Guy is a hypothetical 22-year-old Aboriginal man who has lived a traditional lifestyle in a small community and has been initiated in certain ceremonies.

On this occasion, several members of Guy's family have approached the community clinic, requesting that Guy be evacuated to town. They complain of several days of erratic behaviour, with Guy 'seeing things and hearing voices', and becoming physically aggressive. On that morning he had stormed out of his mother's house after a quarrel. He was followed by brothers and found with a rope around his neck.

The clinic doctor found no obvious physical cause for the behaviour, and has arranged an admission to the inpatient unit in the nearest city for monitoring and treatment. Guy is evacuated by plane, arriving at the inpatient unit on Friday at 7 pm.

There is very little history accompanying Guy. His town-based relatives accompany him and are polite and cooperative with the registrar's admission assessment, but she notes that they are non-communicative. They do say that Guy has been behaving strangely since a large family gathering on the community some weeks ago for 'sorry business' for Guy's grandfather, a strong law man. They say that Guy occasionally binges on grog and ganja (marijuana). On these occasions he has been known to become verbally aggressive, but has never actually harmed anyone or himself.

Because the registrar feels there is not enough information to do otherwise, and because no Aboriginal mental health worker will be available until Monday, she decides to admit Guy as an involuntary patient. A cousin-brother is selected by Guy's relatives to stay with him as a boarder on the unlocked unit.

On Saturday morning after breakfast, Guy leaves the unit. The boarder goes back to his home and says he will bring Guy back if he sees him. As required under the Mental Health Act, the police are notified that Guy is absent from the unit without leave.

On Sunday afternoon Guy walks into the unit, accompanied by his cousin-brother and an auntie. Guy has been at another auntie's house, and has tried to hang himself with a belt after a drinking session and an argument. Answering the registrar's questions, none of the party can explain why Guy was not brought back straight away. They are angry and alarmed that the police visited their house while Guy was at another relative's place. They did not tell the police where Guy was, although they all agree that they know that being 'on a section' means he must be on the unit at all times, for his own safety. Family report that he is still seeing things and hearing things, but give no details and appear largely unconcerned.

The registrar believes that Guy is a continuing danger to himself. He has not been fully assessed, has not had regular medication, and is still making suicidal gestures. She decides to manage him in a locked area until a full team review, including Aboriginal mental health worker involvement, is possible the next day.

The next morning, the nursing staff at handover state that Guy remains polite and quiet, but totally non-interactive with staff, and non-compliant with oral medication. There are no overt signs of suicidal intent or of mental illness, but in the light of two recent potential suicidal episodes, the unit consultant wishes to ensure further assessment. Guy's family are troubled that he has been locked up, and say they want to take him home today. They say that he doesn't need 'whitefella' medicine—they will manage him 'blackfella way, family way'.

Aboriginal mental health workers and senior family and community members in teasing out and managing cultural and social issues for Aboriginal clients, and in assigning meaning to observed behaviours. Nevertheless, the mere presence of Aboriginal mental health workers is not enough, in itself, to guarantee success. Many Aboriginal mental health workers are not from traditional backgrounds. The Aboriginal mental health worker may not be senior enough to advise families with the required level of authority. If the Aboriginal mental health worker is kin to the patient, there may be kin obligations which enhance or impede the health relationship. It is important that the service is flexible enough to allow networking and consultation across the entire Aboriginal mental health worker network to ensure that the appropriate person is on hand, even if he or she is technically assigned to another work unit.

If admission is the preferred option, thought must be given to how this will be managed, to maintain a meaningful connection with family. All clients evacuated to an inpatient unit from remote communities are encouraged to bring a 'boarder'—someone who will stay with them full time to reduce the loneliness and stress experienced. The boarder will also support the client through interviews and investigations. This person should be a family member who has sufficient standing to advise the client, and to lead family opinion. For a young man, the boarder should be a male who has been initiated to a fitting level. A woman would be accompanied by a senior woman with the authority to advise on healing for women's business. Family networks in town should also be mobilised before transfer takes place.

More importantly, it is incumbent on the mental health nurse to think beyond the inpatient treatment model, and look at alternatives. It may be more therapeutic for the client to stay with town family, or at a hostel, and to meet daily with Aboriginal mental health workers and family for ongoing negotiations.

Other options that may be helpful include traditional healing, either as outpatient or inpatient, as decided by patient and family. 'Smoking' by senior women has been employed as a treatment option, as has standard antidepressant medication, by young women diagnosed with postnatal depression. Indigenous patients increasingly choose such use of 'both-way' interventions. Families have also invited 'clever men' and traditional healers to cooperate in treatment on and off the inpatient unit. The success or otherwise of negotiated care and service delivery will be evaluated and articulated by the appropriate family or community elder.

Cultural respect will allow the mental health nurse to value the contribution that culturally appropriate interventions can make to the therapeutic environment. As well as traditional Aboriginal medicine, the authors' experience includes Maori families negotiating traditional treatments as part of an ongoing care package for both community and inpatient care. Similarly, Buddhist ceremonies have been employed as a focal part of a therapeutic plan for patients of Asian background, and attendance at special services has proved beneficial for people of different European Christian groups.

CONCLUSION

Mental health nurses have a responsibility to ensure that they are well informed on current statistics, trends, models and philosophies relating to all areas of mental health. They need to examine their own perceptions and belief systems in regard to mental health issues and behaviours, so they can function effectively in an unbiased manner. Reflective practice and commitment to the understanding of each individual as a person, taking into account and respecting cultural diversity, will enable mental health nurses to work with clients to establish supportive care strategies and valid outcomes.

EXERCISES FOR CLASS ENGAGEMENT

- Make a list of the thoughts you currently have on all issues relating to mental ill health. Discuss your list with other members of your group or class and then re-examine the list as you progress through your study. You should be able to dispel misconceptions and replace them with the facts about mental health and ill health.

- List the most widespread social perceptions of mental illness/people with mental illness. Discuss the ways in which misconceptions about mental illness originate and are perpetuated. Identify how nurses can influence social perceptions of mental illness/people with mental illness.

- In a small group, identify the values that operate in the mental health-care system (you might have an experience from clinical practice that can be examined in analysing the value system). Discuss how the underlying values of mental health services affect individuals from diverse cultures.

- Use your library service or the internet to answer the following questions.
  - What results do you get when you search using the key words 'stigma', 'culture', 'mental health' and 'consumer groups'?

  - What variation in perceptions can you find? Is there variation between consumers and mental health professionals? Between different mental health disciplines? Between countries?
  - Is all the information useful? How do you discriminate?
  - Make a list of useful websites.
  Share your results with your group or class members.

- Considering cultural background as encompassing socio-economic status, migrant/refugee status, gender and age, answer the following questions, and then discuss your answers with your group or class members.
  - What is the 'cultural mix' of your area? City? University? Year group? Hospital catchment area? Home town?
  - Think of the health-care agency you have worked in most recently (or the one with which you are most familiar). How does that agency manifest its culture and ethos? How does the agency's culture affect the ways in which health care is offered to clients? What is the 'fit' between the agency's cultural approach and the catchment area it serves?
  - How do you define yourself culturally? How does this self-definition affect your nursing practice?

REFERENCES

Abdullah SN 1995, Towards an individualized client's care: implication for education. The transcultural approach, *Journal of Advanced Nursing*, 22(4), pp 715–20.

Allen DG 1999, Knowledge, politics, culture and gender: a discourse perspective, *Canadian Journal of Nursing Research*, 30(4), pp 227–34.

Andrews G, Hall W, Teesson M & Henderson S 1999, *The Mental Health of Australians*, Mental Health Branch, Commonwealth Department of Health and Aged Care, Canberra.

Anxiety Disorders Foundation of Australia (NSW Branch) Inc. 1998, Information about Anxiety Disorders. Online: http://www.geocities.com/adfanswinc/.

Australian and New Zealand College of Mental Health Nurses (ANZCMHN) 1995, *Standards of Practice for Mental Health Nursing in Australia*, and *Standards of Practice for Mental Health Nursing in New Zealand*, Greenacres, SA.

Australian and New Zealand College of Mental Health Nurses (ANZCMHN) 2002, *Competencies for Advanced Practice in Psychiatric Mental Health Nursing in New Zealand*, Auckland.

Australian Bureau of Statistics (ABS) 2000, *Australian Demographic Statistics*, ABS, Canberra

Barnett B, Matthey S & Boyce P 1999, Migration and motherhood: a response to Barclay and Kent (1998), *Midwifery*, 15(3), pp 203–7.

Belkin GS 1988, *Introduction to Counselling*, Iowa, WC Brown.

Betancourt JR, Green AR, Carillo JE & Park ER 2002, Cultural competence in health care: emerging frameworks and practical approaches. Online: www.massgeneral.org/healthpolicy/cchc.html.

Blood W 2002, *A Qualiative Analysis of the Reporting and Portrayal of Mental Illness in the Courier Mail and Sunday Mail*, report prepared for the Public Advocates Office, Queensland.

Campinha-Bacote J 2003, Many Faces: Addressing Diversity in Health Care, *Online Journal of Issues in Nursing*, 8(1). Online: http//nursing world.org/ojin/topic20/tpc20_2.htm.

Carroll PJ 1995, Aboriginal languages and effective cross-cultural commu-nication. In: Robinson G (ed.), *Aboriginal Health: Social and Cultural Transitions*, NTU Press, Darwin.

Charonko CV 1992, Cultural influences in 'noncompliant' behavior and decision making, *Holistic Nursing Practice*, 6(3), pp 73–8.

Commonwealth Department of Health and Aged Care 2000, *National Action Plan for Promotion, Prevention and Early Intervention for Mental Health*, Mental Health and Special Programs Branch, Commonwealth Department of Health and Aged Care, Canberra.

Commonwealth Department of Health and Aged Care, Health Services Division 2000, 'Reducing stigma and discrimination'. Online: http://www.health.gov.au/hsdd/mentalhe/mhinfo/cap/stigma.htm, last updated 25 July 2000.

Commonwealth Department of Health and Aged Care and Australian Institute of Health and Welfare (1999), *National Health Priority Areas Report: Mental Health 1998*. AIHW Cat. No. PHE 13. Health and AIHW, Canberra.

Commonwealth Government of Australia (CGA) 2002, *National Review of Nursing Education. Our Duty of Care*, Canberra.

Cooney C 1994, A comparative analysis of transcultural nursing and cultural safety, *Nursing Praxis in New Zealand*, 9(1), pp 6–12.

D'Ardenne P & Mahtani A 1989, *Transcultural Counselling in Action*, Sage, London.

Davies J 2002, *Trapped in the Hell of Their Parents' Suffering*, National Network of Adult and Adolescent Children who have a Mentally Ill Parent/s, Vic. Inc. Australia, http://home.vicnet.net.au/~nnaami/trapped.html.

Dean C & Macmillan C 2002, *Serving the Children of Parents with a Mental Illness: Barriers, Break-Throughs and Benefits*, Australian Infant, Child, Adolescent and Family mental Health Association Ltd, http://www.aicafmha.net.au/conferences/brisbane2001/papers/dean_c.htm.

Dudgeon P, Garvey D & Pickett H (eds) 2000, *Working with Indigenous Australians: a Handbook for Psychologists*, Gunada Press, Perth.

Durie M 2001, *Mauri Ora The Dynamics of Mäori Health*, Oxford University Press, Auckland.

Durvasula RS & Mylvaganam GA 1994, Mental health of Asian Indians: relevant issues and community implications, *Journal of Community Psychology*, 22(2), pp 97–108.

Eades D 1998, They don't speak an Aboriginal language, or do they?. In: Keen I (ed.), *Being Black: Aboriginal Cultures in 'Settled' Australia*, Aboriginal Studies Press, Canberra.

Eisenbruch M 2001, *National Review of Nursing Education: Multicultural Nursing Education*, Department of Education, Science and Training and Department of Health and Ageing, Canberra.

Ferguson B & Browne E (eds) 1991, *Health Care and Immigrants: a Guide for Health Professionals*, McLennan & Petty, Sydney.

Fitzgerald M, Ing V, Heang Ya T, Heang Hay S, Yang T & Duong HL 1998, *Hear Our Voices: Trauma, Birthing and Mental Health among Cambodian Women*, Ausmed, Paramatta.

Flaskerud JH 1984, A comparison of perceptions of problematic behavior by six minority groups and mental health professionals, *Nursing Research*, 33(4), pp 190–2.

Flaskerud JH 1990, Matching client and therapist, ethnicity, language and gender: a review of research, *Issues in Mental Health*, 11, pp 321–36.

Fontaine KL 2003 *Mental Health Nursing* (5th edn), Prentice Hall, New Jersey.

Friedl E 1991, Society and sex roles. In: Podolefsky A & Brown PJ (eds), *Applying Cultural Anthropology: An Introductory Reader*, Mayfield, California.

Fryer D 1995, Unemployment. A Mental Health Issue, *The Jobs*, letter, 24/9, September.

Fullagar S & Gattuso S 2002, Rethinking gender, risk and depression in Australian mental health policy. *Australian e-Journal for the Advancement of Mental Health* (AeJAMH), 1(3).

Fuller J 1995, Challenging old notions of professionalism: How can nurses work with paraprofessional ethnic health workers?, *Journal of Advanced Nursing*, 22(2), pp 465–72.

Gauntlett N, Ford R, Johnson N & Navarro T 1995, Meeting mental health needs of ethnic minority groups, *Nursing Times*, 91(42), pp 36–7.

Harris SG 1995, Yolngu rules of interpersonal communication. In: Edwards WH (ed.), *Traditional Aboriginal Society: A Reader*, Macmillan, Melbourne.

Henderson AS & Jorm AE 1998, *Dementia in Australia*, Commonwealth Department of Health and Family Services, Canberra.

Henderson G & Primeaux M (eds) 1981, *Transcultural Health Care*, Addison Wesley, Menlo Park, Calif.

Jablensky A, McGrath J, Hermann H, Castle D, Gureje O, Morgan V et al. 1999, *National Survey of Mental Health and Well-being, Report 4: People Living with Psychotic Illness: An Australian Study 1997/98*, Mental Health Branch, Commonwealth Department of Health and Aged Care, Canberra.

Jeffs L 2001, Teaching cultural safety the culturally safe way, *Nursing Praxis in New Zealand*, 17(3), pp 41–50.

Kareem J & Littlewood R 1992, *Intercultural Therapy: Themes, Interpretation and Practice*, Blackwell, Oxford.

Leininger M 1995, *Transcultural Nursing: Concepts, Theories and Practices*, Blacklick, Ohio.

Lindberg W 2001, Interview: Warren Lindberg .Online: www.mediawatch.co.nz/archive.

MacKinnon L 1993, Systems in settings: the therapist as power broker, *Australia New Zealand Journal of Family Therapy*, 14(3), pp 117–22.

Martin G 1998, Media influence to suicide: the search for solutions. *Archives of Suicide Research*, 4, pp 51–6.

Mathers C & Schofield D 1998, The Health Consequences of Unemploy-ment: The Evidence. Online: http://www.mja.co.au/public/issues/feb16/mathers/mathers.html.

McAvoy BR & Donaldson LJ 1990, *Health Care for Asians*, Oxford University Press, Oxford.

McLennan A 1998, *Mental Health and Well Being: Profile of Adults*, Australia Bureau of Statistics, Canberra.

Meadows G & Singh B 2001, *Mental Health in Australia, Collaborative Community Practice*, Oxford University Press, Melbourne.

Mental Health Commission 1998, *Blueprint for Mental Health Services in New Zealand: How Things Need To Be*, MHC, Wellington.

Ministry of Health 1996, *Towards Better Mental Health Services: The Report of the National Working Party on Mental Health Workforce Development*, Ministry of Health, Wellington.

Ministry of Health 1997, *Moving Forward: The National Mental Health Plan for More and Better Services*. Online: info@moh.govt.nz, Ministry of Health, Wellington.

Ministry of Health 2000, *Involving Families*, Ministry of Health, Wellington.

Mitchell N 2003, Media Interrupted: Mental Health and the Media. Online: http://www.abc.net.au/rn/science/mind/s788631.htm.

Murray C & Lopez A 1996, *The Global Burden of Disease: A Comprehensive Assessment of Mortality and Disability, Injuries, and Risk Factors in 1990 and Projected To 2020*, Geneva: World Bank, Harvard School of Public Health and World Health Organization.

Nielsen B, Katrakis E & Raphael B 2001, Males and mental health: a public health approach, *NSW Public Health Bulletin*, December.

Northern Territory Government (NTG) 1998, *Northern Territory Aboriginal Mental Health Guidelines and Action Plan*, NTG, Darwin.

Nursing Council of New Zealand 2002, *Guidelines for Cultural Safety, The Treaty of Waitangi and Maori Health in Nursing and Midwifery Education and Practice*, Wellington, Nursing Council of New Zealand, 24.

Pinches A 2002, Recognising not only Consumers' Legal Rights, but also Their 'Community Entitlements', from an address to a Mental Health Legal Centre workshop at the National Conference of the Federation on Community Legal Centres, Melbourne.

Powell G 2002, New Zealand's National Mental Health Strategy: Report on Progress 2000–2001, presented to the MHS Conference, Sydney, 20 August 2002.

Queensland Health 1998, Checklists for Cultural Assessment. Online: http://www.health.qld.gov.au/hssb/cultdiv.

Ramsden I 1997, *Cultural Safety: Implementing the Concept: The Social Force of Nursing and Midwifery*. In: Whaiti PT, McCarthy M & Durie A (eds), *Mai i rangiatea*, Auckland University Press, Auckland.

Ramsden I 2002, *Cultural Safety*: Kawa Whakaruruhau, Massey.

Ramsden IM 2002, *Cultural Safety and Nursing Education in Aotearoa and Te Waipounamu* (doctoral thesis), Victoria University, Wellington.

Regier DA, Farmer ME, Rae DS, Locke BZ, Keith SJ, Judd LL et al. 1990, Co-morbidity of mental disorders with alcohol and other drug abuse: results from Epidemiologic Catchment Area (ECA) Study, *Journal of American Medical Association*, 264, pp 2511–18.

Reser J 1991, Aboriginal mental health: conflicting cultural perspectives. In: Reid J & Trompf P (eds), *The Health of Aboriginal Australia*, Harcourt Brace, Sydney.

Ring IT & Firman D 1998, Reducing indigenous mortality in Australia: lessons from other countries. *Medical Journal of Australia*, 169, pp 528–33.

Robinson C 2003, *Understanding Iterative Homelessness: The Case of People with Mental Disorders*. For Australian Housing and Urban Research Institute, UNSW-UWS Research Centre, New South Wales.

Rose DB 2000, *Dingo Makes us Human: Life and Land in an Australian Aboriginal Culture* (2nd edn), CUP, Cambridge.

SANE Australia 2000, Better Health Channel, Mental Illness and Violence Explained. Online: http://www.betterhealth.vic.gov.au/bhcv2/bhcarticles.nsf/Mental_illness_and_violence_explained?open, last reviewed July 2003.

Sawyer MG, Arney FM, Baghurst PA, Clark JJ, Graetz BW, Kosky RJ et al. 2000, *Mental Health of Young People in Australia*, Child and Adolescent Component of the National Survey of Mental Health and Well-being.

Speight SL, Myers LJ, Cox CI & Highlen PS 1991, A redefinition of multi-cultural counselling, *Journal of Counselling and Development*, 70, pp 29–35.

Spradley JP 1991, Ethnography and culture. In: Worsley P (ed.), *The New Modern Sociology Readings*, Penguin, London.

Statistics New Zealand (SNZ) 2000, *Demographic Trends*, Wellington.

Stein-Parbury J 2000, *Patient and Person*, Harcourt, Sydney

Stern G & Kruckman L 1983, Multi-disciplinary perspectives on post-partum depression: an anthropological critique, *Social Science & Medicine*, 17(15), pp 1027–41.

Sue DW & Sue D 1990, *Counselling the Culturally Different*, John Wiley & Sons, USA.

Sullivan K 1994, *Bicultural Education in Aotearoa/New Zealand*. New Zealand annual review of education/Te arotake a tau o te ao o te mataurangi i Aotearoa. H. Manson, Victoria University, Wellington.

Tatz C 2001, *Aboriginal Suicide is Different*, Aboriginal Studies Press, Canberra.

Transcultural Psychiatry Unit, Curtin University and Royal Australian and New Zealand College of Psychiatrists 2001, *Cultural Awareness Tool: Understanding Cultural Diversity in Mental Health*.

Walker R 1995, *Immigration Policy and the Political Economy of New Zealand. Immigration and National Identity in New Zealand: One People, Two Peoples, Many Peoples*, SW Greif. Palmerston North, Dunmore Press.

World Health Organization 2001, The World Health Report 2001. Mental Health: New Understanding, New Hope. Online: http://www.who.int/whr2001/2001/main/en/chapter2/002h4.htm.

Wright J 1991, Counselling at the cultural interface: is getting back to roots enough?, *Journal of Advanced Nursing*, 16, pp 92–100.

Zubrick SR, Silburn SR, Garton A, Burton P, Dalby R, Carlton J et al. 1995, *Western Australian Child Health Survey: Developing Health and Well-Being in the Nineties*, Australian Bureau of Statistics and the Institute for Child Health Research, Perth, Western Australia.

WEBSITES

http://www.abs.gov.au/ausstats/abs@.nsf/b06660592430724fca2568b5007b8619/3f8a5d

http://www.health.gov.au/hsdd/mentalhe/mhinfo/cap/stigma.htm

http://www.health.gov.au/hsdd/mentalhe/mhinfo/cap/stigma.htm

http://www.mentalhealth.gov.au

http://www.mmhc.com/jgsm/articles/JGSM9906?law.html

http://www.nimh.nih.gov/wmhc/research.cfm

http://www.nzhis.govt.nz/pulications/mhincnews05.htmnl

Australian and New Zealand College of Mental Health Nurses anzcmhn@yahoogroups.com

Australian and New Zealand College of Mental Health Nurses, Inc. www.anzcmhn.org

Australian Bureau of Statistics www.abs.gov.au

Australian Transcultural Mental Health Organisations http://www.atmhn.unimelb.edu.au/organisations/organisations.html

Centre for Ethnic Health http://www.ceh.org.au/.

Commonwealth of Australia, Department of Health and Ageing www.health.gov.au

Congress of Aboriginal and Torres Strait Islander Nurses http://www.indiginet.com.au/catsin/

Department of Health and Aged Care Mental Health Branch of the Commonwealth Government http://www.health.gov.au/hsdd/mentalhe/

Diversity Rx http://www.DiversityRx.org/>

Guide to Mental Health on the Internet in Australia http://www.mentalhealth.org.au/info/links/index.html

Health Promotion Forum of New Zealand www.hpforum.org.nz

Maori Health www.maorihealth.govt.nz/

Maori Mental Health: A Selected Annotated Bibliography (2000) www.hauora.com/downloads/files/ACF30AO.PDF

Maori Organisations of New Zealand www.maori.org.nz

Mental Health Branch—Publications & Resources http://www.health.gov.au/hsdd/mentalhe/resources/index.htm

Mental Health Commission, New Zealand http://www.mhc.govt.nz/

Mental Health Foundation of New Zealand http://www.mentalhealth.org.nz

New Zealand Ministry of Health www.moh.govt.nz

SANE (Schizophrenia Australia) http://www.sane.org/

Statistics New Zealand: Te Tari Tatau www.stat.govt.nz

Transcultural Mental Health On-Line http://www.priory.com/psych/trans.htm

Victorian Transcultural Psychiatry Unit http://www.vtpu.org.au

World Federation for Mental Health http://www.wfmh.com/

WHO, To improve the mental health status of people with severe mental illness. http://www.newhealth.govt.nz/toolkits/mentalpercent20health/background_3.htm

WHO, The World Health Report 2001. Mental Health: New Understanding, New Hope. http://www.who.int/whr2001/2001/main/en/chapter2/002h4.htm

Theories on Mental Health and Illness

Patricia Barkway

KEY POINTS

- Mental health and mental illness are complex, distinct entities that are not necessarily mutually exclusive.
- Various subjective factors influence whether human behaviour is perceived as normal or abnormal.
- Community attitudes about mental health and mental illness contribute to stigma.
- Although personality and human behaviour theories provide explanations for the way in which individuals think, feel and behave, no theory has universal applicability.
- Personality and human behaviour theories underpin psychotherapeutic interventions for mental illness.
- Psychological and sociological theories have influenced the development of nursing theories.
- The answer to the nature versus nurture debate is not simply *either/or*. A more plausible explanation is that personality develops as a consequence of the interaction between nature *and* nurture.

KEY TERMS

- biomedical model
- mental health
- mental illness
- nature versus nurture debate
- nursing theories
- psychological theories
- sociological theories

LEARNING OUTCOMES

The material in this chapter will assist you to:

- describe and critique biomedical, psychological and sociological theories of personality and human behaviour
- outline how the theories explain both normal and abnormal behaviour
- understand the concepts of mental health and mental illness
- identify a preferred theory of personality development
- understand the nature versus nurture debate
- understand the contribution of psychological and sociological theories to the development of nursing theories.

INTRODUCTION

Who are you? How have you come to be who you are? What influences how you think, feel and act? Are your personality and behaviour determined by your genetic make-up and biological events, by thoughts and feelings, by your experiences in the world, or by an interrelationship between some or all of these? Why are some people seemingly more vulnerable to mental illness, while others are resilient despite adversity? Most of us, at one time or another, have pondered these questions. Through attempting to understand why humans behave as they do, a further question arises: are personality and human behaviour determined by genetics and biology (*nature*) or shaped by one's upbringing, experiences and environmental factors (*nurture*)? This question has long engaged the interest and passion of philosophers, healers and health professionals and, in more recent times, scientists. Investigation of these questions has resulted in various theories being proposed to explain *normal* and *abnormal* behaviour, and *mental health* and *mental illness*. These concepts, the theories that attempt to explain them and proposed interventions will be examined in this chapter. The nature versus nurture debate will also be explored.

WHAT IS MENTAL HEALTH?

A succinct, universally applicable definition of mental health has long been elusive. Although contemporary definitions encapsulate the breadth of factors that contribute to mental health, they are wordy and jargonistic. See, for example, the definition proposed by the Australian Health Ministers, which states that mental health is:

> The capacity of individuals within groups and the environment to interact with one another in ways that promote subjective wellbeing, optimal development and use of mental abilities (cognitive, affective and relational) and achievement of individual and collective goals consistent with justice.

(Commonwealth Department of Health and Aged Care 2000, p 127)

In the 1980s Doona suggested that the problem of defining mental health was derived from the fact that the concept of *health* is not a measurable scientific term; she concluded that 'health is probably a value judgement and more amenable to philosophical analysis' (Doona 1982, p 13). Her comment remains pertinent today. Two decades later, Sainsbury (2003) draws a parallel between mental health and happiness. Although this is a seemingly simplistic comparison, Sainsbury does not see happiness as an individual pursuit, but rather a consequence of political and social factors that, in the main, remain outside the direct control of the individual.

Defining mental health

Initial attempts to define mental health have focused on the individual's ability to incorporate external factors. Kittleson cited four major components, namely high self-esteem, effective decision-making, values awareness and expressive communication skills (1989, pp 40–1). Kittleson's depiction of mental health as a positive construct separate from mental illness is welcome but limited. It is welcome because it enables mental health to be viewed as more than merely the absence of the symptoms of mental illness. It is limited because a focus on individual factors implies individual responsibility, which may lead to victim blaming (McMurray 1999, p 327; Wass 2000, pp 67–70). Furthermore, a definition in terms of the individual fails to acknowledge the contribution of social factors and the environment to mental health.

In 1993, Raphael drew attention to contextual and social issues that affect mental health, namely workplace factors, education, macro-economic and other forces. These social forces are acknowledged as contributors to mental health, as are personal qualities such as resilience, coping, physical health and wellbeing (Raphael 1993, pp 15–16). Contemporary definitions of mental health include social determinants such as social connectedness, acceptance of diversity, freedom from discrimination and economic participation (Vic Health 2003; Wilkinson & Marmot 1998). Recognition of social determinants is evident in the United Kingdom Health Development Agency's guidelines for mental health promotion, which are to:

- develop people's coping and general life skills
- promote social support networks—for example, to tackle bullying, support bereaved families, facilitate self-help groups and increase opportunities to participate in the community
- address structural barriers to mental health in areas such as education, employment and housing (Health Development Agency 2003).

The emergence of a definition of mental health that encompasses positive constructs, not just the absence of symptoms, is important because it enables mental health and mental illness to be viewed as distinct from each other, and not as two points at opposite ends of a continuum. Significantly, it means that the two states are not mutually exclusive. A person can enjoy mental health regardless of whether or not they are diagnosed with a mental illness if they have a positive sense of self, personal and social support with which to respond to life's challenges, meaningful relationships with others, access to employment and recreation activities, sufficient financial resources and suitable living arrangements.

'Mental health' as a euphemism for 'mental illness'

Health professionals and the health literature have adopted the practice of using the terms *mental health* and *mental illness* interchangeably. In 1989 Kittleson drew attention to this phenomenon following an examination of undergraduate mental health texts. He found that 'personality development and emotional illness make up the bulk of mental health coverage in the texts' (1989, p 40). A recent perusal of contemporary mental health literature found that this practice is still prevalent in texts and journals (Andrews et al. 1999; Carson & Arnold 1996; Clinton & Nelson 1999; Gray 1999; Forster 2001; Millar & Walsh 2000, *International Journal of Mental Health Nursing* and *Issues in Mental Health Nursing*). Although these publications include 'mental health' in their title, in the main they contain chapters or articles concerning assessment of, and treatments for, mental illness or mental health problems.

The substitution of the term *mental health* when referring to *mental illness* is a twentieth-century phenomenon that has been carried forward into the new millennium. The first references to *mental health* being used as an alternative to 'psychiatry' occurred in the United Kingdom and the United States from the 1920s. Momentum was gained after World War II, when proponents such as Caplan advocated a shift from treatment of mental illness to prevention (Evans 1992, p 55). In the United States, Szasz (1961) argued that mental illness was a *societal ill* and not an individual sickness. Amid this debate, legislators worldwide changed the term 'mental illness' in the names of legislation to 'mental health'. However, this change is nominal because the content of legislation continues to be concerned with mental illness. The *South Australian Mental Health Act (1993)*, for example, identifies the purpose of this legislation as 'providing treatment and protection of persons who have a mental illness' which is [vaguely] defined as 'any illness or disorder of the mind' (*South Australian Consolidated Acts 2002*). Despite the title of the Act, it contains no reference to mental health as a positive concept.

Following legislative name changes, organisations that provided treatment and rehabilitation services to individuals with mental illness also changed their names, replacing words like *psychiatric* and *mental illness/disorder* with 'mental health'—hence the emergence of organisations with titles like 'Southern Districts Mental Health Service'. Nevertheless, despite the change of name there has been little shift in the focus of the services provided, as they continue to address the needs of the mentally ill, with minimal focus on mental health. This is not to suggest that mental illness services should not be provided; clearly there is a demonstrated need for them and they are not under scrutiny here. Rather, the assertion is made that to call them *mental health* services is a misnomer.

A further consequence of using the euphemism 'mental health' when referring to mental illness is that this practice may in fact be contributing to the perpetuation of stigma. Implicit in the avoidance of the term *mental illness* is the notion that mental illness is something to be avoided, hidden or shameful. Ironically, calling mental illness by another name has not reduced stigma; instead it has broadened the application of stigma to now include mental health.

CRITICAL THINKING CHALLENGE 7.1

What is mental health? How does it differ from mental illness?

THEORIES OF PERSONALITY

Personality theories that develop models to explain human behaviours have long been sought. In addition to curiosity and philosophical inquiry, particular emphasis is placed on identifying the causes of *abnormal* behaviour so as to develop models for understanding prevention or treatment of mental illness. Explanations can be broadly divided into three paradigms:

- biomedical or biological/physical models
- psychological models, including psychoanalytic, behavioural, cognitive and humanistic approaches
- sociological models.

Within these paradigms the following are the major viewpoints to offer a theory of personality development or an explanation of human behaviour.

- *Biomedical model*—proposes that behaviour is influenced by physiology, with *normal* behaviour occurring when the body is in a state of equilibrium, and *abnormal* behaviour being a consequence of physical pathology.
- *Psychoanalytic theory*—asserts that behaviour is driven by unconscious processes, and influenced by childhood/developmental conflicts that have either been resolved or remain unresolved.
- *Behavioural psychology*—presents the view that behaviour is influenced by factors external to the individual. Behaviours are learned depending on whether they are rewarded or not, by association with another event or by imitation.
- *Cognitive psychology*—acknowledges the role of perception and thoughts about oneself, one's individual experience and the environment in influencing behaviour.
- *Humanistic psychology*—focuses on the development of a concept of self and the striving of the individual to achieve personal goals.
- *Sociological theories*—shifts the emphasis from the individual to the broader social forces that influence people. This model challenges the notion of individual pathology.

Each of these seemingly disparate perspectives makes a substantial contribution to the understanding of how and why humans behave as they do, and thereby identifies opportunities for prevention and treatment of mental illness. Nevertheless, as a comprehensive theory of human behaviour, each also has major shortcomings. Let us now look at these theories in more detail.

Biomedical model

Also known as psychobiology or the neuroscience perspective, the biomedical model asserts that *normal* behaviour is a consequence of equilibrium within the body and that *abnormal* behaviour results from pathological bodily or brain function. This is not a new notion—in the fourth century BC the Greek physician Hippocrates attributed mental disorder to brain pathology. His ideas were overshadowed, however, when throughout the Dark Ages and later during the Renaissance, thinking and explanations shifted to witchcraft or demonic possession (Alloy, Jacobsen & Acocella 1999, pp 12–15). In the nineteenth century, a return to biophysical explanations accompanied the emergence of the public health movement.

In recent times, advances in technology have led to increased understanding of organic determinants of behaviour. Research and treatment have focused on four main areas:

- *nervous system disorders*, in particular neurotransmitter disturbance at the synaptic gap between neurons—over fifty neurotransmitters have been identified, four of which are implicated in mental illness. These are acetylcholine (Alzheimer's disease), dopamine (schizophrenia), norepinephrine (mood disorder) and serotonin (mood disorder).
- *structural changes to the brain*—perhaps following trauma or in degenerative disorders such as Huntington's disease.
- *endocrine or gland dysfunction*, as in hypothyroidism—this has a similar presentation to clinical depression, and hormonal changes are considered to be a contributing factor in postnatal depression.
- *familial (genetic) transmission of mental illness*—twin studies reviewed by Gottesman found the following lifetime risks of developing schizophrenia: general population 1%, one parent 13%, sibling 9%, dizygotic twin 17%, two parents 46%, monozygotic twin 48% (Gottesman 1991, cited in Alloy et al. 1999, p 388).

Although genetic studies demonstrate a correlation between having a close relative with schizophrenia and the likelihood of developing the disorder, a shared genetic history alone is not sufficient. If genetics were the only aetiological factor, the concordance rate for monozygotic twins could be expected to be 100 per cent. Gottesman's research is important because it supports the diathesis-stress model, a widely held explanation for the development of mental disorder which proposes that constitutional predisposition combined with environmental stress will lead to mental illness (Alloy et al. 1999, p 79).

Critique of the biomedical model

Among treatments that emerge from the biomedical model are medications that alter neurotransmitters. However, evidence that a particular intervention is an effective treatment is not proof of a *causal* link with the illness. Consider a person with insulin-dependent diabetes mellitus, for example. Because this person lacks insulin to metabolise glucose, the condition is managed with regular insulin injections. However, the lack of insulin is a symptom of the disease, not the cause.

Whatever caused the pancreas to cease producing insulin is not known, despite the treatment being effective. Similarly, with schizophrenia the relationship between the use of antipsychotic medications, dopamine levels and symptom management is correlational, not causal. Therefore, although antipsychotic medication affects dopamine receptors and can be an effective treatment to manage the symptoms of schizophrenia, this does not provide evidence that elevated dopamine levels *caused* the disorder.

Psychoanalytic theory

Sigmund Freud developed the first psychological explanation of human behaviour—psychoanalytic theory—in the late nineteenth century. He placed strong emphasis on the role of unconscious processes in determining human behaviour. Central tenets of the theory are that intrapsychic (generally unconscious) forces, developmental factors and family relationships determine human behaviour. Mental illness is seen as a consequence of fixation at a particular developmental stage or conflict that has not been resolved.

Sigmund Freud (1856–1939)

Freud was an Austrian neurologist who, in his clinical practice, saw a number of patients with sensory or neurological problems for which he was unable to identify a physiological cause. In the main these patients were middle-class Viennese women. It was from his work with these patients that Freud hypothesised that the cause of their maladies was psychological. From this assumption he developed a personality theory, which he called psychoanalytic theory.

According to Freud the mind is composed of three forces:

- the *id*—the primitive biological force comprising two basic drives, sexual and aggressive. The id operates on the *pleasure principle* and seeks to satisfy life-sustaining needs such as food, love and creativity, in addition to sexual gratification.
- the *ego*—the cognitive component of personality which attempts to use realistic means (the *reality principle*) to achieve the desires of the id.
- the *superego*—the internalised moral standards of the society in which one lives. It can be equated to a *conscience*.

Freud's theory proposes that personality development progresses through four stages throughout childhood. At each stage the child's behaviour is driven by the need to satisfy sexual and aggressive drives via the mouth, anus or genitals. Failure of the child to satisfy these needs at any one of the stages will result in psychological difficulties that are carried into adulthood. For example, unresolved issues at the oral stage can lead to dependency issues in adulthood, and problems in the anal stage may lead to the child later developing obsessive-compulsive traits. Freud's stages of psychosexual development are:

- *oral*—from birth to about eighteen months, where the primary focus of the id is the mouth
- *anal*—from approximately eighteen months to three years, where libido shifts from the mouth to the anus and primary gratification is derived from expelling or retaining faeces
- *phallic*—from approximately three to six years, where gratification of the id occurs through the genitals
- *genital*—once the child passes through puberty, sexual urges re-emerge, but now they are directed toward another person, not the self as they were at an earlier stage of development
- *latent*—Freud proposed that from approximately six to twelve years, the child goes through a latency phase in which sexual urges are dormant (Alloy et al. 1999; Bond & McKonky 2001; Davison & Neale 2001; Rogers 1951, 1961).

Defence mechanisms

An important contribution of psychoanalytic theory to the understanding of behaviour has been the identification of defence mechanisms and the role they play in mediating anxiety. Defence mechanisms were first described by Freud and later elaborated on by his daughter Anna (Freud 1966). They are unconscious processes whereby anxiety experienced by the ego is reduced. Commonly used defence mechanisms include:

- *repression*—the primary defence mechanism and an unconscious process whereby unacceptable impulses/feelings/thoughts are barred from consciousness (e.g. memories of sexual abuse in childhood)
- *regression*—the avoidance of present difficulties by a reversion to an earlier, less mature way of dealing with the situation (e.g. a toilet-trained child who becomes incontinent following the birth of a sibling)
- *denial*—the blocking of painful information from consciousness (e.g. not accepting that a loss has occurred)
- *projection*—the denial of one's own unconscious impulses by attributing them to another person (e.g. when you dislike someone but believe it is the other person who does not like you)
- *sublimation*—an unconscious process whereby libido is transformed into a more socially acceptable outlet (e.g. creativity, art, sport)
- *displacement*—the transferring of emotion from the source to a substitute (e.g. a person who is unassertive in an interaction with a supervisor at work and 'kicks the cat' on arriving home)
- *rationalisation*—a rational excuse is used to explain behaviour that may be motivated by an irrational force (e.g. cheating when completing a tax return, with the excuse that 'everyone does it')
- *intellectualisation/isolation*—feelings are cut off from the event in which they occur (e.g. after an unsuccessful job interview the person says, 'I didn't really want the job anyway')

- *reaction formation*—the development of a personality trait that is the opposite of the original unconscious or repressed trait (e.g. avoiding a friend's partner because you are attracted to that person).

Critique of psychoanalytic theory

Although the notions of unconscious motivations and defence mechanisms are helpful in interpreting behaviours, Freud's version of psychoanalytic theory has not been without its critics. Fellow psychoanalyst Erik Erikson disagreed with Freud's theory of *psychosexual* stages of development and proposed instead a *psychosocial* theory in which development occurred throughout the lifespan, not just through childhood, as in Freud's model (Erikson 1963; Santrock 2002).

The unconscious nature of Freud's concepts and stages renders them difficult to test and therefore there is little evidence to support Freudian theory. Feminists, too, object to Freud's interpretation of the psychological development of women, arguing that there is scant evidence to support the hypothesis that women view their bodies as inferior to men's because they do not have a penis (Alloy et al. 1999, p 107).

Behavioural psychology

Behaviourism is a school of psychology founded in the United States by JB Watson in the early twentieth century with the purpose of objectively studying observable human behaviour, as opposed to examining the mind, which was the prevalent psychological method at the time in Europe. The model proposes a *scientific* approach to the study of behaviour, a feature that behaviourists argue is lacking in psychoanalytic theory (and in humanistic psychology, which developed later).

Behaviourism opposes the introspective, structuralist approach of psychoanalysis and emphasises the importance of the environment in shaping behaviour. The focus is on observable behaviour and conditions that elicit and maintain the behaviour (*classical conditioning*) or factors that reinforce behaviour (*operant conditioning*) or vicarious learning through watching and imitating the behaviour of others (*modelling*).

Three basic assumptions underpin behaviour theory. These are that personality is determined by prior learning, that human behaviour is changeable throughout the lifespan and that changes in behaviour are generally caused by changes in the environment. The following were prominent figures in the development of behaviourist psychology.

Ivan Pavlov (1849–1936)

Russian physiologist Ivan Pavlov was the first to describe the relationship between stimulus and response. Pavlov demonstrated that a dog could learn to salivate (respond) to a non-food stimulus (a bell) if the bell was simultaneously presented with the food. His discovery became known as *classical conditioning*.

John B Watson (1878–1958)

Watson, who is attributed as being the founder of behaviourism, changed the focus of psychology from the study of inner sensations to the study of observable behaviour. In his quest to make psychology a true science, Watson further developed Pavlov's work on *stimulus–response* learning and experimented by manipulating stimulus conditions. Watson believed that abnormal behaviour was the result of earlier faulty conditioning and that re-conditioning could modify this.

BF Skinner (1904–1990)

Skinner formulated the notion of instrumental or *operant conditioning* in which *reinforcers* (rewards) contribute to the probability of a response being either repeated or extinguished. Skinner's research demonstrated that the contingencies on which behaviour is based are external to the person, rather than internal. Consequently, changing contingencies could alter an individual's behaviour. This is an underlying principle in treatment using an *operant conditioning* approach (Bond & McKonky 2001; Carson, Butcher & Mineka 1996; Skinner 1953).

Critique of behaviourism

Behaviourism provided the first scientifically testable theories of human development as well as plausible explanations of conditions such as depression and anxiety. However, behaviourist explanations are less convincing when applied to psychosis or organic disorders. Furthermore, most behaviourist research has been conducted on animals under laboratory conditions, so to extrapolate findings from this research to humans is mechanistic and does not allow for intrinsic human qualities like creativity or the ability to love, think or solve problems. Finally, behaviourist theory falls short in explaining the success of an individual brought up in an adverse environment, or how mental illness can occur in a person whose environment is apparently healthy and advantaged.

Cognitive psychology

Since the 1950s, interest in the cognitive or thinking processes involved in behavioural responses has expanded. Cognitive theory proposes that people actively interpret their environment and cognitively construct their world. Therefore, behaviour is a result of the interplay of external and internal events. External events are the stimuli and reinforcements that regulate behaviour, and internal events are one's perceptions and thoughts about the world, as well as one's behaviour in the world. In other words, how one thinks about a situation will influence how one behaves in that situation. The following are prominent figures in the development of cognitive psychology.

Albert Bandura (b. 1925)

According to Bandura it is not intrapsychic or environmental forces alone that influence behaviour. Rather, human behaviour results from the interaction of the *environment* with the individual's *perception* and *thinking*. *Self-efficacy*, or the belief that one can achieve a certain goal, is the critical component in the achievement of that goal. Bandura also proposed that consequences do not have to be directly experienced by the individual for learning to occur—learning can occur vicariously through the process of *modelling* or learning by imitation (Carson et al. 1996).

Aaron T Beck (b. 1921)

Problem behaviour, says Beck, results from *cognitive distortions* or *faulty thinking*. For example, a depressed person will selectively choose information that maintains a gloomy perspective. Depression is experienced when one has a negative schema about oneself or one's situation. According to Beck, depression is a behavioural response to an attitude or cognition of hopelessness, as opposed to hopelessness being a symptom of depression; and anxiety is experienced when one has a distorted anticipation of danger. Treatment within Beck's model involves changing one's views about oneself and one's life situation (Alloy et al. 1999, p 110).

Martin Seligman (b. 1942)

Seligman first proposed his theory of *learned helplessness* as an explanation for depression. The theory suggests that if an individual experiences adversity and attempts to alleviate the situation are unsuccessful, then depression follows. Seligman later expanded his model to include *learned optimism*, a process of challenging negative cognitions to change from a position of passivity to one of control (Seligman 1974, 1994).

Critique of cognitive psychology

The therapeutic techniques derived from cognitive (and cognitive behavioural) theory are practical and effective, and can be self-administered by the client under the direction of a therapist. These therapies have an established record in changing problem behaviours such as phobias, obsessions and compulsions, and in stress management (Carson et al. 1996). They also make a contribution in the treatment of depression and schizophrenia (Johnston 1998; Seligman 1994). Nevertheless, cognitive theory is criticised as being unscientific (as are psychoanalytic and humanistic theories) because mental processes cannot objectively be observed and subjective reports are not necessarily reliable (Alloy et al. 1999, pp 115–16). Additionally, the insight that one's thinking is the cause of one's problems will not in itself bring about behaviour change.

Finally, contrary to the proposal that *thoughts* cause *feelings*, which cause *behaviour* (a notion that underpins the cognitive approach), research conducted by Wishman suggests that in the treatment of depression, cognitive changes follow changes in emotion and behaviour

biomedical model, claiming that its purpose is to give control over people's lives to psychiatrists and argues that psychiatrists exercise coercive domination in the guise of protecting the public and the mad from their madness (Szasz 2000, pp 44–5). Contrary to the illusion that psychiatry is coping well with society's vexing problems, Szasz claims that social problems are in fact being obfuscated and aggravated by the disease interpretation of psychiatry (Szasz 2000, p 53).

Critique of sociological models

Sociological models identify vulnerable populations and also biases that influence diagnosis and treatment. It is important to note, however, that although social factors are associated with better or poorer mental health outcomes, the relationships are *correlational* and cannot be assumed to be in themselves *causative*. Nevertheless, the contribution of population statistics and social demographic data remains significant. By demonstrating links between protective factors for mental health and risk factors for mental illness, potential areas for prevention and intervention are thereby identified. For example, the Youth Suicide Prevention Initiative of the National Mental Health Strategy was set up in the 1990s. The initiative was established in response to statistics showing that, at that time, Australia had the highest youth suicide rate in the industrialised world, and that suicide was second only to motor vehicle accidents as the leading cause of death for young men aged 15 to 24 years (Commonwealth Department of Health & Aged Care 2003; Lewis, cited in Mann 1997, p 20).

CRITICAL THINKING CHALLENGE 7.2

■ Identify factors that influence whether a particular behaviour (e.g. hearing voices) would be considered normal or a symptom of mental illness.

■ Compare and contrast two theories of personality development with regard to how each theory explains:
  – mental health
  – mental illness.

■ How do sociological theories differ from psychological theories of personality development and human behaviour?

FROM THEORY TO PRACTICE

Psychological personality theories and sociological perspectives provide plausible explanations of human behaviour in specific situations. These theories inform therapeutic interventions and treatments in mental illness. It must be noted though, that in the main, the theories outlined were developed in Western Europe and the United States, and therefore may not be applicable

outside those contexts. Consequently, caution is recommended regarding the applicability of treatments derived from these theories to other populations, such as Aboriginal and Torres Strait Island or New Zealand Maori cultures, and people of non-English-speaking backgrounds.

Nevertheless, theories have clinical application. For example, the development of agoraphobia (fear of leaving a safe environment) can be explained by classical or respondent conditioning as described by Pavlov and Watson. Consider a situation in which an anxiety-producing event or unconditioned stimulus (UCS) may have occurred in a public place alongside a conditioned (originally neutral) stimulus (CS). Pairing of the UCS and CS can lead to a situation in which the CS alone is sufficient to produce the conditioned response (CR). Hence the anxiety response is learned through the process of classical conditioning (see Table 7.1).

Table 7.1 Production of a conditioned response

UCS	+	CS	=	CR
anxiety-producing event	+	public place	=	anxiety response
		public place	=	anxiety response

Maintenance of the anxiety response, however, cannot be explained by classical conditioning because the theory predicts that the repeated occurrence of the CS in the absence of the UCS will diminish or extinguish the behaviour (Bond & McConkey 2001, p 4.8). Nevertheless, learning theory in the form of operant conditioning does provide an explanation for the continuation of agoraphobic behaviours. Operant or instrumental conditioning predicts that behaviour is controlled by its consequences (Skinner 1953). If a behaviour is rewarded (positive reinforcement) it is likely to be repeated. Also, if a behaviour leads to the removal of an aversive stimulus (negative reinforcement) then it is likely to be repeated. If, however, a behaviour is ignored or punished, the theory predicts that it will lead to extinction of the behaviour.

For example, if an individual experiences anxiety in a public place and that anxiety is reduced by withdrawal to a safe environment (frequently the home) then negative reinforcement is in operation. The likelihood of withdrawal behaviour occurring again is thereby increased because the individual has been rewarded by a reduction in anxiety. This interpretation of agoraphobic behaviour suggests that the disorder is not so much a fear of open or public places, but a fear of the anxiety one might experience away from the safe environment.

Behavioural treatment of agoraphobia can use classical or operant conditioning strategies or both. An example of a classical conditioning strategy is the repeated exposure of the person to the anxiety-provoking situation with the goal of extinguishing the anxiety response. Operant

CASE STUDY: Karin

Karin is a 42-year-old woman who lives in an inner city Sydney suburb with her partner Scott and their three children—Jordan (twelve years), Sally (ten years) and Amelia (five years). Following Jordan's birth Karin continued to work half-time as an accountant. She had not worked since the birth of Sally ten years previously.

Recently, Karin contacted an agoraphobic self-help phone counselling service to seek assistance. Her phone call was prompted by the prospect of the family relocating to Auckland, New Zealand, due to Scott being offered a promotion. Karin is terrified about moving because she has not left the family home for the past three years. Nevertheless, she wants to support Scott because he has unquestioningly been her mainstay over the past five years since she developed agoraphobia.

Karin vividly remembers her first panic attack, although she did not recognise it as such at the time. It was early December; Amelia was a baby, and Karin was Christmas shopping at a large suburban shopping centre. Unexpectedly, she received a call on her mobile telephone informing her that her mother had been involved in a motor vehicle accident and was not expected to live. Karin remembers feeling cold, sweaty and as though her heart would jump out of her chest at the time; she immediately went home.

Karin's next visit to the shopping centre was during the January sales. On entering the crowded mall she was overwhelmed by a sense of foreboding and clamminess, and experienced extreme palpitations. She believed that she was having a heart attack and that she would die. A shopkeeper came to her assistance and called an ambulance. At the hospital Accident and Emergency Department a doctor explained

to Karin that she had experienced a panic attack, not a heart attack. She was advised to breathe into a paper bag if this occurred again, and was prescribed oxazepam to take, should her anxiety become extreme. Karin found that taking the oxazepam prior to an outing helped her to cope, so she continued to obtain prescriptions from her general practitioner.

Karin did not return to this particular shopping centre again. She began shopping at a nearby open mall complex where she knew she could quickly return to her car should the need arise. About six months after the first two panic attacks Karin experienced a further one at her local 'safe' supermarket. Her trolley was full of groceries, the queue was long and there was only one checkout open when, for no apparent reason, Karin suddenly felt she could not breathe and the palpitations returned. She departed immediately, leaving the trolley with the weekly shopping in the aisle. She has not shopped there since, telling Scott she was too embarrassed to return.

Following this event Karin was selective about outings away from home. 'What if it happens again?' she worried. She needed to know that she could leave immediately, if necessary. Consequently, she limited outings away from home to places she knew and could leave quickly. Gradually, over the next eighteen months, Karin stopped going out at all. Currently, Scott and Jordan manage the shopping, Jordan walks the younger children to and from school and Scott attends parent/teacher meetings and other events at the children's school. Their family and friends are always happy to socialise at Karin's and Scott's home because it is centrally located, and Karin is an excellent cook. Everything was fine until Scott was offered a promotion!

---

conditioning involves the person being rewarded for engaging in activities that would normally produce a panic response for that person.

The biomedical model provides an alternative interpretation of agoraphobia and consequently its approach to treatment. This approach identifies the symptoms (anxiety and panic) as the problem. Hence, the focus of treatment from a biomedical perspective is to control the anxiety and panic attack experienced by the individual with less emphasis on identifying the cause. Treatment would include the prescription of anxiolytic or antidepressant medications.

Cognitive theory poses yet another explanation of agoraphobia. It suggests that people who experience panic attacks interpret the physical symptoms of anxiety as catastrophic (palpitations are believed to be a heart attack) and respond accordingly (Bond & McConkey 2001, p 8.32). Intervention would focus on challenging and re-framing these faulty perceptions.

In practice, though, behavioural, cognitive and biomedical interventions are generally used concurrently in

what is referred to as an eclectic approach (Treatment Protocol Project 2000).

CRITICAL THINKING CHALLENGE 7.3

■ After reading Karin's case study (above), consider her experience in the light of cognitive and behavioural theory.

■ How might other theoretical positions explain Karin's experience?

■ What interventions to assist Karin would be indicated within each of these theoretical models?

Theories of psychology, sociology and nursing
During the 1970s and 1980s Australian and New Zealand nursing education moved into the tertiary sector following a similar move by American nurses in the 1950s. As a consequence, teachers of nursing required graduate education in addition to their nursing qualifications. Nurses undertook this study in the already established academic areas

of anthropology, philosophy, education, psychology and sociology. Postgraduate study in these fields subsequently influenced the development of the thinking of many nursing theorists (Condon 2000, pp 104–5).

The first generation of nursing theories to emerge since the 1950s was a synthesis of ideas about nursing practice and psychological/sociological theory. For instance, Madeline Leininger integrated anthropological studies with clinical nursing practice to develop her theory of transcultural nursing (King & Averis 2000, p 181). In psychiatric nursing, Hildegard Peplau acknowledged the influence of the work of psychoanalyst Harry Stack Sullivan on her thinking and clinical practice (Peplau 1988). Jocelyn Lawler developed her nursing theory about the body in nursing from her postgraduate studies in sociology (Condon 2000, p 122).

Also evident in the writing of nurse theorists is the influence of humanistic psychology. Maslow's *human needs* are embraced within models of care such as those proposed by Leininger, Parse, Orem and Watson (Greenwood 2000; Marriner-Tomey & Alligood 2002). So, too, are existentialist and phenomenological thought incorporated in Parse's theory of Human Becoming and Travelbee's model of Human-to-Human Relationship (Daly 2000, p 215; Travelbee 1971). However, it is in the field of psychiatric nursing that the influence of psychological and sociological thought is most obvious, as seen in the theories of the following prominent psychiatric nurses.

Hildegard Peplau (1909–1999)

Peplau is acknowledged as the *mother of psychiatric nursing*, and is also recognised as the first nursing author to use theory from other scientific fields in developing a theory of nursing (Marriner-Tomey & Alligood 2002, p 24). Peplau's Interpersonal Theory of Nursing is specific to practice, making it a mid-range theory, as distinct from a grand theory with broader applicability, like those of Orem and Roy, or a philosophy as espoused by earlier nursing writers such as Nightingale or Henderson (Marriner-Tomey & Alligood 2002).

Peplau's seminal text, *Interpersonal Relations in Nursing,* was first published in 1952 and outlines the therapeutic relationship between the nurse and the client. According to Peplau, the nurse does not perform therapy on the patient, but rather the nurse *is* the therapy. This heralded a shift in nursing practice from *doing to* a patient to *being with* a patient (Doona 1982, p 9). Further legacies of Peplau's theory have been the valuing of teaching and learning about relationship skills in nursing curricula and practice, and a focus on the study of clinical phenomena as a nursing concern (Sills, cited in Werner O'Toole & Rouslin Welt 1989).

In developing her theory, Peplau's thinking was not only influenced by the nursing discourse of her time, but also by several psychological clinicians, including the psychoanalyst Harry Stack Sullivan, humanistic psychologist

Abraham Maslow and the social learning theorist Neal Miller. Sullivan's influence on Peplau's writing can be seen in her valuing of the individual, the intrapersonal (subjective experience) and the interpersonal (relationships). Peplau viewed utilisation of the psychological model as enabling nurses 'to move away from a disease orientation to one whereby the psychological meaning of events, feelings and behaviours could be incorporated in nursing interventions' (Peplau 1996, cited in Howk 2002, p 381).

Joyce Travelbee (1926–1973)

Travelbee's Human-to-Human Relationship model is underpinned by the assumption that the purpose of nursing is achieved through the establishment of a nurse–patient relationship (Travelbee 1971, p 16). Her theory extended the work of Peplau and Orlando on interpersonal relations in nursing and incorporated existential ideas concerning meaning, from the writings of Victor Frankl (Marriner-Tomey & Alligood 2002, p 419). Travelbee viewed the purpose of nursing as not only assisting the patient, family or community to prevent or cope with illness and suffering but also, if necessary, to find meaning in the experience (Travelbee 1971, p 7). Travelbee's emphasis on the emotional and psychological aspects of nursing, such as caring, empathy and rapport, is also consistent with the writings of humanistic psychologist Carl Rogers, in his model of 'client-centered therapy' (Rogers 1951; Travelbee 1971) and is a contemporary influence in the field of palliative care nursing.

Phil Barker (b. 1946)

From his clinical research, psychiatric nurse and psychotherapist Phil Barker developed an interdisciplinary model of care, called the Tidal Model, which seeks to *reveal solutions* rather than *solve problems*. Central tenets of Barker's model include empowerment of the individual and humanistic notions of *being human* and *helping one another*. Underpinning the model are the key principles of:

- active collaboration between the mental health clinician, the individual and family in the planning and delivery of care
- the development and use of a care plan which is centred on the individual's experience, thus empowering the person
- the provision of nursing care in a multidisciplinary context, and
- the use of narrative-based interventions

all of which form the basis of problem resolution and mental health promotion.

Barker acknowledges several influences in the development of the Tidal Model, including: his studies of philosophy and psychology in the 1960s; an initial interest in psychoanalytic, then later behavioural, cognitive and family therapies; and the work of the radical psychiatrist RD Laing. Also significant in the development of the model were the seminal writings and mentorship of Annie Altschul and

Hildegard Peplau from nursing. Together, these influences contributed to Barker's development of an enduring interest in humanistic approaches and ultimately to the development of the Tidal Model, with its focus on assisting the person to find meaning in their experience (Barker 2001; Clan Unity 2002; Fletcher & Stevenson 2001).

CRITICAL THINKING CHALLENGE 7.4

- What role did psychological theories play in the development of psychiatric nursing theories?
- What contribution do psychiatric nursing theories make to nursing practice?

PERSONALITY AND BEHAVIOUR: NATURE VERSUS NURTURE

Who or what is responsible for personality and human development: heredity or the environment? Philosophers have long debated this issue, though scientific interest is more recent, dating from the work of Galton, the nineteenth-century British pioneer in the study of individual differences. Galton is reportedly credited with proposing the immortal phrase *nature versus nurture* (Gottesman 1997; Schaffner 2001, p 2). The ensuing debate resulted in a proliferation of philosophical discussion about, and scientific investigation into, the effects of biological phenomena and inheritance *(nature)* and the individual's environment and experiences in the world *(nurture)*.

Theoretical perspectives on nature versus nurture

The theories discussed in this chapter place varied emphasis on whether hereditary or environmental factors play a more important role in personality development, human behaviour and mental illness. Behaviourism and cognitive psychology advocate for the environment and factors external to the individual, as does the sociological perspective, though for different reasons. The biomedical model argues for a nature explanation, while psychoanalytic theory and humanistic psychology acknowledge the contribution of both. The psychoanalytic concept of the id, for instance, is biological but it interacts with the environment in personality development. In humanistic psychology the need to achieve one's potential is considered to be innate, but the eventual outcome is influenced by one's experiences in the world.

Nature *or* nurture?

There is an abundance of evidence to support an interactive explanation of nature *and* nurture rather than the answer being found in the *either/or* proposal (Azar 1997; Santrock 2002; Schaffner 2001). Despite this, some commentators and theorists continue to advocate for the relative importance of one over the other, notably exponents of the biomedical model for nature, and behaviourism for nurture.

Evidence to support a genetic or nature position can be found in family, twin and adoptee studies. Research over the past twenty years demonstrates that personality, behaviour and mental illness do have a genetic component (Azar 1997; Schaffner 2001). Findings from studies into the heritability of intelligence (IQ) offer the most convincing nurture evidence. An American, British and Swedish study of 240 octogenarian twins found the heritability of IQ to be 62 per cent (Gottesman 1997). In the Colorado Adoption Project a correlation was found between the IQ of adopted adolescents and their birth parents, but no relationship was found between the IQ of adopted adolescents and their adoptive parents. The researchers concluded that the environment in which the young person was reared had little impact on cognitive ability (Azar 1997).

In the case of schizophrenia, however, heredity accounts for less than 50 per cent of the predictability of the disorder. Genetic inheritance is only a partial influence, with the environment accounting for the rest (Plomin, cited in Azar 1997). Gottesman's research found that even when an identical twin had schizophrenia, the likelihood of the other twin *not* developing schizophrenia was 52 per cent (Gottesman 1991). In addition, 63 per cent of people with schizophrenia do not have a first- or second-degree relative with the condition (Schaffner 2001). It is clearly evident therefore, that factors in addition to one's genetic inheritance influence whether the disorder manifests. Such factors, it is assumed, can be found in the environment.

Gottesman's research assumes that siblings reared together share the same environment. Schaffner (2001) recommends caution in presuming this, as different siblings in the same family do not necessarily experience exactly the same environment. Siblings do share many experiences such as the same parents, social class and home environment. However, other experiences are unique to the individual and not shared by siblings. This non-shared environment can include such experiences as birth trauma, illness and different schooling. Significantly, it appears that it is the non-shared environment that accounts for most of the environmental influence on children's personality and mood (Azar 1997; Santrock 2002).

Nature *and* nurture

An individual's personality does not develop without a genetic inheritance, nor can it develop in the absence of influences from experience and the environment. How then can the nature versus nurture debate be resolved?

Gestalt psychology, founded by Fritz Perls (1893–1970) in the 1960s, comprises humanistic and existentialist elements, and offers a model for understanding the nature versus nurture debate—that is, to view personality development as a *gestalt*. There is no exact English equivalent for this German term, but it loosely translates as 'a meaningful, organised whole' that is more than the sum of its parts (Perls, Hefferline & Goodman 1973, p 16). Consider a cake, for example: flour, eggs, milk and sugar are its basic ingredients, but the product or *gestalt* bears no resemblance to any of the original ingredients. Yet each of the ingredients is vital to the final product, as is the process of cooking. Leave out the sugar and it will not taste like a cake; omit the heating process and it will not have the texture of a cake.

Considering human development as a *gestalt* means that neither nature nor nurture can be considered in isolation from the other. The process of their interaction and the context in which they interact are significant. Attributing a relative value of one over the other serves no purpose. Both nature and nurture are vital, inseparable, interdependent components of personality development that also influence human behaviour and whether or not one develops a mental illness.

CRITICAL THINKING CHALLENGE 7.5

- How useful is the nature versus nurture debate in understanding personality development and human behaviour, and why?
- Investigate four contemporary psychotherapeutic interventions. Which theories inform these therapies, and how?

CONCLUSION

The theoretical perspectives discussed in this chapter provide complementary, overlapping and at times contradictory theories of personality development and human behaviour, and explanations for mental health and mental illness. Yet despite individual theories being able to provide plausible explanations for specific behaviours in both normal and abnormal contexts, no theory alone is sufficient to explain all human behaviour, or a single behaviour in all circumstances. Some theories offer a nature, others a nurture, explanation, and yet others incorporate both. Even when a specific theory provides convincing evidence to support a nature or nurture explanation, such evidence is generally correlational, and therefore cannot be considered to be causative. Consequently, in seeking to identify factors that influence personality development and human behaviour, particularly in relation to mental health and mental illness, it is evident that the answer will not be found in asking the *nature or nurture* question, but rather in investigating *how the nature is nurtured.*

EXERCISES FOR CLASS ENGAGEMENT

- In small groups discuss the stigma associated with mental health and mental illness.
  - Identify factors that contribute to stigma.
  - Consider how stigma might affect nursing care.
  - Devise strategies to address stigma.
  Provide feedback to the rest of the class.

- Students should complete Critical thinking challenge 7.1 on p 100 prior to commencing a course of study in mental health. Repeat this activity on completion of the course.
  - Compare and contrast pre- and post-course responses in small groups.
  - If attitudes have changed, identify influences that could account for the changes.

- Re-read the case study on Karin and debate the following statement:
  'Behaviourist theory provides the best explanation of Karin's agoraphobia.'

- In small groups discuss the following questions.
  - What contribution can theories make to mental health promotion?
  - What contribution can theories make to mental illness prevention, early intervention, treatment and rehabilitation?

- What contribution do theories make to nursing practice? Provide feedback and debriefing to the rest of the class.

- Prior to the tutorial, each student should interview either a registered nurse or a person with mental illness regarding their views on:
  - what contributes to the development of mental illness
  - what enables an individual to cope with or overcome mental illness
  - what factors might hinder an individual's recovery from mental illness
  - what advice the person can give to nurses about caring for a person with mental illness.
  Then, in small groups, discuss the following:
  - What key issues emerged in the interview?
  - Compare and contrast professional responses with that of the person who has experienced mental illness.
  - Discuss lay and professional interpretations of mental illness in the light of relevant theories.
  - Identify students' learning with regard to nursing a person with a mental illness.
  Provide feedback and debriefing to the rest of the class.

REFERENCES

Alloy L, Acocella J & Bootzin R 1996, *Abnormal Psychology: Current Perspectives* (7th edn), McGraw-Hill College, New York.

Alloy L, Jacobson N & Acocella J 1999, *Abnormal Psychology: Current perspectives* (8th edn), McGraw-Hill College, New York.

Andrews G, Hall W, Teeson M & Henderson S 1999, *The Mental Health of Australians*, Mental Health Branch, Commonwealth Department of Health and Aged Care, Canberra.

Australian Bureau of Statistics 1997, Mental Health and Wellbeing of Adults, Australia Cat. no. 4326.0. Online: http://www.abs.gov.au/Ausstats/abs@nsf/0/BDAB518304D22FE3CA25688900233CAF?Open, accessed 29 March 2004.

Australian Institute of Health and Welfare 1998, National Health Priority Areas: Mental Health. Online: http://www.aihw.gov.au/publications/health/nhpamh98/index.htm, accessed 29 March 2004.

Azar B 1997, Nature, Nurture: Not Mutually Exclusive, American Psychological Association, Online: http://www.snc.edu/psych/korshavn/natnur02.htm, accessed 14 August 2003.

Barker P 2001, The Tidal Model: the lived experience in person-centered mental health nursing care, *Nursing Philosophy*, 2(3), pp 213–23.

Bond N & McConkey K 2001, *Psychological Science: An Introduction*, McGraw-Hill, Sydney.

Bühler C & Allen M 1972, *Introduction to Humanistic Psychology*, Brooks/Cole, California.

Carson R, Butcher J & Mineka S 1996, *Abnormal Psychology and Modern Life*, Harper Collins College, New York.

Cheek J, Shoebridge J, Willis E & Zadoroznji M 1996, *Society and Health: Social Theory for Health Workers*, Longman, Sydney.

Clan Unity 2002, Phil Barker PhD RN FRCN, Online: http://www.clan-unity.co.uk/philbarkerbiog.htm, 14 August 2003.

Clinton M & Nelson S 1996, *Mental Health and Nursing Practice*, Prentice Hall, Sydney.

Clinton M & Nelson S 1999, *Advanced Practice in Mental Health Nursing*, Blackwell Science, Oxford.

Commonwealth Department of Health and Aged Care 2003, *National Youth Suicide Prevention Strategy*. Online: http://www.mentalhealth.gov.au/sp/nysps/about.htm, accessed 14 August 2003.

Commonwealth Department of Health & Aged Care 2000, *Promotion, Prevention and Early Intervention for Mental Health: a monograph 2000*, Mental Health & Special Programs Branch, Canberra.

Condon J 2000, Changing conceptions in nurse theorising: historical and social perspectives in the United States of America and Australia. In: Greenwood J (ed.), *Nurse Theory in Australia: Development and Application*, Prentice Hall Health, Australia.

Crotty M 1996, *Phenomenology and Nursing Research*, Churchill Livingstone, Melbourne.

Daly J 2000, Parse's Human Becoming School of Thought. In: Greenwood J (ed.), *Nurse Theory in Australia: Development and Application*, Prentice Hall Health, Australia.

Davison G & Neale J 2001, *Abnormal Psychology* (9th edn), John Wiley & Sons, New York.

Doona M 1982, *Travelbee's Intervention in Psychiatric Nursing* (2nd edn), FA Davis Company, Philadelphia.

Erikson, E 1963, *Childhood and Society* (2nd edn), WW Norton, New York.

Evans J 1992, Healthy minds: what is mental health and how can we promote it?, *Nursing Times*, 88(16), pp 54–6.

Fletcher E & Stevenson C 2001, Launching the Tidal Model in an adult acute mental health programme, *Nursing Standard*, 15(49), pp 33–6.

Flinders University, Adelaide 2003, WebCT online notes, HLTH 1001 Health: A Psychological Perspective, https://webct.flinders.edu.au/, accessed 14 August 2003.

Forster S 2001, *The Role of the Mental Health Nurse*, Nelson Thornes, Cheltenham, UK.

Freud A 1966, *The Ego and the Mechanisms of Defense*, International Universities Press, New York.

Gething L 1995, *Lifespan Development*, McGraw-Hill, Sydney.

Gottesman II 1991, *Schizophrenia Genesis: the Origins of Madness*, Freeman, New York.

Gottesman II 1997, Twins: en route to QTLs for cognition, *Science*, 277 (5318), pp 1522–3.

Gray P 1999, *Mental Health in the Workforce: Tackling the Effects of Stress*, Mental Health Foundation, UK.

Greenwood J (ed) 2000, *Nursing Theory in Australia: Development and Application*, Prentice Hall Health, Australia.

Health Development Agency 2003, Mental Health Promotion: Coming In From the Cold. Online: http://www.hda-online.org.uk/hdt/0901/mental.html, accessed 14 August 2003.

Howk C 2002, Hildegard E. Peplau: psychodynamic nursing. In: Marriner-Tomey A & Alligood RM (eds), *Nursing Theorists and Their Work* (5th edn), Mosby, St Louis.

International Journal of Mental Health Nursing (formerly *Australian and New Zealand Journal of Mental Health Nursing*), Blackwell Science, Melbourne 2001–current.

Issues in Mental Health Nursing, Taylor & Francis Health Sciences, London 1978–current.

Ivey A & Ivey M 2003, *Intentional Interviewing and Counselling: Facilitating Client Development in a Multicultural Society* (5th edn), Thompson Brooks/Cole, Pacific Grove, CA.

Johnston B 1998, *Enhancing Recovery From Psychosis: A Practical Guide*, Department of Human Services, Adelaide.

King M & Averis A 2000, The application of Leininger's sunrise model to the culturally appropriate care of indigenous Australians. In: Greenwood J (ed.), *Nurse Theory in Australia: Development and Application*, Prentice Hall Health, Australia.

Kittleson M 1989, Mental health vs mental illness: a philosophical discussion, *Health Education*, April/May, pp 40–2.

McMurray A 1999, *Community Health and Wellness: a Socioecological Approach*, Mosby, Sydney.

Mann L 1997, Youth suicide: can primary health care help?, *Australian Nurses Journal*, 4(7), pp 20–3.

Marriner-Tomey A & Alligood RM 2002, *Nursing Theorists and Their Work* (5th edn), Mosby, St Louis.

Millar E & Walsh M 2000, *Mental Health Matters in Primary Care*, Nelson Thorne, Cheltenham, UK.

New Zealand Health Information Service 2003. Online: http://www.nzhis.govt.nz, accessed 18 November 2003.

Peplau H 1988, *Interpersonal Relations in Nursing*, MacMillan Education, London.

Perls F, Hefferline R & Goodman P 1973, *Gestalt Therapy Now: Experiment and Growth in the Human Personality*, Pelican, London.

Ragsdale S 2003, *Charlotte Malachowski Bühler, PhD (1893–1974)*. Online: http://www.webster.edu/~woolflm/charlottebuhler.html, accessed 14 August 2003.

Raphael B 1993, *Scope for Prevention in Mental Health*, National Health and Medical Research Council, AGPS, Canberra.

Rogers C 1951, *Client-centered Therapy*, Houghton Mifflin, Boston.

Rogers C 1961, *On Becoming a Person: A Therapist's View of Psychotherapy*, Houghton Mifflin, Boston.

Sainsbury P 2003, The pursuit of happiness: the politics of mental health promotion, *Australian e-Journal for the Advancement of Mental Health*, 2(1). Online: http://auseinet.flinders.edu.au/journal/vol2iss1/index.php, accessed 14 August 2003.

Santrock J 2002, *Life-Span Development* (8th edn), McGraw-Hill, New York.

Schaffner K 2001, Nature and nurture, *Current Opinions in Psychiatry*, 14(5), pp 485–90. Online: OVID/Journals @OVID, accessed 14 August 2003.

Seligman M 1974, Depression and learned helplessness. In: Friedman J & Katz M (eds), *The Psychology of Depression: Theory and Research*, Winston-Wiley, Washington.

Seligman M 1994, *Learned Optimism*, Random House, Australia.

Skinner B 1953, *Science and Human Behaviour*, Macmillan, New York.

South Australian Consolidated Acts, *Mental Health Act 1993*. Online: http://www.austlii.edu.au/au/legis/sa/consol_act/mha1993128/, accessed 14 August 2003.

Szasz T 2000, The case against psychiatric power. In: Barker P & Stevenson C (eds), *The Construction of Power and Authority in Psychiatry*, Butterworth-Heinemann, Oxford.

Szasz T 1961, *The Myth of Mental Illness*, Harper & Row, New York.

Thompson J, Barkway P & Saunders L 2001, *Issues & Perspectives in Mental Health: Study Guide*, Flinders University, Adelaide.

Travelbee J 1971, *Interpersonal Aspects of Nursing* (2nd edn), FA Davis, Philadelphia.

Treatment Protocol Project 2000, *Management of Mental Disorder* (3rd edn), World Health Organization Collaborating Centre for Mental Health and Substance Abuse, Sydney.

Vic Health 2003, Together We Do Better. Online: http://www.togetherwedobetter.vic.gov.au/, accessed 14 August 2003.

Wass A 2000, *Promoting Health: The Primary Health Care Approach* (2nd edn), Harcourt Saunders, Sydney.

Werner O'Toole A & Rouslin Welt S 1989, *Interpersonal Theory in Nursing Practice: Selected Works of Hildegard E Peplau*, Springer, New York.

Wilkinson R & Marmot M 1998, *Social Determinants of Health: The Solid Facts*, WHO, Geneva.

Mental Health Across the Lifespan

Debra Nizette

KEY POINTS

- An understanding of human development across the lifespan enhances mental health assessment and the provision of holistic care.
- Self-awareness assists the nurse to better understand the client's experience.
- Mental health vulnerability increases at various times across the lifespan due to a combination of individual and contextual factors.
- The lifespan is generally conceived of as a linear concept, the time from birth to death. Paradoxically, development across this span is more appropriately conceived of as non-linear, multidimensional and contextual.
- The concepts of attachment and resilience play a part in the attainment and maintenance of mental health.
- The promotion of mental health across the lifespan requires a primary health care approach in order to address the social and environmental factors that create vulnerability to mental illness.

KEY TERMS

- adolescence
- adulthood
- attachment
- childhood
- developmental psychology
- human development
- identity
- lifespan
- mental health
- mental health promotion
- older adulthood
- protective factors
- resilience and thriving
- risk factors
- 'self'
- 'stage' theories

LEARNING OUTCOMES

The material in this chapter will assist you to:
- reflect on the relevance of lifespan concepts to your own experience
- understand the relationship of developmental theories and concepts to mental health problems and mental illness across the lifespan
- use these theories and concepts in all phases of the nurse–client relationship, including health promotion.

INTRODUCTION

This chapter provides a foundation for understanding mental health problems and psychopathology within the context of normal human development. It reviews the work of some theorists who have contributed to our understanding of human development, and presents emerging research and perspectives on development. The chapter also explores specific developmental issues at different stages across the lifespan and how they intersect with mental health, creating the potential for mental health vulnerability (potential for illness). Concepts such as attachment, identity and resilience, which inform our understandings of development, are addressed in providing a holistic perspective on mental health issues across the lifespan. Strategies based on health promotion and a primary health care approach are described and proposed as a means to increase protective factors against mental illness across the lifespan.

A LIFESPAN APPROACH

If we consider the period from birth to our current age, we can in retrospect recall physical changes that we have experienced, such as changes in height, weight and appearance. We may also recall changes in our capabilities, skills, relationships, lifestyle and other aspects of our lives. In so doing, we acknowledge multifactorial aspects of ourselves that have evolved over time as a result of experience and change. Developmental psychologists have formulated theories to assist in our understanding of how growth and change affect the personality and how we become 'ourselves'. Developmental theories aim to explain normal growth and development of the personality or 'self'.

A lifespan approach (lifespan developmental psychology) encompasses the sequence of events and experiences in a life from birth until death. Goals of the approach are to describe development, to explain how change occurs throughout the lifespan and to optimise development through the application of theory to real life (Peterson 1996).

Recent conceptualisations of a lifespan approach emerge from the work of Baltes, who proposed a non-linear theory emphasising the multidimensional and non-integrated nature of human development. A non-linear model refutes the idea that there is a definite sequential pathway for development or an ideal end-state or conclusion to development. Baltes challenges the idea that an ideal end-state is ever achieved or desirable. He defines development as 'selective age related change in adaptive capacity' (Baltes, Staudinger & Lindenberger 1999, p 476). Baltes' view supports the idea that development consists of a series of losses and gains. Losses and gains occur throughout the lifespan as new skills are acquired and the individual experiences certain benefits as a result; however, they may also experience a lack of continuity in other skills or abilities. For example, the older adult may not have the memory capacity of a younger person but they may develop pragmatic or problem-solving strategies (such as the use of mnemonics) which result in similar performance, thus compensating for age-related deficits (Baltes & Baltes 1990). An additional gain of development is creativity. Creativity is perceived as essential in our ability to constantly develop new strategies, such as improved problem solving, to compensate for age-related losses.

Box 8.1 A lifespan approach: key points

The tenets that guide an understanding of the lifespan approach include a belief that:

- the potential for growth and development exists throughout the lifespan
- development is multidirectional, with no specific route or direction
- patterns of development vary due to social, historical, cultural and gender variables
- there are numerous dimensions to development and each may follow a different trajectory
- dimensions to development include physical–motor, cognitive–intellectual and personal–social–emotional, and each interacts with the others
- the individual and the environment influence each other
- lifespan development promotes a holistic approach to nursing practice.

A lifespan approach to nursing practice

The nurse has an opportunity to provide information, resources and interventions for clients and families that will support and facilitate emotional development, cognitive growth and psychosocial wellbeing throughout the lifespan. The nurse's ability to use concepts from the developmental theories will enhance his or her understanding of the client and promote individually focused care. As well as equipping the nurse with knowledge to identify disruptions in development, developmental theories can increase the nurse's awareness of the client, their perception of their problem and their responses to it. Moreover, knowledge of the lifespan can facilitate accurate assessment and communication, enhance empathy and promote the development of interventions that are specific and meaningful for the client. It can be useful, for example, to understand why some adolescents and young adults have difficulty relating to others and regulating their own behaviour and emotions.

CRITICAL THINKING CHALLENGE 8.1

Explain what is meant by the lifespan and a lifespan approach for nursing. Discuss how knowledge of lifespan theories and concepts contributes to nursing practice.

Box 8.2 **A lifespan approach: role in practice**

A lifespan approach in practice contributes to:
- communication, in particular development of rapport
- establishment of empathy
- interviewing
- identification of client concerns and general facilitation of therapeutic communication
- risk assessment (self-harm and suicide)
- identification and implementation of appropriate interventions
- appropriate referral
- awareness of boundary issues.

A PRIMARY HEALTH CARE APPROACH

Mental health promotion across the lifespan is most effective in the form of primary health care. A primary health care approach considers the broad contextual (social, family, cultural and environmental) variables that influence a person's health. The elements associated with primary health care as described in the Ottawa Charter (World Health Organization 1986) include:
- promoting supportive partnerships
- creating supportive environments
- developing personal skills
- promotion of public policy
- re-orientation of health services delivery toward promotion, prevention and early intervention.

The Ottawa Charter recognises that the achievement of better health outcomes requires internal and external risk factors to be ameliorated and sustainable, protective factors to be implemented. Governments in both Australia and New Zealand have plans and policies derived from The Ottawa Charter for Health Promotion.

The Australian Government Department of Health and Ageing has a Primary Care Division that focuses on policy development, integration of primary care services in communities, the implementation of prevention strategies and improving access to services. The National Action Plan for Promotion, Prevention and Early Intervention for Mental Health 2000 (Commonwealth Department of Health and Aged Care 2000) recognises the social and economic origins of risk and protective factors that influence mental health. Activities and strategies that aim to positively influence mental health relate to a broad range of aspects of daily life. Home, child care, education and housing are among these. Targeted programs at both national and state level have been implemented as part of this plan.

In New Zealand, primary mental health is being considered alongside the implementation of the National Primary Health Care Strategy and the existing National Mental Health Strategy. It is estimated that the needs of approximately 17 per cent of New Zealanders with mild

to moderate mental health problems would be met through primary mental health-care services (Ministry of Health 2002). While increased costs due to the need for longer appointment times are identified as a barrier to a primary care approach, the report cited a UK study suggesting that nurses employed in a mental health role in GP services benefited the mental health of clients (Corney 1999, cited in Ministry of Health 2002).

A framework that integrates primary health care principles is suggested by Lindsey & Hartrick (1996) for use by nurses. They propose listening to the client, participating in dialogue with the client, working with the client to recognise patterns or themes that may be problematic in maintaining or eliciting health-directed behaviours, discussing and preparing for action and positive change through the identification of relevant strategies or processes. Nurses who are informed of a primary health care approach can access strategies for the clients that are part of primary health care initiatives.

Primary health care approaches are based on sound principles that fit very well with mental health nursing practice. They promote a client-focused approach that is holistic in that social, political and environmental issues are taken into account and placed in the ambit of the nurse's awareness. A primary health care approach also acknowledges the importance of culture in that strategies are generated through engagement with individuals and communities. Primary health care also aims to promote resilience, thriving and healthy, secure attachment in individuals. These concepts deepen our knowledge of development across the lifespan.

MENTAL HEALTH ACROSS THE LIFESPAN

The fundamental elements of mental health are acquired throughout a person's development. Developmental theories emphasise the importance of the early months and years of life in laying a foundation for sound mental health in adulthood. Mental health, like physical health, contributes to a person's quality of life. It enhances our functioning in all aspects of life—work, relationships and social situations—and also enables us to feel that we are worthwhile and acceptable just as we are. Mental health enables us to mediate and manage distress from external events in our life, to cope with the ups and downs, and to be hopeful about the future (see Ch 7). Optimal personal development is related to and dependent upon an individual's mental health.

Mental health problems can occur when there is a disruption to mental health, making the person vulnerable to or less able to manage and mediate distress. 'Mental illness' and 'mental disorder' are terms used when a diagnosis is given to a person experiencing a mental health problem. Not all mental health problems are brought to the attention of a mental health professional and some problems may not meet the criteria for a diagnosis.

Mental health and mental illness exist on a continuum—the person who meets all the criteria for mental health at some stage of their life can nevertheless experience significant mental distress or mental illness at some other stage. Mental health can be assessed via an interview with a client, through observation of client behaviour and from information from partners, friends and family (see Ch 10). Strategies promoting mental health can be implemented at any time throughout the mental health–illness continuum.

As well as describing normal development, developmental theorists propose a set of conditions or criteria necessary for optimal development and subsequent mental health. Each theorist sets out tasks, challenges or milestones that need to be achieved for normal development. Mental health problems can result when developmental tasks and challenges are not met due to some disruption in the internal or external environment. Internal conditions include inherited characteristics and personality characteristics. External conditions include parenting, nurturing in childhood, and positive or negative life events. It is important for the nurse to be aware of the tenets of the lifespan approach (outlined earlier) when considering mental health issues throughout life, as many psychological issues recur repeatedly in different forms.

CRITICAL THINKING CHALLENGE 8.2

How would your own experience affect your ability to understand the significance of events and experiences in the lives of patients?

'Ideal' development

Cognitive, perceptual, emotional and social functioning are dimensions of growth and development that are not well understood even though they are crucial to each individual's wellbeing and mental health. Development itself is difficult to define and hints that 'improvement' is part of a developing state. The literature on ageing (Baltes & Baltes 1990; Bevan & Jeeawody 1998) explores how we can age 'successfully'. The following outcome measurements are proposed:

- length of life
- biological health
- mental health
- cognitive efficacy
- social competence and productivity
- personal control
- life satisfaction.

These criteria demonstrate the multiple influences necessary for overall achievement of 'good ageing'. Multiple criteria take into account objective and subjective measures, so as to incorporate the individual's own definition of success.

'Good' outcomes of development proposed by Maslow (1968), Erikson (1963) and Allport (1961) all describe criteria that are normative; that is, they assume that everyone is the same and that there is a general standard which, if achieved, can lead to an ideal end-state. As noted earlier, this assumption has been challenged. It can be useful, however, to define development as an ideal state so that factors that are barriers to achieving this state can be explored, and ways in which development can be encouraged can be addressed through health-promoting interventions.

Abraham Maslow (1968) outlined a path of motivation to self-actualisation (see also Ch 7) and outlined fifteen characteristics of the self-actualised person. Gordon Allport (1961) defined the mature personality by describing six dimensions, and Erikson's theory (1963) identified 'wisdom' as the ideal end-state of development, but acknowledged that positive outcomes of each stage were contingent upon meeting a challenge or completing a task.

These theorists share a similar philosophy of humanism, yet each has contributed unique insights into the process of development. Erikson's 'stages' differ from Maslow's and Allport's as they more clearly identify a process (stages) that needs to be undertaken whereby one achieves successful outcomes. In Erikson's theory a person may be unable to achieve mastery of one of the developmental tasks due to external factors, such as a loss, or injury, which may disrupt the person's development. Maslow proposed a set of preconditions for self-actualisation that, if unmet, also interfere with development (see Ch 7). Aspects of the human condition that are of interest to developmental theorists include personality as well as psychosexual, cognitive, psychosocial, moral and gender development. Each of these aspects affects behaviour and learning in the developing person.

The ideal outcomes of development (listed in Table 8.1) highlight the characteristics of optimal wellbeing and mental health, but the course of life and significant events can disrupt this ideal. Factors that can disrupt the path of normal development will be discussed further in this chapter.

Stages and theoretical issues in human development

Theories of personality development such as the biomedical, psychological (psychoanalytic, behaviourist, cognitive and humanistic) and sociological (as discussed in Ch 7) assist us to understand human behaviour. Some theorists developed a lifespan approach and devised 'stages' to explain how changes occurred across the lifespan. Stage theories were initiated by the evolutionary perspectives of Charles Darwin, who believed that human development could be understood through the study of childhood. Darwin's work was significant in introducing a scientific approach to the study of development. Stage theories support the idea that individual development can be measured and monitored according to a set of

Table 8.1 Ideal outcomes of development

Characteristics of the self-actualised person (Maslow 1968)	Dimensions of maturity (Allport 1961)	The 'eight stages of man' (Erikson 1963)
■ Accurate perception of reality ■ Acceptance of self and others ■ Spontaneity ■ Problem centring ■ Detachment (emotionally self-sufficient) ■ Autonomy ■ Continued fresh appreciation ■ Mystic or peak experiences ■ Unconditional positive regard for others ■ Characteristic interpersonal relations ■ Democratic character structure ■ Definite moral standards ■ Philosophical sense of humour ■ Creativeness ■ Cultural transcendence	■ Extension of the sense of self (having a life mission) ■ Warm relating of self to others ■ Emotional security ■ Realistic perception, skills and assignments (solves problems as required) ■ Self-objectification (insight or self-awareness) ■ Unifying philosophy on life	■ Basic trust versus mistrust (0–1 year) → Hope ■ Autonomy versus shame and doubt (1–3 years) → Willpower ■ Initiative versus guilt (4–5 years) → Purpose ■ Industry versus inferiority (6–11 years) → Competence and accomplishment ■ Identity versus role confusion (12–18 years) → Fidelity ■ Intimacy versus isolation (early adulthood) → Love ■ Generativity versus stagnation (middle adulthood) → Care and production ■ Ego integrity versus despair (older adulthood) → Wisdom

expected 'norms' at average ages when certain milestones are achieved.

Stages have different meanings depending on the variable being considered. For example, biological stage theories conceive of growth being completed by adulthood, followed by a maintenance period after which physical decline results. A sociocultural/psychosocial conception of stages describes a series of roles and age- or development-related tasks throughout life (Erikson). Cognitive–structural stages (Piaget) are conceived of as an ascending staircase along the lifeline, with later stages integrating and building upon previous cognitive functioning. Stage theories require consideration of normative variables (age or historical influences shared by most people) and non-normative variables (events unique to individuals). Nurses need to be able to use stage theories. During assessment, consideration of general and unique influences ensures that individuals and families are assessed holistically and that the range of issues affecting

development can be examined. Theories help us understand why some people might be more vulnerable to mental health problems or at risk of developing mental illness than others.

Freud, Erikson and Piaget were twentieth-century theorists who, among others, were influential in contributing to a lifespan perspective of development.

Freud

Sigmund Freud (1856–1939) proposed three personality structures, which if functioning in balance, help the person resolve the conflicts of different psychosexual stages of personality development. Maturation is the desired outcome of the individual successfully moving through four psychosexual stages (from infancy to adolescence). Chapter 7 outlined the stages and tasks of each stage. The relevance of Freud's theory lies primarily in its ability to assist the nurse in understanding patient behaviours that appear inconsistent with age or the expected acknowledged, and positive relationships fostered, in order to decrease stress and confusion and to facilitate decision-making and autonomy for the adolescent.

Risk factors

The risks and protective factors of childhood influence adolescence, but it is important to acknowledge that subsequent positive or negative experiences can alter the course of ongoing development. Many opportunities exist to change the balance of risk and protective factors during this time because of the numerous influences the adolescent is exposed to. The risk assessment profile sheet (Fuller 1998) identifies the extensive factors that contribute to risk in this group. Among the risk factors identified are: community factors such as poverty and accommodation; school factors relating to performance and attendance; family factors including the adolescent's connectedness to family, and family violence; peer friendships and the nature of the peer association (for example, delinquent peers); and individual characteristics such as those discussed in 'childhood' including temperament, intelligence, aggression and likeability.

Health promotion

Adolescence is a period of opportunity for prevention and intervention for mental health problems. The extensive number of factors that contribute to risk for the adolescent has been acknowledged previously. Adolescents who have been compromised in meeting earlier developmental tasks or who are at risk can be given opportunities to increase protective factors. Programs that develop assertion skills, crisis management, suicide prevention, identity acceptance and safe sex are all protective against risk.

Skills-building in communication and conflict resolution for families are important in facilitating autonomy in the adolescent. The adolescent gains a sense of self through well-negotiated family conflict. 'Individuality without connectedness is not autonomy, but isolation, and connectedness without self–other differentiation is not interdependence but fusion' (von der Lippe, cited in Skoe & von der Lippe 1998, p 54). Families need skills to facilitate flexibility in problem solving and open communication to manage family conflict. Negotiation and expression of conflict are important in developing coping skills as they provide opportunities for the adolescent to gain mastery of challenging situations.

One of the significant tasks of adolescence, the acquisition of self-confidence and decision-making, can be encouraged in homes and schools. Decision-making is undertaken by people at all stages of the life cycle. It is especially relevant during adolescence, with heightened risk behaviour including self-harm and suicide. Koshar (1999, pp 134–5) proposes a decision-making model that can be used by nurses and families with the adolescent to think through emotional issues. The following steps are proposed:

1 The problem confronting the adolescent is identified and the options to address it are proposed.

2 The consequences of each option are generated and then classified as either positive or negative. The client lists what they anticipate or experience as outcomes of their choices.

3 The client assesses whether the outcomes will be good or bad. The importance and desirability of the consequences are explored.

4 The likelihood of different consequences occurring is assessed and the adolescent makes this assessment according to their unique frame of reference.

5 The decision is outlined and the nurse/parent provides some input for the adolescent to consider.

In this model the focus is on listening to the adolescent and then providing them with input which they can consider (after they have explored the issue as they see it). The model provides a structure that the client can use independently in other situations.

Health-promoting interventions, which acknowledge the adolescent in a holistic way, incorporating their family and community, may assist the adolescent in strengthening attachments (Fuller 1998). Fuller also advocates a system of care that includes a consistent connection with one or more people who provide structure, advocacy and mentorship. Other aspects of the system of care are a comprehensive assessment, coordinated decision-making on managing behaviour and the creation of inter-agency linkages that assist the adolescent with support and resources.

CRITICAL THINKING CHALLENGE 8.4

Andrew loves sport and is on school teams for swimming and football. He likes spending time with his friends, music and going camping. Recently he has been spending increasing amounts of time with Sam, a friend who is in his swimming team. He is disconcerted by sexual feelings that he has been experiencing towards Sam, and is fearful of talking to anyone about it.

Discuss the factors that would support Andrew in understanding his current situation.

ADULTHOOD
Development and theoretical issues

Adulthood can be conceived of as a series of changes that occur after adolescence until the final stages of life. Throughout adulthood there are changes to cognitive, social, psychological and physical development, although by early adulthood many of the brain's functions have stabilised.

Theories that relate to this stage of development include stages four and five of Erikson's theory, which describe early and middle adulthood. These will now be discussed.

Intimacy versus isolation (early adulthood)

A mutually satisfying relationship with another person in which individual identity is sustained is evidence of successful resolution of this stage. This stage also requires 'sacrifices or compromises' (Erikson, cited in Welchman 2000) as a result of a commitment to another person. The risks associated with becoming a couple can be the loss of self-identity from domination of the other, or lack of assertion of one's own desires and needs. Similarly, feelings of aloneness despite being a 'couple' can result from incomplete commitment to the relationship. Early adulthood is a time of greater vulnerability to mental health problems than middle or late adulthood. Stresses associated with new roles at work and in relationships, accompanied by high expectations, are contributors to an increase in mental health problems and illness at this time (Bee & Boyd 2002). The person aged twenty to thirty is struggling with issues of identity and adjusting to increased responsibility as they attempt to establish a career. This period of chaos and pressure to make good decisions for the future can create vulnerability, hence the use of the term 'crisis'. Neugarten (1979) suggested that family and work roles could create conflicts for young adults as they attempt to balance responsibility with possibility and change. Chaos, confusion and change present significant challenges for young adults.

Generativity versus self-absorption (middle adulthood)

According to Erikson, the middle years are the most productive in terms of family, occupational and social contributions. Erikson identifies this stage as characterised by the individual having altruistic tendencies and energies directed at contributing to a better world. While 'generativity' relates to guiding and supporting the next generation it is also about contributing to the enrichment of society. Resolution can be achieved through a realistic appraisal of strengths, limitations and opportunity and identification of appropriate present or future achievements.

Feelings of frustration and unrealised goals and potentials can create dissatisfaction with life in this stage (stagnation), which can affect the next generation if adults place their unrealised expectations on the child (Welchman 2000).

Daniel Levinson's writing on development in women and men (1978, 1996) stemmed from his desire to understand his own adult development. Biographical research on men identified stages or 'transitions' of 'early adulthood' (17–22 years), 'entering the adult world' (between mid-twenties and late thirties) and the 'age 30 transition' (ends at approximately 33 years), the tasks and issues of which resemble Erikson's sixth stage. The mid-life transition (for five years after age 38 or before age 43) is a period from early adulthood into middle adulthood requiring a review of the past and re-evaluation of values and beliefs, which may result in changes to how life is lived. This phase involves evaluation of achievement of the 'dream' or expectations of life. Middle adulthood is a time where a structure for the rest of life is made from the choices available during the transition. In his later study of women's lives, Levinson (1996) interviewed homemakers, women with corporate financial careers and those with academic careers, identifying that women's cycle of adult development mirrored men's in the stages and transitional ages and tasks. However, differences in resources and constraints led to life experience that was self-limiting for the homemaker group. He envisaged a future in society for men and women where differences in life because of gender were minimal, where adult development could focus on meaning and satisfaction from the diversity of experience in life.

Attachment, gender, identity and risk

Theories of women's development emphasise the importance of *connectedness* and positive relationships in maintaining women's mental health throughout the lifespan. An awareness of the work of Carol Gilligan (1982) assists nurses to understand relational issues for women. The concept that Gilligan has named 'voice' is central to this understanding. Gilligan asserts that voice is the 'core of the self' and that we use it to relate to others. Speaking and listening are ways of understanding another. She believes that women's voices need to be heard in order to enhance their personal and social development. Her book *In a Different Voice* asks questions about theories in which men's experiences stand for all 'human experience', excluding the experience of women (Gilligan 1982, p xiii).

Most developmental theories support separation, detachment and autonomy as desirable outcomes of development. Gilligan proposes that 'attachment' in relationships is integral to the successful development of identity in women and that the values of interdependence, nurturing and sensitivity need to be valued as well as independence and autonomy. Unlike men, who need to separate from the mother as they grow in order to achieve a masculine identity, girls develop their identity in the ongoing relationship they have with their mother. Self-in-relation theory was developed by Jean Baker Miller, Judith Jordan, Jan Surrey and Irene Stiver from this early work. This group, from the Stone Centre of Wellesley College, espouses the importance of connection with others in developing a healthy sense of self (Jordan et al. 1991). Self-in-relation theory has been used to explain and understand the origins of mental health problems in women and also to guide appropriate interventions (Nizette & Creedy 1998).

The attachment experience of childhood is important to both sexes, as early childhood experiences of attachment can affect one's sense of self and relationships in adulthood. Research proposes that secure, avoidant or ambivalent attachment in adulthood is associated with childhood relationships and the emotional styles of parents (Hazan & Shaver, cited in Karen 1994). People in

Maslow AH 1968, *Toward a Psychology Of Being* (2nd edn), Van Norstrund, Princeton New Jersey.

Masten A 2001, Ordinary magic: resilience processes in development, *American Psychologist*, 56(3), pp 227–38.

Ministry of Health 2002, *Primary Mental Health: A Review of the Opportunities*, Wellington, New Zealand.

Nakash-Eisikovits O, Dutra L & Westen D 2002, Relationship between attachment patterns and personality pathology in adolescents, *Journal of the American Academy of Child and Adolescent Psychiatry*, 41(9), pp 1111–23.

Neugarten B 1979, Time, age, and the life cycle, *The American Journal of Psychiatry*, 136(7), pp 887–94.

Nizette D & Creedy D 1998, Women and mental illness. In: Rogers Clark C & Smith A (eds), *Women's Health: A Primary Health Care Approach*, McLennan & Petty, Sydney.

Osterlund M 2002, The role of estrogens in neuropsychiatric disorders, *Current Opinion in Psychiatry*, 15(3), pp 307–12.

Park A & Roberts C 2002, The ties that bind. In: *The 19th Report of British Social Attitudes*, National Centre for Social Research, London.

Peterson C 1996, *Looking Forward Through the Lifespan: Developmental Psychology* (3rd edn), Prentice Hall, Sydney.

Phinney JS, 2000, Identity formation across cultures: the interaction of personal, societal, and historical change, *History and Culture*, 43(1), pp 27–31.

Piaget P 1977, *Moral Judgement Development of the Child* (trans. M. Gabain), Penguin, Harmondsworth (original work published 1932).

Pratt M, Golding G & Hunter W 1984, Does morality have a gender? Sex, sex role and moral judgement relationships across the lifespan, *Merrill-Palmer Quarterly*, 30(4), pp 321–40.

Reinke B, Ellicott A, Harris R & Hancock E 1985, Timing of psychosocial changes in women's lives, *Human Development*, 28, pp 259–80.

Rew L, Taylor-Seehafer M, Thomas N & Yockey R 2001, Correlates of resilience in homeless adolescents, *Journal of Nursing Scholarship*, 33(1), pp 33–40.

Salmelainen P 1996, Child neglect: its causes and its role in delinquency, *Contemporary Issues in Crime and Justice*, 33, pp 1–14.

Sanders MR, Markie-Dadds C, Tully LA & Bor W 2000, The Triple P-Positive Parenting Program: a comparison of enhanced, standard, and self-directed behavioral family intervention for parents of children with early onset conduct problems, *Journal of Consulting and Clinical Psychology*, 68(4), pp 624–40.

Shultz TR & Wells D 1985, Judging the intentionality of action-outcomes, *Developmental Psychology*, 21(1), pp 83–9.

Skoe E & von der Lippe A 1998, *Personality Development in Adolescence: A Cross-national and Life Span Perspective*, Routledge, New York.

Stanton A, Lobel M, Sears S & deLuca R 2002, Psychosocial aspects of selected issues in women's reproductive health: current status and future directions, *Journal of Consulting and Clinical Psychiatry*, 70(3), pp 751–70.

Stilwel BM, Galvin M, Kopta SM, Padgett RJ & Holt JW 1997, Moralization of attachment: a fourth domain of conscious functioning, *Journal of the American Academy of Child and Adolescent Psychiatry*, 36(8), pp 1140–7.

Townley M, 2002, Mental health needs of children and young people, *Nursing Standard*, 16(30), pp 38–47.

Wadensten B & Carlsson M, 2003, Theory-driven guidelines for practical care of older people, based on the theory of gerotranscendence, *Journal of Advanced Nursing*, 41(5), pp 462–70.

Waters E, Vaughn BE, Posada G & Kondo-Ikemura K 1995, *Caregiving, Cultural, and Cognitive Perspectives on Secure-Base Behavior and Working Models: New Growing Points of Attachment Theory and Research*, University of Chicago Press, Chicago.

Welchman K 2000, *Erik Erikson: His Life, Work and Significance*, Open University Press; Philadelphia.

Werner E & Smith R 1982, *Vulnerable, but Invincible: A Longitudinal Study of Resilient Children and Youth*, McGraw-Hill, New York.

White F 1996, Parent–adolescent communication and adolescent decision-making, *Journal of Family Studies*, 2(1), pp 41–56.

World Health Organization (WHO) 1986, *Ottowa Charter—Achieving Health for All: A Framework for Health Promotion*, WHO, Copenhagen.

Young K 1996, Health, health promotion and the elderly, *Journal of Clinical Nursing*, 5(4), pp 241–8.

Zeanah CH, Boris NW & Larrieu JA 1997, Infant development and developmental risk: a review of the past 10 years, *Journal of the American Academy of Child & Adolescent Psychiatry*, 36(2), pp 165–78.

Acknowledgment
The author would like to acknowledge Michael Groome for his contribution on moral development.

CHAPTER

9

Crisis and loss
Paul Morrison

KEY POINTS

- Crisis is a normal part of life for all of us.
- A person's ability to cope with a crisis will depend on how much it is perceived as being beyond their ability to function.
- When a person is unable to deal effectively with the situation and the emotions associated with it, they may experience feelings of helplessness, anxiety, fear and guilt.
- Crisis nearly always involves significant losses (primary and secondary) for those involved, and a number of important tasks must be completed for adaptive grieving to occur.
- As people learn to cope effectively with life crises they build a repertoire of skills and competencies that can be used to manage crises that emerge later in life.
- If a crisis is not dealt with effectively it can lead to poor health.
- Nurses are frequently exposed to crisis in families and need to develop therapeutic approaches and skills to enable them to help clients.
- Helping people at times of personal crisis can be difficult and stressful for nurses and other health workers. It can raise issues and conflicts for the helper.
- Nurses need a strong commitment to cultural awareness and sensitivity when caring for clients and families from diverse backgrounds.

KEY TERMS

- abuse
- adapting
- advanced training
- anger
- assessment
- assumptions
- loss
- mourning
- nurse's role
- primary loss
- rape
- rapport
- attempted suicide
- conflict
- coping
- coping strategies
- crisis
- culture
- death
- disclosure
- distress
- emotional reaction
- feelings
- grief
- helping
- life crisis
- life events
- resources
- risk
- secondary loss
- self-harm
- shock
- stress
- sudden death
- suicide
- support
- trauma
- uncertainty
- victim
- violent crime
- vulnerability

LEARNING OUTCOMES

The material in this chapter will assist you to:
- describe some of the types of life crisis that occur and the potential impact these may have on peoples' lives
- understand how people deal with crisis by drawing on the resources available to them to adapt to the crisis situation, and be aware that a failure to cope may indicate a need for professional help
- identify how nurses can help clients and families deal with the types of crisis that may present in a health-care setting
- describe nursing approaches and interventions that may be employed when caring for people and their families at times of crisis
- acknowledge the importance of cultural sensitivity and understanding for professionals when working with clients from diverse cultures at times of crisis and loss
- explain some of the vital constituents needed to establish a positive helping relationship with clients in crisis.

INTRODUCTION

A crisis in life often appears like a bolt out of the blue. The sudden onset of illness, the loss of a job or a death in the family can visit us at any time. These can throw our stable lives into a chaotic state with no apparent positive solution. This chapter examines some of the crises that can erupt without warning. It considers the defining features of a crisis and the potential impact of a crisis on peoples' lives.

While two people can be exposed to the same stressful event, they are likely to construe the event differently; one may be able to adapt and cope well, while the other may feel anxious and 'crushed' by the experience. It is this personal appraisal process that is at the core of coping with a crisis.

When a person is unable to cope, even for a short time, some form of professional intervention may be required. A number of crisis events are broached here including suicide, attempted suicide, self-harm, being a victim of crime, and sudden death, with an emphasis on the important role that nurses can play in helping patients and clients to deal with these effectively. There is also a strong focus on dealing with the loss that usually trails a life crisis. The need for a heightened awareness of cultural considerations in the helping process is also stressed.

The final section of the chapter deals with some of the helping attitudes and skills that are needed to assist people to deal with crisis and loss. These look straightforward enough on paper, but in the 'disordered' environment of a busy casualty department or an acute mental health admission unit they may be much more difficult to practise and sustain. These are nevertheless required competencies for high-quality nurse–patient relationships.

WHAT CONSTITUTES A CRISIS?

Most of us can recall a crisis situation in our lives that made us feel out of kilter with the world, highly anxious and vulnerable, a sense of life being out of control and unpredictable. The death of a friend or parent, being the victim of a crime, physical assault or rape, being part of natural disaster and so on, are some examples of life crises. Some types of crisis are classed as 'situational' crisis (Aguilera 1998): abortion, child abuse, rape, divorce, chronic physical or psychiatric illness, alcohol and drug abuse, suicide and attempted suicide. Others may be termed 'maturational' crisis and are linked to normal stages of development and ageing across the life-span (Aguilera 1998). Some life crises can be anticipated (natural death of a partner), while others are unanticipated (sudden death following a road traffic accident).

A crisis can be distinguished from a stressful event that may pass quickly, such as an exam. Parry (1990) summarised the most common defining features of a crisis as follows:

- There is a triggering stress event or long-term stress.
- The individual experiences distress.
- There is a loss, danger or humiliation.
- There is a sense of uncontrollability.
- The events feel unexpected.
- There is a disruption of routine.
- There is uncertainty about the future.
- The distress continues over time (from about two to six weeks).

CONSEQUENCES OF A PERSONAL CRISIS

A crisis will have a significant impact on the lives of those involved. It can produce great pain, distress and anguish. It can lead to feelings of unreality, uncertainty and isolation. A person in crisis will want to restore the general sense of balance in their life and feel able to cope with life again. The word 'crisis' also implies a sense of urgency, a turning point, a time for major decisions (Parry 1990). People in crisis are often in a state of shock. It is a time when their thinking is muddled and their emotional reactions are characterised by feelings of loss, helplessness and hopelessness. They may try to cope with the situation by denial initially but they need to cope in a more effective way in the long run. The role of helpers is to enable clients to cope with the problem and with the feelings the problem has elicited. The type of support offered may be emotional support, practical help, companionship, advice and information (Parry 1990).

A life crisis will stop people completing daily activities and routines. It causes a huge disruption in their lives and often the lives of those close to them. This usually means that the people involved in a crisis must make behavioural, social and emotional adjustments in their lives. These may be temporary or, in the case of a crisis brought about by the onset of chronic illness, enduring adjustments (Caltabiano et al. 2002). A crisis can change a person's life permanently. It can signal the end of a promising academic career, the end of a close relationship, the inability to get married and have children, or it can heighten personal vulnerability. A crisis brings much uncertainty into peoples' lives because they cannot foresee how it will unfold.

At a time of acute crisis the physical environment too, such as an emergency room, may be a frightening place for patients and their relatives. The level of noise, technical equipment and activity may be daunting. In casualty, the patient who failed in their attempted suicide may feel guilty for wasting people's time. The rape victim may feel further exposed and violated. The abused child may be confused and scared and unsure of who to trust. These reactions are unlikely to be helpful at a time of acute crisis. On the other hand, strong supportive structures (families and friends) have been found to aid coping and adjustment following serious physical illness (Caltabiano et al. 2002) and are likely to play a role in adjusting following other types of crisis too.

Helping people in crisis is not about taking over (although on rare occasions this may be appropriate) and making them dependent. It is more effective to help them to use their own resources and to be supportive. It is about enabling, not disabling (Parry 1990).

A FRAMEWORK FOR COPING AND ADAPTING TO CRISIS

How we deal with change and handle conflict and the demands we face is a form of coping. Our ability to cope and tolerate these life events and incidents will be influenced by many factors which will shape our feelings, thoughts, beliefs, values and actions as well as the responses of others. Crisis nearly always involves some form of significant loss for the person involved and these losses can come in many different forms—the loss of financial or personal security, sleep, appetite or the ability to think clearly; the loss of a sense of identity as a couple, a sense of trust or a sense of belonging.

The coping and adjustment effort required may be significant and people differ in how they respond to these circumstances. The upshot of a crisis will depend on how well the person copes, and the coping process will be influenced by the interaction of 'event' factors, background factors, physical and social environmental factors. For example, an illness can elicit new and distressing signs such as lack of interest in personal hygiene and an inability to communicate effectively with others. Feeling

angry, depressed or guilty after surviving a suicide attempt can be stigmatising for the patient or client and reinforces their desire to hide away from people. Sometimes the disabling effect of medication side-effects (such as drowsiness and drooling mouth) can be very embarrassing (Morrison et al. 2000).

Some people just seem to possess an ability to find a sense of purpose or quality in their lives in spite of the awful things they come up against at a time of crisis. They can resist feeling 'helpless and hopeless' (Caltabiano et al. 2002). Other factors that are important here include age, personal beliefs, gender, personal maturity, social class and the level of religious commitment that a person holds (Moos & Schaefer 1986). These factors will shape the way individuals respond to crises. (See also Ch 7, Theories on mental health and illness).

The complexity of issues, responses and settings in which crises and coping occur can be daunting. Holahan, Moos & Schaefer (1996) devised a framework for coping as a process of adaptation by drawing on earlier research and bringing together the need to consider the person and the context in which coping happens. This more general and inclusive model is depicted in Figure 9.1. It takes account of the personal and situational issues that can affect coping. Panel 1 is made up of the constant stressors in life, such as illness, as well as the supports and aids available to the person, while Panel 2 contains the person's coping strategies and sociodemographic attributes.

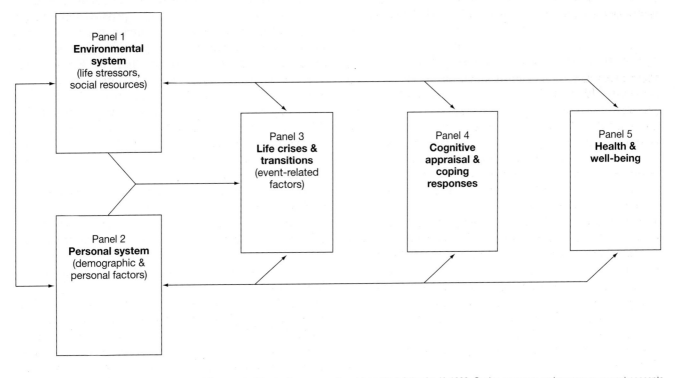

Figure 9.1 A general conceptual framework of the coping process (from Moos RH & Schaefer JA 1993, Coping resources and processes: current concepts and measures. In: Goldberger L & Breznitz S (eds), *Handbook of Stress: Theoretical and Clinical Aspects* (2nd edn), Free Press, New York).

These 'systems' influence the life crises and transitions that occur to all of us (Panel 3). The cognitive evaluation of these (Panel 4) has a direct impact on our health and well-being (Panel 5). According to Holahan et al. (1996), cognitive appraisal and coping responses play a critical role in responses to stress and crisis. It is also notable that the factors in each panel in Figure 9.1 can provide feedback to earlier parts of the framework, giving it a dynamic quality.

Coping strategies have been described within this framework—people typically either 'approach' or 'avoid' stressful events. This illustrates the person's orientation. The approach or avoidance domains are also influenced by the methods of coping people can use. These are 'cognitive' or 'behavioural' methods. When combined, four basic types of coping responses (cognitive approach, behavioural approach, cognitive avoidance, behavioural avoidance) are produced (see Holahan et al. 1996 for details).

Of particular importance here is the fact that the research literature indicates that consistent patterns of relationships have been found to occur using this framework. For example: 'people who rely more on approach coping tend to adapt better to life stressors and experience fewer psychological symptoms. Approach coping strategies such as problem solving and seeking information, can moderate the potential adverse influence of both negative life changes and enduring role stressors on psychological functioning' (Holahan et al. 1996, p 29).

In contrast, people who rely heavily on avoidance coping strategies like 'denial' and 'withdrawal' tend to suffer greater levels of distress after a period of crisis. A significant body of research exploring the relationship between approach/avoidance coping and a range of clinical issues such as depression, physical illness, alcohol use and smoking behaviour, lends considerable support to this framework. It must be noted, however, that these trends might not apply across cultures.

Finally, Holahan et al. (1996) also noted that people exposed to crisis events often emerge stronger and with greater levels of competence. Their ability to cope with future crises may be enhanced. They may be more self-assured and assertive, have developed different views of themselves and their abilities, achieved a new sense of purpose in life and become more resilient, in spite of the fact that they have confronted significant life crises. The framework and the findings provide nurses and other care staff with some guideposts for working with people in crisis. They present a structure to ensure that staff consider the wider canvas of events, experiences, resources and coping styles that may be at the client's disposal with appropriate support and guidance from the nurse.

EVENTS AND PERCEPTIONS THAT CAN LEAD TO PERSONAL CRISIS

Slaikeu (1990) described some of the common precipitating events that can spark a personal crisis, including

pregnancy and the birth of a child, unmarried motherhood, moving from home to school or from home to university, marriage, bereavement, relocation and migration, retirement, surgery and illness, natural disasters and rapid social and technological change. Other devastating events such as the death of a loved one or rape may elicit a crisis response too. Events, even those that most of us are exposed to, can be interpreted as 'the last straw' after a crisis reaction (Slaikeu 1990).

Some time ago Holmes & Rahe (1967) devised a useful way of considering how much stress a person may be exposed to, using the Life Events Scale. The scale lists 41 positive and negative common occurrences that require adjustment and can affect a person's risk of illness. Each occurrence is given a life-change unit score and these can be summed to reflect the level of life-changing events that have occurred to a particular person in the previous twelve months. Some examples include: death of a spouse 100; divorce 73; marriage 50; change in responsibilities at work 29; Christmas 12 and so on. When added together a total score can be arrived at; generally the higher the score the greater the risk of illness in the future.

Even if a person with a very high score seems to be coping with significant life stresses, a major crisis (anxiety, depression, suicide attempt, heart attack) can be just around the corner. Within this model a collection of life-change units that amount to more than 350 in a given year may be a crisis. It is also interesting to note how even positive events (such as a promotion or a marriage) can be stressful and lead to a crisis for some people.

There are no hard and fast rules about what may be deemed a crisis and what may not. A person's perception of events, their culture and life experience, the consequences and losses associated with these and their ability to manage effectively are primary. Scileppa, Teed & Torres (2000) commented: 'Allowing for personal differences in coping styles, it is fair to say that any situation or combination of life occurrence that taxes individuals beyond their typical ability to function can be viewed as a crisis' (p 87).

Levine & Perkins (1997) described crisis somewhat differently, as a time when a person's resources (material, physical, psychological) and those in the person's social network, are overburdened. The person is unable to deal effectively with the emotions surrounding the event. They may experience feelings of helplessness, anxiety, fear and guilt, and their behaviour is ineffective. Most of us cope with crises but sometimes they can lead to other problems such as abuse of alcohol and drugs, or indeed to full-blown psychological or psychiatric illness.

As a nurse your role is to help clients overcome this awful period in their lives, not to judge how bad things seem from your perspective. Losing a pet is something most of us deal with well but for some the loss can be followed by depression or a suicide attempt because that pet may have been the only companion in that person's life.

The nature of any nursing intervention at this time may be centred around giving comfort, helping the person to explore their intense feelings, helping to clarify events, options for the future and sources of support— physical, psychological and social—and trying to enhance the person's coping strategies. If these interventions are helpful then some common outcomes can be expected. The person will feel safe and well supported. Their view of the situation will be couched in reality and they will feel less vulnerable. They will be able to draw on the available sources of support and cope more effectively with the situation.

If the crisis is addressed effectively then this resolution may provide the client with new skills and competencies that can help manage upcoming life crises. If, on the other hand, the crisis is not resolved successfully then this may lead to later problems and issues that have a negative effect on the client's physical and psychological health. For example, unresolved issues may be the source of later problems in living for many victims of childhood sexual abuse who have been found to suffer from a range of negative consequences later on in life, including: depression, guilt, low self-esteem, feelings of inferiority, isolation, loneliness, distrust and poor-quality interpersonal relationships, promiscuity and sexual dysfunction (Johnson 1998).

INTERVENING AT A TIME OF CRISIS

A crisis can present in many different ways and if it is severe enough, professional helpers may be asked to intervene. Aguilera (1998) described two broad approaches to this process. The generic approach is based on the notion that certain common patterns emerge in most crisis situations and that these must be worked through if the person is to adapt in a healthy way. The intervention is aimed at achieving an adaptive resolution by focusing on the typical patterns of response in crisis rather than the distinctive ways in which individuals react (Aguilera 1998). Hence the approach is a general one focusing on the usual steps and stages that might occur following, for example, the sudden death of a partner.

The individual approach is much more psychological and focuses on the client's personal history, needs and responses. There is a greater focus on depth and human understanding, and greater levels of specialist training are required to practise in this way (Aguilera 1998). I suspect that practical reality dictates that professional helpers mingle both approaches. The typical steps in a crisis intervention scenario are outlined in Box 9.1. (See also Ch 23, Therapeutic interventions.)

While these steps may be typical, individuals do not always pass through them in a simple linear fashion. For example, the initial assessment of the problem may be revised as the helper learns more about the client and their life over a period of time. This may change the focus of the intervention, making it more appropriate for the

> **Box 9.1 Steps in crisis intervention**
>
> - **Assessment**: including assessment of the potential risk to the person and others
> - **Planning a therapeutic intervention**: taking account of the impact on the person and the resources available to the person
> - **Intervention**:
>   - Help the person to understand what has happened
>   - Help the person to express feelings openly
>   - Explore coping mechanisms
>   - Re-open the social world
> - **Resolution of the crisis and future planning**
>
> Source: described by Aguilera DC 1998, *Crisis Intervention. Theory and Methodology* (8th edn), Mosby, St Louis.

client's needs. Sometimes the client may set a new direction as they regain a greater sense of personal control over their lives and the coping process. It is notable that a crisis might last between four and six weeks (Aguilera 1998). In addition, many crisis situations are assessed by crisis teams. A fundamental orientation in psychological treatment has been emphasised by Schwartz (2000), who reminds us that however bizarre the client's behaviour might appear, they are human beings first and foremost. The illness is an important *secondary* consideration. This orientation is central to all forms of counselling and helping but it is especially important when helping very vulnerable members of society at times of crisis.

> **CRITICAL THINKING CHALLENGE 9.1**
>
> You are in charge of the Crisis Assessment Team, responsible for taking calls from people who may have a mental illness. It is approaching midnight and only three staff are on duty. One of the staff, a single mother with small children, is due to finish the shift at midnight and collect her children from the babysitter. Three calls come in almost simultaneously.
> - The first call is from your very good friend. She tells you that she had an abortion this afternoon and can't stop crying now. You did not know she was pregnant.
> - The second call comes from the local police, who ask for your immediate attendance at a local hospital where a 22-year-old man is threatening to shoot another resident and then himself.
> - The third call is from Joan, a 38-year-old registered nurse who is well-known to the service and has received treatment for depression in the past. She is obviously drunk but says she has taken 30 paracetamol tablets.
> - What course of action would you recommend in each of these cases?

CRISIS, LOSS AND GRIEF

Worden (2001) described mourning as the 'process which occurs after a loss', while 'grief refers to the personal experience of the loss'. Grief is an emotional response of distress, pain and disorganisation. Mourning involves unravelling the previous bonds between the person and a deceased person (or object or part of the person). A process of mourning is needed to overcome grief.

Grief may be elicited by many different types of loss, such as a loss of self-esteem, loss of job, loss of financial status, loss of freedom, loss of physical abilities, loss of identity. Grief nearly always involves primary losses (death, job, relationship) and secondary losses or losses that result as a consequence of the primary loss (status, security, self-esteem). Secondary losses may not be apparent to the patient or client, and nurses can assist in the grieving process by helping the client to uncover these.

A number of key tasks of mourning have been described by Worden (2001) and these need to be accomplished if the client is to return to a state of stability. These are:

Task 1: To accept the reality of the loss

Task 2: To work through the pain and grief

Task 3: To adjust to a world in which the deceased is not there

Task 4: To relocate the deceased emotionally and move on with life.

When people are in mourning they experience feelings that are common. They may believe these feelings are unique to them, but they are not. Acknowledging this commonality helps people to share the pain and may be facilitated through bereavement groups. Experiencing personal loss is part of what makes us human.

Grieving is a normal process after loss, and involves emotional (sadness, anger), physical (breathlessness, physical weakness) and cognitive (confusion, disbelief) sensations as well as behavioural changes (social withdrawal, crying). It can be helpful to let the client know that these are normal and that it is helpful to express and share these facets of grieving to promote healing.

The conflict within the family about whether a dying relative should have been told they were dying may be a source of guilt and long-lasting family disharmony. Not to tell the person prevents them from getting their house in order and many things may be left unsaid. These sorts of family issues can complicate the grieving and healing process and create additional pressure for the nurse.

Resources are now widely available to ensure that counsellors, professional carers and clients are better informed about issues surrounding death and dying. People with internet access can now study a wide range of information about death and dying, arguments for and against legislation on euthanasia, information about cancer, suicide and AIDS. In addition, there is growing recognition of the need for communities to be aware of the diverse ways of grieving that different communities need to undergo and experience. NSW Health and Queensland Health have developed an online catalogue that outlines how different groups (professional and informal) in the community cope with bereavement, in an effort to provide culturally sensitive health care. Nurses working with culturally diverse client groups would be well advised to become familiar with some of these resources.

SUICIDE AND ATTEMPTED SUICIDE

One crisis situation that most nurses will come across, in both mental health and general settings, is suicide and attempted suicide. Suicide in Australia and New Zealand is a significant mental health problem, especially in young men (15–24 years), older people and people living in rural and remote areas of the country. The respective government web pages dealing with mental health make for grim reading and some strategic initiatives have been developed to address this tragic situation.

People who are seriously depressed or who express feelings of worthlessness, guilt, anxiety and anger, and display severe agitation and irritability, may be at risk of suicide. It is important to note here, however, that 'not all suicides or attempted suicides are by individuals with a clinical diagnosis of depression. Stressful and negative life events can become triggers for suicidal ideation and attempts, such as drug or alcohol abuse' (Sharkey 1999b, p 92). Other illnesses too, such as schizophrenia or bipolar mood disorder, can be prominent. The primary goal of crisis management in many instances is to reduce or eliminate the risk to the clients and/or to others (Doyle 1999) whether in a hospital or community setting.

A key role here for the nurse is to recognise the potential risk and intervene beforehand. Sharkey (1999b) extracted a number of high-risk indicators drawn from the literature in this area. These are outlined in Box 9.2.

Box 9.2 **High-risk indicators for suicide**

- deliberate self-harm
- following admission to a mental health unit, particularly during the first week
- following discharge from a psychiatric setting, particularly during the first month
- drug or alcohol misuse
- recent major life event such as divorce or separation
- being from a particular at-risk group, such as farmer or doctor, or being unemployed
- non-compliance with treatment/medication
- rapid change in treatment type or in accommodation setting
- poor relationship with carers

Source: Sharkey S 1999, Crisis risks associated with depression. In: Ryan T (ed.) *Managing Crisis and Risk in Mental Health Nursing*, Stanley Thornes, Cheltenham, pp 90–104.

If the health-care team has identified a client at risk of suicide, each team member will need to work with the client at a time when the client feels desperate and hopeless and sees no end to the darkness in their lives. (See also Ch 23, Therapeutic interventions.) A good rapport can be established by heeding the advice offered by Wright (1993):

- *Take a threat of suicide seriously.* Individuals who have attempted suicide on a number of occasions can be ignored or dismissed as 'attention-seekers' and later found to have suicided.
- *Try not to be judgmental.* It is very easy to view the client within your frame of reference and assumptions and to judge their feelings and intentions accordingly, perhaps to think, 'What's he/she got to be depressed about with a lovely partner, family, home and a nice car?'.
- *Work with the feelings raised by the client.* Stay with the patient/client's feelings, not yours. Try not to steer the client away from their feelings—'It's not that bad . . . I'm sure you'll feel better in the morning'. Utterances like this may help *you* to feel better, but not the client.
- *Work with positives in a sensible manner.* Even at times of great despair and desperation it may be possible to find glimpses of positive incidents, experiences or perspectives that might be helpful. Remind the client how talking openly about their plans and intentions can be useful.
- *Accept the client's anger.* The client may release strong emotions such as anger and it is best if this is done in a quiet and private setting where others will not be disturbed. When you recognise that it is usual for a client to express negative emotions such as anger or guilt at times of crisis, it can help you to understand and accept these uncomfortable emotional responses, even if they are directed at you.

The major challenge for the nurse here is to provide a supportive relationship through which the client's issues and perspective can be explored and fully understood by the health-care team. This is a basis for establishing a safety framework for the client that involves all the resources at your disposal while treating the client in a respectful manner. This can be a challenge if the client is not very communicative.

Caring for people at risk of suicide or self-harm is emotionally demanding and stressful. It is a source of major anxiety for inexperienced and experienced nurses alike. Despite a relatively common view that talking about suicide with someone at risk is likely to urge them into action, there is no evidence to support this view. In fact, people who are thinking about killing themselves are often relieved that the issue has been broached by staff. It brings it out into the open and allows them to share their sense of dread with another human being. It is okay to ask about their plans, the resources available to the client (knives, ropes, tablets) and their intentions (Wright 1993). A fuller

understanding of the client will help the team to be better able to care for them and decreases the likelihood of suicide.

Griever concerns following suicide

Loss through suicide can evoke certain types of concern in the griever (Cook & Dworkin 1992) including psychological, social and personal concerns. The psychological issues may centre on the need to understand why this has happened. They may feel guilty and display a sense of failure. They may blame others in an angry way and feel totally rejected. The taboo surrounding suicide can interfere with the grieving process and may lead people to withdraw socially, and patterns of communication in families can be disrupted (social concern).

Personal concerns can include the need to deal with a sense of betrayal or a reluctance to get close to people emotionally in the future. These fears will shape the helping process following suicide as the nurse attempts to help the client complete any unfinished business with the deceased, use the support that other people and services provide, and avoid withdrawal from the social world.

SELF-HARM

Some people can harm themselves deliberately (inflicting injury with a sharp object resulting from delusional beliefs) or through neglect (e.g. lack of a proper diet). People with a diagnosis of schizophrenia tend to have a higher risk of self-harm, especially when their symptoms such as delusions and hallucinations are poorly controlled. These clients have a 10 per cent lifetime risk of suicide (Hogman & Meier 1995) and make up one in three hospital suicides (Sharkey 1999a). Some of the key strategies for managing the risk of self-harming clients from this group and those with depression have been outlined by Sharkey (1999b) (see Box 9.3 overleaf and Ch 22 for self-harm).

Sharkey (1999a) also makes the point that there has been a significant shift in the way in which risk in schizophrenia in particular is approached these days. There is a far greater emphasis on the client's experience, community care, the use of formal and informal supportive networks and combination therapies, rather than a sole reliance on medication to control the disease within a constraining environment. Schwartz emphasises that in a crisis:

it is important to remember that, no matter how bizarre their behaviour, people with schizophrenia are human beings with the same feelings, fears, desires, and hopes as everyone else.

(Schwartz 2000, p 371)

Box 9.3 Managing risk of self-harm

Crises in community settings:

- Make frequent contact (home/day centre/outpatients).
- Make rapid follow-up for failed contacts (establish an agreed team plan with clear roles and responsibilities).
- Monitor medication and use optimum dose to lift mood with minimal side-effects and avoiding overmedication.
- Build a therapeutic relationship.

Crises in hospital settings:

- Provide constant supervision through close observation.
- Provide clear notes and communication.
- Clarify responsibilities with the team members.
- Monitor medication and use optimum dose to lift mood with minimal side-effects and avoiding overmedication.
- Use power of detention (if available).
- Build a therapeutic relationship

Long-term management of risk:

- Work to an agreed plan for the future to identify stressors, build esteem and hope.
- Work with family/carers to solve problems, increase or maintain coping strategies.
- Develop structured, safe and meaningful daily activity.

Source: Sharkey S 1999, Crisis risks associated with depression. In: Ryan T (ed.) *Managing Crisis and Risk in Mental Health Nursing*, Stanley Thornes, Cheltenham, pp 90–104.

BEING A VICTIM OF CRIME

A person who has suffered some form of physical and/or psychological harm (rape, sexual assault, domestic violence, incest, assaults on children or old people) at the hands of another is a victim (Wright 1993). In cases where it is obvious what has happened, the police and other agencies will be involved directly. In other cases, when staff suspicions are aroused that a crime has occurred (that a child is being abused, for example), the consequences of raising these suspicions may be devastating for the family and child.

If these suspicions are correct and can be supported by evidence, a child could be spared future episodes of abuse. If incorrect, the child could be removed in error from the home, causing great distress to the child and the family. In other cases a woman may be reluctant to press charges against a partner who assaults her routinely after drinking binges. She may believe that she brought this abuse on herself through her own behaviour and fear that separation from her partner will result in her losing her children because she does not have a job or cannot support them alone.

Emotional and physical abuse are offensive to most people and it is sometimes difficult to imagine how some people can continue to live in these circumstances. Abuse

can raise issues for staff, too, and trigger strong emotional responses (such as anger) that interfere with their ability to care in a professional manner. These personal responses may stem from the staff member's having been abused themselves, or being a child with an alcoholic parent, and being unable to deal with these events in an adaptive way.

In an exploration of the traumas that have been found to occur in the lives of children, Johnson (1998) noted that the professional helper may have to:

- identify specific crisis situations
- recognise who is and who is not affected
- decide who is at risk in a particular situation
- devise options for managing the crisis
- intervene appropriately
- monitor post-crisis recovery
- decide when and how to follow up.

This profile of the professional's role with respect to children is typical of all crisis work. In the case of children, the identification of a crisis poses additional problems and responsibilities. A child turning up at a nurse's clinic for a consultation about head lice may be a victim of assault, rape or incest but be unable to report this due to fear of, or emotional attachment to, the perpetrator. The identification process becomes crucial here and is far from easy. This is why a supportive team approach is vital, as a means of ensuring that assessments are thorough and accurate, and as a means of lending support to other team members. In such cases other agencies (such as the police) are involved.

Abuse can occur in older people too. Kinnear & Graycar (1991) reported that some '4.6 per cent of older people are victims of physical, sexual or financial abuse, perpetrated mostly by family members and those who are in a duty of care relationship with the victim' (p 1). The abuse of older people has been found to occur in residential-care settings as well as private homes (Kinnear & Graycar 1991). An increase in the incidence of abuse in this vulnerable group is also likely to occur as older people comprise a growing proportion of the population as a whole. While most people in this group will live independently, an increasing minority will be dependent on relatives or residential-care providers as their primary support, and in some instances conflict, power relationships and abuse will emerge.

As is the case with other vulnerable groups, the nature and extent of abuse of older people can be very difficult to uncover and validate. The initial contact with these clients may be coincidental (e.g. at a health centre or accident unit) and if the signs are very 'obvious' (bruising, fractures, severe agitation) then suspicions may be raised. However, an older, slightly confused person may be locked in a room all day by relatives to stop them wandering the streets, or not be allowed to drink after 4 pm in case of bed wetting. These restrictions too are forms of abuse and are much harder to spot, unless in the short time that a skilled and attentive nurse has with them these older people can feel safe enough to voice some of their experiences. Then further exploration must follow.

Although the acute phase of the crimes may be seen to be 'sorted out' in a few short weeks, the aftermath may raise long-term issues requiring counselling and therapy over a period of time. A woman who has been raped may be seen by others (or herself) as a 'whore' and be ignored by her partner. A male victim of sexual assault might end up questioning his own sexual identity (Van der Veer 1998). These violations raise significant issues and personal conflicts for the victims. Jurisdictions across Australia have established specialist help lines for sexual assault and rape victims, reflecting the increased need for these expert crisis centres. Time and specialist counselling may be needed to come to terms with these significant events and their impact on all concerned.

It may be worth mentioning here that crime and violence and mental illness tend to be strongly linked in many people's minds, giving rise to unwarranted fear and prejudice about mentally ill people living in the community. This perception can influence health-care staff too. However, most violent crimes occur between people who know each other. Non-psychiatric offenders were five times more likely to focus on people not known to them and therefore present a greater risk to the community than those with a diagnosis of mental illness. In 95 per cent of cases where a psychiatric client has been involved in a violent crime, there has been previous contact with the victim (Pilgrim & Rogers 2003).

In stark contrast, recent research from the United States and Denmark indicates that people with psychotic illness are actually much more likely to become murder victims. One-third of people with serious mental illness were victims of crime. Of these, some 91 per cent were violent crimes including rape and assault. Drug users and alcoholics faced even higher risks (Cuvelier 2002).

However, there will be rare occasions when a person who is mentally ill may try to harm others and the risk must be assessed very carefully. A new mother with severe postnatal psychosis may try to harm the new baby because she feels that the baby is trying to kill her, or an older deluded man may try to harm his wife of forty years because he thinks she is trying to poison him. While not common, these scenarios nevertheless highlight the tension instilled into the nurse's role in assessing and managing a potentially risky situation, and the need to protect potential victims as well as those who might commit such a crime.

SUDDEN DEATH

There will be times when a client commits suicide, especially in mental health care, or when a patient suddenly dies, perhaps in the emergency room following a road accident. A sudden and perhaps unexpected death through suicide will be a source of great stress for staff if they have known the client and then need to support the relatives in their grief. Within the staffing group such events can give rise to strong feelings of guilt and self-blame, personal shame, failure and inadequacy. The shock of such events can be immobilising (Wright 1993). Relatives can be overcome by emotion following unexpected death. In these cases Worden (2001) recommends that the helper begin at the crisis scene (hospital or morgue) to offer help and direction there and then. At this time people may be in a state of shock and disbelief, unable to ask for direct help, and uncertain of what to do.

If as a nurse you are in the emergency room or some other setting to comfort a relative following the sudden death of a child, parent or partner, you can help by being an advocate for the relative, a positive support when they appear lost and uncertain, and help in breaking and accepting bad news. On occasions, you may have to support the relative to view the body and just be there for them when strong emotions and naked human distress are given a free rein (Wright 1993). Traumatic loss may be sudden and violent. It may involve bodily mutilation. It may be seen as preventable. It may be the grieving person's first encounter with a dead person.

While the circumstances of individual crises may vary—suicides, sudden unexpected deaths, accidents and trauma, children and infants, miscarriages and stillbirths—the pain experienced is traumatic and shocking for those who remain. They can be helped to begin to come to terms with this loss in a number of ways. Some of these are outlined in Box 9.4. Of course it is important to be aware that some cultural and religious

---

Box 9.4 What is valued by relatives who have experienced a sudden death

- Clear, unambiguous messages: 'The news is bad. Your daughter has just died'. People need to know the facts quickly.
- Confirmation: you might need to verify the facts of the death several times.
- Try to prepare yourself to answer difficult questions: Why now? Why us? Why could it not be prevented? Why could you not do more?
- It will help if relatives and friends can spend time with the deceased to say goodbye. You might have to help by saying: 'Maybe you would like to see him/her one last time before you go home'. This helps to normalise the viewing.
- Allow the relatives time and space to spend time with the body. Let them sit down. Encourage them to talk and touch the body.
- Before they go home give them some time to go back over what has happened.

Source: Wright B 1993, *Caring in Crisis. A Handbook of Intervention Skills* (2nd edn), Churchill Livingstone, Edinburgh.

140 PART 2 MENTAL HEALTH AND WELLNESS

CRITICAL THINKING CHALLENGE 9.2

Complete the following questionnaire on personal vulnerability.
Answer each question: **Y** = Yes, I agree; **P** = Perhaps, I'm not sure; or **N** = No, I disagree.

	Y	P	N
1 It's hardly worth working hard in your job since most times other people get the benefits of it.	—	—	—
2 I like it when something unexpected happens to break up the routine of the working day.	—	—	—
3 When someone in authority has made a decision there's not much you can do about it.	—	—	—
4 I've found that most of my misfortunes have happened because of mistakes I've made.	—	—	—
5 Life is an interesting adventure.	—	—	—
6 It upsets me a great deal if other people get annoyed with me.	—	—	—
7 If someone has it in for you there's not much point in trying to reason with them.	—	—	—
8 Every problem has a solution.	—	—	—
9 I often feel let down by people I thought I could trust.	—	—	—
10 Most problems will go away if you ignore them.	—	—	—
11 People can avoid problems by planning their lives.	—	—	—
12 I think you can get most things you want if you try hard enough.	—	—	—
13 I've found people are generally very ungrateful for things you do for them.	—	—	—
14 You always have some freedom of choice, even in difficult situations.	—	—	—
15 I enjoy listening to other people and hearing about their experiences.	—	—	—

Score as follows:
Questions 2, 5, 8, 11, 12, 14, 15: Y = 0, P = 1, N = 2
Questions 1, 3, 4, 6, 7, 9, 10, 13: Y = 2, P = 1, N = 0

Results:

Below 5:	You are exceptionally resilient to crisis stress.
5–10:	You manage to face most crises successfully.
11–15:	You may find yourself knocked sideways by stress at times.
Above 15:	You are probably very vulnerable to the effects of crisis.

Source: Parry G 1990, *Coping with Crises*, British Psychological Society in association with Routledge, London, p 53.

practices may need to be observed, so tread carefully and make sure you consult more senior experienced colleagues and, if available, specialist helpers or advisors who know about the accepted customs of a particular cultural group.

It is also important to offer support for family members if possible because they too are often victims of social stigma because of the circumstances surrounding the client's death (suicide, drink driving or drug taking) (Lively, Friedrich & Buckwalter 1995).

Attitudes to death

Dealing with death can be problematic, as attitudes have changed over the years. More and more people die in hospitals and nursing homes, when in the past they died at home. In addition, in Western cultures professional services are hired to look after the dying and the death and this is very different to how things were done years ago. Then, families played a much greater role in these

processes. The attitudes of people and professional health-care staff have changed too, with the growing emphasis on technology in the health system and changing lifestyle patterns. People live longer now, and fewer people are exposed to death or to dying relatives until later in life. Jalland (1997) suggested that the emphasis in medical teams these days is to avoid death through scientific expertise rather than provide comfort to the dying. Yet Kübler-Ross (1981) argued that dying can provide important lessons for professional staff and for the families of the deceased.

CRISIS, LOSS AND CULTURE

Dealing with the losses associated with a life crisis has been referred to as 'grief work' (Levine & Perkins 1997). Moos & Schaefer (1986) described a number of tasks that need to be worked through to help people adapt effectively:

- to find meaning in the event and understand its significance for the person(s)
- to face up to the reality and manage the demands of the situation
- to sustain interpersonal relationships
- to preserve an emotional balance
- to uphold a satisfactory self-image and keep a sense of self-efficacy.

Working through these tasks enhances a person's ability to cope. However, this process is made much more complicated (for carers and clients) when different cultural groups are involved. Culture refers broadly to patterns of attitudes, beliefs, values, behaviours and knowledge that are shared by people from particular social groups and which evolve over time. These become a general blueprint for people's actions and reactions to their experiences and to the crisis points in their lives. In some cultures, for example, community members will feed and support a recently bereaved person (Wright 1993). In some societies, psychotic behaviour can be a sign of special powers and abilities (Helman 1990). Cultural norms dictate how a particular situation or experience is defined and understood (Robbins 1997). (See also Ch 6, Mental health in Australia and New Zealand.)

Being aware of the influence of culture in the person's life will enhance the nurse's ability to care effectively. Indeed, this orientation is a responsibility of all professional mental health workers in Australia today (see, for example, Multicultural Mental Health Australia 2003). If a person is labelled suicidal, depressed or anorexic by professional staff this label may become a badge of shame for the family, who might then hide away. That in itself is bad enough but if the family hail from other parts of the world and English is not their first language then this experience may further alienate them and make successful integration much more difficult and less likely.

Culture has many layers and levels, and nurses cannot be expected to get a good grasp on all the relevant aspects of different cultural groups. However, as nurses we need at least a heightened awareness of the complex nature of culture and an attitude of openness and commitment to help us to learn about it from individual clients. The need for such an attitude is illustrated in a study that explored Aboriginal perceptions of mental health and illness (Turale 1994).

NURSING INTERVENTIONS: ATTITUDES AND SKILLS
Developing enhanced cultural sensitivity
Lorion & Parron (1985) described a number of studies that showed that if helpers or counsellors display low expectations of success with ethnic clients, the outcomes will also be low. Hence it is important for the counsellor or nurse to expect the client to be successful and to move forward. Also, for counselling to be effective, the boundaries for

counselling need to be clearly established. These boundaries may come under close scrutiny when counselling any client but especially one from a different culture, who may expect a friendship outside the formal parameters of the helping relationship.

When counselling clients from a different culture, verbal and non-verbal communication signs may be a major source of misunderstanding. It is important, therefore, for the nurse to spend time checking the accuracy of his or her understanding rather than assuming that they know what the client means. While the need to check for understanding is vitally important with clients from different cultures, it is also a core process in any helping situation. It is all too easy for the nurse to assume that they know what the client means because they were both brought up in the same place. The need to check for understanding should not be overlooked. Poor communication generally tends to be the major source of complaints against health-care staff (Audit Commission 1993).

A nurse from a similar cultural group to the client might be a useful resource, or they might be perceived as a threat to confidentiality, and hinder the development of a trusting relationship in which the client feels comfortable disclosing personal information (d'Ardenne & Mahtani 1989). In time, a trusting rapport could be established and this may not be an issue for the client, but if it continues to be problematic a different nurse should be invited to work with the client. It is important to note, too, that being a member of a professional group may help clients and family members to talk to you as a professional, as the social distance between you and them allows them to feel free to talk. You will of course be bound by professional and ethical rules. The professional relationship allows them the space to talk about issues that could not be broached with relatives or friends.

Helping clients deal with loss
A period of crisis, whatever its nature, often leads to a great sense of personal loss in those affected. A good helping relationship will allow the client to explore the loss and adapt to it more effectively. The primary purpose here is to try and facilitate a normal grief response following a major and significant personal loss. Grieving is a very natural process that all of us must face at some point in our lives. Experiencing grief is part of being human.

The death of a person we loved is perhaps the most striking loss that most of us will experience. When caring for a person who has experienced such a loss it may be helpful to use the assessment framework outlined in the article by Cook & Dworkin (1992) that can be found on the References list. They recommend that the nurse collect factual data about a person's particular situation, their social context and coping styles as well as more subtle aspects of the interaction such as non-verbal behaviour and the nurse's personal reactions to the client's story.

background of the survivor' (p 34). For example, if a client has been socialised not to speak ill of the dead, they may be unable to express the anger they feel towards a deceased relative, and the counsellor will have to work with the client to help them to arrive at and express a 'balanced' perspective.

People from other (non-Western) cultures may be less likely to seek out professional help for fear of 'losing face' in their own community. Even if they do, they may be less trusting of the helper because their culture has taught them not to rely on outsiders. In contrast, a helper who is close to the client culturally may be perceived as a threat to confidentiality and this may have a negative impact on the process, making it difficult to establish a trusting relationship in which the client feels comfortable disclosing personal information (d'Ardenne & Mahtani 1989).

It is important also to note that the relationship aspects of the process will remain crucial whatever cultural factors come into play. Horvath (1995) described a meta-analysis that explored the relationship between the quality of the alliance the therapist has with their client and the outcome of therapy, over a fifteen-year period. He noted that the quality of the alliance was a 'robust predictor of therapy outcome' (p 12). Nurses who expand their counselling role will need to ensure that relationships with their clients have an appropriate affective/emotional bond. This may be harder to establish and maintain when caring for someone with a different cultural background to your own.

Finally, it is all too easy to find yourself very committed to clients and then overwhelmed and emotionally exhausted by despairing clients and families in crisis. As a result, you will not be able to help clients effectively and your own health will suffer. To guard against this you will need to work with colleagues who can provide some form of supervision so that you can establish suitable boundaries between you and those you seek to help. This will also help you to achieve greater clarity in the helping process and ensure that the client's issues are being addressed. (See also Ch 1 for supervision.)

Exploring opportunities for advanced training

Dealing with crisis requires great skill, and nursing interventions can be enhanced with advanced training. Some of the theoretical frameworks developed in other areas, notably psychology and counselling, are very well suited to the nursing practice context (see, for example, Barker 2003 and Watkins 2001). Some approaches that offer great scope in this area are the person-centred approach to counselling following Carl Rogers (Merry 2000), the gestalt approach developed by Frederick Perls (Ellis & Leary-Joyce 2000) and the narrative approach espoused by Michael White (Payne 2000).

The use of a suitable theoretical approach will help you to provide comfort to the client (and their family) and to address the intense feelings associated with a crisis. They will also help the client to clarify events and preferred options in their lives, and to identify the primary resources and sources of support available to them. In short, they will help the client to be the author of their own life and to strive to live in the way that they prefer. Nursing interventions that are underpinned by appropriate counselling and therapy theory can be of great help to the client as they strive to adapt effectively to a crisis in their lives.

CONCLUSION

Dealing with crisis is a normal part of life for all of us. As a nurse, however, you will be exposed to crisis and its aftermath on a regular basis, no matter what area of nursing you specialise in. Nursing exposes us to the pain

---

CRITICAL THINKING CHALLENGE 9.3

Careen (42 years old) is a qualified architect and partner in a busy city office. She is an attractive woman with an intermittent history of bipolar disorder and has been happily married to James for twenty years. They have two daughters: Siobhán (17) and Oonagh (15). It is clear that the family love Careen very much and when she has been ill, they have coped admirably. On this occasion, Careen has had to be admitted to hospital because she has not been sleeping and her behaviour has become more erratic and unpredictable— driving recklessly and putting people at risk, threatening to kill a shop assistant when he responded rudely to her, turning up for work at 3.30 in the morning with no clothes on, and being sexually provocative with strangers. The level of dis-inhibition she displayed was such that she was assessed by the crisis team as being a risk to herself and others and was admitted to the acute unit on a short-term basis.

David is a registered mental health nurse of some years' experience. He is very conscientious and has a very good rapport with clients, their families and other health-care professionals. He is currently studying for a Master's degree and is in charge of the unit on night duty. When doing his rounds of the unit at 5.30 am he found Careen having unprotected sex with Nick in her room. Nick has a long history of mild depression, alcohol and intravenous drug abuse.

- What should David do to care for Careen and her family in the coming weeks?
- Who should be informed about the incident? What guidelines could he use to structure his choices and decisions?

and suffering that unfolds daily in other people's lives. It does so in an intense way and sometimes over a very short and compressed period of time. This level of exposure will elicit attendant emotional reactions and upset in you and others. You will also have to learn to cope with the stressful events in your own life that emerge from time to time. These can interfere with your ability to help others, so it is important to make sure that you deal with these and limit their impact on the way you deal with work-related issues.

Learning to cope with crisis and respond positively through enhanced self-awareness, the development of specialist counselling skills and increased cultural sensitivity will not only help you to function more effectively at work, it will also help you to stay healthy. To conclude, it is important to remember that people do survive even the most harrowing of experiences and existences. It might help to do further reading in the area, such as the most remarkable account of survival found in Dave Pelzer's *My Story*—three books in one describing his journey of survival from the most horrifying abuse by his alcoholic mother (Pelzer 2002). These stories are inspiring reading for any health professional.

EXERCISES FOR CLASS ENGAGEMENT

■ *When written in Chinese the word 'crisis' is composed of two characters. One represents danger and the other represents opportunity.*

John F. Kennedy

You gain strength, courage and confidence by every experience in which you really stop to look fear in the face. You are able to say to yourself, 'I lived through this horror. I can take the next thing that comes along.' You must do the thing you think you cannot do.

Eleanor Roosevelt

Take a pencil and a sheet of paper. Write a short summary of a particular crisis in your life. Describe the event or time and recall how you felt and how you responded to it. See if you can name the people who were most helpful. What did they do or say that helped you to get through? What particular skills, competencies or personal qualities did you find in yourself that helped you to get through this crisis period? How has the experience enhanced your coping skills since then?

Share this story with your group, and together consider how your experiences might help or hinder your ability to help people in crisis.

■ Seán and Conor were brought up in a small, staunchly Catholic and conservative town where everyone went to Mass on Sunday and most families knew each other well. They had known since their early teens that they were both gay but had not disclosed this to family members or teachers. Feeling greatly burdened and out of step with the community they decided to speak to the Parish priest and told him about their sexual orientation. The priest chased them out of his house and told them that they would both 'roast in Hell'. Seán and Conor stopped going to Mass and soon after left the town for city life, returning only for occasional visits to their families.

● How might this reaction to their disclosure have affected the lives of Seán and Conor?

● Consider how you might respond if a close friend or relative made this type of disclosure to you.

■ Briefly describe a few changes and losses other than the death of someone close to you, that you have experienced in the past few years.

● With your group, discuss some of the ways in which each type of loss is similar to and yet different from the other. List commonalities and unique aspects of each loss.

● See if you can identify any secondary losses.

■ *Two cars were being driven fast and in opposite directions along a winding country lane. It was late summertime, and the hedgerows on either side of the lane were lush and high. It was impossible to see around any of the corners.*

Both drivers, because of the heat of the day, had their windows wound down, and their minds were focused on the road ahead and their destination. And, as it happened, the driver of one of the cars was a man and the other was a woman.

They approached the final bend at speed, and they only just managed to see each other in time. They slammed on their brakes and just managed to slide past each other without scraping the paintwork.

As they did so, the woman turned to the man, and through the open window she shouted, 'PIG!'.

Quick as a flash the man replied, 'COW!'.

He accelerated around the corner . . . and crashed into a pig.

(Source: Rabbi Lionel Blue, on 'Thought for the Day', BBC Radio 4, Today
Programme. Cited in: Owen N 2001, The magic of metaphor,
Crown House Publishing, Carmarthen.)

● Can you think of a time when you assumed something to be the case and found out later that you were wrong? How did you cope with that?

■ What kinds of assumptions might you make when caring for someone from a different cultural background to yours? Or that they might make about you? What difficulties might arise as a result? How could such issues be managed effectively by nurses and other health-care workers? Share your findings with your group.

REFERENCES

Aguilera DC 1998, *Crisis Intervention. Theory and Methodology* (8th edn), Mosby, St Louis.

Audit Commission 1993, *What Seems to be the Matter: Communication Between Hospitals and Patients*, National Health Service Report 12, HMSO, London.

Barker P (ed.) 2003, *Psychiatric and Mental Health Nursing. The Craft of Caring*, Arnold, London.

Bowlby J 1980, *Attachment and Loss. Volume 3, Loss—Sadness and Depression*, Hogarth Press, London.

Caltabiano ML, Byrne D, Martin PR & Sarafino EP 2002, *Health Psychology: Biopsychosocial Interactions*, John Wiley & Sons, Australia.

Cook AS & Dworkin DS 1992, *Helping the Bereaved: Therapeutic Interventions for Children, Adolescents and Adults*, Basic Books, New York.

Cuvelier M 2002, The mentally ill are six to seven times more likely to be murdered, *Psychology Today*, May/June, 23.

d'Ardenne P & Mahtani A 1989, *Transcultural Counselling in Action*, Sage, London.

DeSpelder LA & Strickland AL 1992, *The Last Dance: Encountering Death and Dying*, Mayfield, Mountainview, CA.

Doyle M 1999, Organizational responses to crisis and risk: issues and implications for mental health nurses. In: Ryan T (ed.), *Managing Crisis and Risk in Mental Health Nursing*, Stanley Thornes, Cheltenham, pp 40–56.

Ellis M & Leary-Joyce J 2000, Gestalt therapy. In: Feltham C & Horton I (eds), *Handbook of Counselling and Psychotherapy*, Sage, London, pp 337–42.

Geldard D 1998, *Basic Counselling Skills* (3rd edn), Prentice Hall, Sydney.

Helman CG 1990, *Culture, Health and Illness. An Introduction for Health Professionals*, Butterworth-Heinemann, London.

Hogman G & Meier R 1995, *One in Ten: A Report by the National Schizophrenia Fellowship into Suicide and Unnatural Deaths Involving People with Schizophrenia*, National Schizophrenia Fellowship, London.

Holahan CJ, Moos RH & Schaefer JA 1996, Coping, stress resistance and growth: conceptualizing adaptive functioning. In: Zeiderner M & Endler NS (eds), *Handbook of Coping. Theory, Research and Applications*, John Wiley & Sons, New York.

Holmes TH & Rahe RH 1967, The Social Readjustment Rating Scale, *Journal of Psychosomatic Research*, 11(2), pp 213–18.

Horvath AO 1995, The therapeutic relationship: from transference to alliance, *In Session: Psychotherapy in Practice*, 1(1), pp 7–17.

Jalland P 1997, *Death in the Victorian Family*, Oxford University Press, Oxford.

Johnson K 1998, *Trauma in the Lives of Children. Crisis and Stress Management Techniques for Counsellors, Teachers and Other Professionals*, Hunter House, Alameda, CA.

Johnson SE 1987, *After a Child Dies: Counselling Bereaved Families*, Springer, New York.

Kinnear P & Graycar A 1991, Abuse of older people: crime or family dynamics, *Trends & Issues in Crime and Criminal Justice*, 113, Australian Institute of Criminology, Canberra.

Kübler-Ross E 1981, *On Death and Dying*, Macmillan, New York.

Levine M & Perkins DV 1997, *Principles of Community Psychology. Perspectives and Applications* (2nd edn), Oxford University Press, New York.

Lively S, Friedrich RM & Buckwalter KC 1995, Sibling perception of schizophrenia: impact on relationships, roles, and health, *Issues in Mental Health Nursing*, 16(3), pp 225–38.

Lorion RP & Parron DL 1985, Countering the countertransference: a strategy for treating the untreatable. In: Pedersen P (ed.), *Handbook of Cross Cultural Counselling and Therapy*, Greenwood Press, Westport.

McKissock M 1992, *Coping with Grief* (rev. edn), ABC Books, Sydney.

Merry T 2000, Person-centred counselling and therapy. In: Feltham C & Horton I (eds), *Handbook of Counselling and Psychotherapy*, Sage, London, pp 348–52.

Moos N 1995, An integrative model of grief, *Death Studies*, 19(4), pp 337–64.

Moos RH & Schaefer JA 1986, Life transitions and crises: a conceptual overview. In: Moos RH (ed.) *Coping with Life Crisis: An Integrated Approach*, Plenum, New York, pp 3–28.

Morrison P, Gaskill D, Meehan T, Lunney P, Lawrence G & Collings P 2000, The use of the Liverpool University neuroleptic side-effect rating scale (LUNSERS) in clinical practice, *Australian and New Zealand Journal of Mental Health Nursing*, 9, pp 166–76.

Multicultural Mental Health Australia 2003, *Synergy*, 3, pp 1–24.

Parry G 1990, *Coping with Crises*, British Psychological Society in association with Routledge, London.

Payne M 2000, *Narrative Therapy. An Introduction for Counsellors*, Sage, London.

Payne S, Horn S & Relf M 1999, *Loss and Bereavement*, Open University Press, Oxford.

Pelzer D 2002, *My Story*, Orion, London.

Pilgrim D & Rogers A 2003, Mental disorder and violence: an empirical picture in context, *Journal of Mental Health*, 12(1), pp 7–18.

Robbins RH 1997, *Cultural Anthropology. A Problem-based Approach* (2nd edn), FE Peacock, Itasca, Illinois.

Schwartz S 2000, *Abnormal Psychology. A Discovery Approach*, Mayfield, California.

Scileppa JA, Teed EL & Torres RD 2000, *Community Psychology. A Common Sense Approach to Mental Health*, Prentice Hall, New Jersey.

Sharkey S 1999a, Crisis and risks associated with schizophrenia. In: Ryan T (ed.), *Managing Crisis and Risk in Mental Health Nursing*, Stanley Thornes, Cheltenham, pp 59–74.

Sharkey S 1999b, Crisis risks associated with depression. In: Ryan T (ed.) *Managing Crisis and Risk in Mental Health Nursing*, Stanley Thornes, Cheltenham, pp 90–104.

Sherr L 1989, *Death, Dying and Bereavement*, Blackwell, Oxford.

Slaikeu KA 1990, *Crisis Intervention. A Handbook for Practice and Research* (2nd edn), Allyn & Bacon, Boston.

Turale S 1994, Ballarat Koorie life experiences: learning about Koorie perceptions of mental health and illness, *Australian Journal of Mental Health Nursing*, 3(1), pp 16–28.

Van der Veer G 1998, *Counselling and Therapy with Refugees and Victims of Trauma. Psychological Problems of Victims of War, Torture and Repression* (2nd edn), John Wiley & Sons, Chichester.

Watkins P 2001, *Mental Health Nursing. The Art of Professional Care*, Butterworth-Heinemann, Oxford.

Worden JW 2001, *Grief Counselling and Grief Therapy. A Guide for the Mental Health Practitioner* (3rd edn), Springer, New York.

Wright B 1993, *Caring in Crisis. A Handbook of Intervention Skills* (2nd edn), Churchill Livingstone, Edinburgh.

Assessment and Diagnosis

Jan Barling

10

KEY POINTS

- Assessment and diagnosis are critical in ongoing care delivery for people with a mental disorder.
- Comprehensive biopsychosocial assessment requires specific interviewing skills.
- A biopsychosocial model of assessment gathers information based on psychiatric, physical, spiritual and cultural data.
- Risk assessment is essential in triage assessment.
- A range of measures are available to determine patient status and outcome.
- The ICD-10-AM and the DSM-IV-TR are current classification systems used in mental health.
- The use of classification systems for the diagnosis of mental disorders has raised cultural, social and professional issues.

KEY TERMS

- biopsychosocial comprehensive assessment
- classification of mental disorders
- cultural assessment
- diagnosis of mental disorders
- DSM-IV-TR
- ICD-10-AM
- mental health outcome measures
- mental status examination
- physical assessment
- risk assessment
- spiritual assessment
- triage assessment

LEARNING OUTCOMES

The material in this chapter will assist you to:
- explain the rationale for assessment, diagnosis and classification of mental disorders
- critically examine issues related to assessment, diagnosis and classification of mental disorders
- understand assessment as it relates to the Australian National Standards for Mental Health (1996)
- understand current diagnostic and classification systems in mental health
- develop an understanding of triage assessment
- identify essential interviewing skills required for the assessment process
- identify information required to conduct a comprehensive biopsychosocial assessment
- conduct a mental status examination
- explain risk assessment
- gain knowledge of observations, tests and procedures required to complete a comprehensive physical assessment
- identify appropriate outcome measures for use in mental health services.

INTRODUCTION

The cornerstone of mental health nursing is an accurate and thorough biopsychosocial and spiritual assessment. The initial assessment determines whether the person has a mental health problem, what the problem is, what the most suitable treatment may be and if there are any concurrent social or health problems that may also need attention or treatment. Therefore, a comprehensive assessment is essential in determining the patient diagnosis and developing an appropriate treatment plan.

This chapter introduces the skills and knowledge that will assist you in performing a comprehensive and accurate biopsychosocial assessment and in developing a plan of care in collaboration with the patient. This individual plan of care will determine future treatment interventions that will contribute to the patient achieving their determined goals. This chapter also introduces the diagnostic classification systems used in mental health services, along with critiques of these systems.

CLASSIFICATION SYSTEMS

The nineteenth century saw the establishment of asylums for the treatment of people suffering from a mental disorder. This period corresponded with the beginnings of scientific methodology and the classification of mental disorders through experimentation and observation.

Emil Kraepelin developed the first comprehensive classification system. Kraepelin classified all mental disorders known at the time into thirteen categories. He grouped the disorders according to common aetiology and descriptive categories based on symptom similarities. The descriptive diagnostic classification systems we use today are based on the one devised by Kraepelin (Schwartz 2000).

Classification systems provide a functional, standardised and validated means of grouping objects or phenomena (Weir & Oie 1996). A mental health professional classifies mental disorders according to patterns of behaviour, thought and emotion. Research has led to the development of a universal system of classifying mental disorders: the *Diagnostic and Statistical Manual of Mental Disorders*, 4th edition (text revision) (DSM-IV-TR) (American Psychiatric Association 2000); and the *International Statistical Classification of Diseases and Related Health Problems* (ICD-10-AM) (WHO 1992).

An understanding of classification systems enables mental health nurses to communicate effectively and professionally with other health disciplines, to participate collaboratively in patient care, to contribute to clinical research, and to organise and use data in clinical problem solving and in choosing effective interventions (Clinton & Nelson 1996). McMinn (1995) discusses the dilemma of having two classification systems when working in multidisciplinary teams; that is, the nursing diagnostic system (which is used in some settings) and the more widely accepted classification systems for mental disorders, the

DSM-IV-TR and the ICD-10-AM. The Australian National Standards for Mental Health (Australian Health Ministers Mental Health Working Group 1996) advocate the introduction of universally accepted classification systems, which will be discussed in this chapter.

ASSESSMENT

Assessment is the first step in the diagnosis of mental disorders. A mental health assessment 'is a complex intellectual activity that includes formulating hypotheses about a person, deciding what data are necessary to confirm or disconfirm these hypotheses, gathering the required data, interpreting them and finally drawing conclusions' (Schwartz 2000, p 96). Mental health assessment occurs in conjunction with a full clinical assessment: 'clinical assessment is the systematic evaluation and measurement of psychological, biological, and social factors in an individual presenting with a possible psychological disorder' (Durand & Barlow 2000, p 61).

A broader definition of assessment is:

gathering, classifying, categorising, analysing and documenting patient information about health status. It starts with the process of establishing a therapeutic alliance between the patient and the mental health worker and forms the basis of care planning. The process of assessment should be approached with empathy and compassion to support the development of trust between the patient and/or client and the mental health worker.

(NSW Health 2001, p 21)

Performing thorough, accurate and ongoing assessment is a major part of the role of the mental health nurse. Assessment is a complicated process, as the diagnosis arrived at from assessment determines the treatment for the person presenting with a mental health problem. A thorough assessment gives the opportunity to gauge consumer strengths as well as needs.

In Australia, The National Mental Health Policy (Australian Health Ministers 1992), National Standards for Mental Health (Australian Health Ministers Mental Health Working Group 1996) and the Second National Mental Health Plan (Australian Health Ministers 1998) all emphasise the importance of a thorough and comprehensive assessment for consumers accessing mental health services. Standard 11.3 of the National Standards relates to assessment and review, and provides criteria for mental health services to ensure that consumers and carers receive a comprehensive, timely and accurate assessment with a regular review of progress (Australian Health Ministers Mental Health Working Group 1996). A summary of the criteria for achieving this standard is provided in Box 10.1.

In accordance with these standards, most mental health services have developed standardised assessment protocols which staff in all health disciplines are familiar with and have been trained in. The assessment of patients presenting

---

Box 10.1 **Criteria for national standards on assessment**

- Assessments are conducted by appropriately qualified and experienced mental health professionals.
- Assessment is conducted wherever possible in settings chosen by the consumer, considering the safety of mental health staff and the consumer.
- The mental health system follows up appropriately those who decline to participate in assessment.
- Assessment records are commenced during the first contact with the service.
- Assessment is comprehensive and includes the carers and other people involved with the consumer, with the consumer's consent.
- Assessment is conducted using accepted methods and tools.
- Documented protocols and procedures within the mental health system describe the assessment process.
- Assessment is recorded in an individualised clinical record in a timely and accurate manner.
- There is an opportunity for the assessment to be conducted in the preferred language of the consumer and their carers.

- Assessment is conducted with sensitivity to cultural and language issues which may affect assessment.
- Diagnosis is made using international standards by an appropriately qualified and experienced mental health professional.
- Consumers and carers, with the consumer's consent, are provided with information on diagnosis, options for treatment and possible prognoses.
- Assessment by telephone and video technology is acceptable where face-to-face contact is not possible due to distance or the consumer's preference.
- Assessments are continually reviewed throughout the consumer's contact with the service.
- New assessments are subject to clinical review by the mental health service.
- All active consumers are re-assessed and reviewed every three months by a multidisciplinary team and recorded in the individual's clinical record.
- Staff of the mental health service involved in assessment undergo specific training in assessment and receive supervision from a more experienced colleague.

Source: Australian Health Ministers National Mental Health Working Group 1996, *National Standards in Mental Health Services*, Department of Health and Family Services, Canberra, p 31.

---

to mental health services is standardised across all disciplines, with corresponding accurate documentation. The NSW Mental Outcomes and Assessment Training Tool (NSW Health 2001) provides a standard format for documentation, with a set of expectations including:

- the domains covered in assessments and care plans at triage
- comprehensive clinical assessments
- review during ongoing care and discharge planning
- how these assessments should be recorded in the medical record
- routine outcome measures.

Similar expectations with regard to assessment and documentation in other States and Territories have been or are being implemented as part of the Second National Mental Health Plan (Australian Health Ministers 1998).

This direction in mental health services results in all health disciplines performing and documenting a standard mental health assessment that provides clear communication for all those involved in a person's care.

ESSENTIAL NURSING SKILLS

The assessment process is the first step in developing a therapeutic nurse–patient relationship. The therapeutic relationship 'represents a time-bound alliance between the nurse and patient which is consciously entered into' (Carson 2000, p 202). This relationship depends on communication skills, the most important being *empathy* and *presencing*.

Empathy represents a mutual interpersonal process in which the nurse is able to capture the inner struggle of the patient, bring together different aspects of the patient's situation in a meaningful way, and communicate that understanding in a way that is understood as truth by the patient.

(Zderad 1969, cited in Carson 2000, p 217)

Egan has expressed empathy in the following stylised formula:

You feel . . . (name the correct emotion expressed by the client) . . . because or when . . . (here indicate the correct experiences and behaviours that give rise to the feelings.

(Egan 1998, p 84)

This formula allows the patient to feel heard and understood. 'Presencing' has been defined as 'attempting to be non-judgmental and non-defensive while creating a conducive environment for an open constructive conversation and allowing the experience of the client to affect you' (Glass 2003, p 55). Glass also states (p 55) that 'presencing concerns a head and heart shift, it involves suppressing your own concerns and moving from your own space/happenings to the client's space/happening'. As such, presencing involves 'being in the moment' with the patient and giving your undivided attention. This skill has also been referred to as *immediacy* (refer to Ch 22).

Chapter 22 addresses the communication skills that are needed to achieve empathy and immediacy when interviewing a patient. The following issues also need to be considered:

- Where possible the nurse should interview the patient in a location where the patient's dignity, privacy and comfort are respected. A quiet, private setting where patient and nurse can interact at eye level provides the structure for the formation of a therapeutic alliance.

- Consider the patient's developmental stage. Major crises that occur in life are often related to the transition required through each stage. For example, is a young mother's depression related to the transition from 'independent' career woman to 'dependent' mother? Is the sixteen-year-old's antisocial behaviour related to the transitional period of childhood to adolescence? A developmental perspective can assist the nurse in understanding the client's perspective (refer to Ch 8).

- Be aware of apprehension in the patient. Most people presenting for assessment are fearful or confused about symptoms they have experienced. They may also be embarrassed about the stigma surrounding mental illness. In addition, some believe that professionals working in mental health can 'read' people's minds or at least have remarkable powers of insight into the individual. Some inexperienced nurses are apprehensive about communicating with people with a mental disorder. Being aware of the patient's apprehension may facilitate understanding of the problem.

- Explore general issues first, then be more specific. The nurse should take a broad, holistic approach at the beginning of the interview. The first three to ten minutes should be the most open-ended of the interview. Using open-ended questions will help the patient to begin to feel respected and listened to, and be more willing to focus on specific issues. The nurse's responses during the initial assessment phase should be focused on building rapport, and should consist of empathetic silences, repeating the patient's last words, identifying the patient's affect ('That must have made you very sad') and requesting clarification.

- As the nurse begins to develop an overall picture of the patient, questions become more specific and direct: 'Tell me more about this depression, Mr Jones'.

- As the assessment interview progresses, the nurse should ask more focused questions: 'How long have you been feeling that life is hopeless?', 'How many kilos have you lost in the past month?'. At this stage of the interview the nurse is trying to collect information related to when the symptoms appeared, whether they have been getting better or worse, what the symptoms are like, how severe they are and their relation to other symptoms. Collecting this information enables the nurse to formulate a diagnosis related to diagnostic criteria for specific mental disorders.

- Finally, the nurse should focus on closed questions— that is, questions with a yes or no answer: 'Have you ever had blackouts?', 'Have you found yourself thinking that everyone is against you?'.

The development of interviewing skills will ensure that the nurse and the patient can enter into a therapeutic relationship where problems are identified and a plan of care is established.

BIOPSYCHOSOCIAL MODEL OF ASSESSMENT

A biopsychosocial assessment involves a comprehensive assessment of all aspects of the patient's problem—biological, psychological, sociological, developmental, spiritual and cultural—with information derived from interviews with the patient and their family, or others as appropriate. Concerns need to be addressed in terms of how they may have led to the illness developing and how they may be maintaining the problem behaviour for the patient (Onyett 1992).

Assessment is completed with all patients, regardless of the setting. The forms used and details sought may vary, but the principal information gathered is similar. Broadly speaking, the information gathered in an assessment interview provides the framework for a comprehensive biopsychosocial assessment of the patient's current presentation to mental health services.

When assessing a person for the first time, information needs to be gathered in order to answer the following questions:

- Does the person have a mental health problem? If so, what is the problem?
- What is the most suitable treatment for the individual?
- Can the team provide appropriate treatment? If not, to whom can the individual be referred?
- If the individual is accepted for treatment, are there concurrent social or health problems that need urgent attention before psychiatric treatment commences?
- What effect might the intervention have on the individual's health status? (Adapted from Treatment Protocol Project 2000, p 9.)

Psychiatric assessment

The purpose of the psychiatric assessment is to develop an understanding of the person presenting for help. It involves taking a basic psychiatric history and a mental status assessment. The following information is required in conducting a comprehensive psychiatric assessment:

- identifying information
- reason for referral
- presenting problem and/or precipitating factors
- previous mental health history/medical history/drug history
- developmental/psychosocial/ relationship history
- risk factors
- assessment of strengths
- assessment of mental health status.

Identifying information

Identifying information includes: name, age, sex, present address, telephone number, languages spoken, general practitioner, marital status, occupation and next of kin. Some forms will require additional information about children, education level attained and family of origin, for example.

Example

Mary Jones is 32 years old, married, with four children, lives at 22 Brown St, telephone number 8888 888. She speaks English and is working part time in a real estate office. Her regular GP, Max Smith, is aware of her coming to the Cowan Mental Health Clinic today.

Reason for referral

This should include:

- who has asked for the patient to be seen and why
- the nature of the problem
- events that led to this presentation
- any recent suicide attempts
- any recent episodes of self-harm.

Example

Mary presented to a community mental health clinic with her husband. She was referred by her GP, who was concerned about Mary's deteriorating mental state over the last three months and requested a mental health assessment. There have been no recent suicide attempts or episodes of self-harm.

Presenting problem

Obtain a brief description of the principal complaint and the time frame in the patient's own words. Listening to the patient facilitates the development of a therapeutic alliance.

You will need to obtain the following information:

- specific symptoms that are present and their duration
- time relationships between the onset or exacerbation of symptoms and the presence of social stressors/physical illness
- any disturbance in mood, appetite, sexual drive or sleep
- any treatments given by other doctors or specialists for this problem
- the individual's response to treatment.

The following narratives provide examples of how the mental health nurse can maximise the quality of information sought.

First, determine the consumer's perception of the situation.

Example

Nurse: Mary, Dr Smith asked me to see you today because he is concerned about some of the things you have been saying and doing. Can you tell me what you think has been going on?

Mary: I have been feeling really confused and upset for the last few months and just not right.

Nurse: What are some of the things that may be making you feel just not right?

Mary: I don't seem to be able to cope with everyday living and lately I have been hearing voices, which are really upsetting me.

Nurse: How are the voices upsetting you?

Mary: They are in my head all the time and they keep telling me to kill myself. It's horrible.

Second, get an overview of the precipitating factors/ events. Ensure that the chronology of the events and the emergence of the symptoms are clear. The context of the presenting problem is also important. Box 10.2 details the social and environmental precipitating events that may have triggered the episode or be maintaining the behaviour.

Example

Nurse: How long have you been feeling 'not right'?

Mary: It seemed to happen soon after Jenny was born. At first, I would cry all the time and couldn't manage any of the housework. It was really difficult trying to look after Jenny and the other kids. Sometimes I would go to bed because I just didn't want to face the day. I thought there was something really wrong, because I wasn't sleeping or eating and I kept getting headaches, muscle aches and pains and

---

Box 10.2 Precipitating environmental and social problems

- **Problems with primary support**: death of family member, health problems in family, disruption of family by separation, divorce or estrangement, removal from home, remarriage of parents, sexual or physical abuse, parental overprotection, neglect of child, inadequate discipline, discord with siblings, birth of siblings.
  Note: In most States, reporting of suspected child abuse is mandatory for health-care professionals.
- **Problems related to social environment**: death of family member, inadequate social support, living alone, difficulty with acculturation, discrimination, adjustment to life-cycle transition, care of animals if admission required.
- **Educational problems**: literacy, academic problems, discord with teachers and classmates, inadequate school environment.
- **Occupational problems**: unemployment, threat of job loss, stressful work schedule, difficult work conditions, job dissatisfaction, job change, discord with boss or co-workers.
- **Economic problems**: extreme poverty, inadequate finances, insufficient welfare support.
- **Problems with access to health care**: inadequate health-care services, transportation to health-care facilities unavailable, inadequate health insurance.
- **Problems related to interaction with the legal system**: arrest, incarceration, litigation, victim of crime.
- **Other psychosocial and environmental problems**: exposure to disasters, war, other hostilities, discord with non-family caregivers such as counsellor, social worker or physician, unavailability of social service agencies.

Source: adapted from New South Wales Health, 2001, *NSW Mental Health Outcome and Assessment Training (MH-OAT) Facilitator's Manual*, NSW Health, Sydney, p 93.

an upset stomach. I have been seeing Dr Smith a lot, hoping he could fix me up.

Nurse: When was Jenny born?

Mary: June the 18th. She will be three months old tomorrow.

Nurse: You said you told Dr Smith about the voices this morning. Have the voices been bothering you ever since you felt not right, after Jenny was born?

Mary: No, the voices only started about a month ago, but they are getting worse and I don't know what to do. It feels like I'm going mad.

The nurse would have to ask more open-ended questions to determine whether any other social or environmental problems may have precipitated or be contributing to the problem.

Mental health/medical/drug history

Mental health history—Information required includes the number of admissions to mental health inpatient units, number of episodes of self-harm, attempted suicide or occasions of assault, and an indication of any mental health treatments received. This information is usually obtained from the patient, previous clinical notes, a letter from the doctor, or history provided by relatives or friends.

Example

Nurse: Mary, what you are experiencing must be pretty scary. Has this ever happened before?

Mary: No, this is the first time I have ever felt like I have been going mad and the voices really frighten me.

Nurse: What about after the other three kids were born. How did you feel then?

Mary: I had no problem at all. Everyone has always said how together I am. That's why this is really freaking me out.

Medical history—Information includes major medical and surgical history. If relevant, the patient's consent should be sought to obtain a detailed medical history from the treating doctor.

Example

Nurse: Have you ever been in hospital for an operation or a medical complaint?

Mary: No, I was just in hospital for the birth of the kids. The last one was pretty tiring and hard.

Nurse: Did you have any medical problems after the birth?

Mary: No, I just have long births and lots of pain.

Nurse: Do you have any physical problems for which the doctor is treating you?

Mary: No, apart from the last three months with the headaches and stomach aches.

Nurse: To help us obtain a better picture of your health, will you give us your consent to obtain information from your doctor if we need to?

Drug history—Gather information related to the current medications the person is taking. This includes prescription and non-prescription medication, including complementary medication.

Other important information includes:

- the medication regimen
- all prescribed and non-prescribed medications, including natural remedies
- an indication of dosage, frequency and prescriber
- when drugs were last used
- any compliance problems with taking the medication
- whether the patient has ever had any adverse reactions to any drugs
- whether the patient is allergic to any drugs.

Example

Nurse: Are you taking any medication that the doctor has prescribed for you?

Mary: Not that I can remember.

Nurse: So, you are not taking any medication to help with things that have been happening in the last three months?

Mary: Just over the last month I have been taking Valium to help me sleep at night.

Nurse: Can you remember how much?

Mary: Yes, 5 mg.

Nurse: How often do you take it?

Mary: Every night.

Nurse: Can you think of any other medications the doctor has prescribed?

In some areas, specific assessment charts are provided in order to obtain detailed information on drug and alcohol intake.

Psychosocial/relationship history

This outlines circumstances that are significant for understanding current issues and covers many aspects of the individual's life, such as relationships, family background, work or school history and, possibly, developmental stages.

Obtain information about:

- infancy (especially important if the presenting patient is a child)
- childhood and adolescence
- work history
- marital history
- relationships with others
- children
- illegal activities.

Example

Mary is the middle of three children, both siblings being males. Her parents are alive, retired and living 100 kilometres away. Mary remembers that her parents' relationship was tense (when she was young) but seemed to improve as she and her brothers grew older. She believes her relationship with John, her husband (of ten years), is 'okay' and that with four children and her job there is no time for arguments.

The children are aged eight years, six years, five years and three months, and Mary says she enjoys the company of the older children. She enjoys her part-time work, twelve hours per week, although it has been more difficult since her youngest child was born.

Determining risk factors

Several risk factors need to be assessed for each patient:

- harm to others
- harm to self
- suicide
- absconding
- vulnerability to exploitation or abuse (sexual)
- vulnerability to exploitation or abuse (violence).

Assessment of the above risk factors is documented in the triage section of this chapter.

Example

Nurse: You mentioned that the voices were frightening and that they were telling you to kill yourself. How do they do this?

Mary: They tell me to do certain things like jump in front of a train. It's awful.

Nurse: Are the voices so strong that you think you might try and kill yourself?

Mary: No, I am managing to stay in control, but it is a constant battle.

Nurse: How do you stay in control?

Mary: I just think of what it would do to the family. But at times I think I would be better off dead.

Nurse: So you have no plan to kill yourself?

Mary: No, I have never thought about how I would kill myself. I'm just concerned about the voices.

Nurse: Do the voices say anything else?

Mary: Sometimes they tell me to take Jenny with me as she would be better off dead. They say things like, 'Take the baby and go and stand on the road'.

Assessment of strengths

There is little within any of the formal assessment tools that assesses the strengths of the consumer. In Mary's case, noting that she has financial or family support can be seen as a positive feature in this regard.

Examples of strengths and resources include:

- intelligence
- education
- support systems
- religious and spiritual beliefs
- motivation
- physical health.

Mental status examination

The mental status examination (MSE) is a semi-structured interview used mainly as a screening tool to assess a person's current neurological and psychological status along several dimensions. The exam involves observations as well as an interview.

Example

Mary presents as neatly dressed with make-up applied and hair combed. She does not make eye contact and sits with her hands clenched in her lap. She speaks quietly using full sentences. Mary states that she feels depressed, and her affect is flat. She states that she feels suicidal and has auditory hallucinations. Mary is orientated to time and place and says that it is 'not normal' to hear voices. She is prepared to have treatment and appreciates the reassurance of safety.

Nurse: It sounds like you have been having a rough time of it since Jenny was born. What are some of the things that have been bothering you?

Mary: I don't seem to be able to enjoy things anymore ... It is a real struggle for me to get out of bed in the morning and day-to-day chores are very difficult ... I feel very sad and I cry all the time ... It is so bad that I sometimes feel life is not worth living.

Nurse: You sound depressed and unhappy ... You mentioned that you sometimes think life is not worth living. Have you ever thought of killing yourself?

Mary: Sometimes I think about it but I manage to talk myself out of it. I know I would never do anything as drastic as that but I feel so low sometimes that I think about it a lot.

Nurse: Do you know why you are here today?

Mary: Yes, Doctor Smith referred me to the community mental health centre because he was worried about the voices I have been hearing for the last month.

Nurse: Are you worried about the voices as well?

Mary: Yes. I know this is not normal and they are starting to frighten me.

Nurse: You mentioned thinking about killing yourself and that the voices are telling you to kill yourself and maybe Jenny. Do you believe the voices are powerful enough to convince you to run in front of a train or to take Jenny out on the road?

Mary: They are very scary, and I am frightened they may take control. That is why I really need help.

Nurse: It concerns me that you are frightened by the voices which are telling you to kill yourself and that you sometimes think about killing yourself. I think we may need to put a plan of action in place that ensures that you and Jenny are safe. Is that okay with you?

Mary: Yes, anything so I can start feeling normal again.

Nurse: Would you be willing to see the psychiatrist and see where to go from there, maybe start some medications?

Mary: Yes, if it will stop the voices and start making me feel better, I'll do anything.

Following are the components of the MSE and relevant observations for each component (Treatment Protocol Project 2000, pp 13–18).

Appearance and behaviour

The aim of this section is to observe and describe the manner and appearance of the individual at the time of assessment.

- Describe the individual's physical appearance (grooming, hygiene, clothing (including shoes), nails, build, tattoos and other significant features).
- What is the individual's reaction to the present situation and the examiner (hostile, friendly, withdrawn, guarded, cooperative, uncommunicative, seductive)?
- Describe the individual's motor behaviour (psychomotor retarded, restless, repetitive behaviours, hyperactive, tremor, hand-wringing, bizarre) (include description).

Speech

The physical aspects of speech can be described in terms of rate, volume and quantity of information (slow, rapid, monotonous, loud, quiet, slurred, whispered). Some particular characteristics of speech you might consider are:

- mutism—total absence of speech
- poverty of speech—replies to questions are brief and monosyllabic
- pressure of speech—speech is extremely rapid, difficult to interrupt, loud and hard to understand.

Mood and affect

Mood describes internal feeling or emotion, which often influences behaviour and the individual's perception of the world. *Affect* refers to the external emotional response. Both aspects can provide useful diagnostic information.

- Describe the individual's mood (depressed, euphoric, childish, silly, labile (alternating between extremes), suspicious, fearful, hostile, anxious, irritable, self-contemptuous).
- Describe the individual's affect. Note whether the emotional response is appropriate given the subject matter being discussed. Some terms you may need to be familiar with are:
    - *normal*—expected variations in facial expression, voice, gestures and movements that are congruent with the context or topic of discussion
    - *restricted*—decreased intensity and range of emotional expression
    - *blunted*—severe decrease in intensity and range of emotional expression
    - *flat*—almost complete or complete absence of emotional expression with accompanying expressionless face and monotonous voice.

Form of thought

This is assessed according to:

- amount of thought and its rate of production (poverty of ideas, flight of ideas, slow or hesitant thinking, vague)

- continuity of ideas (the logical order or flow of ideas). Individuals may or may not be able to stick to the topic of conversation. They may digress into irrelevant conversation, completely lose their train of thought, or talk 'around' the topic.
- disturbance in language (the use of words that do not exist or conversations that do not make sense). Some important terms that indicate disturbance in form of thought are listed in the glossary.

Box 10.3 Types of delusions

Delusions associated with schizophrenia

- **Delusions of persecution:** beliefs that centre on the theme that one is being deliberately wronged, conspired against, or harmed by another person/agency.
- **Delusional mood:** the individual feels that his or her familiar environment has changed in some way that is puzzling. The individual may not be able to describe this change clearly.
- **Delusions of reference:** the belief that events or other people's actions or words refer specifically to the individual and have a special meaning for the individual. Does not include being overly self-conscious as in social phobia. (Note: ideas of reference are false beliefs which are not as firmly held as delusions, and for which the individual may be persuaded to see an alternative point of view.)
- **Delusions of control, influence or passivity:** the belief that one's feelings, impulses, thoughts or actions are not one's own, but are controlled by an external force. The individual must acknowledge that they no longer have a will of their own but are being controlled by another force (other than God or fate).

Delusions not necessarily associated with schizophrenia

- **Religious delusions:** the individual believes they have a special link with God/Christ. Excludes intense religious or cultural beliefs.
- **Nihilistic delusions:** the individual believes that the self or part of the self does not exist, or is dead, or that others or the world do not exist. Often associated with depressive episodes.
- **Fantastic delusions:** the belief that the individual has had an amazing adventure or experience. Often associated with manic episodes.
- **Delusions of jealousy:** belief, without good reason, that one's partner is unfaithful. May be associated with a delusional disorder.
- **Grandiose delusions:** exaggerated belief of one's importance, power, knowledge or identity. Often associated with manic episodes or schizophrenia.

Source: Treatment Protocol Project 2000, *Management of Mental Disorders*, Vol. 1 (3rd edn), World Health Organization, Collaborating Centre For Mental Health And Substance Abuse, Sydney, p 15.

Thought content

Assessment is of:

- *delusions*—false beliefs that are firmly held despite objective and contradictory evidence, and despite the fact that other members of the culture do not share the same beliefs. There are numerous types of delusions, some of which tend to be associated with different disorders. For definitions of the types of delusions that nurses need to be familiar with, refer to Box 10.3.
- *suicidal thoughts*—these will be dealt with in more detail when examining the assessment of risk factors in the context of a comprehensive biopsychosocial assessment.
- *other*—this includes obsessions, compulsions, antisocial urges, phobias, intentions, hypochondriacal symptoms and preoccupations (perhaps with illness).

Perception

Assess for hallucinations. A hallucination is a false sensory perception in which the individual sees, hears, smells and senses or tastes something that other people do not. The hallucination occurs in the absence of appropriate external stimulus. Hallucinations are not necessarily associated with a psychotic disturbance and can occur when falling asleep (hypnogogic hallucinations), when waking up (hypnopompic hallucinations) or in the course of an intense religious experience. The type of hallucination and the content should be described. Some types of hallucinations and perceptual disorders are described in Box 10.4.

Sensorium and cognition

Level of consciousness—Impairment of consciousness usually indicates organic brain disease.

Memory—The three main areas of memory are: immediate, recent and remote. The clinician often obtains most of the information about the individual's memory through responses to other questions during the course of the interview.

Orientation—Obvious disturbances in orientation usually indicate organic brain disease. The commonly used categories for assessment of orientation are time, place and person. Impairments usually develop in this order and, if treatable, usually clear in the reverse order.

Concentration—Concentration may be assessed by asking the individual to subtract serial 7's from 100. This task is only necessary if you suspect that there is some degree of impairment. Performance anxiety, mood disturbance, an alteration of consciousness, or a lack of education may interfere with this task.

Abstract thought—Abstract thinking involves the ability to:
- deal with concepts
- extract common characteristics from groups or objects
- juggle more than one idea at a time
- interpret information.

Abstract thinking may be assessed by asking the individual to interpret the meaning of common proverbs (e.g. a bird in the hand is worth two in the bush). Care needs to be taken when using proverbs

---

Box 10.4 Types of hallucinations and other perceptual disorders

- **Auditory hallucinations:** may be non-verbal (tapping, humming, music, laughing) or verbal (conversation, accusatory; often associated with depression). An auditory hallucination is probably the most common type of hallucination.
- **Visual hallucinations:** being able to see objects, people or images that others cannot see. Most commonly occurs in organic mental disorders.
- **Olfactory hallucination:** smelling things that do not exist. Most commonly occurs in organic mental disorders.
- **Gustatory hallucination:** relate to a sense of taste. Most commonly occur in organic mental disorders.
- **Tactile hallucination:** the false perception of touch or surface sensation, such as from an amputated (phantom) limb, or crawling sensations on or under the skin.
- **Somatic hallucinations:** the false perception that things are occurring in or to the body.

Other perceptual disturbances
- **Derealisation:** the external world appears different and unfamiliar. The individual feels distanced from the world

and things may seem colourless and dead. Derealisation may be associated with extreme anxiety, stress, fatigue and affective disorder, or with hyperventilation, which is a symptom of panic disorder.
- **Depersonalisation:** the perception of the self seems different or unfamiliar. The individual may feel unreal, or that their body is somehow distorted, or may have a sense of perceiving themselves from a distance. In its severe form the individual may actually feel as if they are dead. May be associated with extreme anxiety, stress or fatigue.
- **Heightened perception:** perceptions are extremely vivid. For example, sounds are unnaturally loud, clear or intense, colours are more brilliant or beautiful, and details of the environment tend to stand out in an interesting way.
- **Dulled perception:** perceptions are experienced as dark, uninteresting and flat. For example, tastes are blunted, colours muddied or dirtied, and sounds are impure or ugly. Excludes the individual lacking interest in things.

mental disorder. These tests are ordered by the medical officer. A few investigations, such as a full blood count and general biomedical indices (renal, liver function, electrolytes and thyroid function) are almost universally indicated. Table 10.1 lists the laboratory tests and their relevance to psychiatric disorders.

Table 10.1 Haematological tests related to psychiatric disorders

Test	Possible results	Possible cause or meaning
Full blood count (FBC)		
Leukocyte count (WBC)	■ Leukopenia (decrease in leukocytes) ■ Agranulocytosis (decrease in the number of granulocytic leukocytes) ■ Leukocytosis (increase in leukocyte count above normal limits)	■ May be produced by: phenothiazines, clozapine, carbamazepine ■ Lithium causes a benign mild-to-moderate increase ■ Neuroleptic malignant syndrome (NMS) also associated with an increase
WBC differential	■ 'Shift to the left' from segmented neutrophils to band forms	■ Shift often suggests bacterial infections ■ Has been reported in about 40% of cases of NMS
Red blood cell count (RBC)	■ Polycythemia (increased RBCs) ■ Anaemia (decreased RBCs)	■ *Primary form*: caused by several disease states ■ *Secondary form*: compensation for decreased oxygenation, such as chronic pulmonary disease ■ Blood is more viscous, and the patient should not become dehydrated ■ Related to some form of anaemia which requires further investigation
Haematocrit (Hct)	■ Increase ■ Decrease (related to anaemia)	■ May be due to dehydration ■ May be associated with a wide range of mental health changes including asthenia, depression and psychosis ■ 20% of women of child-bearing age have iron deficiency anaemia
Haemoglobin (Hb)	■ Decrease	■ Another indicator of anaemia
Erythrocyte indices: red cell distribution width (RDW)	■ Elevated RDW	■ Suggests a combined anaemia related to chronic alcoholism, resulting from vitamin B_{12}, folate and iron deficiencies
Other haematological measures		
Vitamin B_{12}	■ Deficiency	■ Neuropsychiatric symptoms such as psychosis, paranoia, fatigue, agitation, marked personality change, dementia and delirium may develop ■ Oral contraceptives decrease B_{12}
Folate	■ Deficiency	■ Alcohol, phenytoin, oral contraceptives and oestrogens may be responsible
Platelet count	■ Thrombocytopenia—decrease	■ Psychiatric medications such as carbamazepine, phenothiazines, clozapine, or other non-psychiatric medications ■ Several medical conditions
Serum electrolytes		
Sodium	■ Hyponatremia—low serum sodium	■ Significant mental state changes may ensue ■ Associated with: Addison's disease, syndrome of inappropriate secretion of antidiuretic hormone (SIADH), polydipsia (water intoxication) and carbamazepine use
Potassium	■ Hypokalemia—low serum potassium	■ Produces weakness, fatigue, electrocardiogram changes, paralytic ileus and muscle paresis. ■ Associated with: bulimia, psychogenic vomiting, use and abuse of diuretics and laxative abuse ■ Can be life threatening
Chloride	■ Increase ■ Decrease	■ Increases to compensate for lower bicarbonate ■ Associated with: bingeing/purging behaviour and repeated vomiting
Bicarbonate	■ Increase ■ Decrease	■ Associated with bingeing and purging, excessive use of laxatives, psychogenic vomiting ■ May develop in some patients with hyperventilation syndrome and panic disorder

Table 10.1 Haematological tests related to psychiatric disorders (*continued*)

Test	Possible results	Possible cause or meaning
Renal function tests		
Blood urea nitrogen (BUN)	■ Increase	■ Cause may be dehydration ■ Associated with mental status changes, lethargy and delirium ■ Toxicity of medications cleared by the kidney (such as lithium) may increase
Serum creatinine	■ Increase	■ Does not usually become elevated until 50% of the nephrons in the kidney are damaged
Serum enzymes		
Amylase	■ Increase	■ Associated with: bingeing/purging behaviour in eating disorders
Alanine aminotransferase (ALT)	■ ALT > AST	■ Common in acute forms of viral and drug-induced hepatic dysfunction
Aspartate aminotransferase (AST)	■ Increase ■ AST > ALT	■ Use of sodium valproate ■ Severe elevations in chronic forms of liver disease and in some myocardial infarctions
Creatine phosphokinase (CPK)	■ Increase	■ Muscle tissue injury ■ Neuroleptic malignant syndrome ■ Repeated intramuscular injections e.g. depot antipsychotics
Thyroid function		
Serum triiodothyronine (T3)	■ Decrease	■ Hypothyroidism ■ Individuals with depression may convert less T4 to T3 ■ Lithium and sodium valproate may suppress thyroid function
Serum thyroxine (T4)	■ Increase	■ Hyperthyroidism, T3 toxicosis, may produce mood changes, anxiety and symptoms of mania
Thyroid stimulating hormone (TSH)	■ Increase ■ Decrease	■ Hyperthyroidism as a cause, symptoms as in increase of T3 ■ Hypothyroidism—symptoms similar to depression, except for cold intolerance, dry skin, hair loss and bradycardia ■ Lithium may also cause increase ■ Considered non-diagnostic—may be hyperthyroidism, pituitary hypothyroidism

Source: Boyd M 2002, *Psychiatric Nursing: Contemporary Practice*, 2nd edn, Lippincott, New York, pp 203–4.

Spiritual assessment

The spiritual dimension is often overlooked in assessment. It is important because it provides a deeper understanding of the patient, their social setting and the possible origins of the problem. Carson proposes that 'the presence and intensity of faith in God, degree of religious commitment, and sense of purpose and meaning along with basic life values, strongly affect the patient's potential for recovery' (Carson 2000, p 253).

Elkins et al. (1998) identify the following characteristics of spirituality:

- provides a transcendental dimension, possibly but not necessarily experienced as a personal god
- acts as a source of meaning in life, filling an existential vacuum
- creates a sense of mission or vocation and the sacredness of life
- enables experiences of awe, reverence and wonder
- promotes an awareness and acceptance of the tragic as part of life
- frequently challenges material values

- usually promotes altruism and idealism
- may change all aspects of being and living
- may be experienced without formal religion.

Spirituality is often neglected in the understanding of mental health problems. Meadows (2001) believes that patients may be hesitant in talking about their spiritual experiences as they believe that the experience is interpreted as abnormal or 'crazy' by the clinician. Even if the clinician accepts the reality of the patient's experience, team and organisational factors may hinder further discussion. It is important to realise that each individual has their own unique spiritual interpretation of the universe and as such none of us can claim to understand the correct spiritual nature of things (Post, Puchalski & Larson, cited in Meadows & Singh 2000). It is therefore important that the spiritual dimension of an assessment is not overlooked. Creating a setting where the person feels safe to talk about the spiritual dimension of their being is important to facilitate this form of assessment. Table 10.2 provides questions that may be of benefit in conducting a spiritual assessment.

Table 10.2 Questions to use in spiritual and philosophical assessment

Concept of God	Is religion or God important to you? If so can you describe how?
	Do you use prayer in your life? If so, does prayer benefit you in any way?
	Do you believe that God or a deity is involved in your personal life? If so how?
	What is your God or deity like?
Sources of strength and hope	Who are your support people?
	Who is the most important person in your life?
	Are people available to you when you are in need?
	Who or what provides you with strength and hope?
Religious practices	Is your religious faith helpful to you?
	Are any religious practices meaningful to you?
	Has your illness affected your religious practices?
	Are any religious books or symbols helpful to you?
Meaning and purpose	What gives your life meaning and purpose?
	What makes you get up out of bed every morning and do what you have to do?
	Do you feel that your life makes a difference? If so in what ways?
	In what ways has your illness had an impact on your meaning and purpose?

Source: Carson V 2000, *Mental Health Nursing: The Nurse–Patient Journey* (2nd edn), WB Saunders, Sydney, p 253.

Cultural assessment

Cultural assessment is a complex issue. Given the diversity of cultures in the Australian community it would be impossible for the mental health nurse to understand all cultures. Despite this, mental health nurses need to engage the patient and the family so that appropriate care can be given. Adoption and application of the underlying principles of cultural safety (see Ch 6) by nurses in Australia and New Zealand will enable appropriate assessment.

Attitudes that interfere with appropriate assessment include:

- *ethnocentrism*: the belief that our world view, based on the values and norms of our culture, is superior to others and is the only valid world view (Frisch & Frisch 2002, p 115)
- *stereotyping*: the failure to identify individual variations and differences within cultural groups. It results in expectations that all individuals within certain cultural groups will have the same values, beliefs, customs and behaviours. Individuals within these cultural groups are labelled according to this stereotype (Frisch & Frisch 2002, p 116).
- *cultural blindness*: an attempt to treat all people fairly by ignoring differences within a culture and acting as though the differences do not exist. Such cultural blindness can be seen as insensitivity just as much as stereotyping and ethnocentrism (Frisch & Frisch 2002, p 117).

Being aware of these attitudes in ourselves and others is the first step in developing awareness of our values and how they affect practice.

Failure to communicate effectively with clients can cause delays in diagnosis and treatment and can have tragic results (Crisp & Taylor 2001). Crisp & Taylor (2001, p 132) identify some barriers to communication of which nurses and other health-care workers should be aware:

- the formal use of one national language (such as English)
- institutional racism and prejudice
- racist and prejudicial attitudes of both nurse and clients towards each other
- ethnocentrism and stereotyping
- cultural differences
- differences in class and education between clients and nurses
- different experiences
- different perceptions of health and illness
- unfamiliar health-care systems
- different expectations of health care
- culture shock.

Box 10.5 highlights the communication skills that may assist when communicating with people from different cultural backgrounds.

Narayan (2003) has developed a cultural assessment checklist that may assist nurses during the first interview to develop a rapport and an understanding of the particular patient's culture—see Table 10.3 (on p 162).

Triage assessment

A triage assessment refers to the decision-making process that occurs when alternatives for acute care are being considered. The factors that influence the decisions made need to be based on a holistic system of care. A thorough biopsychosocial approach, where all relevant aspects of the person's symptoms and current situation are considered, is most appropriate. The principle of any triage

> **Box 10.5 Communication skills for communicating with people from different ethnic backgrounds**
>
> - Speak slowly, audibly and distinctly and use terminology that patients from other cultures can understand.
> - Use simple words and avoid jargon.
> - Listen as much as you speak; do not interrupt, because this can be seen as rude.
> - Allow extra time to communicate with someone whose language is not your own. Trying to understand one another may take extra effort and time.
> - Respect silence; do not fill every gap in the conversation.
> - When you experience frustration or sense conflict or mis-understanding in a cross-cultural situation, stop and ask yourself whether the conflict is due to cultural differences. Try to see a common basis or understanding.
> - Adapt your style to the demands of the situation. Speak the patient's language.
> - Do not make judgments about people based on their accent or language fluency.
> - Be open and sensitive about how you give feedback.
> - Know who in the family is the appointed head or decision-maker.
> - Understand the 'hot buttons' that can lead to conflict.
> - Avoid using slang.
> - Do not use racial or ethnic epithets.
> - Avoid verbal and non-verbal behaviour that does not meet accepted cultural norms, including definite pro-nouncements about a culture that is not your own.
> - Identify and network with the traditional brokers and healers.
> - Ask the patient if he or she uses herbs and what the expected benefits are.
> - Learn to identify culturally relevant rituals.
> - Stress the patient's strengths and demonstrate respect and caring.

Source: Carson V 2000, *Mental Health Nursing: The Nurse–Patient Journey* (2nd edn), WB Saunders, Sydney, p 278.

system is for the right person to be directed to the right place at the right time for the right reasons (NSW Health 2001).

A triage assessment is completed at a face-to-face presentation at an emergency department or mental health acute-care service. Key questions that need to be asked at the presentation of the patient are as follows:
- Is this an acute medical or surgical rather than psychiatric emergency?
- Is this patient an acute risk for assaulting staff or other patients?
- Is the patient at acute risk of serious harm to self?
- Should the patient be able to leave if he or she wishes to?
- Does the patient need to be seen straight away or can he or she safely wait a while?
- Does the patient need to be seen at all? (Treatment Protocol Project 2003, p 40)

A Crisis Triage Rating Scale (CTRS) (Bengelsdorf et al. 1984) has been developed to screen emergency psychiatric patients rapidly. The scale evaluates patients according to three factors. A descriptive statement accompanies each score.
- Dangerousness (1 = most dangerous to self or others, 5 = least dangerous)
- Support system (1 = poor or absent, 5 = excellent)
- Motivation and cooperation (1 = least likely to cooperate, 5 = most likely).

This scale is useful in predicting whether hospitalisation is required. The three scores are added to give a minimum of 3 and a maximum of 15. A score below 9 indicates a need for hospitalisation, above 9 indicates that another form of intervention is required (Treatment Protocol Project 2000; Bengelsdorf et al. 1984). A critical

appraisal of the client's risk status is essential in triage. Risk status is rated on a four-point scale from low to extreme, and is assessed in four domains:
- harm to others
- harm to self
- suicide
- absconding.

Risk of harm to others
Patients rated as low on the scale would present with no indication of violence or aggression prior to assessment, while consumers who rated at the extreme end of the scale would be engaging in aggressive behaviours such as verbal abuse and physical aggression. They may be openly threatening harm and have access to weapons. Behaviours related to the moderate and high risk of harm to others would include a previous history of violence, poor impulse control, being in a delusional state, and the content of the delusions, evidence of substance abuse and/or withdrawal, and body language consistent with potential aggression, such as fist clenching, pacing, restlessness, agitation and disruptive behaviour (NSW Health 2001).

Risk of harm to self
Patients rated low on the scale would have had no indication of self-harm prior to assessment, while those rated as extreme would be engaging in self-harm or self-mutilating activities. Some patients may be engaging in self-mutilating activities as a result of demand hallucinations (auditory hallucinations that tell the person to perform acts that they do not want to), or acting on delusional beliefs that involve self-harm activities. Behaviours equating to moderate and high-risk status include a history of previous self-harm behaviour, intrusive thought of self-harm behaviour,

Table 10.3 Cultural assessment checklist

Degree of acculturation	■ How strictly does the patient adhere to the beliefs and values of their culture of origin in comparison to internalisation of new cultural norms?
Language and communication	■ What language is the patient most comfortable speaking and reading? ■ Does the patient require an interpreter?
Non-verbal patterns of communication ■ Eye contact ■ Tone of voice ■ Personal space ■ Facial expressions, gestures ■ Touch	■ Is eye contact considered polite or rude? ■ Is special meaning attached to loud or whispered conversations? ■ Is personal space wider or closer than in your culture? ■ What is the meaning behind certain facial expressions and hand/body gestures? ■ When, where and by whom can a patient be touched?
Etiquette and social customs ■ Typical greeting ■ Social customs before business ■ Direct or indirect communication patterns	■ How would you like to be greeted/addressed by our staff? ■ What behaviour is expected of guests? Taking off shoes, accepting food and drink? ■ Is it polite to engage in small talk before getting down to business? ■ Should discussion be direct and forthright or subtle and indirect?
Patient's explanation of the problem ■ Diagnosis ■ Onset ■ Cause ■ Course ■ Prognosis ■ Treatment	■ What do you call this problem? How would you describe this problem? ■ When and how did the problem begin? Why then? ■ What caused the problem? Why do you think you developed this problem and not someone else? What might other people think is wrong with you? ■ What are the chief problems this condition has caused you? ■ What do you fear most about the problem? How serious is the problem? Do you think it is curable? ■ How have you treated the problem so far? What have you done to feel better? ■ Who in your family/community/religious group can help you? Are you consulting other healers?
Nutrition assessment ■ Pattern of meals ■ Sick food ■ Food intolerance and taboos	■ What is eaten? When are meals eaten? Perform a two-day diet recall. Could this pattern interfere with plan of care? ■ What foods are thought to promote health? What foods are considered good for sick people? ■ Is there potential for food/drug interactions with traditional foods? ■ Are there religious food prescriptions and restrictions?
Pain assessment ■ Cultural patterns of coping with pain ■ Patient's perception of severe pain ■ Appropriate treatments	■ Does the patient tend to be stoic or expressive when in pain? ■ What does pain mean to the patient? ■ What is the worst pain you have ever had? How did you cope with it? How well did the treatment work? ■ What is the patient's attitude towards taking pain medication?
Medication assessment ■ Patient's perception of Western medication ■ Possible pharmacogenetic variation	■ Is the patient's attitude towards Western medication valued or distrusted? ■ Could there be a genetic variation in the way the patient responds to medication? ■ Are there traditional remedies, such as herbs, teas or ointments that the patient uses? ■ In past experiences with the health-care system, what has the patient found helpful? Offensive? Confusing?
Psychosocial assessment ■ Family structure ■ Family resources ■ Community resources	■ Who do you consider family? What impact does the illness have on your family? ■ Who is the head of the family? With whom should we discuss your care? Is there someone who helps you make decisions? ■ Who helps when you are sick? How do they help you? How would you like them to help you? ■ What health/support services are available through the patient's cultural community?

Source: adapted from Narayan MC 2003, Cultural Assessment Checklist, *Home Health Care Nurse*, 21(9), pp 611–18.

attempting to reduce stress by such behaviours as picking and pinching skin or pulling hair, seeking instruments to induce self-harm, and having a delusional belief system that involves self-harm (NSW Health 2001).

Risk of suicide
Patients assessed as low suicide risk would present with no indication of suicide prior to assessment, while those

rated as extreme are intent on committing suicide, with access to the means and a well-developed plan. The person has limited social support or has disengaged from social supports. The person has no future orientation and may have experienced a recent loss. Those assessed as moderate may have some suicidal thoughts with no plan or intent, while those people deemed to be at high risk may have intrusive thoughts of suicide that are difficult to be distracted from. They may feel hopeless and helpless and lack the problem-solving ability to change the situation. The person may be thinking about how they will commit suicide, including where to obtain the means. The person may be disengaging from social supports and have a past history of suicide attempts (NSW Health 2001).

The chapter on crisis and loss (Ch 9) provides a more in-depth assessment of self-harm and suicide.

Risk of absconding
Assessing for a person's risk of absconding is related to the person's ability or willingness to accept treatment. The person deemed to be at moderate risk of absconding has ambivalence about being in hospital or continuing their relationship with community services. Staff find they are regularly encouraging the person to stay in treatment.

Those at high risk have had a previous history of absconding and are expressing their reluctance to stay in the healthcare facility or to continue to live in the present community.

The information obtained from the assessment of the patient's risk status and the patient's CTRS score results in the patient being assigned to one of five categories. The categories represent how urgently the patient needs to be assessed by a mental health professional. Table 10.4 provides an example of the categories and management guidelines.

Vulnerability to exploitation or abuse
Some people living with a mental disorder are vulnerable to exploitation or abuse through sex or violence. It is therefore important that in any triage assessment the person's vulnerability to exploitation and abuse be

Table 10.4 Triage guidelines

	Description	Observation/ treatment acuity	Typical presentation	General principles of management
1	■ Immediate life-threatening illness ■ Immediate danger to self or others	■ Immediate intervention (life-threatening—immediate)	■ Cardiorespiratory arrest ■ Actively violent, aggressive behaviour ■ Actively self-destructive behaviour ■ Possession of weapon	■ Continuous visual surveillance ■ Provide safe environment for patient and others ■ Ensure adequate personnel to provide restraint/detention ■ Consult mental health specialist
2	■ Probable danger to self or others ■ Severe behavioural disturbance	■ Constant observation (emergency—within 10 minutes)	■ Extreme agitation/restlessness ■ Aggressive ■ Confused/unable to cooperate ■ Threat of self-harm ■ Threat of harm to others ■ May have police escort	■ Continuous visual surveillance ■ Provide safe environment for patient and others ■ Ensure adequate personnel to provide restraint/detention ■ Consult mental health specialist
3	■ Possible danger to self or others ■ Patient is very distressed or psychotic ■ Patient is experiencing a situational crisis and is very disturbed	■ Close observation (urgent—within 30 minutes) ■ Confusion/withdrawn	■ Presence of psychotic symptoms ■ Presence of affective disturbance ■ Suicidal ideation ■ Agitation/restlessness ■ Bizarre/disorganised/intrusive behaviour	■ Consult mental health specialist ■ Re-triage if evidence of increasing behavioural disturbance (restlessness, intrusiveness, increasing distress)
4	■ Patient has a longstanding, semi-urgent mental disorder/problem ■ Moderate distress	■ Periodic observation (semi-urgent—within 60 minutes)	■ No agitation/restlessness ■ Irritability without aggression ■ Cooperative ■ Gives coherent history ■ Symptoms of anxiety or depression without suicidal ideation	■ Re-triage if evidence of increasing behavioural disturbance (restlessness, intrusiveness, increasing distress)
5	■ Patient has a longstanding, non-acute mental disorder/problem ■ No danger to self or others ■ No acute distress ■ No behavioural disturbance	■ General observation (non-urgent—within 120 minutes)	■ Cooperative, communicative ■ Complaint with instructions ■ Request for medication ■ Financial/social/accommodation/relationship problems	■ Referral to mental health specialist/team ■ Mobilise or establish support network ■ Known patient

Source: NSW Health 2001, *NSW Mental Health Outcome And Assessment Training (MH-OAT) Facilitator's Manual*, NSW Health, Sydney, Overhead 44.

behaviour. Studies have demonstrated that variation in mental illness is a function of cultural misunderstanding and treatment opportunities. Cultural differences have been found to affect both diagnosis and treatment. Instruments designed to assess psychiatric disorder lack accuracy in cross-cultural situations even when questionnaires are stringently translated. Studies have also demonstrated that the language of interviews has a strong effect on self-assessments of mental health. Communication difficulties clearly contribute to the problems of over-diagnosis, under-diagnosis and incorrect diagnosis. They may also affect the treatment provided—for example, patients diagnosed with schizophrenia were more likely to receive electroconvulsive therapy if they were NESB (Easthope & Julian 1998).

Studies based on clinical and community samples suggest that pre-migration experiences have a profound effect on mental health (Krupinski & Burrows 1986, cited in Gribich 1996). For example, a study of Vietnamese refugees in the United States found that the number of traumatic events prior to immigration, the length of time spent in refugee camps, low income and poor proficiency in English all influenced the development of mental disorder (Chung & Kagawa-Singer 1993, cited in Easthope & Julian 1996). Migrants who experience traumas (normally refugees) are more likely to suffer from mental disorders.

Post-migration events also affect mental health. Migrants with low family income, receiving benefits and with poor English-speaking skills, are more likely to suffer from anxiety or affective disorders than other migrants. Both pre and post migration, women and the elderly are more likely to show anxiety symptoms than men and the young (Gribich 1996).

Migrants' social location can also influence the incidence of mental disorder. Many NESB migrants are forced to take jobs that are stressful and exhausting. Many of these migrants may have had high-status positions in their country of origin. The lack of English may also make it more difficult to access support services, both medical and welfare, that could prevent the development of mental disorders (Easthope & Julian 1998).

Aboriginality

Australian Aborigines are the most disadvantaged group of people in Australian society in terms of socioeconomic status, morbidity and mortality. Statistics drawn from the 'Health and Welfare of Australia's Aboriginal and Torres Strait Islander People's Report' (McLennan & Madden 1997) highlight increased morbidity and mortality figures for indigenous people.

People of Aboriginal descent have a greater risk of poor health, shortened life expectancy, imprisonment, drug and alcohol abuse, violent death, poverty, low standards of education and of their behaviour being labelled psychotic (Smallwood 1996). All these factors contribute to the potential development of a mental disorder, or a label leading to institutionalisation. Smallwood (1996) states that cultural identity is a primary factor in wellbeing. Acknowledgment of the losses (of land, freedom, control over lives and environment) experienced by Aboriginal people needs to be considered in any discourse about the mental health and mental wellbeing of Aboriginal people. Swan (1995) states that mental illness has been absent from discussion on Aboriginal health issues. (Chapter 6 explores issues of culture and mental health in more detail.)

CRITICAL THINKING CHALLENGE 10.3

- Interview a patient in your care to identify areas of strength in the patient. How does the recognition of strength influence your final treatment plan?
- Does the multiaxial assessment system in the DSM-IV-TR provide a comprehensive assessment of factors that may be contributing to a person's mental disorder? Can you think of any factors that may have been excluded?
- As a result of the critique of DSM-IV-TR you may be left with the dilemma of 'to diagnose or not to diagnose'. Reflect on the pros and cons of classification and diagnosis of people with abnormal or different behaviour.
- What would you see as being problematic if a universal classification system were not used?

CONCLUSION

This chapter has overviewed the assessment process initiated when a consumer presents to the mental health-care system and other areas such as emergency departments. The view of the consumer is of paramount importance. If nurses understand the meaning that the consumer assigns to the situation, development of integrative, collaborative care planning is likely to occur. The DSM-IV-TR and ICD-10-AM diagnostic systems have a common meaning and interpretation within the mental health system. The diagnosis and assessment of mental disorders is not without bias—the values, expectations and beliefs of what constitutes abnormal behaviour can influence the mental health professional with respect to the diagnostic category applied to a person. In addition, many social factors influence the likelihood of a person experiencing a mental disorder. It is hoped that as mental health professionals you will consider these aspects when you are caring for people with a diagnosed mental disorder.

EXERCISES FOR CLASS ENGAGEMENT

■ David is a 17-year-old student studying for his Year 12 school certificate. Five months ago his mother noticed that he was spending more time in his room and spending little time with friends. In recent weeks he has started listening to loud music with lyrics associated with violence and suicide. When his mother asked him about this he stated that there was nothing wrong, that he just needed time on his own and that this is the music that most of his friends are listening to. His room is always dark with the blinds drawn, with dirty clothes, magazines, books and stale food over the floor and bed. He rarely showers and has been wearing the same clothes for the last two weeks. On Friday night when he was called to dinner, he yelled, 'Get out of my head! If you don't leave me alone you'll be sorry!'. Later that night David's parents were woken by David yelling and punching the wall and screaming, 'I can't take it any more!'. His father has called the after-hours crisis team for an assessment interview.

Have three members of the class role play David.
- In the first role play, David has a substance use disorder.
- In the second role play, David has a depressive disorder
- In the third role play, David has a psychotic disorder.

Ensure that other members of the class are unaware of the disorder David is role playing.
- Have other members of the class conduct an assessment interview with David.

- Those not involved in the role play should form a fishbowl around those in the role play.
- Have the students forming the fishbowl observe:
  - the non-verbal and verbal behaviour of David and the assessor
  - appropriate nursing skills for an assessment interview
  - questions that assist in the formulation of the diagnosis.
- At the end of the interview, have those in the role play give feedback to the group on what they thought went well and what they thought didn't go well.

■ There are many issues associated with assessment and diagnosis of mental disorders. Divide the class into three. Each group should discuss one of the following issues:
- social issues
- professional issues
- issues related to diagnosis and classification.

Each group should then report back to the rest of the class.

■ If you are interested in the pros and cons of the DSM-IV-TR you might want to visit the following website, which provides arguments for and against labelling and classifying human behaviour as it relates to the DSM-IV-TR: http://www.apa.org/journals/nietzel.html

REFERENCES

American Psychiatric Association 2000, *Diagnostic and Statistical Manual of Mental Disorders* (4th edn, text rev.), International Version, APA, Washington DC.

Andrews G, Peters L & Teeson M 1994, The measurement of consumer outcome in mental health: a report to the national mental health information strategy committee, Clinical Research Unit For Anxiety Disorders, Sydney.

Australian Health Ministers 1992, *National Mental Health Policy*, AGPS, Canberra.

Australian Health Ministers 1998, *Second National Mental Health Plan*, Commonwealth Department of Human Services and Health, Mental Health Branch, AGPS, Canberra.

Australian Health Ministers National Mental Health Working Group 1996, *National Standards in Mental Health Services*, Commonwealth Department of Health and Family Services, AGPS, Canberra.

Bengelsdorf H, Levy L, Emerson R & Barile F 1984, A crisis triage rating scale: brief dispositional assessment of patients at risk of hospitalisation, *Journal of Nervous and Mental Disease*, 172(7), pp 424–30.

Bootzin R, Acocella J & Alloy L 1993, *Abnormal Psychology: Current Perspectives* (6th edn), McGraw-Hill, New York.

Boyd M 2002, *Psychiatric Nursing: Contemporary Practice* (2nd edn), Lippincott, New York.

Burgess AW 1998, *Advanced Practice: Psychiatric Nursing*, Prentice Hall, Sydney.

Carson V 2000, *Mental Health Nursing: The Nurse–Patient Journey* (2nd edn), WB Saunders, Sydney.

Clinton M & Nelson S 1996, *Mental Health and Nursing Practice*, Prentice Hall, Sydney.

Crisp J & Taylor C 2001, *Potter and Perry's Fundamentals of Nursing*, Mosby, Sydney.

Davies A, Sherbourne C, Peterson J & Ware J 1988, *Scoring Manual: Adult Health Status and Patient Satisfaction Measure used in RAND's Health Insurance Experiment*, RAND Corporation, Santa Monica.

Derogatis L, Lipman R, Rickels K, Uhlenhuth E & Covi L 1974, The Hopkins Symptom checklist (HSCL): a self-report symptom inventory, *Behavioural Science*, 19(1), pp 1–15.

Durand M & Barlow D 2002, *Abnormal Psychology: An Introduction*, Wadsworth, Sydney.

Easthope G & Julian R 1998, Mental Health and Ethnicity. In: Clinton & Nelson (eds), *Mental Health & Nursing Practice*, Prentice Hall, Sydney.

Egan G 1998, *The Skilled Helper: A Problem-Management Approach to Helping* (6th edn), Brooks/Cole, Melbourne.

Eilkens D, Hedstorm L, Hughes L, Leaf J & Saunders C 1988, Towards a humanistic-phenomenological spirituality. In: Meadows G & Singh B (eds), 2001 *Mental Health in Australia: Collaborative Community Practice*, Oxford University Press, Melbourne.

Eisen S, Dill D & Grob M 1994, Reliability and validity of a brief patient report instrument for psychiatric outcome evaluation, *Hospital and Community Psychiatry*, 45(3), pp 242–7.

Follete W & Houts A 1996, Models of scientific progress and the role of theory in taxonomy development. A case study of the DSM, *Journal of Consulting and Clinical Psychology*, 64(6), pp 1120–32.

Folstein M, Folstein S & McHugh P 1975, Mini Mental State: a practical guide for grading the cognitive state of patients for the clinician, *Journal of Psychiatric Research*, 12(3), pp 189–98.

Frisch N & Frisch L 2002, *Psychiatric Mental Health Nursing: Understanding the Client as Well as the Condition*, Delmar, Melbourne.

Glass N 2003, *Interpersonal Relating: Study Guide*, School of Nursing and Health Care Practices, Southern Cross University, Lismore.

Goodman S, Sewell D, Cooley E & Leavitt N 1993, Assessing levels of adaptive functioning: the role functioning scale, *Community Mental Health Journal*, 29(2), pp 119–31.

Gribich C (ed) 1996, *Health in Australia: Sociological Concepts and Issues*, Prentice Hall, Sydney.

Hall B 1996, The psychiatric model: critical analysis of its undermining effects on nursing in chronic mental illness, *Advances in Nursing Science*, 18(3), pp 16–26.

Hofling C, Leininger M & Bregg E 1976, *Basic Psychiatric Concepts in Nursing* (2nd edn), JB Lippincott, Philadelphia.

Horsfall J, Stuhlmiller C & Champ S 2000, *Interpersonal Nursing for Mental Health*, McLennan & Petty, Sydney.

Kleinman A 1998, How do professional values influence the work of psychiatrists?. In: Castillo R (ed.), *Meanings of Madness*, Brooks/Cole, Melbourne.

McLennan W & Madden R 1997, *The Health and Welfare of Australian Aboriginal and Torres Strait Islander Peoples*, Australian Bureau of Statistics, Canberra.

McMinn B 1995, Diagnostic classification systems and nursing diagnosis of collaborative problems, *Australian and New Zealand Journal of Mental Health Nursing*, 4(3), pp 124–31.

McPheeters H 1984, Statewide mental health outcome evaluation: a perspective of two Southern States, *Community Mental Health Journal*, 20(1), pp 44–55.

Meadows G 2001, The importance of spirituality. In: Meadows G & Singh B 2001 (eds), *Mental Health in Australia: Collaborative and Community Practice*, Oxford University Press, Melbourne.

Meadows G & Singh B 2001 (eds), *Mental Health in Australia: Collaborative and Community Practice*, Oxford University Press, Melbourne.

Narayan MC 2003, Cultural Assessment Checklist, *Home Health Care Nurse*, 21(9), pp 611–18.

New South Wales Health, 2001, *NSW Mental Health Outcome and Assessment Training (MH-OAT) Facilitator's Manual*, NSW Health, Sydney.

Newman F 1980, Strengths, uses and problems of global scales as an evaluation instrument, *Evaluation and Program Planning*, 3(4), pp 257–68.

Onyett S 1998 *Case Management in Mental Health*, Chapman and Hall, London.

Parker G, Rosen A, Emdur N & Hadzi-Pavlovic D 1991, The life skills profile: psychometric properties of a measure assessing function and disability in schizophrenia, *Acta Psychiatricia Scandinavica*, 83(2), pp 145–52.

Peterson A & Waddel C (eds) 1998, *Health Matters: a Sociology of Illness, Prevention and Care*, Allen & Unwin, Sydney.

Rosen A, Hadzi-Pavlovic D & Parker G 1989, The life skills profile: a measure assessing function and disability, *Schizophrenia Bulletin*, 15(2), pp 325–37.

Rosenhan D 1973, On being sane in insane places, reprinted from *Science*, 179(70), pp 250–8.

Schwartz S 2000, *Abnormal Psychology: A Discovery Approach*, Mayfield, London.

Short S, Sharman E & Speedy S 1998, *Sociology for Nurses: An Australian Introduction* (2nd edn), Macmillan, Hong Kong.

Smallwood G 1998, Aboriginality and mental health. In: Clinton M & Nelson S (eds), *Mental Health & Nursing Practice*, Prentice Hall, Sydney.

Stedman T, Yellowlees P, Mellsop G, Clarke R & Drake S 1997, Measuring consumer outcomes in mental health, Department of Health and Family Services, Canberra.

Stein G 1999, Usefulness of the health of the nation outcome scales, *British Journal of Psychiatry*, 174(5), pp 375–7.

Swan P 1995, Aboriginal Mental Health: an Indigenous and Cultural Perspective, *Proceedings of Celebrating a New Era: An International Conference on Mental Health Nursing*, 21st Annual Conference, Australian and New Zealand College of Mental Health Nurses Inc., Canberra.

Trauer T, Callaly T, Hantz P, Little J, Shields R & Smith J 1999, Health of the Nation Outcome Scale: results of the Victorian field trial, *British Journal of Psychiatry*, 174(5), pp 380–8.

Treatment Protocol Project, 1999, *Acute Inpatient Psychiatric Care: A Source Book* (2nd edn), World Health Organization Collaborating Centre For Mental Health and Substance Abuse, Sydney.

Treatment Protocol Project, 2000, *Management of Mental Disorders*, Vol. 1 (3rd edn), World Health Organization, Collaborating Centre for Mental Health and Substance Abuse, Sydney.

Tucker G 1998, Putting DSM-IV in perspective, *American Journal of Psychiatry*, 155(2), pp 159–61.

Veit C & Ware J 1983, The structure of psychological distress and well being in general populations, *Journal of Clinical and Consulting Psychiatry*, 51(5), pp 730–45.

Ware J & Sherbourne C 1992, The MOS 36-Item short-form health survey (SF 36): 1. Conceptual framework and item selection, *Medical Care*, 30(6), pp 473–81.

Ware J, Snow K, Kosinski M & Gandek B 1993, *SF-36 Health Survey Manual and Interpretation Guide*, The Health Institute, New England, Boston, Massachusetts.

Weir D & Oei T 1996, Mental disorder: conceptual framework, classification and assessment. In: Clinton M & Nelson S (eds), 1996, *Mental Health and Nursing Practice*, Prentice Hall, Sydney.

Wing J, Curtis R & Beevor A 1996, *Health of the Nation Outcome Scales: Report on Research*, Royal College of Psychiatrists, London.

World Health Organization 1992, *ICD-10: International Statistical Classification of Diseases and Related Health Problems* (10th rev.), WHO, Geneva.

Understanding Mental Illness

11

Intellectual Disabilities

Charles Harmon, Philip Petrie,
Norma Cloonan and
Irvin Savage

KEY POINTS

- Definitions and systems of classification exist for mental retardation/intellectual disability.
- Mental health nurses need to liaise effectively with disability support services.
- Dual disability and dual diagnosis should be differentiated.
- People with an intellectual disability can fail to receive mental health services.
- Nurses are involved with the acute nursing assessment and management of individuals with a dual disability.
- Assessment and communication issues need to be considered.
- Pitfalls in the assessment process need to be negotiated.
- Continuous care for the dual disability client needs to be facilitated.
- Discharge planning and mental health support plans are significant nursing responsibilities.

KEY TERMS

- carer
- challenging behaviour
- continuity of care
- disability services
- dual disability
- intellectual disability
- mental health services
- mental retardation

- normalisation
- nursing assessment
- nursing management
- social inclusion
- stakeholders
- support
- support worker

LEARNING OUTCOMES

The material in this chapter will assist you to:
- analyse factors that contribute to difficulties in the diagnosis and management of persons with a dual disability (i.e. persons with an intellectual disability who also have a mental illness)
- discuss the definitions and features of mental retardation according to the DSM-IV-TR and the American Association on Mental Retardation
- outline reasons why the term 'intellectual disability' has replaced the term 'mental retardation' in the Australian and New Zealand contexts
- outline the service philosophy pertinent to services for people with an intellectual disability
- discuss the factors that contribute to a thorough mental health nursing assessment for individuals with a dual disability
- discuss the nursing management appropriate for individuals with a dual disability who have acute care requirements due to mental illness
- discuss the nursing strategies relevant to ensuring continuity of care for people with a dual disability in the first month after their discharge from the care of a mental health service.

INTRODUCTION

This chapter provides information on the nursing care and management of clients who have a dual disability— that is, a diagnosis of a mental illness co-morbid with an intellectual disability—in the context of mental health services. To assist readers who have little first-hand experience with people with an intellectual disability, a number of case studies are included.

Essentially, quality mental health nursing care for clients with an intellectual disability is the same type of care offered to any other member of the community, with some important differences.

- It might be necessary for the mental health nurse to modify the way in which she or he communicates with the client in order to accommodate a level of understanding appropriate to the client's disability.
- A modification of the assessment process may provide the nurse with information vital to the management of the client.
- The process of forming a therapeutic alliance with the client will be greatly enhanced by promoting a cooperative relationship between the relevant mental health professionals and the client's usual carers and/or service providers.
- The client should be supported upon discharge from mental health services via the design and implementation of a mental health support plan.

THE LANGUAGE OF DISABILITY SERVICES

In order to fully appreciate the subject of intellectual disability and mental illness, it is necessary to learn some of the language used by disability professionals (see also the list of key terms at the beginning of this chapter). Much of the literature, particularly regarding definition of terms and the prevalence of dual disability, has been written by British or American authors, and so some guidance is provided here on interpreting the varied terminology used in these sources and applying the information in an Australian or New Zealand context.

Terminology

The term 'dual diagnosis' is most often used by mental health professionals in reference to clients who have a diagnosis of mental illness as well as a substance abuse problem. (This form of 'dual diagnosis' is addressed in Ch 19.) There is, however, another form of 'dual diagnosis' that provides a label for people with a mental illness who have a co-morbid intellectual disability. To avoid confusion, the term 'dual disability' (rather than 'dual diagnosis') is used in this chapter.

Many terms have been used to describe people who in some way represent a departure from the usual. Labels such as 'feebleminded' and 'mentally subnormal' have been used in the past to describe people with an intellectual disability but these terms have, thankfully, been superseded. Indeed, terms such as 'idiot', 'imbecile' and 'moron' were once used by the scientific community to describe people with an intellectual disability but these terms are no longer in everyday professional use because of the way in which their meaning has altered over time. Internationally, the terms *mental retardation* and *intellectual handicap* remain in use, depending on the country or jurisdiction. In the Australian and New Zealand contexts, however, the descriptor *intellectual disability* is preferred by consumers and disability service professionals, mainly because it is felt that terms such as 'mental retardation' are stigmatising.

Systems of classification

The term *mental retardation* is defined in the *Diagnostic and Statistical Manual of Mental Disorders*, fourth edition (DSM-IV-TR) as:

significantly subaverage general intellectual functioning . . . accompanied by significant limitations in adaptive functioning in at least two of the following skill areas: communication, self-care, home living, social/interpersonal skills, use of community resources, self-direction, functional academic skills, work, leisure, health, and safety . . . occur[ring] before age 18 years.

(American Psychiatric Association 2000, p 41)

Subaverage intellectual functioning is defined as below an intelligence quotient (IQ) of 70 and is principally subdivided into four levels of increasing severity from mild (IQ range 50–55 to 70), moderate (IQ range 35–40 to 50–55), severe (IQ range 20–25 to 35–40) to profound (IQ below 20–25). According to this system of classification, of the 2–3 per cent of the general population who might be diagnosed with mental retardation, about 85 per cent are thought to belong to the *mild* category, 10 per cent in the *moderate* category and approximately 5 per cent in either the *severe* or *profound* category (American Psychiatric Association (APA) 2000, pp 42–4). In a similar vein, the tenth edition of the *International Classification of Diseases* (ICD-10) (World Health Organization 1993) employs a system of categorisation that emphasises IQ.

The American Association on Mental Retardation (AAMR) (2002, p 39) defines mental retardation as 'a disability characterized by significant limitations both in intellectual functioning and in adaptive behaviour as expressed in conceptual, social, and practical adaptive skills . . . [that] . . . originates before age 18'. This definition is similar to the DSM-IV-TR definition because it maintains that mental retardation occurs below a threshold IQ score of around 70 but differs in that it emphasises levels of functioning based on adaptive behaviour rather than IQ. Furthermore, the individual is assessed according to their support requirements and categorised according to 'the intensity of needed supports'—that is, intermittent, limited, extensive or pervasive (AAMR 2002, p 152).

It is important to note that although IQ is still used as a determinant for the granting of pensions and other services by funding bodies, adaptive behaviour is regarded as a far more practical basis for individual assessment by professionals working in services for clients with an intellectual disability. Thus the AAMR definition has most application within disability services in Australia and New Zealand. As a description of adaptive behaviour assessment is beyond the scope of this chapter, you may wish to refer to the AAMR text (AAMR 2002, pp 73–91) for more information.

Although there is no such thing as the 'typical' person with an intellectual disability, the following stories are nevertheless intended to give you a general idea of the characteristics of individuals who might fit into the AAMR intensity-of-support categories.

- Ruth is a woman who has intermittent support needs. She is twenty years old and lives in a suburban apartment in a manner much like the rest of the community. Ruth used to attend a supported employment facility but has recently graduated to open employment in a manufacturing business, having learned the necessary vocational skills at an evening college. She lives a fairly independent life with the support of her family but receives one or two visits each month from her key worker, who assists her in planning meals and budgeting. Ruth has limited numeracy skills but she can competently manage money transactions and perform everyday mathematical calculations. She reads slowly and hesitantly but can read an article in her local paper with few difficulties.

- Barry is twenty-five years old and has limited support needs. He lived at home with his parents until he was twenty but now shares a suburban house with two other men. Barry works in a supported employment facility but occasionally works on weekends as a labourer with his uncle's landscape-gardening business. Although he makes friends easily and is well known at his local community soccer club, Barry has difficulty budgeting and using his money wisely. He also has a history of trouble with the police because he has occasionally gotten into fights following drinking sessions. Consequently Barry receives five hours of contact per week with a disability worker who assists him in learning financial management skills and in conducting himself responsibly when socialising.

- Jan is a forty-year-old woman who has extensive support needs. She has a hearing impairment and regularly takes medication due to her epilepsy. After the death of her parents when she was twelve, Jan was institutionalised in a large state-owned residential facility, where she lived with thirty other individuals in a dormitory-style unit. At age twenty-five she was placed in a home in the community with four other people with similar support needs. The home is staffed by residential support workers and the clients attend day programs where they are provided with opportunities to participate in community activities and improve their living skills. Jan has a limited spoken vocabulary but with the assistance of a hearing aid can understand much of what is said to her. She can read important words like her own name, 'hot', and 'danger', but cannot read a newspaper or the captions in a television program. She can perform many tasks associated with self-care and personal hygiene, and assists in the preparation of meals and other domestic chores around the house.

- Petra is a ten-year-old girl who has pervasive support needs. Apart from her intellectual disability, she has cerebral palsy (a disorder that limits her ability to move and coordinate her limbs) and epilepsy. These disabilities greatly limit her developmental opportunities and her independence. Petra lives at home with her parents and attends a school that caters for her specific needs. She has great difficulty speaking because of her cerebral palsy but can indicate her needs using sounds and gestures that her parents understand and with the aid of a 'pointer board', which she uses to point to symbols to indicate a range of things from concrete needs (such as food or drink) to emotions (such as happy). Petra also has a computer device that has a keyboard featuring the symbols on her pointer board and the capacity to electronically 'speak' for her. Petra is unable to walk independently but has a 'walker', a complex mechanical device that assists in mobilisation, and a motorised wheelchair. Petra's parents hope that she can one day lead an independent life away from her family home just like any other young adult.

CAUSES OF INTELLECTUAL DISABILITY AND ASSOCIATED DISORDERS

Intellectual disability may result from impediments to intellectual development and/or neurological damage caused by factors that include:

- heredity (e.g. genetic causes such as Down syndrome and fragile X syndrome)
- alterations in embryonic development (e.g. fetal alcohol syndrome)
- familial and environmental influences (including deprivation of learning/developmental opportunities due to an unstimulating home environment)
- autistic spectrum disorders (e.g. autistic disorder)
- pregnancy and perinatal problems (including hypoxia or viral infections)
- general medical conditions after birth (including infections and traumas) (APA 2000, p 45).

The best known are genetic causes such as Down syndrome, which occurs in approximately one in 700–1000 births (Dykens, Hodapp & Finucane 2000, p 61). According to Dykens et al. (2000, p 5), however, only about 50 per cent of people with an intellectual disability have known 'organic' causes for their condition, with an estimated one-third of all cases being due to genetic abnormalities. This statistic is indicative of the problem of disabilities as an under-explored field for researchers, but this situation may well change, given the prominence of the human genome project and the wealth of data it is generating.

Intellectual disability may also be accompanied by other types of impairment such as hearing impairments, visual impairments and epilepsy (Gilbert, Todd & Jackson 1998). In addition, people with an intellectual disability often lack the ability to make healthy lifestyle choices and are especially prone to developing preventable medical disorders in adulthood (e.g. cardiovascular diseases, nutritional disorders and endocrine disorders), including mental health problems (Barr et al. 1999).

SERVICES FOR PEOPLE WITH AN INTELLECTUAL DISABILITY

In New Zealand and Australia, most people with an intellectual disability live at home, either with their families or in single or shared accommodation in the general community. A smaller proportion of people with higher support needs live in supported accommodation either in group homes or, more rarely, in large residential institutions. The proportion of individuals living in institutions has gradually diminished over the past two decades in response to government policies aimed at the de-institutionalisation of services and the movement of residents into community homes and other services more appropriate for their needs (e.g. aged-care facilities).

In Australia, the most recent set of blueprints for the process of de-institutionalisation has been legislated via the Disability Services Acts of the Commonwealth, State and Territory governments devised between the mid-1980s and early 1990s. The latest New Zealand Disability Strategy: *Making a world of difference: Whakanui Oranga* (2001) is less explicit in its reference to the creation of a vision for disability services and tends to network with other departmental policies.

Estimates from the New Zealand Ministry of Health revealed that there are approximately 400 people remaining in large residential institutions in that country, which is less than one per cent of the population of New Zealanders with an intellectual disability. Of the two institutions that remain open, one was expected to have closed by the end of 2003 and the other is expected to close by the end of 2006 (D Hughes, project manager, Disability Services Directorate, New Zealand Ministry of Health, personal communication, 28 July 2003). According to Bostock et al. (2001), the situation is similar in Australia, with approximately 6200 people with an intellectual disability living in large institutions—about 1.6 per cent of the population of people with an intellectual disability.

In 2001, the Australian States had different targets and schedules for the de-institutionalisation of services:

- Queensland—10 per cent reduction in its current institutional bed numbers ($n = 1284$) by 2011
- New South Wales—total closure of its institutional beds ($n = 2500$) by 2010
- Victoria—56 per cent reduction in current bed numbers ($n = 822$) by 2011
- Western Australia—35 per cent reduction in bed numbers ($n = 735$) by the end of 2003
- South Australia—10 per cent reduction in bed numbers ($n = 688$) by the end of 2002
- Tasmania, the Australian Capital Territory and the Northern Territory have no large-scale institutions (Bostock et al. 2001, p 24).

As institutions have diminished there has been a corresponding growth in community-based services for people with an intellectual disability. Non-government organisations play an emerging role in direct service provision. Increasingly, however, services have become more specialised within the disability support model and few staff employed by these services have the relevant experience or education to work with people who have a mental illness. These factors can create difficulties for the person with a dual disability in that their acute and/or long-term mental health needs might not be met effectively.

Service philosophy in disability services

Over the past thirty years the principles of *normalisation*, first fully articulated by Wolfensberger (1972), have been a driving force behind the creation and design of services for persons with an intellectual disability. This set of principles accounts, to some degree, for the various Disability Services Acts instituted by the Australian Commonwealth, States and Territories, the New Zealand Disability Strategy, and the various Guardianship Acts. More recently, O'Brien's model (1987) has provided direction with respect to the normalisation of services. O'Brien identifies measures to ensure that people with an intellectual disability have:

- an increased physical presence in the community
- choice about the way in which they live their lives
- the opportunity to acquire and develop skills that promote independent living
- respect as citizens
- the opportunity for community participation (O'Brien 1987, p 182).

This model emphasises a humanist perspective in which citizens with an intellectual disability are given the same rights and opportunities as any other citizens, even if they need the support of appropriate services. Importantly, proponents of this model advocate the use of generic services (i.e. services that any citizen would use, such as public transport, private banking services or general hospitals), rather than specialist disability-based services, in the quest for integration between the disabled and non-disabled populations.

PREVALENCE OF DUAL DISABILITY

It is difficult to accurately determine prevalence rates for dual disability, for a number of reasons. Historically, a belief that people with intellectual disabilities could not experience mental illness in the same way as the general population (Borthwick-Duffy 1994; Raghavan 1996) probably contributed to the dearth of information on dual disability by preventing research activities. Many early studies concentrated on residents in institutional settings where rates of mental illness would be expected to be higher than for most people living in the community. In addition, it has not always been easy to estimate the number of people with an intellectual disability as many individuals with relatively minor problems remain undiagnosed. Difficulties in conversing with intellectually disabled individuals with communications deficits and the prevalence of autism and behavioural disorders among this population have also contributed to the problem by confounding diagnostic procedures.

Unfortunately, there appears to have been no research conducted in the Australian or New Zealand contexts that provides accurate information about the prevalence of dual disability in the general population. In a survey of service providers for clients with an intellectual disability conducted in Queensland, however, Edwards & Lennox (2002) estimated that between 7.4 per cent and 20.2 per cent of clients ($n = 7196$) had a dual disability. The validity of this study was, however, compromised to some extent by the failure of 33 per cent of the surveyed agencies to provide data to the researchers.

Prevalence studies among broader populations generally indicate higher rates of mental illness among the intellectually disabled population than among the general population (Benson 1985; Borthwick-Duffy 1994; Jacobson 1990). Unfortunately, many of these studies have methodological differences and do not examine the same types of populations, so the respective data are not easily comparable.

Some authors have theorised that people with an intellectual disability have a higher probability of developing a mental illness than the general population because their deficits with respect to communication, processing skills, cognitive functioning and social skills cause them to be more vulnerable to stress (Reiss 1994; Sovner 1996). Gilbert et al. (1998) noted that intellectual disability may be accompanied by other types of impairment that have been associated with mental health problems in the general population, such as hearing impairments, visual impairments and epilepsy, and that socioeconomic factors such as unemployment and poverty may also contribute to higher rates of mental disorders in this group.

A study of intellectually disabled people living in community settings in Wales (Deb, Thomas & Bright 2001) found that some 4.4 per cent of the sample ($N = 90$) met ICD-10 criteria for schizophrenia, 2.2 per cent for depressive disorder, 2.2 per cent for generalised anxiety disorder, 4.4 per cent for phobic disorder and 1 per cent for delusional disorder. According to Deb et al.:

> the overall rate of functional psychiatric illness (point prevalence) was similar to that found in the general community (16%). However rates of schizophrenic illness and phobic disorder were significantly higher in the study cohort compared with those in the general population (0.4% and 1.1% respectively).

(Deb et al. 2001, p 495)

FALLING THROUGH THE CRACKS

McIntyre, Blacher & Baker (2002) reported on the negative impact of mental illness on individuals with an intellectual disability and their families. Because of a range of difficulties, however, people within the intellectually disabled population who also have a mental illness remain undiagnosed, are often ignored, or do not have equitable access to mental health services (Fletcher & Poindexter 1996). The Australian Second National Mental Health Plan identified people with an intellectual disability as one of the 'target groups for whom improved service access and better service responses are essential' (Australian Health Ministers 1998, p 10).

Part of the problem appears to be that carers and disability service personnel tend to lack the skills required to meet the additional mental health needs of these people (Coyle 2000). Equally, however, health professionals lack skills in dealing with this population (Naylor & Clifton 1994; McConkey & Truesdale 2000) and many may even be unwilling to treat them (McConkey & Truesdale 2000, p 159). Given these problems, much can go wrong in the care of people with dual disabilities, as the case studies of Roy and John illustrate.

CASE STUDY: Roy

Roy had his first admission to a psychiatric hospital at the age of fifteen and by the age of twenty he was a permanent inpatient with a diagnosis of mental retardation and manic depression (see Ch 15 for manic depression, now known as bipolar disorder). After considerable trial and error, his mental illness was successfully treated with the assistance of the mood stabiliser, lithium carbonate, and the 'typical' antipsychotic medication, thioridazine. By the age of twenty Roy was living in Mimosa Lodge, a large residential facility run by a charitable organisation, where he was seen initially by a community mental health nurse and a general practitioner (GP).

CASE STUDY: Roy (continued)

Roy continued his liaison with his GP for the remaining thirty years of his residency at Mimosa Lodge but at the age of fifty moved to a group home run by a non-government agency. Staff noted that he was an amiable man who spoke very little but was capable of working in supported employment. Roy was able to feed and dress himself but required reminders to perform hygiene tasks. Initially, Roy appeared to settle in well and was regarded as a bit of a joker, always attempting to cuddle the female staff. However, very little documentation accompanied him to the new service and there was a minimum of information regarding the history and management of his mental illness. Without records, there was nothing to indicate when he had commenced antipsychotic medication, or why the treatment was started. The staff presumed that his medication had been initiated to manage challenging behaviours that were no longer in evidence. There were also concerns about Roy's shuffling gait and sleep difficulties, perhaps medication-related, and so his new GP halved the quantity of thioridazine.

Roy's sleep pattern deteriorated rapidly, his speech and movements became accelerated, he became more insistent on cuddling both male and female staff and these physical contacts became more overtly sexual. Pre-existing behaviour management techniques (such as identifying and avoiding triggers for Roy's behaviour, ignoring Roy's inappropriate behaviour, redirecting him to more appropriate tasks and asking him to spend time in the garden when he was otherwise unmanageable) became ineffective and Roy began to initiate low-level physical assaults upon staff. Additional staff were needed to support Roy at night and the overall support structure started to fracture. After six weeks nurses from the local community mental health team arranged for Roy's admission to a psychiatric inpatient unit, where he spent eight weeks being stabilised on a regimen of lithium carbonate and the 'atypical' antipsychotic medication, quetiapine. Nursing management consisted of the standard practices for a person with bipolar disorder (see Ch 15).

CASE STUDY: John

John is a twenty-year-old man who has limited support needs. He uses little verbal language but understands much of what is said to him and augments his limited speech with gestures and hand signs similar to those used by some people with severe hearing impairments. He can perform most self-care activities but is unable to read and write, except for a few words including his own name.

John was seventeen when his mother died and this event marked the occurrence of challenging behaviours including sudden displays of aggression directed towards others as well as himself. Because his father could not cope with these behaviours, John was subsequently moved from his family home to a respite house for people with an intellectual disability. John displayed a range of problem behaviours including high-level verbal and physical assaults, theft from staff and other residents, lying, monopolisation of staff time and self-abusive behaviours such as pulling his own hair out and picking the scabs off cuts and abrasions. The house manager sought a full physical examination because blood had been noted in the toilet bowl after John had used it. John became angry and abusive when he was asked about it, but investigations found no physiological cause for the blood in the toilet.

In his assessment, the psychologist identified a grief reaction to the loss of John's mother and 'attention seeking' as the primary cause of his difficult behaviours. A range of behaviour support strategies were subsequently designed and implemented by nurses, including educative programs designed to provide him with more independence in leisure skills, and outings and other activities that John enjoyed.

Enjoyable activities were approved on the proviso that he had not stolen property or displayed aggression towards others, and John was distracted and redirected to other activities if he engaged in inappropriate behaviours (see Ch 23 for behaviour therapy and other therapeutic nursing interventions).

Nevertheless, over the next six months, the behavioural programs appeared to be having little impact and John's behaviour continued to deteriorate. At the request of the house staff, John was seen by the mental health team but was uncommunicative, and although staff provided written and verbal information to the assessing psychiatrist describing John's behaviours and their possible motivation, it was determined that John did not have a mental illness.

John's behaviours continued to be highly problematic and ten months after his placement at the respite house, he was taken by ambulance to the local base hospital for the emergency surgical removal of a length of fencing wire that was lodged in his urethra. The surgeon noted that there was evidence of repeated trauma to the urethra and the neck of the bladder and that it was probable that these were self-inflicted injuries that had been sustained over a number of months (see Ch 22 for self-harm, and Ch 9 for grief and bereavement). Concerns about the extent and apparent duration of the self-injurious behaviours resulted in a request by the surgeon for an assessment of John by the base hospital mental health liaison nurse. Further assessment by a psychiatrist resulted in John receiving a provisional diagnosis of major depression. Community mental health staff were subsequently engaged to assist disability staff with his ongoing management.

Comments on case studies 'Roy' and 'John'

It is clear that the outcomes in both cases above could have been catastrophic, particularly if either Roy or John had sustained more serious permanent injury. In Roy's case, changing his antipsychotic medication (thioridazine) dose had unfortunate consequences that could have been avoided if adequate documentation had accompanied him in his move from one service to the next. Such documentation would have advised the new service of Roy's long-term mental health diagnosis and alerted personnel to the need to consult a specialist psychiatrist rather than generalist medical services when seeking a review of his medication. Similarly, the management of his behaviour immediately after the halving of his thioridazine dose was not informed by standard mental health management practices and, indeed, mental health professionals were not engaged until his behaviour had reached crisis point.

In John's case the mental health staff were consulted at an appropriate time but he did not receive appropriate management until his depression was severe and he had engaged in potentially serious self-harm activities. What was required in both instances was effective communication between disability and mental health services accompanied by a thorough mental health assessment of the clients and the creation of a management plan understood and implemented not only by mental health services but also carers in the clients' home settings (see acute assessment and management, below).

One explanation for the lack of communication between services in these cases may be that mental health and disability services operate from different paradigms and therefore encounter problems in working together.

- Disability services operate according to the notion that its clients are not ill, but are citizens of a society that has not been adequately prepared to accept them as valued citizens. The activities of disability services are, therefore, based on the creation of a more inclusive society and the preparation of disabled persons, via educational technologies, for greater participation. Intellectually disabled clients who exhibit aberrant behaviours accordingly need greater acceptance and education, via behaviour management strategies, in order to take their place in society.
- Mental health services, on the other hand, take the view that their clients behave in a disturbed fashion because they are either mentally disordered or mentally ill and may, as a consequence, require medical and nursing interventions based on diagnosis in accordance with the DSM-IV-TR. In some cases, the mental health client is deprived of their liberty via involuntary admission to an admission unit or psychiatric intensive care unit.

It is, therefore, not surprising that personnel in disability services are poorly prepared for clients with a mental illness who may not respond to behavioural interventions and that personnel within mental health services lack understanding about what disability staff are trying to achieve.

CRITICAL THINKING CHALLENGE 11.1

- How might the mental health nurse obtain an adequate history regarding Roy's mental illness?
- What information should mental health nurses obtain from Roy's usual disability service carers in order to ensure a thorough assessment of his mental status?
- How likely is it that Roy had had previous episodes of mental illness during his stay at Mimosa Lodge?

CRITICAL THINKING CHALLENGE 11.2

- Analyse possible factors that may have contributed to the delays in treatment for John's mental illness.
- How might the mental health nurse establish communication with John given his limited vocabulary?
- List the ethical considerations that should be taken into account when nursing John in an acute-care setting. Discuss how each of these problems might be addressed.

ACUTE ASSESSMENT

Acute assessment here refers to assessment of an individual with a diagnosis of a mental illness co-morbid with an intellectual disability.

Just like the rest of the community, people with an intellectual disability can display a range of unusual or disturbed behaviours in response to adversity. Unlike most of the community, however, people with an intellectual disability often have difficulty communicating the reasons for their maladaptive behaviour, which might range from stereotypical (or repetitive) behaviours (such as hand flapping or body rocking), to 'acting out' behaviors (such as displays of yelling and violent body movements), self-injurious behaviours (such as scratching at their skin or old wounds), or aggression towards others.

Sovner (1996) proposed that people with an intellectual disability might develop disturbed behaviours as part of their usual behavioural repertoire because they had limited developmental opportunities and/or inappropriate learning situations when they were young. Equally, however, disturbed behaviours may develop as a response to the pain and discomfort of general medical conditions or the distress associated with mental health disorders. The mental health assessment of clients with an intellectual disability can thus become something of an art when one is faced with the task of sorting out the origins of behaviour and its meaning in relation to the client's mental illness.

Assessment and communication issues

Further difficulties arise for the mental health nurse because clients with an intellectual disability often have limited capacity for conversation because of their primary disability or because of concurrent disabilities such as

NURSE'S STORY

Using augmentative forms of communication can be a difficult task for the novice but basic communication can be achieved quite quickly with the aid of motivation and some basic education. I had the pleasure of supervising a group of nursing students at a clinical placement that was both a residential facility and a school for children and adolescents with cerebral palsy. Very few of the children had speech that could be understood by the nursing students and so we commenced the process of teaching the students to communicate via pointer board, which displays symbols that can be used to indicate meaning. Needless to say, the students were daunted by the task ahead of them, particularly when they entered the classrooms and were confronted by children seated at desks decorated with symbols and enthusiastically gesturing to them to come over and 'have a chat'.

I'd tried to plan for this experience by giving the students some prior reading and a brief demonstration of the use of pointer boards. Essentially, however, the classroom teachers and I had contrived the learning environment so that the children would teach the students how to communicate via this medium. This was very exciting for me as I watched the students struggle with the new information and the pressure exerted on them by their eager 'teachers'. Within about ten minutes, however, you could see progress being made. One nursing student yelled: 'She went to the movies with her mum, in her mum's car, and saw a movie with a handsome actor—Tom Cruise!'. The child smiled proudly. When the nursing student guessed the title of the movie the young child was absolutely delighted. The two had struck up a rapport and communication flowed much more quickly from this point.

Charles Harmon, RN

hearing impairment. In addition, clients with higher support needs may experience problems in generalising (or transferring) communication skills from familiar environments, such as their home, to less familiar environments, such as psychiatric emergency centres. Another common problem is that the client may become shy or confused and, as a consequence, use regressed or echolalic speech (i.e. repeating what has been said), as in this example:

Nurse: How are you today, Robyn? You look a bit sad.
Robyn: A bit sad.

The client may also tend to answer 'Yes' to questions in order to please the interviewer or because they have interpreted questions literally:

Nurse: Do you hear voices, Robyn?
Robyn: Yes, I hear voices all the time.

Employing the assistance of carers, family members and significant others to assist with the communication process is most advisable, particularly if the client has a significant communication impairment (e.g. is semi- or non-verbal) and uses augmentative forms of communication such as sign language (signing), pointer boards (also known as communications or symbol boards) or computer devices.

Further information on augmentative and alternative communication is beyond the scope of this chapter but is available in the literature (Abudarham & Hurd 2002; Cockerill & Carroll-Few 2001; Linfoot 1994; von Tetzchner & Grove 2003). In addition, a useful Australian website on sign language can be found at: http://www.ispdr.net.au/~johnw/. Note that sign languages may vary from one country to the next, just as with spoken languages. Having said this, Australian, New Zealand and British hand signs are similar, but US signs are often quite different.

Coombs & Martin (2002) have shown that mental health clinicians typically obtain information during the assessment and review processes either directly from the

client or from their own observations of the individual, rather than using other sources of information such as the client's family or usual carers. However, Silka & Hauser (1997) assert that, in the case of clients with an intellectually disability, it is necessary to gather information from all possible sources to obtain a full clinical picture, especially if the client has significant communications deficits and cannot participate in an assessment process that relies on their ability to respond verbally to questions.

In all instances the approach to obtaining information about a client should be calm and non-threatening, using concrete, open-ended questions, avoiding jargon, complex technical terms or abstract questions (Hamer 1998). For clients with an intellectual disability, the mental health nurse will need to use skills in both observation and communication, verbal and non-verbal, in carrying out the assessment. If the client's usual carers are willing to participate in this process it is helpful to interview them to obtain information about the client's usual behaviour patterns (Moss & Lee 2001). It is also important to ask the carer how the client's presenting behaviour is a departure from the usual. This information may help to identify the 'typical' signs that indicate mental illness as well as 'atypical' signs, which are behaviours peculiar to the client following the onset of the mental illness, including stereotypical (or repetitive) behaviours, 'acting out' behaviours and self-abusive behaviours (Ross & Oliver 2002).

Other data pertinent to the assessment process should include information that may assist in developing the client's history, including information from other service providers such as their GP, medical specialists and behavioural specialists. In particular, a medication history should be established.

One of the first questions asked during the initial assessment should be whether the client has recently undergone a full medical examination. As outlined in the

CASE STUDY: Robert

Robert is a 22-year-old man with an intellectual disability and extensive support needs. He understands much of what is said to him and has some spoken language but communicates mostly with gestures and a vocabulary of about twenty hand 'signs' because he has difficulty articulating words. Robert presented to the emergency department with his carers, who reported that he was 'hallucinating' and that they believed him to have schizophrenia. Robert refused a medical examination, attempting to hit anyone who came near him. He was then referred to the mental health nurse in the emergency department.

The mental health nurse gathered a history from Robert's carers, who reported that his behaviour had deteriorated over the past three weeks. They stated that Robert had been a good communicator but had become increasingly non-compliant, poking objects in his ears and hitting the side of his head, and when they asked him why he did it he indicated that he had noises in his head. Although he had no previous history of mental illness his carers believed that he was responding to hallucinatory 'voices'. During the past week he had stopped eating and sleeping and mumbled to himself all the time. He had become aggressive towards his carers, lashing out when they approached him, and they could no longer cope with him in the group home. During the interview Robert appeared preoccupied, mumbling to himself and occasionally slapping the left side of his head.

Due to Robert's distressed state he was admitted to a mental health unit for further observation and investigations. Over the next twelve hours nursing staff assessed Robert's behaviour using the JOMAAC assessment tool (see Box 11.1). They reported that Robert did not appear to be hallucinating but did appear to be distressed, holding and occasionally hitting the left side of his head. When asked by the staff why he hit his head he signed 'noise' and would then mumble to himself. Robert was administered paracetamol and appeared more settled. He was then given a physical examination and was found to have a quantity of severely infected dirt and foreign matter in his left ear. Robert was commenced on antibiotics and pain-relief medication and discharged three days later with his behaviour and symptoms resolved.

In this case the client did not have a dual disability and was not hallucinating, and comprehensive mental and physical examination and assessment averted further pain and disturbance for the client and his carers.

case study of Robert, a deterioration in skills or behaviour can be due to an undiagnosed physical complaint or exacerbation of an existing one. Barr (1998) has asserted that physical illness in this group of people is often not detected and that many conditions are diagnosed too late, making treatment less effective.

Enhancing the assessment process

Where possible, standard assessment formats such as the mental status assessment and self-harm and/or risk assessment should be used in the assessment of all mental health clients (see Ch 10 for mental status examination, Ch 23 for risk assessment and Ch 22 for self-harm).

There are other tools available, however, to assist with the assessment of adult clients with intellectual disabilities when the standard tools are considered ineffective because of the client's limitations in cognition and communication. Three such instruments are as follows:

- The Psychiatric Assessment Schedule for Adults with Developmental Disabilities (PAS-ADD) is a diagnostic tool suitable for the mental health nurse or other mental health professional adept at clinical interviewing (Moss et al. 1993).
- The Mini Psychiatric Assessment Schedule for Adults with Developmental Disabilities (Mini PAS-ADD) is a relatively more accessible tool for most nursing staff, although specific training is required for its effective use. Essentially, the Mini PAS-ADD consists of a life events checklist as well as a four-point scale upon which clinicians may 'rate' the client's symptoms of depression, anxiety, expansive mood, obsessive compulsive disorder, psychosis and autism (Prosser et al. 1998).
- In addition to the above, Hamer (1998) recommends the use of the JOMAAC assessment tool (see Box 11.1), in which the adult client is assessed according to observations of their judgment, orientation, memory, affect, attitude and cognition. The main advantage of this form of ongoing assessment is that the nurse can draw some conclusions about the client's current mental status based on direct observation, with minimal reliance on the client providing dialogue.

For the assessment of children and adolescents with an intellectual disability, the Developmental Behaviour Checklist (Einfeld & Tonge 1995) is a 96-item checklist that allows carers (including nurses) to rate the severity of a child's behavioural and emotional problems on a scale.

Other pitfalls in the assessment process

There are other difficulties that may occur from the perspective of the mental health nurse who is assessing a client with a dual disability.

- The client may display uncharacteristically impoverished or regressed social and communication skills, which might mask the signs of mental health disorder.
- The client may give unreliable or inappropriate responses to questions asked by clinicians at the time of assessment due to their lack of understanding of the abstract terms and concepts used in the assessment process (Hamer 1998).

Box 11.1 **JOMACC assessment at a glance**

Judgment
- Perception of events or stimuli
- Appropriateness of appearance, such as grooming, touching and language
- Interpretation of vulnerable situations (observations such as hitting a bigger, stronger client)
- Aggression towards self
- Aggression towards others
- Aggression towards property
- Suicidal gestures
- Responses to recent significant life events
- No behavioural improvement despite consistent, high-quality behavioural programming
- Awareness of surroundings
- Awareness of internal stimuli
- Awareness of name, location and reason for hospitalisation
- Impaired level of consciousness

Orientation
- Awareness of surroundings
- Awareness of internal stimuli
- Awareness of name, location and reason for hospitalisation
- Impaired level of consciousness

Memory
- Recent memory tests (What did you have for breakfast? What activity did you just do?)
- Ability to repeat what was said
- Remote memory tests (the name of community caregiver)

Affect
- Acting-out behaviour
- Emotional status (laughing, crying, flat, constricted)
- Verbalisation of fear
- Withdrawal behaviour
- Reluctance to perform a learned skill
- Reluctance to be with familiar people
- Multiple complaints, somatisation
- Reluctance to be in familiar surroundings
- Response to known upcoming event
- Response to current or near-current event
- Temper tantrum
- Change in activity level
- Facial expression, tone
- Aggression
- Hand or body gestures
- Appropriateness of emotional state
- Range of emotional state
- Sleep disturbance
- Changes in eating patterns
- Decreased concentration
- Loss of interest
- Statements regarding self-worth, suicide, hurting self or others
- Changes in person's behaviour or mood that occurs in all settings, versus just some settings
- Hypersexuality

Attitude
- Uncooperative
- Sarcastic
- Perplexed
- Hostile
- Apprehensive
- Unfeeling

Cognition
- Ability to keep thoughts focused
- Speech patterns (echolalic, mutism, intonation, pressure, rate, deterioration)
- Displays beliefs that are obviously false
- Gestured hallucinations
- Voiced hallucinations
- Poor interpersonal relationships
- Decreased ability to perform activities of daily living (feeding, dressing, toileting)
- Poor eye contact
- Bizarre rituals
- Emotional dissociation (including mood variability and impulsiveness)
- Catatonia
- Paranoid behaviour

Source: Hamer BA 1998, Assessing mental status in persons with mental retardation, *Journal of Psychosocial Nursing & Mental Health Services*, 35(5), pp 27–31.

- Ross & Oliver (2002) asserted that the presence of atypical signs in response to mental illness, such as the challenging behaviours exhibited by John and the stereotypical (or repetitive) behaviours exhibited by Margaret (see p 184), may add another potentially confusing dimension to the assessment process.
- A related impediment is *diagnostic overshadowing* (Reiss, Levitan & Szyszko 1982), in which important indicators of mental illness are simply attributed to the client's intellectual disability rather than being interpreted as signs of mental illness—that is, the client's behaviour is overshadowed by their diagnosis of intellectual disability (see the case study of Margaret on p 184 for an example).

ACUTE NURSING MANAGEMENT
The key to managing clients who have a mental illness co-morbid with an intellectual disability lies in establishing effective communication with them, their carers and/or their families, combined with a thorough assessment.

CASE STUDY: Margaret

Margaret is a 35-year-old woman who normally lives with her mother and has limited support needs. Margaret has a small vocabulary but is able to understand much of what is said to her. She can perform self-help tasks and has developed competencies in occupational, leisure and social skills. Diagnostic overshadowing played a large part in the delay between the onset of severe symptoms and diagnosis for this client.

The police brought Margaret into the emergency department late one Sunday after local residents reported that she had been lying on the road outside a shopping centre. Margaret was very distressed and crying, and when asked why she lay on the road replied: 'You will get run over lying on the road and go to heaven, sorry Mr Policeman'. She was able to give her name, phone number and address to the attending mental health nurse and a subsequent phone call found that Margaret lived at home with her mother and had gone to the local shops for bread. The mental health nurse and the duty psychiatrist decided that Margaret could go home to the care of her mother as there was no history of mental illness and she was able to say where she lived. Lying on the road was dismissed as 'behaviour' due to her intellectual disability. This proved to be *diagnostic overshadowing*.

Two days later Margaret's mother Jean telephoned the mental health service staff to say that a local shopkeeper had brought Margaret home after he had found her lying on the road. Jean was told that someone from the mental health team would visit in the next couple of days, but this was not regarded as high priority, as the behaviour was seen as part of Margaret's intellectual disability. The following afternoon, community mental health nurses visited and questioned Margaret, who became tearful and repeated: 'I'll get run over and go to heaven'. Jean told the staff that she had heard Margaret crying at night and that she had been awake early in the morning and needed to be told to shower. This was unlike Margaret but Jean said that she had been sad since her grandmother died three months ago and seemed to lack motivation.

On their way back to the community mental health centre the nurses called in to the local shops and discovered that Margaret had been lying on the road intermittently for the past four weeks. At first she would get up as soon as someone called out to her but over the past two weeks she would cry: 'No I'll get run over and go to heaven'. The staff, recognising her behaviour as suicidal, arranged for Margaret to be admitted to the mental health unit as an involuntary patient (i.e. she was deprived of her right to discharge herself from hospital on the grounds that there was a reasonable risk that she would harm herself). (See Ch 22 for suicide and self-harm, and Ch 4 for mental health legislation.) Margaret's subsequent nursing care is described below.

There is ample evidence that clients with a dual disability can benefit from a range of physical interventions, such as pharmacological treatments (Jenkins 2000) and electroconvulsive therapy (Ruedrich & Alamir 1999), in much the same way as do other members of the community who suffer from a mental illness (see Ch 23 for a range of therapeutic interventions).

Collins (1999) points out that psychotherapy for clients with a dual disability was often not used, based on the belief that their intellectual capacity and limited communications repertoire rendered them ineligible. There is now evidence that a range of 'talk therapies' such as psychodynamic, behavioural and cognitive therapies are effective for those with functional language skills, albeit in an abridged form (McKee 2001; Raghavan 1998). Similarly, Raghavan (1998) has commented on the reported efficacy of various relaxation techniques used to manage anxiety states for clients with a dual disability. The nursing interventions described in Chapter 23 can be employed in much the same way as they are for the remainder of the population, with the addition of more comprehensive discharge planning.

The case study of Margaret (above) provides an example of the acute nursing care that would be provided for the dual disability client following their admission to an inpatient unit.

In Margaret's case, nursing and medical staff found that she was uncommunicative upon admission to the mental health unit and that she sat gently rocking and averting her gaze from staff. Fortunately, the staff were able to engage Jean (Margaret's mother) in the process of taking a history and for some of the assessment process. After medical staff had performed a physical examination of Margaret, it was decided to take her to her bedroom and continue the assessment process once she had familiarised herself with her new environment. In the interim, a nurse was able to commence brief conversations with Margaret using gentle open-ended questions. Margaret was subsequently asked to unpack her suitcase and engage in self-care activities independently.

Margaret lived at home, and in such cases it is important to work with the family, to gain their trust and to ensure the optimal outcome for the client, and to obtain a reliable history of the client's mental and physical status. Over the course of the next hour, the nurse was able to ascertain from Jean that Margaret was uncharacteristically withdrawn and that her movements were much slower than usual. Jean also revealed that Margaret's concentration had deteriorated in recent weeks, and Margaret was able to add that she felt terrible and that she didn't 'want to live anymore'. Apart from these typical signs of clinical depression (see the diagnostic criteria in Ch 15), staff noted that Margaret's rocking had continued and that she made low, barely audible noises. Jean confirmed that rocking and moaning were atypical signs of Margaret's depression as they were not normally part of her behavioural repertoire.

Having gained the confidence of the new patient, the nurse was able to interview Margaret alone and, after some encouragement, found that she had retained her plan to kill herself by lying down in the middle of a road and being run over by a car. She did not have any other plans for her own death but repeated that what she really wanted was to die and go to heaven to see her grandmother. Eventually, the nurse was able to complete the initial assessments for Margaret, including mental status assessment and a risk assessment and was able to write admission notes that described her signs and symptoms, including the atypical signs, of depression. Margaret was subsequently placed on half-hourly general observations with fourth-hourly observations using the JOMAAC tool as a format for further assessment of mental status. Although primary nursing was not a part of the unit's policy on patient care, Margaret was allocated a single nurse for each subsequent morning and afternoon 'shift' on the first two days of her admission in order to facilitate communications and to assist in the process of ongoing assessment. Despite these arrangements, Margaret remained largely uncommunicative and chose to speak only with a few of the staff.

Apart from the interventions outlined above, the management of Margaret's depression was much like that afforded to other patients (see Ch 15). While she was being stabilised on an antidepressant (in this case venlafaxine), Margaret was offered grief counselling (see Ch 9) to help her to cope with the loss of her grandmother. Although Margaret was quick to understand that she needed to take her medication with her morning and evening meals until her doctor said to stop, she was unable to grasp education given to her by staff about the physiology of her depressive illness and the need to be vigilant regarding the symptoms of relapse. She also had a very limited understanding of the way in which her medication was helping her.

At the suggestion of Margaret's mother, and with Margaret's permission, it was decided to devise a mental health support plan (see p 186) in order to disseminate information about Margaret's management strategies to her carers when she had been discharged. The plan featured possible relapse signs (such as social withdrawal and 'rocking') and management strategies should Margaret again decide to harm herself (such as removing Margaret from harmful circumstances, clarifying Margaret's intentions, and contacting the community mental health team if Jean required assistance). It was also possible to use behaviour modification techniques (see Ch 23), which meant that treats or activities might be withheld to penalise undesirable behaviour such as lying on the road, or rewards given to reinforce desirable behaviour.

FACILITATING CONTINUOUS CARE
According to Yamada, Korman & Hughes (2000), the achievement of lasting positive outcomes for clients with a dual disability and the avoidance of unnecessary hospitalisations due to acute relapse of illness is highly dependent on the commitment of staff to the discharge planning process. The following discussion about the long-term, ongoing care of clients with a dual disability recognises that these clients typically access a range of services for their ongoing or continuous care and support (Accordino, Porter & Morse 2001; Barlow 1999; Silka & Hauser 1997). It is also important to recognise that those individuals living with their family or in their own home typically have contact with some form (or many different types) of disability support service and that those clients who live in supported accommodation services frequently maintain a high level of contact with and support from their family members. In addition, the role of the family, apart from providing typical family relationships, is often to fulfil the role of substitute decision-maker or advocate.

Understanding disability support services
Although it is difficult to outline all the salient features of disability services, one common component of these services that is vital to this discussion is the process of individual planning. Individual plans, also known by a variety of other names such as individual care plans, individual program plans and general service plans, are considered the core documents that guide disability service providers in planning for and delivering a service that endeavours to meet the individual needs and aspirations of each service user. The plan is usually developed on initial entry to the service, monitored regularly, and reviewed at least annually. The development of the plan typically involves assessment of the client and consultation with other stakeholders, with prioritised goals forming the key performance indicators for the service.

Individual plans, while varying in the scope of outcomes targeted, are based on the needs of the client, and may also guide the client's support network in assisting them to attain a preferred lifestyle and living environment. Individual plans may include an array of behaviour intervention and support plans (Whitworth, Harris & Jones 1999), including:

- *ecological interventions*—changing the client's environment to help them to achieve a quality of life while minimising toxic stimuli
- *positive skill development programs*—teaching the client diverse skills such as social or leisure skills
- *focused interventions*—using behaviourist approaches based on reinforcement of positive behaviours and the non-reinforcement of inappropriate behaviours
- *reactive strategies*—plans aimed at minimising harm when the client exhibits inappropriate behaviours (LaVigna, Willis & Donnellan 1989).

In disability services, holistic support is attained through the development of documented individual (multi-elemental) support plans, which can direct support services in assisting the client to achieve some level of personal success, self-esteem and quality of life (Fletcher & Poindexter 1996).

Another feature of many disability support services that should be discussed is the professional background of the people they employ. There is often a misconception among mental health professionals that all disability support services, particularly those providing primary support through accommodation and case management services, are equipped to fully manage people with a mental illness. This is often far from reality. Many disability support organisations do not specifically employ staff with mental health nursing backgrounds but traditionally draw their staff from the fields of social welfare, disability nursing, aged-care nursing, or any number of unrelated and various employment backgrounds (Holt, Costello & Oliver 2000). Where a client requires a specialist service for addressing their specific needs (e.g. health needs), the role of disability service personnel is to assist the client to access appropriate generic community services (i.e. the services used by any member of the community).

When a client with a dual disability is discharged back into the care of a disability accommodation support service, the mental health nurse needs to have a clear understanding of the service, its service features, the skills of the staff and the function it is funded to provide within the disability support network. This understanding should minimise confusion or misunderstandings in the implementation of management programs and ensure that the client does not get caught in any voids created by inter-agency disputes over roles and responsibilities. Of course this level of understanding must be afforded to the family and carers of the client living at home, as they may or may not have the skills, knowledge and experience required to effectively support the individual through the treatment process.

Discharge planning

The purpose of discharge planning is, ideally, to return the client to his or her prior environment or other suitable community-based setting. Effective discharge planning should commence at the time of the client's initial presentation to the mental health service and should include elements such as a schedule for outpatient follow-up and the provision of any other additional services as required (Silka & Hauser 1997).

In facilitating the discharge planning process, the mental health nurse should first identify the client's support network and establish effective communication with the relevant personnel. The two services should then work together to facilitate the inclusion of the discharge plan in the client's individual plan as a mental health support plan (MHSP), an important phase of which is identifying the roles and responsibilities of each of the members of the client's support network, as well as resources required. The plan should be documented (including monitoring and review phases) in a functional format that all personnel can follow and implement. Information about the client's mental illness and its management should then be supplied as necessary to the client, their family, carers, support staff and/or advocacy personnel.

Silka & Hauser (1997) recommend that, before discharge, a conference be held between all members of the support network to ensure that the relevant responsibilities and processes of support are articulated, negotiated, agreed to, understood and documented, including: steps to be taken that may avoid future inpatient stays; further tests or assessments and any appropriate additional referrals for further support; and criteria for and processes of responding to critical incidents.

The general practitioner plays a significant role in the continuous care process. As Coughlan (2000) clearly identified, many families and carers of people with a dual disability often rely on ongoing support with regard to medication, not through the prescribing psychiatrist but more often through their GP. This phenomenon is more obvious in rural settings, where mental health services may be scarce but occur in urban areas where families and individuals prefer to trust the GP they have known for many years. Therefore, identifying and liaising with the client's GP should ensure that the latter is aware of prescribed treatments and other relevant interventions.

Information sharing

Holt et al. (2000) suggest that the ability of clients, family members, carers and others to respond quickly and early to an episode of acute illness is diminished if they have little insight into or training about mental illness and how it affects the client. Family members, carers and disability support workers who are educated in the issues of dual disability, or who are supported in identifying and accessing information resources, are more likely to provide effective support to the client and work more effectively with (other) service professionals. Additionally, the inclusion of psycho-educational strategies (such as providing information about the signs, such as poor sleep patterns or agitation, which may indicate that the person is going to become acutely ill, or the effects, side-effects and protocols for administration of neuroleptic medications) in the client's treatment plan has been demonstrated to have positive results in treatment compliance and the overall wellbeing of the client (Coyle 2000; Pekkala & Merinder 2002).

Mental health support plans

Many support services, as part of the individual planning process, are now developing a broad array of specific health-care plans to ensure that the medical and health needs of the client are planned, implemented and monitored by appropriate health professionals. Examples include mealtime support plans, epilepsy management plans and diabetes management plans. Specific to the discussion here is the emergence of the mental health support plan (MHSP), also known as mental health plans or mental health care plans. An example of an MHSP that relates to the 'Sophie' case study opposite is shown in Figure 11.1 (on pp 188–9). Often developed by nurses and others with specific mental health training and experience who work within the disability service network, the MHSP is increasingly being implemented by disability services and welcomed by families.

The MHSP provides staff, carers, families and individuals with clearly documented guidelines that can be used for a number of purposes, including:

- providing a forum for the inclusion of significant others in the development, implementation and review of the client's treatment
- ensuring that prescribed treatments are provided as directed by the psychiatrist and/or other related health professionals
- the clear documentation of strategies, routines and programs
- ensuring that early intervention strategies are identified (including understanding the early signs of acute illness and the appropriate use of medications), thus minimising the need for acute admissions.

In order to ensure that an effective MHSP is devised, it is the responsibility of mental health nurses to make themselves available to provide input during the planning process, either through attending individual planning meetings held by the disability service personnel supporting the client, or by providing information as required to the author of the individual plan. It should also be recognised that the MHSP is an appropriate clinical tool for families and other non-professional or unpaid carers to ensure that treatment goals are achievable in the less formal environment of the family home and also to assist carers in their preparation for crises that may arise from exacerbation of their family member's mental illness.

Providing resources for clinicians and clients

At the time of writing, some of the health regions across Australia had begun to develop policies and practices to assist clinicians in their attempts to provide quality services for clients with a dual disability, and New Zealand appears to have made even more progress in this area.

- The Victorian Department of Health has created the Victorian Dual Disability Service, which provides support for clinicians and personnel from disability and mental health services. However, this unit is mainly centre-based in Melbourne and has limited capacity to provide 'outreach' facilities to regional areas.
- The South Australian Department of Human Services has a division known as the Intellectual Disability Services Council, which is responsible for the Dual Disability Program, a centre-based service.
- The Queensland Department of Health has formed alliances with Disability Services Queensland and the University of Queensland Developmental Disability Unit, with the aim of improving service delivery to people with a dual disability. This alliance has produced several reports and appears to be a promising source of reform within the Queensland mental health-care system.
- Otherwise, there exists a more patchy approach throughout the rest of Australia, although the South-Western Sydney Area Mental Health Service has taken a bold and imaginative step in employing a Clinical Nurse Consultant Dual Diagnosis (Intellectual Disability and Mental Illness) to facilitate the development of services for clients and also to ensure inter-agency cooperation and the development of mental health support plans.

CASE STUDY: Sophie

Sophie is a nineteen-year-old woman with an intellectual disability and extensive support needs who normally lives at home with her family. She was admitted as an involuntary patient to a psychiatric admission unit after she was provisionally diagnosed with a first-episode psychotic illness.

Mental health personnel had obtained a history of Sophie's recent mental status changes from Sophie's parents and initially communicated with her with the assistance of her brother, who she trusted. During her initial assessment, Sophie explained that she was afraid of her parents and that she believed them to be evil. She indicated that she had 'voices' in her head but was unable to communicate what these voices were telling her. Her parents added that, in the months before her admission, Sophie had been reluctant to shower, spent a lot of time in her room and could be heard talking to herself. When asked if anything was wrong, she became evasive, stating that she was just singing to herself. Sophie became more withdrawn and

disorganised in her behaviour, eventually becoming aggressive when approached by her parents. Her personal hygiene deteriorated, she refused to change her clothes and remained in her room, coming out only for meals. Staff noted that, apart from her aggression, Sophie displayed 'atypical' signs such as making strange noises and hitting the side of her head when she became stressed.

In the weeks after her admission, staff used the JOMAAC tool to assess Sophie's progress until some of the nursing staff managed to build up a rapport with her. She continued to take her prescribed antipsychotic medication (risperidone) and otherwise received the nursing care afforded to a person with a psychotic illness (see Ch 14). As Sophie's condition stabilised in the protective environment of the admission unit, mental health staff commenced discharge planning including the preparation of a mental health support plan. An example of a mental health support plan as it might have been designed for Sophie is provided in Figure 11.1.

MENTAL HEALTH SUPPORT PLAN

Name: Ms Sophie Jones

Date commenced:
Review date:

Written by: Norma Cloonan (Clinical Nurse Consultant)

Rationale and aims

This plan is designed to give Sophie's parents and support service personnel guidance in how best to support her in managing her mental illness, including preventative strategies for when her symptoms are acute and difficult for her to self-manage.

Sophie has experienced an acute psychotic episode with an associated functional disability, and has a moderate intellectual disability. She lives at home with her parents and works as an Electronic Components Assembler. There is no known family history of mental illness, and Sophie's condition, whilst it is unclear when it began, only became a problem for her and her family about four months ago. After a period of inpatient assessment and stabilising of her condition, she was discharged back into the community, with Mental Health Services continuing to monitor her progress.

This Mental Health Support Plan has been developed through consultation with Sophie and the people in her support network and will be reviewed at least three-monthly.

The aim of the Mental Health Support Plan is to support Sophie to maintain her place in the community, including her living arrangements and her employment, through preventative treatments and strategies, and through early response and intervention should her psychosis re-occur.

Signs and symptoms of Sophie's psychosis

When Sophie is in an acute phase of her psychosis she will be exhibiting the following signs:

- Sophie will sit and talk to herself, often looking at one place near her as she speaks (note that her speech will be conversational, as if she is talking to and listening to another person).
- Sophie will refuse to change her clothes as she believes that her mother has been putting 'bad things' in her clothing.
- She will talk repetitively about her mother and father being 'bad'.
- She will be suspicious of other people, particularly if they are known friends of her parents.
- She will be easily distracted, often not listening to speakers or simply ignoring them, or she will need questions to be repeated several times before she answers them.
- She will isolate herself in her bedroom, coming out only for meals.
- She may become aggressive towards her family or towards herself (striking the side of her head).

Triggers: things that may make the symptoms worse

The following situations and events have been identified as having possible influence on triggering an exacerbation of her psychosis. These are listed to draw your attention to ensuring that they are avoided where possible:

1 **Missed medication and medication non-compliance**—Sophie has been observed spitting her medication out when she thinks no one is looking.
2 **Alcohol consumption**—although she does not seek out alcohol, it has been noticed that even light beer on a special occasion has a negative effect on her mental state.
3 **Lack of sleep**—Sophie has been more withdrawn and guarded when she has not had adequate sleep.
4 **Stress**—extra pressure at work, other people pressuring her, being picked on, etc.

Prevention strategies

The following strategies are to be implemented in the effort to prevent further acute episodes of psychosis in Sophie:

1 **Supervise her taking her medication**—make sure she has a drink with her medication and that she takes it before a meal. Keep an eye out for discarded medication and report any incidents of medication non-compliance to her Community Mental Health Nurse.
2 The Community Mental Health Nurse is to **monitor Sophie's progress** by meeting with her weekly and responding to calls from the family or employer as required.
3 Sophie is to be seen by her **psychiatrist once a month (initially)** for a medication review. The Community Mental Health Nurse will attend each appointment.
4 Sophie's parents and support workers are to **report any signs or symptoms** of Sophie's psychosis as listed above immediately to the Community Mental Health Nurse.

Responding to a crisis

Sophie may require more assessment and support with her psychosis than can be offered by those in her community support network. The following procedures are to be followed if the signs and symptoms of Sophie's psychosis are observed:

1 **Give her one dose of her PRN medication**—she may go to sleep within 20 minutes, although when she is very ill the medication may appear to have little effect.
2 **Contact the mental health nurse** (during business hours) **or the mental health team** after hours (phone: 5555 5555) and inform them of Sophie's condition.
3 **Follow instructions**—a decision about how to manage the situation will be made after consultation with the psychiatrist.
4 **If she is to be taken to the local hospital for admission**, this will be done by the mental health team or the police. Make sure you pack a bag for her and send any records or notes that may assist the psychiatrist in assessing her condition and reviewing her treatment.

Note: If Sophie is admitted to the local hospital, this plan must be reviewed before discharge.

Signatures of agreement

Author's signature: _____ Date: _____

Signatures of agreement to this plan:

Name: _____ Signature: _____ Date: _____
Name: _____ Signature: _____ Date: _____
Name: _____ Signature: _____ Date: _____
Name: _____ Signature: _____ Date: _____
Name: _____ Signature: _____ Date: _____
Name: _____ Signature: _____ Date: _____

Plan review date:

Note: This sample mental health support plan (MHSP) has been designed to demonstrate the presentation of information for this textbook chapter. The information in this sample has been kept to a minimum and is not to be considered a clinical model for the management of any individual client who has a psychotic illness.

Figure 11.1 Example of a mental health support plan

In New Zealand, the Ministry of Health contracts dual diagnosis teams to work with clients with a dual disability. Although these teams are based mostly in hospitals via referral through the Needs Assessment and Service Coordination agency (NASC) (and thus are centre-based), outreach services are also available (D Hughes, project manager, Disability Services Directorate, New Zealand Ministry of Health, personal communication, 28 July 2003). As this service arrangement has been in place for about four years, New Zealand services for people with a dual disability appear to be more advanced than their Australian counterparts.

CONCLUSION

Providing nursing management for clients with a dual disability is a challenging task that requires mental health nurses to alter their practice to accommodate the specific needs of the client and also to liaise with carers and disability service personnel. The nurse must also anticipate that not all health professionals can work effectively with this client group, sometimes because of a lack of specific skills and knowledge and sometimes because of personal prejudices. With the improvement of support services and the greater availability of information, however, it is anticipated that future mental health nurses will be better informed about this important issue and that they may be better prepared and motivated to address the specific needs of clients with a dual diagnosis.

EXERCISES FOR CLASS ENGAGEMENT

■ Prepare a list of derogatory terms you have heard used to describe people with an intellectual disability. Prepare a list of non-discriminatory terms used to describe people with this form of disability. Compare your lists with those of your group members. Which is the longest list? What are the reasons for this discrepancy?

■ How do individual group members feel about working with people who have an intellectual disability? Identify the impediments to providing care for these people.

■ What factors might interfere with the achievement of a positive outcome for the client with dual disability within mental health services and within disability services? Outline strategies to overcome these barriers.

REFERENCES

Abdurman S & Hurd A (eds) 2002, *Management of Communication Needs in People with Learning Disability*, Whurr, London.

Accordino MP, Porter DF & Morse T 2001, Deinstitutionalization of persons with severe mental illness: context and consequences, *Journal of Rehabilitation*, 67(2), pp 16–21.

American Association on Mental Retardation (AAMR) 2002, *Mental Retardation: Definition, Classification and Systems of Supports* (10th edn), American Association on Mental Retardation, Washington DC.

American Psychiatric Association (APA) 2000, *Diagnostic and Statistical Manual of Mental Disorders* (4th edn, text rev.), APA, Washington DC.

Australian Health Ministers 1998, *Second National Mental Health Plan*, Commonwealth Department of Health and Family Services, Canberra.

Barlow C 1999, Issues in the management of clients with the dual diagnosis of learning disability and mental illness, *Journal of Disability Nursing, Health, and Social Care*, 3(3), pp 159–62.

Barr O 1998, Responding to the health needs of people with learning disabilities. In: Thompson T & Mathias P (eds), *Standards and Learning Disability* (2nd edn), Bailliére-Tindall, London.

Barr O, Gilgun J, Kane T & Moore G 1999, Health screening for people with learning disabilities by a community learning disability nursing service in Northern Ireland, *Journal of Advanced Nursing*, 29(6), pp 1482–91.

Benson BA 1985, Behaviour disorders and mental retardation: associations with age, sex and level of functioning in an outpatient clinic sample, *Applied Research in Mental Retardation*, (6), pp 79–85.

Borthwick-Duffy SA 1994, Epidemiology and prevalence of psychopathology in people with mental retardation, *Journal of Consulting and Clinical Psychology*, 62(1), pp 17–27.

Bostock L, Gleeson B, McPherson A & Pang L 2001, *Deinstitutionalisation and Housing Futures: Final Report*, Australian Housing and Urban Research Institute, Sydney.

Cockerill H & Carroll-Few L (eds) 2001, *Communication Without Speech: Practical Augmentative & Alternative Communication*, MacKeith, London.

Collins S 1999, Treatment and other therapeutic interventions: psychological approaches, *Tizard Learning Disability Review*, 4(2), pp 20–7.

Coombs T & Martin C 2002, Information and Risk Assessment: What do Nurses Think is Important?, paper presented to the conference of the Australian and New Zealand College of Mental Health Nurses, Sydney, 15–18 October.

Coughlan BJ 2000, Psychopharmacology in the treatment of people with learning disabilities: a review, *Mental Health Care*, 3(9), pp 304–7.

Coyle D 2000, Meeting the needs of people with learning disabilities and mental health problems: a review, *Mental Health Care*, 3(12), pp 408–11.

Deb S, Thomas M & Bright C 2001, Mental disorder in adults with intellectual disability. 1: Prevalence of functional psychiatric illness among a community-based population aged between 16 and 64 years, *Journal of Intellectual Disability Research*, 45(6), pp 495–505.

Dykens EM, Hodapp RM & Finucane BM 2000, *Genetics and Mental Retardation: A New Look at Behaviour Interventions*, Paul Brookes, Baltimore.

Edwards N & Lennox N 2002, Dual Diagnosis Project, University of Queensland, Brisbane. Online: http://www.sph.uq.edu.au/QCIDD/, accessed 28 July 2003.

Einfeld SL & Tonge BJ 1995, The Developmental Behaviour Checklist: the development and validation of an instrument to assess behavioural and emotional disturbance in children and adolescents with mental retardation: 1 Rationale and methods, *Journal of Autism and Developmental Disorders*, 25(2), 81–104.

Fletcher RJ & Poindexter AR 1996, Current trends in mental health care for persons with mental retardation, *Journal of Rehabilitation*, 63(1), pp 23–6.

Gilbert T, Todd M & Jackson N 1998, People with learning disabilities who also have mental health problems: practice issues and directions for learning disability nursing, *Journal of Advanced Nursing*, 27, pp 1151–7.

Hamer BA 1998, Assessing mental status in persons with mental retardation, *Journal of Psychosocial Nursing*, 36(5), pp 27–31.

Holt G, Costello H & Oliver B 2000, Training direct care staff about the mental health needs and related issues of people with developmental disabilities, *Mental Health Aspects of Developmental Disabilities*, 3(4), pp 132–9.

Jacobson JW 1990, Do some mental disorders occur less frequently among persons with mental retardation?, *American Journal on Mental Retardation*, 94(6), pp 596–602.

Jenkins R 2000, Use of psychotropic medication in people with learning disability, *Learning Disability Nursing*, 9(13), pp 844–50.

LaVigna GW, Willis TJ & Donnellan AM 1989, The role of positive programming in behavioral treatment. In: Cipani E (ed.), The treatment of severe behavior disorders: behavior analysis approaches. *Monographs of the American Association on Mental Retardation*, (12), pp 59–83.

Linfoot K (ed.) 1994, *Communication Strategies for People with Developmental Disabilities: Issues from Theory to Practice*, McLennan & Petty, Sydney.

McConkey R & Truesdale M 2000, Reactions of nurses and therapists in mainstream health services to contact with people who have learning disabilities, *Journal of Advanced Nursing*, 32(1), pp 158–63.

McIntyre LL, Blacher J & Baker BL 2002, Behaviour/mental health problems in young adults with intellectual disability: the impact on families, *Journal of Intellectual Disability Research*, 46(3), pp 239–49.

McKee R 2001, Therapeutic interventions in the support of people with learning disabilities who present mental health problems, *Assignment: Ongoing Work of Health Care Students*, 7(3), pp 4–8.

Minister for Disability Services 2001, *The New Zealand Disability Strategy: Making a World of Difference*, Whakanui Oranga, New Zealand Ministry of Health, Wellington.

Moss S & Lee P 2001, Mental health. In: Thompson J & Pickering S (eds), *Meeting the Health Needs of People who have a Learning Disability*, Bailliére Tindall, London.

Moss SC, Patel P, Prosser H, Goldberg DP, Simpson N, Rowe S et al. 1993, Psychiatric morbidity in older people with moderate and severe learning disability (mental retardation). Part 1: Development and reliability of the patient interview (the PAS-ADD), *British Journal of Psychiatry*, 163, pp 471–80.

Naylor V & Clifton M 1994, People with learning disabilities: meeting complex needs, *Health and Social Care*, 1(6), pp 343–53.

O'Brien J 1987, A guide to lifestyle planning: using the activities catalogue to integrate services and natural support systems. In: Wilcox B & Belamy GT (eds), *A Comprehensive Guide to the Activities Catalogue*, Paul H Brooks, Baltimore.

Pekkala E & Merinder L 2002, *Psychoeducation for Schizophrenia*, The Cochrane Library, Oxford.

Prosser H, Moss S, Costello H, Simpson N, Patel P & Rowe S 1998, Reliability and validity of the Mini-PAS-ADD for assessing psychiatric disorders in adults with intellectual disability, *Journal of Intellectual Disability Research*, 42, pp 264–72.

Raghavan R 1996, Confusing diagnosis, *Nursing Times*, 92(23), pp 59–63.

Raghavan R 1998, Anxiety disorders in people with learning disabilities: a review of literature, *Journal of Learning Disabilities for Nursing, Health and Social Care*, 2(1), pp 3–9.

Reiss S 1994, *Handbook of Challenging Behaviour: Mental Health Aspects of Mental Retardation*, IDS, Columbia.

Reiss S, Levitan GW & Szyszko J 1982, Emotional disturbance and mental retardation: diagnostic overshadowing, *American Journal of Mental Deficiency*, 86(6), pp 567–74.

Ross E & Oliver C 2002, The relationship between levels of mood, interest and pleasure and 'challenging behaviour' in adults with severe and profound intellectual disability, *Journal of Intellectual Disability Research*, 46(3), pp 191–7.

Ruedrich SL & Alamir S 1999, Electroconvulsive therapy for persons with developmental disabilities: review, case report and recommendations, *Health Aspects of Developmental Disabilities*, 2(3), pp 83–91.

Ryan J & Ryan A (n.d.) Hands can talk. Online: http://www.ispdr.net.au/~johnw/, accessed 8 July 2003.

Silka VR & Hauser MJ 1997, Psychiatric assessment of the person with mental retardation, *Psychiatric Annals*, 27(3), pp 162–9.

Sovner R 1996, Six models of behaviour from a psychiatric perspective, *The Habilitative Mental Healthcare Newsletter*, 15(3), pp 51–4.

von Tezchner S & Grove N 2003, *Augmentative and Alternative Communication and Developmental Issues*, Whurr, London.

Whitworth D, Harris P & Jones R 1999, Staff culture and the management of challenging behaviours in people with learning disabilities, *Mental Health Care*, 2(11), pp 376–9.

Wolfensberger W 1972, *Normalization: the Principle of Normalization in Human Services*, National Institute on Mental Retardation, Toronto.

World Health Organization 1993, *International Statistical Classification of Diseases and Related Health Problems* (10th edn), WHO, Geneva.

Yamada MM, Korman, M & Hughes CW 2000, Predicting rehospitalisation of persons with severe mental illness, *Journal of Rehabilitation*, 66(2), pp 32–9.

USEFUL WEBSITES

Australian National Council on Intellectual Disability (NCID) (the national association representing people with intellectual disability and their families in Australia http://www.dice.org.au/

IHC New Zealand Inc (counterpart to NCID and the largest provider of services to New Zealand people with intellectual disabilities and their families) http://www.ihc.org.nz/

University of Queensland Centre for Intellectual and Developmental Disability http://www.sph.uq.edu.au/QCIDD/

Victorian Dual Diagnosis Service http://www.vdds.org.au/default.htm

Information on the Mini PAS-ADD http://www.biomed2.man.ac.uk/ugrad/medicine/hester-adrian/MINIPAS.HTML

Information on the Developmental Behaviour Checklist http://www.med.monash.edu.au/psychmed/units/devpsych/dbc.html

Acknowledgment

The authors wish to acknowledge Mr Philip Petrie (Disability Support Consultant) for the individual mental health support plan format in Figure 11.1.

Disclaimer

Names, characters, places and incidents mentioned in the scenarios contained within this chapter have fictitious origins or are an amalgam of incidents recorded in the literature. Any resemblance to actual events, locales or persons is purely coincidental.

12

Disorders of Childhood and Adolescence

Mike Groome, Kristin Henderson and Jem Masters

KEY POINTS

- The prevalence of emotional problems in the earlier years of life ranges from ten to twenty per cent within developed countries, including Australia and New Zealand.
- Mental health problems cannot be seen as operating in isolation from other aspects of young people's lives.
- A child or adolescent experiencing behavioural or emotional problems may be indicative of problems within the family.
- Working with children and adolescents can be challenging but very fulfilling.
- It is essential to clarify the young person's perception of the problem and their goals for 'treatment', as well as that of the parents.
- 'Engagement' is the establishment of a therapeutic alliance, or rapport, to achieve desired outcomes and goals. This occurs from the initial interview. Understanding young people's language and communicating effectively is integral to engaging with them and vital to the success of their ongoing treatment.
- Young people can appear to be more guarded, sensitive or aggressive than adults with similar disorders.
- Nurses involved in the care of children and adolescents admitted to mental health facilities often have to deal with legal issues relating to duty of care, child protection and mental health legislation.

KEY TERMS

- engagement
- Gillick competence
- internalising and externalising problems
- medication compliance
- psychoeducation
- resocialisation

LEARNING OUTCOMES

The material in this chapter will assist you to:
- develop an introductory understanding and overview of childhood and adolescent mental health problems and disorders
- obtain insight into the extent of childhood and adolescent mental health problems and disorders internationally and in Australia
- gain an awareness of the range of services provided to children and adolescents
- explore the role of the nurse in child and adolescent mental health services.

INTRODUCTION

Just as in everyday life children and adolescents cannot simply be considered little adults, so within the field of psychological problems there are differences between early life and adulthood. This chapter introduces the field of child and adolescent mental health nursing. It explores the role of the nurse and then, using case studies from clinical practice, gives some examples of disorders experienced by children and adolescents and interventions that the nurse can use to help them.

Although some disorders are shared across generations, they may differ in their form of presentation at different developmental stages. Some problems common to adults may start in childhood or be influenced by events that occurred early in life. Some problems may resolve with neurological development or emotional maturity, or with a stable, supportive environment. Likewise, with effective intervention and treatment there may be other problems from which the young person can achieve a complete recovery.

Over the past decade, discoveries in neurological research have reinforced the idea that the human brain is quite 'plastic' and that some areas are influenced during development by the environment, including such factors as the level of stress or anxiety a young person experiences. There is also greater awareness of the interaction between genetic endowment and the surrounding world. These developments are helping to provide new understanding of how individual children cope with emotional difficulties and gain control over their lives. They have also reinforced the effectiveness of a wide range of therapeutic interventions (Hoagwood & Serene 2002).

An important factor in considering the effect of any kind of illness on young people is the disruption it may bring to every aspect of development and education. Although in adulthood our lives can be dramatically changed through illness, we have usually completed the basic developmental tasks of life and have finished the foundations of education. For the child or adolescent, however, various problems may develop simply due to the interruption caused by illness. Bowlby & Robertson (cited in Payne & Walker 2000) illustrated the effects on young children of their being separated from their family during hospitalisation. It is largely due to their efforts that in most general hospitals we now have liberal attitudes to parents and siblings being able to maximise contact with the sick child. In addition, in most major centres, consultation liaison services provided by teams of mental health professionals, including mental health nurses, give expert opinion and support for children and young people and their families when dealing with severe or prolonged physical illness.

Specialised child and adolescent mental health services are frequently not available in many areas of Australasia (Sawyer et al. 2000). If one takes the view that there are critical periods in life when particular development tasks

can be achieved, it is possible that these problems may have a long-term effect on people's lives (Brannon & Feist 2000). It is important therefore that services be developed and extended to more young people and that issues of equitable access to services be pursued vigorously.

DIAGNOSIS IN CHILD AND ADOLESCENT MENTAL HEALTH CARE

The American Psychiatric Association, in its *Diagnostic and Statistical Manual of Mental Disorders*, fourth edition (DSM-IV-TR, APA 2000) lists the disorders usually first diagnosed in infancy, childhood or adolescence (see Box 12.1). The major categories within child and adolescent services are listed, with some examples of specific diagnoses. The list in Box 12.1 is not exhaustive—for complete descriptions, refer to the DSM-IV-TR. Because some disorders are not unique to this stage of life, they are not included in the DSM-IV-TR list. Depressive disorders are an example, although depression is becoming increasingly common in children and adolescents (Sawyer et al. 2000).

Box 12.1 Common DSM-IV-TR diagnostic categories for disorders usually first diagnosed in infancy, childhood or adolescence

Learning disorders
Motor skills disorder
Communication disorders:
- stuttering

Pervasive developmental disorders:
- autistic disorder
- Rett's disorder
- Asperger's disorder

Attention-deficit and disruptive behaviour disorders:
- attention-deficit/hyperactivity disorder NOS
- conduct disorder
- oppositional defiant disorder

Feeding and eating disorders:
- pica
- rumination disorder

Tic disorders:
- Tourette's disorder
- chronic motor or vocal tic disorder

Elimination disorders:
- encopresis
- enuresis

Source: American Psychiatric Association 2000, *Diagnostic and Statistical Manual of Mental Disorders* (4th edn, text rev.), APA, Washington DC.

The diagnostic categories described in Box 12.1 are internationally recognised, although, in a national Australian survey (Sawyer et al. 2000), mental health problems were assessed using the Child Behaviour Checklist developed by Achenbach (1991). The checklist is used in many services in Australia and is shown in Box 12.2. As you can see, this checklist places stronger emphasis on behaviour and problems than categories of disorders. Problems are categorised into two general and eight specific areas, as shown here.

Box 12.2 Child behaviour checklist

General areas

- *Internalising problems*: inhibited or over-controlled behaviours, such as anxiety or depression
- *Externalising problems*: antisocial or under-controlled behaviours, such as delinquency or aggression

Specific areas

- *Somatic complaints*: recurring physical problems that have no known cause or cannot be medically verified. These may include headaches, or a tendency to develop signs and symptoms of a medical disorder.
- *Delinquent behaviour*: behaviour where rules set by parents and/or communities are broken, such as property damage, theft of cars and other items
- *Attention problems*: concentration difficulties and an inability to sit still, including school performance problems
- *Aggressive behaviour*: bullying, teasing, fighting and temper tantrums
- *Social problems*: where individuals have impairment of their relationships with peers
- *Withdrawal*: where the individual is specifically inhibited by shyness and being socially isolated
- *Anxious/depressed behaviour*: a range of feelings of loneliness, sadness, feeling unloved, a sense of worthlessness, anxiety and generalised fears
- *Thought disorders*: or what might be seen as bizarre behaviour or thinking

Source: adapted from Sawyer MG, Arney FM, Baghurst PA, Clark JJ, Graetz BW, Kosky RJ et al. 2000, *Child and Adolescent Component of the National Survey of Mental Health and Well-Being*, Mental Health and Special Programs Branch, Commonwealth Department of Health and Aged Care, Canberra.

Viewing problems within such a framework helps us to understand young people as having issues related to predominant personality traits, developmental factors, or incidents and influences within their family and wider social environment.

By contrast, static diagnostic systems can tend to lose the fluid, changing and reorganising nature of young people's experience as they progress towards adulthood, and may also run the risk of encouraging a focus on one 'problem' in isolation (Hoagwood & Serene 2002). For this reason, this chapter describes mental health problems in the context in which symptoms are observed, rather than in relation to categorical diagnostic criteria.

INCIDENCE

Writers in various Western countries have often expressed concern about the prevalence of emotional problems in the earlier years of life. Within countries surveyed, the incidence ranges from ten to twenty per cent. The World Health Organization has predicted that these figures will double by 2020, making emotional problems one of the more common causes of illness and disability in children (WHO 2001). This pattern is reflected in Australasia, with a current incidence of 14 per cent (Sawyer et al. 2000). Interestingly, on average, roughly the same number of children had externalising problems (12.9 per cent) as internalising problems (12.8 per cent) (Sawyer et al. 2000). Externalising problems are more noticeable and may therefore demand and receive more attention. Conversely, introversion and depression may go undetected because the child is often well behaved and sometimes what may be considered 'too good' by family members or 'overly compliant' by professionals.

MENTAL ILLNESS IN CONTEXT

Mental health problems can affect many other aspects of young people's lives and therefore the problems must be seen in context. The more significant the mental health problem an individual has, the greater the possibility of problems in other areas of their lives. Furthermore, parents and other family members may often see these problems as affecting their own lifestyles and activities. Not enough is known about the long-term outlook for these young people, but it is important for professionals to see young people in the context of their everyday experience. Help may be needed across a broad range of life issues—with family functioning, social skills or school problems, for example. While the mental health problem may have caused these difficulties, it is equally important to consider that the life issue may have been the cause *or* an aggravating factor in the disorder (Sawyer et al. 2000). A balanced view is required, so that causal factors are not attributed to one area without adequately observing what is happening in other aspects of the young person's life. It may be that the child or adolescent is acting as a 'barometer' for problems existing in the family—the young person may be presenting with symptoms that reflect problems in the family or between parents. This may not be recognised initially and may only be revealed after some time. An important aspect of assessment includes an evaluation of the family's functioning and coping skills.

SERVICES AVAILABLE TO CHILDREN AND YOUNG PEOPLE

In most Western countries, specialised services are usually called Child and Adolescent Mental Health Services (CAMHS) or Child and Youth Mental Health Services (CYMHS). Previously known as Child Guidance Clinics and as Paediatric Psychiatry, the services have expanded their scope considerably, offering a range of specialist assessment and treatment options. These services are usually found only in main centres.

It is believed that one in five young people suffering from mental health problems throughout the Western world will receive the expert help they need (NIMH 2002). In Australia, most children aged between four and twelve years with mental health problems are seen by paediatricians, whereas most teenagers are seen by school-based counsellors. On average, three per cent of children and adolescents with mental health problems have attended a mental health clinic, while two per cent were seen in a hospital psychiatric service. Approximately fifty per cent of Australian parents either think help for their child is too expensive, or do not know where to access it; forty-six per cent believe they can manage the problems themselves (Sawyer et al. 2000). Clearly, doctors and schools play an important role. It is a recommendation of the 2000 Australian survey that the help provided by the different services be better explained to local communities and that specialised mental health services provide strong support for these other services (Sawyer et al. 2000).

CRITICAL THINKING CHALLENGE 12.1

- Why do GPs, paediatricians and schools have such a vital role in early detection of mental health problems in children and young people?
- What interventions might GPs, paediatricians and schools provide?

For adolescents in particular, simply providing a traditional outpatient or inpatient service may not be enough. Many teenagers worry about what others would think if they asked for help. Even more say they prefer to take care of their own problems, as they struggle with their sense of identity and relationships with adults. Unlike children, because of the adolescent's striving for increasing autonomy, a family approach may not be useful. A variety of unhealthy or 'at-risk' behaviours may be present. Half of adolescents with mental health problems also smoke or drink and a third report binge drinking. There is also a close link between mental health problems and suicidal behaviour or thinking (Sawyer et al. 2000). Many health services and programs tend to focus on single issues, such as drugs and alcohol, or medical treatment, with insufficient attention paid to co-morbidity (Andrews et al. 1999). There is need for more collaboration and more funding for generalised adolescent health services and reach-out programs. In some centres in Australia, there are adolescent health centres where no appointment is needed and teenagers can go unaccompanied. These provide a wide range of services and programs for all health and lifestyle matters.

There is variation between regional services in the type of intervention and treatment available from specialised child and adolescent mental health services. As with adult services, there are usually a range of walk-in clinics and mobile crisis and support teams, backed up by separate residential units for children and adolescents.

The treatment provided also varies from centre to centre, depending on the major problems presenting locally, age range, treatment philosophy, theoretical models, expertise available and the living circumstances of the young person and their family. Interventions may include behaviour therapy, cognitive behavioural therapy, couples therapy, parenting programs, play therapy, psychodynamic individual or group work, socialisation and social skills programs, systems-based family therapy, or individual therapy for a parent. Sometimes approaches are combined to achieve better outcomes. For example, a child may benefit from behaviour therapy to help them deal with problematic behaviour, but the family may also require assistance to enable them to develop positive styles of functioning together. As with adult services, nurses have a range of roles, often developing expertise in various modes of therapy.

THE NURSING ROLE

Working with children and adolescents can be challenging but fulfilling and rewarding. As children and adolescents are still developing as individuals, an intervention in their young lives can often make a dramatic difference for the rest of their life and often is more effective than it would have been if it had happened in adulthood. With adequate care and a conducive environment, young people can grow stronger emotionally, psychologically and physically. Working with a child and adolescent mental health team provides the opportunity to use a wide range of dynamic, clinical treatment strategies and therapies. A multidisciplinary team approach is frequently used. Nurses often play a significant role in various aspects of care, including that of therapist, with children, adolescents and families. It is usually expected that a nurse wishing to enter this field will have some years of experience as a mental health (psychiatric) nurse and further education, thus possessing a solid grounding in theory and clinical practice.

Depending on the nature and philosophy of a particular service, nurses who wish to extend their skills and knowledge base are encouraged to do so. Some services have tended to use a generic model in which different professionals do much the same work. In fact, as with adult services, generic positions may be advertised in child and adolescent services. These positions can provide good opportunities for individual nurses to further their career by advancing their education and experience. For example, apart from graduate nursing programs, child and adolescent mental health nurses have options available for advanced studies in specialist areas of mental health, through postgraduate and Masters programs. In addition, nurses can enter a variety of psychotherapy training programs available for all professional disciplines. However, development of these roles often depends more on the individual nurse's personality, experience or education than on a clear definition of the nursing role (Limerick & Baldwin 2000). Such a practice can lead to a situation where nurses see themselves as psychotherapists rather than nurses. This appears to be an issue in several other countries, including the United Kingdom and the United States (Baldwin 2002). A variety of solutions have been proposed to address this issue, including seeking to identify the uniqueness of the nursing role (Limerick & Baldwin 2000). This is an ongoing debate for the profession and this chapter does not attempt to discuss the issues involved. It is, however, a matter that individual nurses may need to explore as they consider their developing expertise in the field.

The following list of core knowledge and traits regarded as fundamental for all professionals working in child and adolescent mental health services has been generated from unpublished English research by Limerick (1999, cited in Limerick & Baldwin 2000).

- child development theories
- theories that support child and adolescent mental health practice
- first session/interview skills
- therapeutic interventions
- evaluating skills
- professional management skills
- communication skills
- professional development skills
- practitioner qualities, such as trust, confidence and support.

With these attributes, mental health nurses can become a significant resource for their clients. However, to be able to intervene effectively with clients, the nurse needs to master the art of engaging with children and young people, both as individuals and in the context of their families.

CRITICAL THINKING CHALLENGE 12.2

Either individually or in a group, have a brainstorming session: list all the skills that a child and youth mental health nurse would require. Subdivide these into skills that you think may be specific to either a community mental health nurse or a mental health nurse working in an inpatient setting.

ENGAGING WITH CHILDREN AND ADOLESCENTS

One of the most useful skills the mental health nurse can acquire and refine is the ability to engage clients and

establish rapport. Engagement between nurses, young people and their families is fundamental to developing a relationship based on trust. A relationship founded on trust will foster a willingness to work together towards change. Faber & Mazlish (1999) identify the outcome to which the beginning mental health nurse working with young people should aspire as essentially: to master communicating so that children and teenagers will listen, but also being so good at listening that the young person is more likely to communicate.

Mental health nurses working with children and adolescents also need to develop and refine the skill of discreet observation of the young person's mood and behaviour, and their interactions with their peers, family, friends and others. Observation of these factors, considered in the broader psychosocial context, will enable the nurse to achieve a comprehensive assessment of the factors contributing to the current difficulties experienced by the young person and their family.

Ongoing discussion with parents (carers) should clarify an understanding about which specific factors may be contributing to current problems. With a more specific diagnosis, the nurse and family may then begin the process of exploring solutions (planning). Any solutions agreed upon with the family are best implemented with the family's support and commitment, so as to maximise the probability of positive change. Constant monitoring (evaluation) of behavioural interventions and responses by family members is essential to ensure that the mental health team, the young person and their family continue to share a common understanding about the management of the problem and a commitment to recovery.

Children

As outlined previously, a myriad of factors contribute to and affect the mental health of young people. Familial or genetic predisposition to mental illness, the presence of a coexisting medical or neurological problem, developmental problems or growing up in a chaotic or deprived environment, are just a few of the considerations of which the beginning mental health nurse should be mindful during assessments of young people and their families. Furthermore, these factors will also affect the direction taken with goal planning and nursing interventions. It should be remembered that the nursing care plan is in fact a recovery plan for the young person and family; therefore the goals must be achievable and the strategies must be practical when implemented by the child and family (with nursing support). If the plan is based on what the nurse can achieve rather than what the family can realistically accomplish, then the medium- to long-term success for recovery may be severely impaired and continuity of care lost. A case study and exploration of the issues discussed thus far will illustrate some key concepts.

CASE STUDY: Adam

A mother contacts the community child and youth mental health service, unsure whether it is appropriate to seek help regarding her nine-year-old son, Adam, who she describes as 'becoming increasingly anxious and who has developed a fixation with tidiness', so much so that it is causing disruption in the family. The family consists of two female siblings, aged eleven and seven, and a father who is an accomplished musician who frequently travels for extended periods performing nationally and internationally. The mental health nurse receiving the call assures the mother that her concerns warrant a further assessment by a member of the mental health team, as her child appears to be highly anxious. He is unable to relax and appears to be developing maladaptive behaviours (excessive tidying). Furthermore, his anxiety is having an adverse effect on his relationship with his siblings. The nurse gathers more specific information by phone and explains to the mother that this referral will be discussed at the next team meeting and that she will receive a call within a week regarding an appointment for her, her husband and their son, for further assessment.

Discussion of case study: Adam

Within the first minutes of the mother's description of her son's problem, the mental health nurse was able to predict a role for the mental health team in assisting this family. The mother was assured that her concerns were well founded. The nurse spent a little more time gathering only the information necessary to discuss the case (assessment) with the team, so a plan for a further 'face-to-face' interview could be made. Thus the mother feels reassured by the prospect of an appointment (implementation). A therapeutic alliance has been initiated between the family and the mental health service.

This early process reflects the beginning of the nurse's role in engaging the family in the therapeutic alliance and emphasises how important each team member's role is in promoting a positive impression on the family (even before meeting them personally). The impression the family gains from an initial phone call can colour their perception of further interactions with the mental health team. Furthermore, the parents' feeling of confidence in the mental health nurse and other team members will likely have an impact on the confidence that the child and siblings have. This is important, as all family members will be involved in the child's recovery.

The foundation and building of a therapeutic relationship with the young person and the family will usually begin at the time of the initial phone call or face-to-face interview. This interview can be difficult for the young person, who may not fully understand why they are attending an assessment at the mental health service, or may not perceive that there is a problem. The skilled mental health nurse will use this opportunity to establish the young person's understanding of their need for an appointment. If the young person seems unsure (or unwilling to concede), they can often be encouraged to describe what difficulties were occurring at home that led to their needing an appointment for assessment.

It is essential to clarify the child's perception of the problem and their goals for treatment, as well as those of the parents. The nurse's role is to facilitate expression of the difficulties and to make explicit the goal that the client and family have regarding recovery. This is necessary so that all parties (client, family and mental health team) can agree on the treatment plan.

Another case study will illustrate these key issues. While a diagnosis such as attention-deficit hyperactivity disorder might possibly be indicated in this situation, the case illustrates that it is important to concentrate on the presenting problems and any associated difficulties, rather than giving priority to diagnostic classification. Involvement in diagnostic controversies can potentially misdirect the focus of care from the individual needs of the child and family.

CRITICAL THINKING CHALLENGE 12.3

Imagine you are contacting a health service about worries and concerns you have for a family member. What nursing attributes and skills would you find reassuring during the first phone contact?

CASE STUDY: Tim

Tim is a six-year-old boy who is attending his first appointment at a community child and youth mental health service, accompanied by his parents. He is the oldest of three children and has a young brother and baby sister. His parents report an escalation in Tim's behaviour just before he turned three: 'It's like he never grew out of the 'terrible twos'. He just kept on going at a hundred miles an hour,' reported his mother. Tim's father concurred: 'The more limits I set, the worse he gets'. Tim's reply when asked if he knew why he was here was simply: 'I've been naughty'.

Discussion of case study: Tim

The skilled mental health nurse will attempt to clarify these comments using objective language and will eventually identify some very specific behaviours that the parents regard as priorities for change. The nurse will attempt to match the parents' goals with those of their son.

The nurse's response to Tim's perception that he has been 'naughty' might be: 'Naughty—what does that mean?'. The aim for the nurse is to guide Tim to use specific words to tag specific behaviours, and if these match those identified by his parents, a simple goal may be developed to achieve an outcome that is satisfying to both parties. Tim's descriptions of how he sees 'the problem' may also assist the nurse to establish more accurately what the problem might be. Consider this further exchange between Tim and the nurse:

Nurse: 'Naughty'—what does that mean?

Tim: When I run away or squeal.

Nurse: So you run away?

Tim: My brother . . . he's three . . . he runs away too . . . When he runs away from Mummy, she chases him.

Nurse: And does your brother squeal?

Tim: No, but when my baby sister squeals, Daddy helps Mummy play with her.

This exchange demonstrates how, through active listening, the nurse has gathered some very specific information about the family dynamics that provides a possible explanation for some of Tim's behaviour. It could be that he is mimicking the behaviours of his younger siblings to receive the same attention from his parents that he perceives his brother and sister receive when they run away or squeal.

Encounters with children and adolescents and their families as illustrated in these case studies demonstrate how the nurse and other team members can engage young people in ongoing treatment, and how treatment will be influenced by further findings. The initiation of a sound therapeutic alliance with the child and family is an achievement, although the alliance also requires nurturing.

Generally, a therapeutic alliance is accomplished when respect is paramount in the nurse–client relationship. Like adults, young people respond most positively to

being treated with genuine respect. Young people feel respected when they are listened to and given opportunities to make choices and contribute to solving problems. As Faber & Mazlish (1999) identify, making choices gives the child valuable practice in making decisions; opportunities for problem solving give them courage to follow things through independently. A commitment by the mental health nurse to facilitating choice and promoting problem-solving opportunities for young people will be further enhanced by a belief in the humanistic idea that all behaviour has meaning. If we as mental health nurses explore the meaning behind the behaviours we observe, we can plan appropriate strategies to modify behaviour and promote positive change.

Within Australia and New Zealand, child and youth mental health services work with many young people who present in acute emotional distress. Some will internalise their distress and may become withdrawn and depressed. Others may externalise their emotional pain. When this occurs, the child will demonstrate altered behaviours, which may include rigid thinking, compulsive patterns of behaviour, agitation, impulsivity and, in severe cases, aggression. If the nurse has established a therapeutic alliance with the child, the shared trust and respect will provide a foundation for choice-giving and problem solving. An example from practice will best illustrate this concept.

Discussion of case study: Fiona

Skills required—In the case study below, even though Fiona is refusing to be involved in the initial assessment, her behaviours and her brief interjections are a valuable source of assessment information. The nurse will document Fiona's behaviours and her comments. In context, this will reflect some family dynamics and give some indication of how Fiona currently feels about her life. The challenge for the nurse will be to initially engage Fiona in a shared interest of hers that is non-emotional and therefore less threatening.

Rather than attempting to engage Fiona too early, the nurse wisely chooses to wait for an opportunity. This does not arise until the very end of the initial interview, when the nurse announces that the assessment is almost

CASE STUDY: Fiona

Fiona is twelve years old and is attending the child and youth mental health service for the first time, accompanied by her mother, with whom she lives. Her younger brother has lived with her father since their parents separated three years ago. Fiona's mother is extremely concerned about a gradual change in Fiona's mood over the past two years. She has reportedly become angry and unpredictable, a dramatic change from the quiet but confident child she used to be. Her mother describes instances where Fiona

will impulsively run from home and engage in risky behaviours such as riding her bike recklessly on their busy street. When met by members of the mental health team, Fiona is at first passive, refusing eye contact, seeming to ignore the conversation between her mother and the nurse and refusing to respond when spoken to directly. Several times during the conversation, however, Fiona interrupts with a hostile comment, countering information provided by her mother.

complete. 'About time,' Fiona grumbles, 'I just want to get in the car and listen to my new CD'. The nurse grasps this opportunity:

Nurse: Ah, a new CD . . . which group?

Fiona: No-one *you'd* know.

Nurse: Try me.

To Fiona's surprise, the nurse has recently bought the same CD and although Fiona feigns horror that an adult would even know the band, she cannot completely disguise her admiration.

Nurse: See you in a fortnight then?

Fiona: If I'm not too busy with my music.

Fiona's choice of words ('If I'm not too busy . . .') indicates that she is trying to sound uninterested while still leaving her options open.

Approach taken and outcome achieved—Troubled children and adolescents are not always easily engaged. Often the factors contributing to their need for mental health support have affected their ability to trust others; in many cases they have felt let down by adults. The nurse who recognises this will allow time for the young person to engage, initially on his or her own terms, so the fragile therapeutic alliance can gradually strengthen. Fiona's hostility was ignored; the nurse chose instead to preserve Fiona's fragile sense of dignity. Respecting Fiona's ability to make sound decisions, the nurse did not assume that she would be returning in a fortnight, but rather posed it as a question; this approach was aimed at reassuring Fiona that she had a choice. Her choice to return in a fortnight would demonstrate her courage in recognising that a problem exists, and her willingness to explore some supports.

CRITICAL THINKING CHALLENGE 12.4

- What might the outcomes have been if the nurse had persisted in asking Fiona questions early in the interview?
- What assumptions could be made regarding Fiona's need to interrupt while her mother and the nurse were speaking?

Adolescents

When adolescents and their family (carers) present to a health-care facility, there is an expectation on their part that treatment will achieve the desired outcomes, in terms of the physical, emotional and mental state of the young person. However, it is possible that these outcomes may not be achieved, because of many situational factors. One such factor may be the young person's lack of willingness to be part of the referral, assessment and treatment process due to their not recognising or acknowledging that they have a significant problem. Mental health nurses providing mental health care for adolescents need to acknowledge that possible influencing factors such as poor insight, resistance to treatment or challenging of authority may be part of normal adolescent behaviour.

NURSE'S STORY

As an experienced mental health nurse, I'd regarded myself as a spontaneous, reflective clinician, confident that my responses to and interactions with patients were at all times respectful, helpful and kind. I was taken by surprise then, when I began working with young people in a mental health setting—surprised that I now felt hesitant and unsure of the appropriate response. My confidence and spontaneity had given way to feeling stilted and unsure . . . until a defining moment, when I realised that I should open my senses to messages from others, and that taking time to (literally) look in the mirror could deepen my understanding of how others see themselves. This is my story . . .

With his bath finished and his pyjamas on, eight-year-old Cobey and I stand in front of the full-length mirror looking straight at ourselves, occasionally glancing across at each other's reflection, then back to our own, and as we look into this mirror I wonder what it is that we each see.

I see myself: casually dressed, complete and unchanging, honest . . . and oh, so tired! I suspect that Cobey, like me, sees himself; but I speculate that the self that he observes might be a fragmented self, like looking into a broken mirror—lots of small pieces, together, but not quite. Coincidentally,

I note a small crack in the glass near where Cobey is standing. The mirror has been damaged, but because of the safety component of the glass, it has not shattered but simply absorbed the knock, leaving three fractures darting out from the one puncture point.

I kneel down beside Cobey to try to observe his reflection as he might be seeing it. As I had anticipated, his image is disjointed, and the symbolic implications momentarily tug at me.

'What do you see?', I ask quietly.

No answer. He moves bodily up and down and sideways, all the time trying to piece together his reflection in a harmonious union. But it is not to be—whichever position he views himself from, he is in several pieces, a fragmented whole.

'I'm in pieces . . . nothing fits together properly', he eventually says, giggling. Then for a few more minutes he moves about, trying to find where he might place himself so that the pieces of him do come together as they should. In a short while, in frustration, he curses the mirror and leaves the room.

I stand stunned. So much about us both reflected in this brief encounter.

Kristin Henderson

CASE STUDY: Julie

Julie is a fourteen-year-old who, over the past year, has become increasingly withdrawn from her peer group. She was previously an A-grade student in a select school, but over the past four months her school grades have dropped noticeably and she is not completing her homework. She no longer has an interest in playing netball or attending her athletics club. Julie's mother states that Julie has been aggressive towards her and has been harming herself by cutting her wrists with any sharp object available. Julie was commenced on antidepressant medication by her GP six weeks prior to admission but there has been minimal change in her mental state.

further engage the young person and further develop the therapeutic relationship. Establishing a confidante may be the turning point in the young person's treatment.

Discussion of case study: Julie

In the case study above, Julie requires intensive therapy, which may include cognitive behavioural therapy, family therapy, individual psychotherapy and a review of her medication. Psychosocial issues also need to be considered during Julie's treatment. This may include exploring school issues, as well as whether there is any risk of Julie having been physically, emotionally or sexually abused. Also, there may have been significant losses that have contributed to her depression.

In assisting young people like Julie, the mental health nurse will need to establish rapport and maintain engagement. It will be important to gain the client's confidence from the initial meeting, as there will be many sensitive issues to address. Adolescents seeking help from adults will not always commit time for a therapeutic relationship to grow, if they doubt in any way the sincerity of the person in whom they are confiding.

In some instances, the action of inflicting harm upon oneself can provide a sense of relief from severe emotional distress and psychic pain. It is therefore essential that the nurse recognises this possibility and, while working with the young person, makes every effort for them to feel respected and not judged on the behaviour that has led to them seeking help. Medical care, such as attention to a wound, should be addressed discreetly and professionally. The key aspect of providing care for the young person is establishing their current level of safety and working with them on how this can best be achieved. It will be helpful to ensure that the young person has adequate support networks, so they can strengthen these connections with a view to obtaining help in more adaptive ways in the future.

CRITICAL THINKING CHALLENGE 12.6

List the potential barriers to establishing a therapeutic alliance with Julie.

CONFIDENTIALITY

An important issue for young people is understanding how the information shared during interactions with team members is documented and knowing who has access to these records. It is important to them that their need for confidentiality be maintained. However, when there are risk factors involved, the young person must know that nurses and their colleagues are bound to impart information that has a direct effect on their safety or the safety of others.

Interviews with adolescents should not be restricted to the formality of interview rooms. As long as safety can be assured, some adolescents may prefer to be interviewed in a more public place, such as a courtyard. Flexibility (and not a small dose of ingenuity!) is the key to providing a quality service that will encourage young people to return in crisis.

MEDICATION COMPLIANCE

As stated previously, medication compliance is a major issue for adolescents, regardless of their condition. Many young people do not want to be different from their peer group. This may include not wanting to be seen as different by needing tablets. The rationale for taking medication should be explained and adverse effects discussed, together with how to reduce the complications of medication therapy. Problem solving with the young person about ways to discreetly include the taking of prescribed medication in their daily lifestyle pattern will be of benefit. The risk of taking non-prescribed medications should be highlighted. This can be achieved by maximising therapeutic interventions. In adolescent mental health, engagement through developing rapport and trust are key elements to achieving change. Without these elements, minimal change can be achieved.

The above case studies have sought to reinforce the importance of engagement. Demonstrating empathy and performing with absolute sincerity are important factors in caring for children and adolescents. It is important that young people feel that they are the priority for the nurse at this particular time.

A further important consideration for nurses working with children and adolescents is legal issues related to the treatment of mentally ill young people.

LEGAL ISSUES

Nurses involved in the care of young people admitted to mental health agencies often have to deal with legal issues relating to duty of care, child protection and mental health leglislation.

In the developed world, children and younger adolescents must have their parents' or guardian's consent to seek treatment for any form of medical intervention, including mental health assessments and treatment. Young people in Australia can give their own consent to receive medical or nursing treatment, as long as their parents are aware and the health professionals believe that the young person is competent to give consent. The ability for young people to consent to medical treatment or seek medical consultations is referred to as 'Gillick competence' (Gillick v. West Norfolk and Wisbech Area Health Authority 1986). Medical and nursing staff may question whether the young person is 'Gillick competent' or has the cognitive ability to make an informed judgment to give their own consent for treatment. The legal precedent is the case where a parent took the local health authority to court after one of her children received treatment from a GP without her consent. This case has had a major impact on the provision of paediatric health care and is cited across legal and health-care systems in the Western world as a basis for establishing how consent is obtained from young people (NSW College of Nursing 2000). In mental health as with general health care, consent could be challenged by parents and doctors; however, to ensure the safety and wellbeing of young people, mental health legislation provides strong guidelines and rights of appeal. Mental health nurses who treat young people should be aware that it is unethical and legally unsafe to engage a young person in treatment without informing their parent(s). Health-care agencies and inpatient units tend to have specific protocols and policies to address this issue.

The legal process by which young people can be admitted to mental health agencies is similar to that for adult patients. This ensures that the legal processes are consistent and that due process is followed in regard to human rights issues as well as protecting others. Many inpatient facilities that admit young people prefer to admit voluntarily, rather than through the Mental Health Act. If the safety of an adolescent is at risk and they are unable to consent to voluntary treatment, the Mental Health Act can be enacted. Younger people are usually regarded as voluntary if their parents have provided consent. The other main legal issues that need to be observed in child and adolescent mental health are child protection and statutory orders in regard to custody.

The States and Territories of each country have their own legislation governing child protection and guardianship. However, the overriding principals are those of the World Health Organization and the United Nations Convention on the Rights of the Child (Parliament of the Commonwealth of Australia, 17th Report 1998). In theory all children and adolescents have legal rights to education, health and wellbeing.

CONCLUSION

This chapter has highlighted skills that a beginning nurse practitioner requires when working for the first time with children and adolescents in the mental health field. It has focused primarily on engagement: establishing a therapeutic relationship and forging a therapeutic alliance. It is believed by the authors that nurses must first master strategies for engaging young people and their families before more advanced skills in mental health nursing can be consolidated effectively. Engaging young people and families early and initiating a therapeutic relationship will enhance the quality of assessment information provided by the clients. Furthermore, a sense of trust shared between parties will promote commitment to a shared treatment plan created in partnership between the young person, their parents and the mental health team.

EXERCISES FOR CLASS ENGAGEMENT

- Contact your nearest child and youth mental health service and request information on the services available to children and young people. Share this information with your group.
  - Are these services proactive and responsive?
  - Does the service actively promote early intervention?

- Contact a nurse working in a community setting and another from an inpatient unit, and ask them to speak to your group about their roles. Note any differences between the mental health nursing of young people in the community and that of young people in an inpatient setting.

- In small groups, nominate one person to act as a mental health nurse and another to play the role of a sullen, guarded adolescent. Remaining group members are to observe and document the difficulties presented in establishing rapport.

- Contact a child and youth mental health agency or community youth shelter and arrange to speak with a person who has experience with depressed or suicidal youth. Then clarify your responses to critical thinking challenge 12.2 on page 196.

- Seek out the mental health and child protection Acts applicable in your State, Territory or region. Summarise key points in the application of these to establishing safety for young people. Share your findings.

REFERENCES

Achenbach TM 1991, *Manual for the Child Behavior Checklist*, Burlington VT Department of Psychiatry University of Vermont, Vermont.

American Psychiatric Association 2000, *Diagnostic and Statistical Manual of Mental Disorders* (4th edn, text rev.), APA, Washington DC.

Andrews G, Hall W, Teeson M & Henderson S 1999, *The Mental Health of Australians*, Mental Health Branch, Commonwealth Department of Health and Aged Care, Canberra.

Baldwin L 2002, The nursing role in outpatient child and adolescent mental health services, *Journal of Clinical Nursing*, 11(4), pp 520–5.

Brannon L & Feist J 2000, *Health Psychology*, Wadsworth, Belmont.

Faber A & Mazlish E 1999, *How To Talk So Kids Will Listen & Listen So Kids Will Talk*, Avon, New York.

Green J & Jacobs B 1998, *In Patient Child Psychiatry*, Routledge, London.

Hoagwood K & Serene OS 2002, The NIMH Blueprint for Change Report, *Research Priorities in Child and Adolescent Mental Health*, 41(7), pp 760–7.

Limerick M & Baldwin L 2000, Nursing in outpatient child and adolescent mental health, *Nursing Standard*, 15(13–15), pp 43–5.

Loff B & Cordner S 1998, Suicide in Australia prompts action, *The Lancet*, 352(9128), pp 633–4.

National Institute of Mental Health 2002, Brief Notes on the Mental Health of Children and Adolescents. Online: http://www.nimh.nih.gov/.

New South Wales College Of Nursing 2000, *Mental Health Nursing Interventions And Management*, Course Material, Burwood.

New South Wales Department of Health 1990, *New South Wales Mental Health Act 1990*, Sydney.

Parliament of the Commonwealth of Australia Joint Standing Committee on Treaties 1998, *United Nations Convention on the Rights of the Child*, 17th Report, Commonwealth of Australia, Canberra.

Payne S & Walker J 2000, *Psychology for Nurses and the Caring Professions*, Open University Press, Buckingham.

Sawyer MG, Arney FM, Baghurst PA, Clark JJ, Graetz BW, Kosky RJ et al. 2000, *Child and Adolescent Component of the National Survey of Mental Health and Well-Being*, Mental Health and Special Programs Branch, Commonwealth Department of Health and Aged Care, Canberra.

Sharman W 1997, *Children and Adolescents with Mental Health Problems*, Bailliere Tindall, London.

World Health Organization 2001, *Fact Sheet No. 265*, December 2001. Online: http://www.who.int/.

Disorders of Old Age

Wendy Moyle

13

KEY POINTS

- The Australian and New Zealand populations are ageing and it is older people that nurses will most likely be providing care for in the future.
- Most older people are healthy and do not require health and social support.
- Staff attitudes are important in influencing the delivery of care to older people.
- Nursing management of mental illness in older people should include listening to the individual, encouraging an active and healthy lifestyle, and cultivating an interactive therapeutic nurse–patient relationship.
- In assessing an older person the nurse should avoid making ageist assumptions, such as assuming that dementia is the cause of changes in behaviour and activity.
- Mental health nursing staff should not assume that deterioration in function is a normal part of ageing.
- Mental health disorders in old age include depression, anxiety, delirium, dementia and schizophrenia. The most common disorder is depression.

KEY TERMS

- ageing
- ageism
- assessment
- delirium
- dementia
- depression
- mental disorders

LEARNING OUTCOMES

The material in this chapter will assist you to:
- demonstrate an understanding of the common mental disorders that occur in older adults
- explore management of the following mental disorders in older people: depression, anxiety disorders, suicide, substance misuse, delirium, dementia and schizophrenia
- explore strategies to promote mental health in older people
- reflect on your own and others' attitudes towards older people.

INTRODUCTION

Australia and New Zealand are ageing societies. It is imperative that nurses understand and can work with older people, as they are likely to be the population that nurses will predominately be required to provide health care for in the future.

This chapter provides an overview of mental disorders that are common in the older adult population, and explores the issues and principles underlying their assessment and treatment, including a number of general strategies to promote mental health. In addition, some negative attitudes towards older people are discussed, along with the implications of these negative attitudes for attempts to enhance the quality of care for older people.

DEMOGRAPHY OF AGEING IN AUSTRALIA AND NEW ZEALAND

In 1998, 2.3 million (12 per cent) of the 18.8 million people in Australia were aged 65 years or older (AIHW 1999). The number of older adults in this population continues to grow, with almost a quarter of older Australians aged over 80 years. The proportion of older adults in New Zealand is similar. In the year 2002, in both New Zealand and Australia, 15 per cent of males were over the age of sixty, as were 17 per cent of New Zealand women and 18 per cent of Australian women (NZ Statistics 2003a).

There are current trends for New Zealand Maori and Australian Aboriginal populations that health-care practitioners should incorporate into their practice. For example, both groups have poor health as they age and a lower life expectancy than non-Maori and non-Aboriginal populations (Lewis 2002). The New Zealand Maori population is increasing as a proportion of the New Zealand population and the proportion of older Maori people is also increasing, with projections being that this group will increase from the current 4 per cent of New Zealand's older population to 11 per cent in 2051. When making a diagnosis of mental illness, cultural concepts related to physical and mental well-being must be considered. The common mental status screening instruments such as the Mini Mental Status Examination (MMSE) are of particular concern as they do not take into consideration an individual's education attainment, language or culture. Cultural considerations must be taken into account when a mental health assessment is undertaken (see Ch 6 for more information).

Although older people may not necessarily be dependent on others, ageing brings with it an increase in certain disease processes (Walker 2001). Mental illness is not, however, a normal occurrence of ageing, although the risk of developing mental illness does increase with age (Evans & Katona 1993). The predicted increase in the older population is therefore expected to multiply the numbers of adults with mental illness (Bartels & Smyer 2002).

It is difficult to have a firm sense of how many older people have a mental illness as prevalence figures vary considerably according to the populations surveyed and the methodologies used (Lawlor & Radic 1994). In addition, there are also a number of negative stereotypical perceptions of age and older people that may inhibit the diagnosis and treatment of physical and mental illness. In 1969 Butler coined the term 'ageism' to define the systematic stereotyping of and discrimination against people because they are old (cited in Butler 1975). We have come to realise that ageism can apply to any age group, not just the aged. Thus, ageism has more recently been defined as discrimination against people on the grounds of their age alone, as a consequence of which stereotypical assumptions are made about how people are viewed throughout life (Behrens 1998).

Unfortunately, health professionals are not immune to ageist attitudes (Moyle 2003a; Stevens & Crouch 1992). Over the past decade a number of studies have investigated how health-care professionals feel about caring for older people. Nursing students' attitudes to elderly people have frequently been found to be negative (Fagerberg & Ekman 1997, 1998; Martell 1999; Stevens & Crouch 1992). Ageist views may in turn also affect the prevalence rates of mental illness in the older population through misdiagnosis or an unwillingness to diagnose individuals because they are seen as 'old'.

Although the exact numbers of older people with mental disorders in the community are not known, we do know that there are higher rates of mental illness in populations who are institutionalised in residential-care settings (AIHW 1998; Ames 1994). Older people living alone are 3.3 times more likely to be depressed than those residing in a household with others (Schulman et al. 2002).

It is important, however, not to stereotype older people as being unwell, and to remember that not all older adults require hospital services and assistance. Most older people in Australia and/or New Zealand live in their own home (91 per cent of people over 65 years), and only one in twenty people aged 65 to 69 report that they require assistance with self-care activities (AIHW 1998). The need for assistance rises to one in ten in those aged 70 to 79, and one in three in adults aged 80 or over (AIHW1998).

ASSESSMENT OF OLDER PEOPLE

All staff working with older people should begin by learning about normal older people, as the moment a problem appears, abnormality becomes the priority. The world is full of active and healthy older people and most older people do not require additional health and social support.

The main reasons for assessing older people are:

- to obtain a baseline assessment of function—this can assist in avoiding unrealistic goals
- to demonstrate positive changes to clients and to gather evidence for relatives, nurses and other health professionals

- for selection purposes—for example, in research—to ensure that groups of people are of similar levels
- to evaluate a new approach, treatment program or service
- for legal purposes (e.g. complications following a head injury)
- to assist diagnosis and prognosis.

Most of the time nurses are involved with obtaining a baseline assessment of function and assisting with diagnosis and prognosis. However, when a client is experiencing psychological distress there may be little time to conduct a full assessment. The use of observation skills and a brief assessment of the client's mental status provide valuable baseline data on which to base subsequent observations and care. An MMSE pro forma based on an abbreviated form of the mental status examination described in Chapter 10 can be used during client interviews to ensure that all areas are covered, and to organise and communicate observations when writing progress notes.

The MMSE is based on observable behaviour and includes:

- general appearance
- behaviour (motor) patterns
- form of speech
- content of speech
- mood

- intellectual functioning
- insight and judgment.

An easy way of memorising the various aspects of the tool is to recall the mnemonic: 'Great Britain Finds Cows' Milk In Ireland'.

Ageism in assessment

Although there are many safe ways to investigate the reasons behind a change in behaviour and ability, conclusions are often drawn too quickly. It is too easy to assume, because a seventy-year-old person fails to recognise familiar faces, and rambles and behaves strangely, that a dementing condition is the cause. There could be any number of reasons for this behaviour, from delirium to depression, and therefore it is important that nurses spend time with clients and their spouse or carers, to ensure a through and accurate assessment and to reduce the influence of ageist staff attitudes.

CRITICAL THINKING CHALLENGE 13.1

Reflect upon the nurse's story below. Consider why the conclusion of dementia was so readily presumed and how you might ensure, when assessing older clients, that this does not happen in practice.

NURSE'S STORY: Dolores

I was working in Accident and Emergency when Dolores was brought into the department in an unkempt and confused state. She was initially assumed by staff to be suffering from a dementing syndrome such as Alzheimer's disease, as she was aged, incoherent and lay chanting on the stretcher.

On examination Dolores was found to be wearing several layers of clothing, each soiled with excrement. While one nurse undressed Dolores, another asked her husband Jack for information about her condition, how long she had been in this state and whether there was any underlying condition or medication that may have contributed to the situation. Jack indicated that his wife had been coherent, with clarity of thought, up until the previous week. She had not recently had an operation or ingested any medication or substance that might have caused a chemical-induced delirium.

The nurses were alerted to the possibility of a toxic delirium as Jack informed them that Dolores had a large chest wound and that she had not been receiving medical care. Under the many layers of clothing Dolores was found to have a fungating breast cancer. Early in her illness she had asked her elderly husband to nurse her at home and to promise that he would never take her to see a doctor. As her

illness progressed she would not allow Jack to undress her and as she became cold and soiled he placed new clothing over her existing clothing.

Dolores did not have Alzheimer's disease. She was suffering from delirium as a result of a chemical imbalance due to her physical deterioration. Unfortunately, her condition deteriorated quickly and she survived only another five hours in hospital.

Nursing staff were distressed by the sight of Dolores in her many layers of wet and dirty clothing, and some staff felt that Jack had not cared for or about her. They assumed that a caring husband would have taken her for medical treatment earlier. But this assumption was incorrect—a neighbour and another relative spoke of Jack's devotion to Dolores and his desire to carry out her every wish, even if it meant caring for her without medical and nursing assistance. It was during a debriefing, at the end of the day, that several staff came to recognise that despite their knowledge and education they had all too quickly jumped to an incorrect diagnosis because on initial observation Dolores was seen as being elderly and confused. It was timely to initiate continuing education sessions in the department to concentrate on such issues.

MENTAL HEALTH DISORDERS IN THE OLDER POPULATION

Although a number of conditions—such as depression, anxiety disorders, suicide, substance misuse, delirium, dementia and schizophrenia—fall within the context of mental illness in old age, they do not occur *because of* ageing. Each of these disorders is explored in the following sections.

Depression

The most common mental illness of old age is depression (Bagley et al. 2000; Schulman et al. 2002). Depression in older adults has often been found to be associated with vascular brain changes (Snowdon 2001).

Presentation

The presentation of depression (see Ch 15) in older age is often less obvious than in younger people as older people will often focus attention on their physical symptoms (see Ch 20) and are less likely to acknowledge feeling depressed (Snowdon 2001). Although they may exhibit the cardinal features of depression, such as lowered mood and loss of interest (DSM-IV-TR, American Psychiatric Association 2000), older people will often attribute these feelings to their physical condition rather than to a psychological state.

It is important to interview a spouse or carer as both a corroboration of the client's history and to substantiate a professional assessment, as well as to gather additional information to assist in the assessment. A spouse or carer will commonly report changes that the individual has not recognised, such as social withdrawal, irritability, avoiding family and friends, poor hygiene and memory change. Losses such as status, income and bereavement can contribute to feelings of dejection (see Ch 9).

Diagnosing depression in an older population is compounded by the difficulty of differentiating it clinically from dementia and delirium (explored later in this chapter). Depression and dementia may both present with psychomotor slowing, apathy, impaired memory, fatigue, sleep disturbance and poor concentration.

Prevalence

There are varying accounts of the prevalence of depression among people over the age of sixty-five. Prevalence rates are estimated to be between 1.5 and 25 per cent (Blazer 1997) with the higher rate being attributed to an institutionalised population (Ames 1994). Variance in prevalence rates also results from epidemiologists generally only recording cases of major depression and dysthymia. They commonly have not included individuals with minor depression, which is common in old age as a result of a depression arising from functional decline and medical symptoms. Individuals with minor depression may have significant depressive symptoms but not fulfil all the DSM-IV-TR criteria for major depression or dysthymia (see Ch 15 for diagnostic criteria). Prevalence rates for depression are approximately 50 per cent higher in women than in men (Bagley et al. 2000).

Aetiology

There is a common perception that older people become depressed as a part of the normal ageing process. This is not so, but older people are vulnerable to developing a depressive illness because of age-related biochemical changes and psychological factors. Depression is frequently associated with many common medical conditions found in later life such as stroke, cancer, myocardial infarction, diabetes, rheumatoid arthritis and Parkinson's disease (Snowdon 2001). Psychological risk factors are bereavement, medications and losses related to physical illness, financial security, accommodation and independence (Bruce 2002; Norman & Redfern 1997; Snowdon 2001). Furthermore, older adults who are institutionalised face a number of adjustment changes to their normal routine as they often struggle with living in an environment where there are a lot of people, noise, rituals and habits that seem strange to them. Such factors may make them vulnerable to mental illness (Manion & Rantz 1995). See Chapter 8 for more information about mental health across the lifespan.

Assessment

It is essential that nurses are involved in the assessment of older clients and their psychosocial situations to assist in an early intervention nursing care plan. It can be very difficult, especially in older clients, to distinguish between depression and dementia because both conditions share common features such as poor concentration, low mood and social isolation. To make this distinction even more difficult, depression often coexists with dementia. Furthermore, the diagnosis may be hindered where the person also has a physical illness which leads health professionals to believe that the person's depressive symptoms are understandable given their physical status. Undiagnosed and untreated depression places the person at risk of mental suffering, poor physical health, social isolation and suicide.

A depression screening instrument such as the Geriatric Depression Scale (GDS) (Yesavage, Brink & Rose 1983) may assist in making the diagnosis, referral for treatment and in providing a baseline assessment against which to measure the effect of treatments. The GDS consists of thirty questions, which focus on the individual's thoughts and feelings of depression experienced over the previous week. Unlike other screening instruments, the GDS avoids asking questions about physical symptoms, as this generation of people traditionally tends to concentrate on physical symptoms and avoids discussing emotional symptoms. They may also regard the presence of depressive symptoms as a part of their ageing process and neither ask for nor expect help with such symptoms.

Where a differential diagnosis cannot be made, psychiatric consultation and/or a trial of antidepressant therapy may be warranted. While cognitive deficits are common in dementia and depression in older people, they will normally resolve with recovery from depression.

The possibility of a depressive illness should be considered in older people if they develop cognitive impairment or anxiety. To assist with the diagnosis of depression in an older person, keep in mind the following when caring for older individuals:

- Check for the presence of depressive symptoms using a screening instrument for this age group, such as the GDS.
- Individuals can suffer from depression, a physical disorder and/or dementia, all at the same time.
- Do not assume that symptoms can be easily related to the individual's life circumstances or their age.

Anxiety disorders

Anxiety disorders and alcohol abuse and dependence are common psychiatric co-morbidities associated with depression in late life (Devanand 2002) (see Ch 17). Symptoms of anxiety are commonly associated with major depression, and in older depressed adults there is considerable variability in the severity of the illness (Flint & Rifat 1997a). The most common anxiety disorders associated with depression in older adults are generalised anxiety disorder and phobias (Devanand 2002). Although treatment for depression may reduce anxiety this is not always the case, with anxiety symptoms persisting despite the resolution of other depressive symptoms (Flint & Rifat 1997b). Co-morbid anxiety disorder in clients with major depression lowers the rate of client recovery and is also associated with a higher rate of suicide (Coryell, Endicott & Winokur 1992).

Nursing management of depression

Most depressive and anxiety disorders in older adults respond to treatment (Snowdon 2001). However, in older clients with severe depression associated with dementia, the prognosis is poor.

Psychotherapeutic support

The most effective treatment for depression is early intervention. Nurses are in a unique and important position within the health-care team as they have more contact with a client in hospital and community settings, which makes the early recognition of depressive symptoms and early intervention possible. Nurses are invaluable in giving psychotherapeutic support to enable clients to talk about their feelings. Psychosocial therapies such as cognitive therapy (CT), cognitive behavioural therapy (CBT), interpersonal therapy (IPT), group therapy and counselling are useful, especially when the depressive illness is loss-related. Cognitive therapy and CBT identify distorted or illogical thinking processes and maladaptive patterns of behaviours and then attempt to replace them with more reality-based thinking and adaptive behaviours (Beck et al. 1979). Interpersonal therapy identifies and modifies interpersonal problems resulting from grief, role disputes and transitions, or interpersonal deficits (see Ch 23 for more information about these treatment modes).

Pharmacotherapy and electroconvulsive therapy

Pharmacotherapy (e.g. antidepressants, antipsychotics) and electroconvulsive therapy (ECT) may be prescribed

CASE STUDY: Linda

Linda is a 67-year-old married woman. She has spent all her married life helping her husband run a small business in a country town. She has adult children living in the country who she sees frequently. Linda's family brought her to the family GP although Linda had not wanted to come as she stated she was too tired to go out of the house. Linda's family reported to the GP that Linda had recently lost interest in everything that she had once enjoyed, such as visiting her grandchildren and entertaining friends and family at home. She had taken to staying in bed until late, not showering and refusing to partake in family activities. Linda was eating very little and had lost a significant amount of weight, and she appeared severely emaciated, her clothes appearing to be several sizes too large for her. Limited communication and retarded motor functioning made communication with Linda difficult.

The GP made an urgent referral to a psychiatrist, who admitted Linda to a city psychiatric hospital where she was diagnosed with major depression with severe psychomotor retardation. She had had an admission thirteen years

previously for the same diagnosis. She was prescribed antidepressants and commenced a course of ECT, as ECT had proved helpful in her previous admission.

The nursing care plan for Linda included spending time with her to establish rapport and trust, and allowing Linda time to respond (this was imperative because of Linda's severe psychomotor retardation). Nurses employed CBT to assist Linda to talk about her feelings and helped her to identify distorted or illogical thinking processes such as her fear that the family business would not be sustainable. CBT helped Linda to replace these illogical ideas with reality-based thoughts and assisted her with new coping strategies. Linda responded well to the treatment and was discharged after six weeks into the care of a GP and a community mental health nurse. The long-term plan was for Linda to stay on antidepressants, to undertake regular consultation with her health care team and for Linda or her family to report if she again started to feel anxious and depressed, as early intervention was important in keeping Linda well and out of hospital.

and used alone or in conjunction with the psychosocial therapies (see Ch 23 and Ch 24). Although depression may be greatly improved with pharmacotherapy it is imperative that older clients are monitored for medication side-effects that can have adverse effects on their cardiac condition. For example, tricyclic antidepressants and mono-amine oxidase inhibitors are known to affect cardiac conduction, rate, contractility and rhythm and may also cause orthostatic hypotension (Glassman, Roose & Bigger 1993). Thus, physical functioning monitoring should be incorporated into the nurse's daily routine and results that deviate from the person's baseline results must be reported. In recent years, selective serotonin reuptake inhibitors (SSRIs) have been prescribed, as they are known to have fewer cardiac side-effects. However, there is always an increased risk of drug interactions when clients are on multiple medications, and older clients who have been associated with the health-care sector are highly likely to be on a number of medications. It is also important to establish whether clients are on complementary and alternative medications, as some of these (e.g. St John's Wort) can cause potentially fatal reactions when taken with antidepressant medication.

The case study on the previous page provides an example of how a depressive illness affects an individual and their family. It also demonstrates the importance of an individualised nursing care plan that focuses not only on the condition but also on preparation for discharge, future rehabilitation and prevention.

CRITICAL THINKING CHALLENGE 13.2

Reflect on the case study and determine the priorities for Linda's care in the acute stages of her illness and upon admission to hospital. How would the priorities change prior to discharge, so that recovery and the prevention of future episodes of depression can be addressed?

Suicide

The older client should be assessed to determine whether they are suicidal at the time of assessment for depression. The risk of successful suicide in the older population is very real and should never be discounted as a possibility. Any talk of suicide by an older individual should be taken seriously and reported to a medical practitioner or specialist services if the client is in the community, or to senior nursing staff and specialist services if the client is hospitalised. Never assume because a client is elderly and hospitalised, or in a nursing home, that they are not capable of hoarding medications to use in a suicide attempt. If the client offers information about their intended suicide, identifying how, when and by what means will enable the level of risk to be assessed (see Ch 23 for risk assessment).

Prevalence

Older adults tend to use more violent methods in their suicide attempts and this generally accounts for their high success rates (Snowdon 1997). Suicide rates for males show two peaks: one in younger males (ages 20–39) and the other in the oldest age group (80 years and over) (AIHW 1998). Although adults aged over 65 years in Australia make up only 12 per cent of the population, they account for 15 per cent of successful suicides (Snowdon 1997). In New Zealand the suicide rates in 1998 showed a similar preponderance of males (77 per cent); one in five were Maori deaths. The highest number of deaths in New Zealand occurred in the 25–44 year age group (246 deaths) and 63 deaths occurred in the 65+ years age group (NZ Statistics 2003b),

Substance misuse

Substance misuse involving illicit drugs is rare in older adults, but dependence on prescription medications such as benzodiazepines is not uncommon (Blixen et al. 1997), as a high proportion of older people experience sleep disturbances for which they seek medication. In Australia there is a steady decline in substance abuse disorders with age; substance abuse for Australians over 65 years has been reported at around three per cent (AIHW 1998). However, as substance misuse in older clients is reported to be under-recognised and under-treated (Weintraub et al. 2002), the figures may actually be higher. The 1996/97 New Zealand Health survey found that although older people were less likely to have had a drink than those aged under 60 years, they were more likely to be drinking more often. This survey identified that 68 per cent of people over 65 years said they had drunk alcohol in the last year. One-third of this group drank four or more times per week, compared with 27 per cent of 45–54 year olds and 13 per cent of 25–44 year olds (Ministry of Health 1999)

People who abuse alcohol are likely to suffer from major depression (Devanand 2002). We also know that alcohol and drug misuse are associated with a variety of medical problems and high rates of medical treatment (Moos, Mertens & Brennan 1994; Weintraub et al. 2002) and that undiagnosed substance use in older clients may lead to serious withdrawal syndromes during hospitalisation (Foy, Kay & Taylor 1997).

It is imperative that nurses assess clients for substance misuse during their preliminary assessment, especially when older clients are admitted for surgery. Rather than asking if a client drinks alcohol, ask them, 'How much alcohol do you drink per day?'. If they state 'not much' or 'I only drink socially', ask the client to tell you exactly how much alcohol this involves. From personal experience, older clients could relate that they don't drink 'much', but consider that six stubbies of beer and two whiskies a day constitutes being a social drinker! (See also Ch 19.)

Delirium

Delirium may be defined as 'a disturbance of consciousness . . . manifested by a reduced clarity of awareness of environment [in which the] ability to focus, sustain, or shift attention is impaired' (DSM-IV-TR, APA 2000, p 136). Delirium is a syndrome that constitutes a characteristic pattern of signs and symptoms and can be caused by anything that rapidly damages the brain. The condition is very common in older people, especially those people in hospital or a nursing home. Delirium is also associated with high rates of morbidity.

Differentiating between delirium and dementia can be more difficult in elderly people (see Table 13.1 on p 212). Delirium develops over a period of hours to days and tends to fluctuate during the course of a given day. Dementia, on the other hand, is progressive and presents as a gradual failure of brain functioning. The exact nature of the pathophysiology of delirium is unknown. Both cortical and brainstem functions are impaired in delirium, the cortex mediating cognitive function and the brainstem wakefulness. Delirium is ruled out if a dementing syndrome accounts for the disturbance in consciousness. However, it is not unusual for delirium to coincide in people with dementia as a result of a medical condition. In this case the person may present with additional symptoms of short duration that are above and beyond that which can be accounted for by the dementia.

There is little data on the time course of delirium in older clients, possibly because it is often missed unless family or nursing staff are in constant contact with the individual. Most clients have a prodromal stage lasting from a few hours to a day or so. This refers to a change in the person's habitual behaviour and cognitive functioning (sleep disturbance, restlessness and irritability, general malaise and anxiety).

It is important to establish early recognition of delirium because if the disease or damage that is causing it can be treated, the confusion will resolve. If the client is aged there is a tendency for nursing staff to pass off behavioural changes as part of ageing and they may therefore avoid carrying out a thorough assessment. This may result in no treatment or inappropriate treatment being given, whereas if the delirium is related to biochemical changes due to an infection, for example, this could be resolved by a course of antibiotics (see the nurse's story on Dolores earlier).

Risk factors

Being older places individuals at risk of delirium. There are also a number of other risk factors that predispose older people to delirium:

- pre-existing brain damage
- pre-existing dementia
- sensory impairment.
  Additional risk factors are:
- infections, especially urinary tract or chest
- cardiac failure and other major heart conditions
- respiratory failure resulting in raised carbon dioxide levels

- kidney failure resulting in raised levels of protein and urea
- constipation (although the reason for this has not been established)
- medications
- drug withdrawal, including alcohol (delirium tremens, DTs).

Prior to an older person undergoing surgery it is important that the nurse assesses the client to ensure that any changes in behaviour following surgery can be detected and early intervention given. There are two established risk factors for older people undergoing surgery: previous alcohol or drug abuse, and prolonged operating time under a general anaesthetic.

Dementia

Prevalence

Dementia is not a normal part of life or ageing. However, the number of people with dementia is increasing in Australia and New Zealand as more people live longer and the prevalence of dementia increases exponentially with age. The prevalence rate for Australian people aged between 60 and 80 is estimated to be approximately 2.6 per cent and 11.5 per cent for those between 80 and 84 years. The prevalence rate for the population aged over 85 years is estimated to be 24 per cent (Williams 2000). The New Zealand prevalence statistics are similar, with estimates of 1 per cent prevalence of dementia in those aged 60–64 years and rising each year of life to around 30 per cent of those aged 85 years and older. The prevalence rate for those in New Zealand aged over 65 years is estimated to be approximately 8 per cent. (Lewis 2002). People in the early stage of dementia usually live in the community. People with higher levels of cognitive loss as a result of dementia are usually accommodated in residential-care facilities.

Aetiology

The major types of dementia are Alzheimer's disease (50–60 per cent) and vascular dementia (20–30 per cent). Many of the remainder suffer from a mixed dementia. As well as Alzheimer's disease and vascular dementia there are other causes of dementia, such as: Lewy body type, Parkinson's disease, frontal lobe dementia, physical or toxic damage, genetic disorders, infections, vitamin deficiencies and endocrine disorders. Many older adults with dementia exhibit significant depressive symptoms, and depression may be an early symptom of Alzheimer's disease (Jacques & Jackson 2000).

Clinical features

The following features should be observed for, monitored and treated where appropriate.
- cognitive abnormalities:
  - *memory impairment*
    - demonstrable evidence of impairment of both short- and long-term memory
    - impairment in abstract thinking

- *impaired judgment*—inability to deduce the consequences of their actions or to make appropriate judgment on how to organise their lives
- *impaired higher cortical function*—aphasia (loss of ability to identify objects by their proper names), apraxia (inability to perform movements when asked), agnosia (difficulty in recognising parts of one's own body), deficits in constructional ability (inability to assemble objects in their correct spatial relationship to each other)
- *personality change*—exaggeration of previous character traits, or a complete change from the individual's former habitual 'state of being'
■ non-cognitive abnormalities:
- *disorders of mood*—depression, anxiety and, rarely, mania
- *disorders of perception*—hallucinations (visual or auditory), mis-identifications
- *delusions*—seen in the earlier stages of disease as one requires relatively intact cognitive functioning for delusions
■ disorders of behaviour:
- *wandering*—movement without purpose, or semi-purposeful
- *aggression*—verbal or physical, generalised or focal
- inappropriate social or sexual behaviour
- *restlessness*—generalised, constant, purposeless movement.

The above features and in particular the disorders of behaviour often result in behavioural problems that are challenging for care staff to manage. An increase in behaviour problems occurring in the evening hours and beginning at a time near sunset has been termed 'sundowning' (Bliwise 1994). Staff and relatives often report that the individual exhibits an increase in disorientation, restlessness and aggressive behaviour during the evening hours. This increase in disorientation has been attributed to diurnal variations in hormone and light, as well as to fatigue and a search for familiar surroundings in which to rest. However, in some individuals this pattern is reversed—they are found to be more disoriented in the morning. There is also an argument that this could be a socially constructed syndrome created by people around the individual.

Although the cause of sundowning is not known, it is important to assess individuals to help guide the formulation of an individualised care plan. People with dementia are often highly responsive to the environment they find themselves in. Therefore, the environment needs to be made safe, and made familiar with objects that have meaning for the individual (e.g. family photographs). Unnecessary changes to routines should be avoided.

In the mid-1980s Dr Tom Kitwood and colleagues at the Bradford Dementia Group in the United Kingdom commenced work on a theory of caring for people with dementia that was underpinned by the need to rebalance the 'technical framing' of dementia and complement it with a philosophy that was constructed from 'personhood'

Table 13.1 Comparison of dementia, delirium and depression

	Dementia	Delirium	Depression
Onset	Chronic	Rapid onset, usually hours or days	Often abrupt and may coincide with life events such as death of a loved one
Course	Slow, progressive cognitive failure; symptoms may be worse in evening (sundowning)	Short, diurnal fluctuations in symptoms	Diurnal fluctuations, worse in morning
Duration	Months to years	Hours to days	Six weeks to years
Signs and symptoms	Conscious	Clouding of consciousness	Conscious
	Sleep disturbance is not usually a feature but the sleep–wake cycle may be set at the wrong time frame	Sleep disturbance	Sleep–wake disturbance
	Behaviour tends to be worse in the evening	Fluctuations noted during the course of the day	Selective disorientation
	Aimless wandering or searching	Restless and uneasy	May appear to be 'slowed up'
	Hallucinations are rare	Visual hallucinations that are usually disturbing	Delusions and hallucinations are rare
	Mood may be flattened or labile	Emotional lability and distress	Sad, with feelings of hopelessness and helplessness

and 'person-centred values' (Kitwood 1988; Kitwood & Bredin 1992). Kitwood (1988) argued that dementia is not the problem—rather, it is our inability to accommodate the dementia sufferer's view of the world. Kitwood & Bredin (1992) suggested that this created a 'them and us' dialectic tension, which is sustained by the devalued status of someone who has demented. Kitwood (1988) argued that the limitations of care environments produced what he termed a 'malignant social psychology'. As a means of addressing this, Kitwood & Bredin (1992) reconceptualised the dementing process along the following lines:

SD (senile dementia) = P + B + H + NI + SP.

Senile dementia is viewed as the product of the following elements:

P = personality, which includes coping styles and defences against anxiety

B = biography and responses to the vicissitudes of later life

H = health status, including acuity of the senses

NI = neurological impairment, separated into its location, type and intensity

SP = social psychology, which constitutes the fabric of everyday life.

Comparing delirium, dementia and depression
It is important to differentiate between delirium and dementia so that early intervention for delirium can take place, and to differentiate whether features displayed by an individual are a result of dementia or depression. Any of these conditions may present with very similar features. Table 13.1 provides an overview of the different facets of these conditions. However, clients require adequate assessment in order to establish a diagnosis (see also Ch 10).

Schizophrenia
Although usually apparent before age 45 years, schizophrenia may be of late onset (Palmer et al. 2002). There is evidence that about 20 per cent of older adults with schizophrenia develop schizophrenia in middle-age, known as 'late-onset schizophrenia' (Harris & Jeste 1988). Clients with psychotic disorders have been shown to have a high prevalence of aggressive behaviour (Bowie et al. 2001), which makes the nursing care of these clients challenging.

Antipsychotic medications are generally effective in managing psychotic symptoms, but they are not a cure for this disorder. In recent times, non-pharmaceutical support through therapies such as CBT and social skills training has proved useful to older clients with schizophrenia (Granholm et al. 2002; McQuaid et al. 2000). Although further research is required, nurses may be able to assist older clients with schizophrenia using these therapeutic interventions.

The move to reduce the number of long-stay psychiatric facilities has resulted in a greater number of older clients with schizophrenia being discharged to nursing homes

CASE STUDY: Lorraine

Lorraine is a 76-year-old woman who was recently admitted to a new residential aged-care facility. She has a psychiatric diagnosis of paranoid schizophrenia and medical diagnoses including diabetes mellitus and ischaemic heart disease. She has had a number of long-term psychiatric admissions and has required community support whenever she is out of hospital. Her medical and psychiatric conditions have made it difficult for Lorraine to self-care and she was considered to be at risk if left in the community. She was happy to be admitted to the nursing home, as she felt unsafe in her unit.

Lorraine proved to be a challenge for the nursing home staff, who were not used to having a resident with a diagnosis of schizophrenia. Staff identified that Lorraine lacked insight and that she provoked staff and other residents with inappropriate comments and verbal outbursts. She wanted constant staff attention and if she did not receive this she screamed and demanded attention. Her screaming made staff and residents very uncomfortable, as she would not stop until a staff member paid attention to her and spent time either walking or talking with her. Staff complained that they did not have the time that Lorraine demanded they spend with her. After a week in the facility Lorraine refused to get out of bed, crouching under the bed clothes and stating that no one liked her and that she wanted to go home, where she had friends.

Staff complained that Lorraine was manipulative and they asked not to be her nurse. They openly expressed their dislike of Lorraine, and there were occasions where it appeared that they were either deliberately avoiding her or provoking her as a form of punishment. This resulted in Lorraine's withdrawing from staff and other residents. Following an assessment of the situation by the care manager, a mental health assessment team was asked to assess Lorraine and to suggest strategies to manage her behaviour.

The mental health team suggested the following strategies:
- Give Lorraine firm guidance on appropriate behaviours.
- Provide her with reassurance that her needs would be met as soon as possible.
- Reward her for good behaviour.
- Remove her from situations where she distracted other residents.
- Distract her with activities such as walking, music and art.

A staff education program was commenced with a focus on mental health disorders such as schizophrenia, conflict resolution, cognitive behaviour therapy and needs-centred care. As staff began to respond more favourably to Lorraine, she also responded more appropriately and there were fewer episodes of inappropriate behaviour.

and other aged-care settings. It is therefore important for nurses working in long-term care to understand this condition and how the client might react to the transition.

The case study on the previous page demonstrates the difficulties for aged-care staff when they have limited mental health education and resources to assist the client, staff and other residents with the transition.

CRITICAL THINKING CHALLENGE 13.3

Reflect on the case study. Explore in more detail how you would plan, implement and evaluate Lorraine's care. Finally, describe strategies that could be used to help staff adjust to Lorraine's challenging behaviours.

NURSING MANAGEMENT

Mental health initiatives for older people are often vague and unspecific or tend to concentrate on dementia to the exclusion of other mental disorders. There also appears to be a need for greater cohesion of services for older people. A number of nursing interventions have been identified as being of assistance to older people.

- It is important to listen to the individual in an active way, in particular to listen to the feelings and emotions behind the words.
- Encourage older people to participate in physical and social activities that invite them to focus on aspects of their life apart from illness.
- Assist older people to understand disease processes, how to take medications and to maintain a physically and mentally active lifestyle.
- Help them to select coping strategies to assist them with any losses such as a decline in health or financial status or bereavement.
- If bereavement is a problem, help the person to work through the pain of grief and to adjust to an environment where the deceased is no longer available (see Chs 8 and 9).

These interventions are generalised, and so it is important to evaluate care processes regularly to ensure that the interventions are appropriate for the situation. It is also imperative that health-care professionals consider the individual's culture, as decisions about care may be affected by cultural differences. For example, some cultural groups may not be willing to seek institutional care for family members as such services may appear to be culturally inappropriate for their needs. At present there are very few services delivered by Maori or Aboriginal people, for Maori or Aboriginal people. The care and treatment of people with mental illness needs addressing in culturally sensitive ways.

The nurse–patient relationship

An interactive therapeutic nurse–patient relationship, where the nurse brings a positive approach and attitude to the client, and nurtures the therapeutic interaction between nurse and patient, will assist the client's health and wellbeing (Beeber 1998; Moyle 1997, 2003b; Thelander 1997). This is a trusting relationship where values are respected as the nurse listens to client's concerns, provides information and advice, relieves distress by encouraging the expression of emotion, improves patient morale through review of their capacities or satisfaction, and encourages the client to practise self-help (Beeber 1998; Stuart & Sundeen 2001). If the nurse–patient relationship develops well it can play a large part in sustaining the client in the face of their emotional difficulties (see Ch 2).

The nurse–patient relationship should remain professional. Identification of the nurse–patient relationship with emotion is viewed as being 'over involved' and not therapeutic. Such an involved relationship may result in the client being overly dependent on the nurse and losing their self-reliance. However, research findings (Moyle 1997, 2003b) have identified that the therapeutic relationship is a learned skill that does not come instinctively to nurses, and that attention to establishing a therapeutic nurse–patient relationship is required. Nurses will therefore benefit from an education process that both teaches them about the importance of such a relationship and encourages its development.

Maintaining health and function

Finally, nurses can assist older clients in maintaining function by ensuring that clients have small, frequent meals, are well hydrated, and maintain bowel function through a high-fibre diet, hydration and exercise. Clients should be encouraged to mobilise and be independent, and the nurse should ensure that they have undisturbed rest and relaxation. Other therapies that nurses may find therapeutic for older clients are hand and back massage, and pet therapy.

STAFF ATTITUDES

Health-care professionals as well as the public often have negative images of ageing (Moyle, 2003a) as well as poor attitudes to and tolerance of mental illness. It is this negative image of old age and mental health that may prevent the provision of a quality mental health service for older people. It is imperative that staff counter the belief that deterioration in cognitive functioning is a normal part of ageing. This requires a refocusing of attention from disease towards education that promotes older people as skilled and valued human beings.

The term 'confusion' is often used by nurses to describe any number of client behaviours from inattention to inappropriate vocalisation, and the term is used most often towards uncooperative clients (Stuart & Sundeen 2001). The following case study demonstrates how poor attitudes can influence both the assessment of

CASE STUDY: Joan

Joan is an 83-year-old woman who has been widowed for ten years. She lives with her son and daughter-in-law in a granny flat in a section of a large house. Joan has always been active both physically and mentally and has contributed to the running of the household, organising meals and driving the grandchildren to school or extracurricular activities. Joan is on medication for hypertension, which has been well controlled for the past three years.

While taking the youngest granddaughter shopping, Joan had a car accident, hitting a car as she pulled out of the shopping centre car park. Joan was taken to the local hospital accident and emergency department where she was diagnosed with whiplash, a fracture of the lumbar spine and concussion. She was admitted to a medical ward for a period of rest and recuperation. Following admission Joan became agitated and complained that she felt 'locked up' and started calling out loudly for her son to take her home. She was also incontinent of urine. As this was now late at night and Joan's calling out was disturbing other patients, the nurse organised for Joan to be prescribed 500 mcg of haloperidol PRN. This medication appeared to calm Joan, and she soon slept peacefully. Unfortunately, upon waking and in trying to get to the bathroom she fell and suffered a fractured femur of the left leg.

Joan was moved to the orthopaedic ward where she spent several weeks recuperating. During the time in the orthopaedic ward Joan appeared to become more confused and staff complained that she was uncooperative, particularly when bathing and eating. Joan was reluctant to eat the hospital food and was rapidly losing weight. Staff feared that

Joan would fall again and nursed her either in bed with bed rails up or in a chair that she was unable to get out of. She was given sedation regularly to keep her settled. Joan had not undergone a mental health assessment during her hospital stay. The health professional focus was on whether her femur was 'mending'. Little consideration was given to a rehabilitation program as staff had by this stage decided that Joan had a dementing illness and that she would require nursing-home care. Joan's family did not accept this diagnosis and were concerned to see Joan in such a frail and confused state since her hospital admission. Joan's physical and mental status deteriorated while she was hospitalised until upon discharge she demonstrated a poor ability to self-care, poor mobility and low motivation and cooperation.

When Joan was admitted to the nursing home, an assessment of the documentation that arrived with her brought into question whether she had been adequately assessed during her hospitalisation. It also appeared that little attention had been paid to developing a rehabilitation plan. It seemed that staff had decided that Joan had a dementing syndrome and felt that there was no chance of her re-entering the community outside a nursing home. At the time of the nursing-home admission Joan was given a diagnosis of depression, adjustment reaction and anxiety.

Conclusion

The outcome for Joan may have been different if an adequate assessment had been carried out throughout the time of her hospitalisation and if a rehabilitation and discharge plan had been encouraged.

and care planning for older clients. The case study also demonstrates the importance of mental health education for nurses working in all settings.

CRITICAL THINKING CHALLENGE 13.4

Reflect on the case study. Examine the care Joan was given and develop a nursing care plan that would allow for the setting of priorities for her rehabilitative process (see Ch 2 for partnership, self-help, recovery, rehabilitation and consumer issues).

CONCLUSION

As people age they experience psychosocial factors such as bereavement and loss of physical and mental functioning. This may place older people at risk of mental disorders and in particular depressive illness. However, mental disorders are not a normal part of ageing and clients require adequate assessment and diagnosis to ensure that their symptoms are not related to, for example, adverse effects of medications.

The diagnosis and treatment of mental disorders in older adults can be difficult. Furthermore, co-morbid conditions and negative stereotypical ageist assumptions make treatment and diagnosis especially difficult. Although mental disorders are not a normal part of ageing, older people have a high success rate for suicide, and therefore it is imperative that they are assessed and treated effectively.

Nurses have an important role to play in both assessment and treatment of mental disorders in the elderly. Their skills in establishing a therapeutic nurse–patient relationship and in using psychotherapeutic support such as CBT and IPT to assist the older client to recognise distorted or illogical thinking processes and maladaptive patterns of behaviours resulting from grief, role disputes and transitions, or interpersonal deficits, can, along with pharmacotherapy and at times ECT, improve the older client's quality of life. Although depression is the most prevalent mental disorder in the aged, it is also a treatable condition. The establishment of a nurse–patient relationship provides the opportunity for nursing staff to recognise the symptoms of depression and to suggest further assessment and treatment if required.

EXERCISES FOR CLASS ENGAGEMENT

Discuss the following questions with your group or class members.

- Document and discuss the differences between delirium and dementia in relation to time course, cause and clinical features.
- Identify the risk factors for delirium and discuss how you might assess for delirium.

- Why is it important to consider the diagnosis of delirium and dementia when care planning?
- Explore the reasons that it is difficult to differentiate depression clinically from dementia and delirium.
- How might the symptoms of depression affect the relatives and friends of the depressed older person?

REFERENCES

American Psychiatric Association 2000, *Diagnostic and Statistical Manual of Mental Disorders* (4th edn, text rev.) (DSM-IV-TR), APA, Washington DC.

Ames D 1994, Depression in nursing and residential homes. In: Chiu E & Ames D (eds), *Functional Psychiatric Disorders of the Elderly*, Oxford University Press, Oxford.

Australian Institute of Health and Welfare 1998, *Mental Health. A Report Focusing on Depression*, Commonwealth Department of Health and Ageing, Canberra.

Australian Institute of Health and Welfare 1999, *Older Australians at a Glance* (2nd edn), Commonwealth Department of Health and Ageing, Canberra.

Bagley H, Cordingley L, Burns A, Mozley C, Sutcliffe C, Challis D et al. 2000, Recognition of depression by staff in nursing and residential homes, *Journal of Advanced Nursing*, 9(3), pp 445–50.

Bartels SJ & Smyer MA 2002, Mental disorders of aging: an emerging public health crisis?, *Generations*, 26(1), pp 14–20.

Beck AT, Rush AJ, Shaw BF & Emery G 1979, *Cognitive Therapy of Depression*, Guilford Press, New York.

Beeber LS 1998, Treating depression through the therapeutic nurse-client relationship, *Nursing Clinics of North America*, 33(1), pp 153–72.

Behrens H 1998, Ageism: real or imagined?, *Elderly Care*, 10(2), pp 10–13.

Blazer D 1997, Depression in the elderly: myths and misconceptions, *Psychiatric Clinics of North America*, 20(1), pp 111–19.

Bliwise DL 1994, What is sundowning?, *Journal of American Geriatric Society*, 42(9), pp 1009–11.

Blixen CE, McDougall GJ & Suen LJ 1997, Dual diagnosis of elders discharged from a psychiatric hospital, *International Journal of Geriatric Psychiatry*, 12(3), pp 307–13.

Bowie CR, Moriarty PJ, Harvey PD, Parrella M, White L & Davis KL 2001, Aggression in elderly schizophrenia patients: a comparison of nursing home and state hospital residents, *Journal of Neuropsychiatry and Clinical Neuroscience*, 13(3), pp 357–66.

Bruce ML 2002, Psychosocial risk factors for depressive disorders in late life, *Biological Psychiatry*, 52, pp 175–84.

Butler R 1975, *Why Survive? Being Old in America*, Harper & Row, New York.

Coryell W, Endicott J & Winokur G 1992, Anxiety syndromes as epiphenomena of primary major depression: outcome and familial psychopathology, *American Journal of Psychiatry*, 149(1), pp 100–7.

Devanand DP 2002, Comorbid psychiatric disorders in late life depression, *Biological Psychiatry*, 52(3), pp 236–42.

Evans S & Katona C 1993, Epidemiology of depressive symptoms in elderly primary care attenders, *Dementia*, 4(6), pp 327–33.

Fagerberg I & Ekman S 1997, First-year Swedish nursing students' experiences with elderly patients, *Western Journal of Nursing Research*, 19(2), pp 177–89.

Fagerberg I & Ekman S 1998, Caring for elderly patients: a longitudinal study of Swedish nursing students' narratives, *Health Care in Later Life*, 3(4), pp 258–71.

Flint AJ & Rifat SL 1997a, Anxious depression in elderly patients: response to antidepressant treatment, *American Journal of Geriatric Psychiatry*, 5(2), pp 107–15.

Flint AJ & Rifat SL 1997b, Two-year outcome of elderly patients with anxious depression, *Psychiatry Research*, 66(1), pp 23–31.

Foy A, Kay J & Taylor A 1997, The course of alcohol withdrawal in a general hospital, *QJM*, 90(4), pp 253–61.

Glassman AH, Roose SP & Bigger JT 1993, The safety of tricyclic antidepressants in cardiac patients, Risk-benefit considered, *JAMA*, 269(20), pp 2673–5.

Granholm E, McQuaid JR, McClure FS, Pedrelli P & Jeste DV 2002, A randomised controlled pilot study of cognitive behavioural social skills training for older patients with schizophrenia, *Schizophrenia Research*, 53(1/2), pp 167–9.

Harris M & Jeste D 1988, Late-onset schizophrenia; an overview, *Schizophrenia Bulletin*, 14(1), pp 99–113.

Jacques A & Jackson GA 2000, *Understanding Dementia*, Churchill Livingstone, Edinburgh.

Kitwood T 1988, The technical, the person and the framing of dementia, *Social Behaviour*, 3, pp 161–80.

Kitwood, T & Bredin, M 1992, Towards a theory of dementia care: personhood and well-being, *Ageing and Society*, 12, pp 269–87.

Lawlor B & Radic A 1994, Prevalence of mental illness in an elderly community dwelling population using Agecat, *Irish Journal of Psychological Medicine*, 11(4), pp 157–9.

Lewis H 2002, *Dementia in New Zealand: Improving Quality in Residential Care*, report to the Disability Issues Directorate. Online: www.moh.govt.nz/moh.nsf, accessed November 2003.

Lipowski Z 1983, Transient cognitive disorders in the elderly, *American Journal of Psychiatry*, 140(11), pp 1426–34.

Manion, PS & Rantz, M 1995, Relocation stress syndrome: a comprehensive plan for long-term admissions, *Geriatric Nursing*, 16(3), pp 108–12.

Martell R 1999, Students shun elderly care despite enjoying placements, *Nursing Standard*, 14(8), p 8.

McQuaid JR, Granholm E, McClure FS, Roepke S, Pedrelli P, Patterson TL et al. 2000, Development of an integrated cognitive-behavioural and social skills training intervention for older patients with schizophrenia, *Journal of Psychotherapy Practice Research*, 9(3), pp 149–56.

Ministry of Health, New Zealand 1999, *Taking the Pulse: the 1996/97 New Zealand Health Survey*, Wickliffe Press, Dunedin.

Moos RH, Mertens JR & Brennan PL 1994, Rates and predictors of four-year readmission among late-middle aged and older substance abuse patients, *Journal of Studies of Alcohol*, 55, pp 561–70.

Moyle W 1997, On Being Nurtured While Depressed, unpublished PhD thesis, Centre for Mental Health Nursing, QUT, Brisbane.

Moyle W 2003a, Nursing students' perceptions of older people: continuing society's myths, *Australian Journal of Advanced Nursing*, 20(4), pp 15–19.

Moyle W 2003b, Nurse–patient relationship: a dichotomy of expectations, *International Journal of Mental Health Nursing*, 12(2), pp 103–9.

New Zealand Statistics 2003a, Quick Facts: People. Online: www.stats.govt.nz/, accessed 18 November 2003.

New Zealand Statistics 2003b, Suicide Deaths, 1998. Online: www.stats.govt.nz/stats/suicidestats-p.html, accessed 18 November 2003.

Norman I & Redfern S 1997, *Mental Health for Elderly People*, Churchill Livingstone, New York.

Palmer BW, Folsom D, Bartels S & Jeste DV 2002, Psychotic disorders in late life: implications for treatment and future directions for clinical services, *Generations*, 26(1), pp 39–43.

Schulman E, Gairola G, Kuder L, & McCulloch J 2002, Depression and associated characteristics among community-based elderly people, *Journal of Allied Health*, 31(3), pp 140–6.

Snowdon, J 1997, Suicide rates and methods in different age groups, Australian data and perceptions, *International Journal of Geriatric Psychiatry*, 12(2), pp 253–8.

Snowdon J 2001, Late-life depression: what can be done?, *Australian Prescriber*, 24(3), pp 65–7.

Stevens J & Crouch M 1992, Working with the elderly: do student nurses care for it?, *The Australian Journal of Advanced Nursing*, 9(3), pp 12–17.

Stuart G & Sundeen SJ 2001, *Principles and Practice of Psychiatric Nursing* (7th edn), Mosby, St Louis.

Thelander BL 1997, The psychotherapy of Hildegard Peplau in the treatment of people with serious mental illness, *Perspectives in Psychiatric Care*, 33(3), pp 24–32.

Walker J 2001, Health and productive ageing. In: Chiva A & Stears D (eds), *Promoting the Health of Older People*, Open University, Buckingham, pp 73–85.

Weintraub E, Weintraub D, Dixon L, Delahunty J, Gandhi D, Cohen A et al. 2002, Geriatric patients on a substance abuse consultation service, *American Journal of Geriatric Psychiatry*, 10(3), pp 337–42.

Williams S 2000, Drugs offer muted hope in Alzheimer's, *Australian Medicine*, 20(Nov.), p 8.

Yesavage JA, Brink TL & Rose TL 1983, Development and validation of a geriatric depression rating scale: a preliminary report, *Journal of Psychiatric Research*, 17, p 27.

Further reading

Arnold DT 2002, *Better Elder Care. A Nurse's Guide to Caring for Older Adults*, Springhouse Co., Springhouse.

Beales D, Denham MJ & Tullock A 1998, *Community Care of Older People*, Radcliffe Medical Press, Abingdon, UK.

Jacques A & Jackson GA 2000, *Understanding Dementia*, Churchill Livingstone, Edinburgh.

Keltner NL 1999, *Psychiatric Nursing*, Mosby, St Louis.

Nussbaum P 1997, *Handbook of Neuropsychology and Aging*, Plenum Press, New York.

Waughfield CG 2002, *Mental Health Concepts*, Delmar/Thomson Learning, Clifton Park, NY.

Youngkin EQ 1999, *Pharmacotherapeutics. A Primary Care Clinical Guide*, Appleton & Lange, Stamford.

Zarit SH 1998, *Mental Disorders in Older Adults. Fundamentals of Assessment and Treatment*, Guilford Press, New York.

CHAPTER

14 | Schizophrenic Disorders

Murray Bardwell and Richard Taylor

KEY POINTS

- Schizophrenia is considered one of the most debilitating disorders in the range of mental disorders prevalent in society.
- Schizophrenia as a mental disorder is poorly understood, although current and future research may shed greater light on its causation in terms of a neuroanatomical condition.
- Stress can be viewed as a trigger for those predisposed to a mental illness.
- Recognising and understanding the impact of the pro-dromal phase of schizophrenia may enable better clinical outcomes for future management of this disorder.
- Treatment regimens that include behavioural and cognitive therapies combined with pharmacological therapies are likely to have better outcomes in terms of the management of this disorder.
- The burden of disease combined with the burden associated with stigma in schizophrenia makes this one of the most socially debilitating disease conditions.
- Homelessness and schizophrenia are closely intertwined and prevalent in our society.

KEY TERMS

- affect
- agranulocytosis
- akathisia
- ambivalence
- hallucination
- loose associations
- incoherence
- neologism
- apathy
- autism
- avolition
- blunted affect
- catatonia
- concrete thinking
- delusion
- dystonia
- echolalia
- echopraxia
- extrapyramidal side-effects
- ideas of reference
- negative symptoms
- paranoid
- positive symptoms
- premorbid
- psychosis
- regression
- relapse
- schizophrenia
- tardive dyskinesia
- thought blocking
- thought disorder

LEARNING OUTCOMES

The material in this chapter will assist you to:
- define the term 'schizophrenia'
- discuss biological and environmental theories on the development of schizophrenia
- distinguish the presentations of schizophrenia in terms of prodromal, acute and chronic phases
- identify the major pharmacological strategies in the treatment of schizophrenia, their target symptoms and their major adverse effects
- identify non-pharmacological strategies in the treatment of schizophrenia
- distinguish the role of the nurse in the management of individuals with schizophrenia
- identify education strategies that may be employed in psychoeducation of the individual and family.

INTRODUCTION

Schizophrenia is one of the most debilitating and mis-understood disorders within the spectrum of mental illnesses. Throughout history, schizophrenia has been feared, despised and misunderstood—people experiencing the effects of what we now know as schizophrenia have been burned at the stake as witches, imprisoned or held up for ridicule. Although our society no longer burns witches at the stake it could be argued that very little else has changed. It is still common in a society rich in health information for people to erroneously equate schizophrenia with split personality or multiple personality. It is not uncommon for mental health professionals to be asked whether they think a person may have schizophrenia because they are agreeable one minute and hostile the next. Our prison population continues to have a disproportionate number of individuals incarcerated because of behaviours arising from schizophrenia (Commonwealth of Australia 1993). The popular film industry occasionally features a character with schizophrenia, but such characterisations fail to accurately depict the manifestations of this illness and its painful effects.

Gaining an understanding of schizophrenia can be a challenging and frightening experience. This chapter attempts to provide some insight into the condition and articulate the role of nurses in helping the individual with schizophrenia to reach their optimal level of health.

PREVALENCE

Schizophrenia is a disorder characterised by a major disturbance in thought, perception, cognition and psychosocial functioning and is one of the most severe mental disorders. Schizophrenia is found in approximately one per cent of the population worldwide. It currently affects 200,000 people in Australia and has been attributed with causing a loss in earnings of up to $488 million, with a further $88 million incurred by carers of individuals with schizophrenia. In addition, the direct cost to the health system is currently $661 million and is projected to exceed one billion dollars on current trends (Access and Economics 2001).

Schizophrenia is not spread evenly throughout the population. Its onset tends to occur among those between the late teenage years and early adulthood (approximately 18–24 years of age). The condition also tends to be more prevalent among socially disadvantaged groups. The homeless population are one example where there are higher rates of the condition (Caton 1997). Caution needs to be observed in interpreting these social patterns. There is debate over whether the experience of the illness results in a decline in the individual's social condition or whether the social disadvantage increases the likelihood of experiencing the illness (Caton 1997).

For many, especially the homeless and the destitute, access to much-needed health care remains a major issue. Of those who can access mental health services, many experience difficulties arising from the often serious and debilitating side-effects of medications required to manage their illnesses. Compliance with treatment is often problematic and many choose to cease taking medication, which often results in a return to severe mental illness and repeated admissions. This tragic pattern is often referred to in mental health contexts as the revolving-door syndrome. There is room for optimism, however, brought about by greater emphasis on treatment of people living with schizophrenia in the community and on advances in drug technology. Schizophrenia should not be thought of as a single disease process or as personality deficit. Schizophrenia is a complex syndrome with many varieties and symptoms that remains poorly understood within the community.

AETIOLOGY

Research has yet to determine the exact cause of schizophrenia. Researchers are increasingly turning to neurobiological explanations and away from psychodynamic explanations (Birtwistle & Baldwin 1998; Sharma & Murray 1993). Put simply, schizophrenia is more commonly viewed as an illness of neurological functioning than as a disorder of the mind. In all probability the cause of schizophrenia lies in a complex interaction between multiple combinations of genetic and environmental factors—for example, exposure to infection during gestation or birth, which may interfere with normal brain development and function. This complex interplay results in the constellation of behaviours collectively known as the schizophrenias (Andreasen 1999; Geddes & Lawrie 1995; Levinson et al. 1998; Munk-Jorgensen & Ewald 2001).

The fact that the brains of those with schizophrenia differ from those without the illness is now largely undisputed (Coffey 1998; Cotter & Pariante 2002). How or why these aberrations in brain biochemistry and anatomy affect the functioning of the brain remains a mystery, as does the reason that these abnormalities appear to remain dormant until late adolescence in most individuals (Cotter & Pariante 2002).

Biological theories

The three most commonly discussed biological causative factors are genetics, brain anatomy and brain biochemistry. It would be erroneous to consider these three factors as mutually exclusive. Far more likely is the existence of a relationship between the three; for example, some as-yet unidentified pattern of inheritance may predispose an individual to differences in anatomy or fluctuations in neurotransmitter biochemistry (Lewis & Murray 1987, cited in Coffey 1998).

Neuro-anatomical abnormalities

Schizophrenia is often referred to as a neuropsychological disorder, which implies that the origins of the psychological

CHAPTER

15

Mood Disorders

Jan Horsfall

KEY POINTS

- The assessment of mood disorders requires attending to the five domains: behaviour, cognition, communication, mood and physical functioning.
- While each person is unique, there are key nursing principles and interventions for working with people experiencing a mood disorder.
- Depression is associated with an increased risk of attempting and completing suicide.
- The establishment of a therapeutic relationship is critical to treatment success.
- Mood disorders are responsive to a variety of psychological, sociocultural and biological interventions.
- Theories relevant to nursing people with depression and bipolar disorder do not fully explain mood disorders, but serve to guide and support nursing interventions.
- The major classes of medication used in the treatment of mood disorders are antidepressants and mood stabilisers.

KEY TERMS

- affect
- bipolar disorder
- catastrophising
- cognitive restructuring
- egocentrism
- euphoria
- hypomania
- limit-setting
- major depressive disorder
- mania
- mood
- psychomotor retardation
- rumination
- somatisation

LEARNING OUTCOMES

The material in this chapter will assist you to:
- identify behaviours associated with mood disorders
- describe cognitive/thinking changes associated with mood disorders
- understand communication changes associated with mood disorders
- identify mood changes associated with major depression and bipolar disorders
- describe changes in physical functioning associated with mood disorders
- explain nursing principles for use with people experiencing mood disorders
- explain the reasons for nursing interventions and the expected client responses
- outline cognitive, social and biological theories that contribute to the understanding of the aetiology of mood disorders
- understand the basic mechanisms of antidepressants and mood stabilisers
- recognise some of the personal challenges arising for nurses working with people who are experiencing major depression.

INTRODUCTION

This chapter explores the mental health nursing assessment and intervention skills, knowledge and attitudes required to work effectively with clients with mood disorders. The focus is holistic: any aspects of a client's life can affect depression and mania, and a person's thoughts, feelings and behaviours are altered by mood disorders. Hence, the person of the nurse, the life history of the clients, aspects of their lives such as gender and culture, as well as the basic requirements of eating, sleeping and communicating, have to be addressed.

MAJOR DEPRESSIVE DISORDER

Indicators and symptoms

Major depressive disorder is a condition involving seriously depressed mood and other symptoms defined by the Diagnostic and Statistical Manual of Mental Disorders (4th edn, DSM-IV-TR) criteria. Symptoms of major depressive disorder affect all aspects of a person's bodily systems and interfere significantly with a range of daily living activities, with noticeable changes in behaviour, cognition, communication, mood and physical functioning. All five domains must be considered for a nurse to make a holistic assessment of a person with a mood disorder. The DSM-IV-TR (American Psychiatric Association 2000) diagnostic criteria for major depressive disorder are listed in Box 15.1.

In the descriptions below, the symptoms marked with an asterisk (*) are those designated in the DSM-IV-TR (APA 2000) as diagnostic symptoms for major depression.

Behavioural changes

Behavioural changes in depression include social and emotional withdrawal and markedly decreased interest in, and pleasure from, previously enjoyable activities*. The person is often less effective in areas of work or family relations (Horsfall, Stuhlmiller & Champ 2000). Substance abuse may precede, occur with, or result from depression; and overall alcohol dependence and depression co-morbidity is high (Kirchner et al. 2002).

Cognitive changes

The depressed person becomes increasingly egocentric—that is, they focus on self to the degree that other people's needs are beyond their awareness. Classically, the person's thoughts about self, others and the world become increasingly negative. The person thinks of themself as incompetent, faulty, unloveable and a failure—these are examples of catastrophic thinking or catastrophising and inappropriate guilt* (Fontaine 2003). Others are viewed as uncaring and unhelpful. The world is perceived as a place of despair and desolation, and the future as gloomy.

Many depressed people have difficulty concentrating* on activities such as reading that had previously been effortless or rewarding. Some people become immobilised by cognitive difficulties involved in ordinary decision-making processes (Keltner & Warren 2003). The depressed person's cognitive spectrum usually narrows, with some negative thoughts and ideas being frequently ruminated over. These ruminations, which become repetitive and increasingly intrusive, can eventually interfere with other thought processes. Self-deprecating beliefs, negative expectations of others and a sense of doom may contribute to thoughts of death and suicidal ideation*.

Communication changes

Commonly, depressed people's communication mirrors the narrowing and repetitive focus of their thoughts.

Box 15.1 Diagnostic criteria for major depressive episode

Five (or more) of the following symptoms have been present during the same two-week period and represent a change from previous functioning; at least one of the symptoms as either (1) depressed mood or (2) loss of interest or pleasure. (Do not include symptoms that are clearly due to a general medical condition, or mood-incongruent delusions or hallucinations.)

(1) depressed mood most of the day, nearly every day, as indicated by either subjective report (e.g. feels sad or empty) or observation made by others (e.g. appears tearful). (In children or adolescents, can be irritable mood.)

(2) markedly diminished interest or pleasure in all, or almost all, activities most of the day, nearly every day (as indicated by subjective account or observation made by others)

(3) significant weight loss when not dieting or weight gain (e.g. a change of more than 5% of body weight in a month), or decrease or increase in appetite nearly every day. (In children, consider failure to make expected weight gains.)

(4) insomnia or hypersomnia nearly every day

(5) psychomotor agitation or retardation nearly every day (observable by others, not merely subjective feelings of restlessness or being slowed down)

(6) fatigue or loss of energy every day

(7) feelings of worthlessness or excessive or inappropriate guilt (which may be delusional) nearly every day (not merely self-reproach or guilt about being sick)

(8) diminished ability to think or concentrate, or indecisiveness, nearly every day (either by subjective account or observed by others)

(9) recurrent thoughts of death (not just fear of dying), recurrent suicidal ideation without a specific plan, or a suicide attempt or a specific plan for committing suicide.

Source: American Psychiatric Association 2000, *Diagnostic and Statistical Manual of Mental Disorders* (4th edn, text rev.) (DSM-IV-TR), APA, Washington DC.

Negative self-absorption in combination with insufficient energy and interest in others means they are unlikely to initiate a conversation, and when asked a question may take a long time to answer, and give a short reply (Keltner & Warren 2003).

Mood changes

For major depression, the mood has to have been significantly lower than usual for at least two weeks*. Sadness, anguish and misery, along with a feeling of separation from others, and feelings of hopelessness and powerlessness, constitute the pain of depression. Many depressed clients cry a lot. These feelings of sadness and hopelessness and the behaviours they give rise to, such as crying and looking dejected, are referred to as affect. *Affect* is the observable behaviours associated with changes in a person's mood.

Alterations in physical functioning

Sleep disturbances*, particularly insomnia, are common concomitants of depression. Fatigue* is frequently associated with depression: it seems that the depressed mood, disturbed sleep and negative thinking deplete the person's energy levels. Sexual desire diminishes. The person's appetite for food is disturbed*, usually decreasing, with a subsequent loss of weight and constipation. Very depressed people may experience psychomotor disturbances*, such as psychomotor retardation. Some people do not notice, or mention, their low mood as their distress is expressed via pain or other symptoms across a range of body systems (see Ch 20). Such somatisation may be more prevalent in adolescents than adults, and more prevalent in Asian people than in Europeans (Choi et al. 2002).

Principles for effective nursing

Although every depressed person is unique, expert RNs working in mental health come to recognise key nursing principles over time. A *principle* is 'a general law or rule as a guide [for] action; a fundamental motive or reason [for] action, especially one consciously recognised and followed' (Little, Fowler & Coulson 1992).

As well as individualised care, nursing people with a mood disorder always begins with a holistic assessment that is ongoing and therefore continues throughout the continuum from hospital to community. Holistic assessment takes account of the present and the past, and considers feelings, culture, communication, relationships, spirituality and behaviours (Barker 2001).

In this section, principles that have learning potential for undergraduate nurse readers are presented. These principles were derived from interviews with four expert mental health nurses. The nursing principles are not presented in order of priority, nor are they the only possible ones, but they constitute guidelines that students and new graduates can draw on, practise and improve.

The first of four expert nurses interviewed for this chapter, Belinda, worked for many years in a setting that specialised in treating clients with mood disorders. The following dot points constitute the nursing principles she outlined and which, in combination, contribute to nurses' understanding of people with depression and assist their recovery. They are divided into principles that help nurses to understand the client who is depressed, and principles that guide nurses' care of the client who is depressed.

- Understanding the client:
  - Many people who are depressed have not expressed their sadness at deaths, other tragedies and losses in their lives.
  - Behind apparently minor losses there are often significant prior deaths and separations that the person has not grieved for.
- Principles of care:
  - **Honesty with self** is the starting point for working with others in distress.
  - Self-awareness allows the nurse to **listen and hear** the depressed person's story.
  - Interpersonal **imagination** and creativity enable the nurse to work out how this person will be able to tell the story she or he needs to tell.
  - All clients require **individualised care**. Nurses must not think they know what a person needs because they have worked with many depressed clients.
  - The client's **loss should be acknowledged** by saying, for example, 'You've had a terrible time', when this is clearly what has happened.
  - **Clients need feedback** (positive and negative, but always constructive) about their communications and behaviours.
  - As negativity is contagious, creating an interpersonal environment where pain and trauma can be shared needs to be balanced with a few appropriate laughs.
  - The **common humanity** of nurses and clients enables nurses to offer empathy and hope.
  - Mental health **nurses need to lead balanced lives** themselves.
  - Sometimes the client's loss seems small—the death of a budgerigar, for example—but **no loss should be trivialised**. The budgie may have been the person's only reliable, constant and undemanding companion and confidante over many years.
  - Interaction with a depressed person, careful listening, and observation of subtle communications, allow the nurse to **pick up cues** about how best to work with the client.

The highlighted parts of the above principles are most important. According to student levels of self-awareness and interpersonal skills (Stuart 2001a), some of these approaches are reasonably straightforward, but others will need much practice. The last four principles from this list are briefly explained below.

Shared humanity

The issue here is that even though nursing principles can provide guidance, the nurse's personality, life experience and emotional intelligence are also crucial (Stuart 2001a). Nurses and clients have a common humanity and the person of the nurse is an important ingredient in effectively nursing a depressed client. Kind but unskilled people can be detrimental to the wellbeing of a depressed person. Likewise, a knowledgeable, technically well-skilled communicator without heart, empathy and respect for humankind will not be able to support a depressed person through a healing trajectory. Personality, care, skills and a hopeful attitude work constructively in combination to improve outcomes for depressed clients.

Life balance

There is no guaranteed cure for depression, only a repertoire of treatments, a combination of which benefits most clients. Depressed people often require a range of interventions including hospitalisation, counselling, medication, electroconvulsive therapy, stress management strategies, relaxation techniques, and making changes at home or at work. They can benefit from reducing stimulant use (e.g. coffee), diet change (e.g. lowering refined sugar intake, which affects the adrenal production of cortisol) and reducing central nervous system depressant use (e.g. alcohol). Brugman (2002) describes the implementation of a nurse-led walking group in response to previous research that shows that taking up or maintaining exercise improves mood by enhancing serotonin transmission, activating endorphins and distracting depressed people from negative thoughts. Given that nurses work as health educators and role models, it is incumbent on them to manage their own stress well and to lead a balanced life (Stuart 2001a).

No loss is trivial

Loss is the involuntary separation from someone close or an important value or symbol: the consequence of loss is that something significant and personal has gone. Grief is the expression of thoughts and feelings about who and what has gone, and the process of grieving is an essential part of healing (Jacik 1996). Obvious loss in Western society is associated with recent death; however, painful losses include shattered hopes, broken faith or ideals, decreased social status, unemployment and childhood separations. One nurse recalled a depressed client mourning the death of her pet budgie.

NURSE'S STORY: A depressed woman by Christine

After Carmen's husband committed suicide, a community nurse of the same ethnic background as Carmen had visited her for a month. She was offered counselling and practical assistance, but declined, saying that she could manage on her own, and would contact the Community Health Centre (CHC) if she needed to. Eighteen months later her general practitioner referred her to a private psychiatrist, who again referred her to the CHC. I became her community mental health nurse. Carmen was in a severely depressed state and was prescribed antidepressants.

In her early thirties and with young children, Carmen had been surviving in Sydney without adult support as she and her husband had immigrated to Australia alone. I recognised the severity of her depression, her **social and cultural isolation** and the fact that her primary school children were dependent upon her.

My first priority was to visit her regularly to keep reliable contact with her and to **patiently develop a therapeutic relationship**. This progressed very slowly. I also felt a keen responsibility towards the children, the eldest obviously having to help her mother get through some day-to-day activities. Each time I visited I accepted her drink and food offerings, I would sit with her, talk a little to allow her to feel comfortable with me at **her own pace**. I was aiming to 'be with her', **develop trust** and engage her so that she would eventually be able to talk about her distress.

A few months after I began home visits, her sister arrived from their country of origin. The arrival of an adult family member seemed to allow Carmen to stop forcing herself to keep going. She appeared more depressed and I thought that she **might be suicidal** (even though there was no unambiguous evidence that this was the case); and I was concerned about the **children's safety** under the circumstances.

I organised for her to be admitted to a psychiatric hospital and explained to her and the hospital that it was important that she rest and recover, given her responsibilities on top of a major depression. During her two-week hospitalisation I visited her and reminded the staff that she sorely needed rest, given what she had been through. This was a turning point. Her medication was changed. When she returned home she was able to take **more appropriate responsibility for herself and the children**.

During her hospitalisation she decided that she would do a **TAFE course**. She had university qualifications from her own country that were not accepted in Australia and opted for a course that would not be too demanding, but which would give her future employment opportunities. She completed the course during the period I visited.

Carmen had blamed God for her husband's death and abandoned her religion. Her husband's suicide had been so traumatic that she could not remember the funeral clearly, or where he was buried. I offered to take her to the cemetery, and there she wept and wailed inconsolably. This was another turning point. She **re-found her faith**, and began taking the children to their church. She became angry with her husband for deserting her and their children when the going was tough. Her healing was very individual and **the grieving phases were not predictable**.

signs of deteriorating mood and behaviour show that this decreases the likelihood of a future manic episode (Baker 2001). It may take an individual with a bipolar disorder many years, depending on the interval between episodes and their acknowledgment of the illness, to be ready to learn about relapse triggers and symptom indicators. Symptom recognition can be included with problem-solving strategies in nurse-initiated psychoeducation programs that also address client concerns about medication side-effects and other drug-adherence issues.

THEORIES ON MOOD DISORDERS

All theories relating to the aetiology of mood disorders, whether biological, psychological or social, are hypotheses. No theory is fully explanatory and they only offer partial guidance, or support for, specific nursing interventions. Five theories that throw some light on the Carmen, Charles and David vignettes are outlined here.

Life events

For the purpose of understanding mood disorders, life events are psychosocial stressors and interactions that are very distressing or traumatic for an individual (Varcarolis 2002). Loss is a prime example of such a life event. All three clients described by Adam, Christine and Philippa experienced significant loss. Carmen had been separated from her country of origin; her husband had died prematurely, unexpectedly and by his own hand; she was isolated from her culture and extended family; and her religious beliefs had failed to provide solace. Charles was separated from his parents for two years as a child; he was taken from those he loved again; he had left friends in Australia and in his country of origin; and he felt he had lost the unconditional love of his father, who was living vicariously through his academic success (c.f. Choi et al. 2002). David's wife had left him, but his perfectionist behaviour may have alienated her before that; he was distant from his adult children and felt that they had not excelled at school; things went wrong at work; and ultimately he felt himself to be a failed husband, father and businessman.

Experiencing sexual assault, physical abuse or emotional abuse commonly has negative outcomes for mental health. Women experience higher rates of interpersonal violence than men; and research reveals that higher rates of depression, suicidality and anxiety are significantly associated with such trauma, especially sexual violence (Coker et al. 2001).

Learned helplessness

Learned helplessness is 'both a behavioral state and a personality trait of one who believes that control has been lost over ... the environment' (Stuart 2001b, p 354). This model arose out of Seligman's (1975) experimental torture of dogs, which became depressed when they learned that no matter what they did, they could not avoid electric shocks. Learned helplessness also relates to hopelessness and powerlessness—that is, the inability to escape an intolerable situation leads to the ultimate mode of adaptation: subjugation and acceptance. In combination this means that the person comes to believe that they cannot do anything to change their circumstances—and are therefore trapped. By and large, children have less autonomy and power within their families than parents do. Charles was not in charge of his life: he was sent away twice without any say in the matter, and was on an academic treadmill not of his own choice. Carmen had lost control of her life: after her husband suicided she was compelled to raise her two children alone without access to family supports that would have been 'natural' in her country of origin. The consequence of this theory for practice is the importance of supporting and encouraging the person to reclaim realistic control of some aspects of their life.

Gender

In Australia, according to a large survey of a nationally representative sample of adults, the National Survey of Mental Health and Wellbeing (NSMHW), women experience depression at 1.8 times the rate of men (Australian Bureau of Statistics 1998). This preponderance of depression in women has been evident for many decades. One possible consequence of this is gender stereotyping whereby health professionals make inappropriate assumptions that result in over-diagnosing depression in women and under-diagnosing men's depression (Horsfall 2001).

Researchers have noted that the emotional dependence, over-responsibility, passivity, non-expression of anger, and low self-esteem associated with depression, are considered 'normal' female characteristics in some families and cultures (Horsfall 1994). When daughters are socialised to be subservient and comply with family customs in ways that boys do not have to, then teenage girls (the age when female rates of depression increase) and young women are unable to gain autonomy and feel in charge of their lives, and feelings of hopelessness and depression can ensue. 'Rigid expectations about gender roles continue to linger [after teenage years] and contribute to higher rates of depression among women' (Fontaine 2003, p 367). Carmen's life opportunities narrowed from her perspective after her husband died. This related to her gender and single-mother status within a specific cultural and religious context.

CRITICAL THINKING CHALLENGE 15.3

How might the socialisation of girls within the family and school system lead, to some extent, to passivity, self put-downs and non-assertiveness?

Given the differing needs of Carmen and David, for example, how do you understand the relevance of gender to recovery from depression? (See Horsfall 2001 for further discussion.)

Cognitive factors

This model posits that people become depressed because their thinking is negatively distorted (Stuart 2001b). Cognitions are disturbed in depressed people; however, this may be a consequence, not a cause. Depressive thinking involves the triad of negative views of self, others and the world; it is pessimistic and clients often overgeneralise, catastrophise, and think superstitiously and dichotomously (viewing everything as either black or white). David revealed catastrophic thinking when he falsely concluded that he was a failure because things went wrong at work, even though some factors were beyond his control. Superstitious thinking is also exemplified by David when he considered that one family decision was the cause of his wife's departure, his children's perceived inadequacies and his business problems. Dichotomous thinking may be evidenced by David's suicide attempt, in that after his wife left him he believed everything was going wrong and would continue to do so, and therefore he would be better off dead. This model pertains to cognitive restructuring, especially with clients like David, who tend to overgeneralise, catastrophise, and think superstitiously and dichotomously.

Neurotransmitter involvement

'There is much evidence to support [the view] that depression is a biologically heterogeneous disorder' (Varcarolis 2002, p 458). This indicates that many neurotransmitters are implicated and the mechanisms of their interactions are not fully understood. Neurotransmitter dysregulation may result from environmental stressors, drug use, some medical conditions and/or an inherited vulnerability.

The three neurotransmitters that have attracted most medical research attention in relation to mood disorders are the catecholamines—serotonin, norepinephrine and dopamine. Also, acetylcholine and gamma-aminobutyric acid are likely to have modulating effects on those biogenic amines (Keltner & Warren 2003). It is known that stressful events overtax norepinephrine, serotonin and acetylcholine systems and lead to depletion of these neurotransmitters (Varcarolis 2002).

Serotonin is an important regulator of sleep, appetite and libido; and decreased levels may account for lowered energy levels, concentration difficulties and the inability to feel pleasure (Varcarolis 2002). Keltner & Warren (2003) conclude, given the research evidence available thus far, that to 'conceptualize depression as a decreased level of serotonin and norepinephrine . . . oversimplifies both the problem [of depression] and the solution [its treatment]' (p 348).

MEDICATIONS FOR TREATMENT OF MOOD DISORDERS

The major classes of medication used in the treatment of major depressive and bipolar disorders are the antidepressants and the mood stabilisers. In this section these classes of medication are briefly discussed.

Antidepressants

There are four types of antidepressants: selective serotonin reuptake inhibitors (SSRIs); tricyclic antidepressants (TCAs); novel antidepressants such as bupropion, venlafaxine and nefazodone; and mono-amine oxidase inhibitors (MAOIs). Antidepressant medications target the following symptoms of depression:

- sleep disturbances
- appetite disturbances
- fatigue and lack of energy
- decreased libido
- psychomotor retardation, or agitation
- worsening mood in the morning (diurnal mood variation)
- concentration difficulties
- inability to experience pleasure (anhedonia) (Varcarolis 2002, pp 469–70).

Antidepressant medication takes approximately ten to twenty days for the therapeutic effects to be felt. At present the preferred first-line antidepressant drugs are SSRIs, TCAs or the new products; the MAOIs are prescribed as a last resort because of their dangerous interactions with many pickled, smoked, brewed, dried, fermented, cured or otherwise aged foodstuffs that contain tyramine (Varcarolis 2002).

The SSRIs block serotonin uptake and their advantage in comparison to TCAs is their decreased anticholinergic side-effects such as dry mouth, blurred vision, constipation and urinary retention, as well as less cardiotoxicity. Common SSRI side-effects include the following:

- sexual dysfunction (anorgasmia)
- nausea
- tension headache
- sleep disturbance
- agitation
- anxiety
- tremor
- weight gain (Varcarolis 2002, p 471).

Some of these unwanted effects are especially problematic—for example, sexual and sleep disturbances can be part of depression at the outset. However, their side-effects profile is an improvement on the TCAs and they are much less toxic in overdose (Buckley & McManus 2002). About thirty per cent of clients who take antidepressants do not experience mood relief. When a client starts an antidepressant regimen and they begin to feel better, suicidal ideation can remain strong, and with increased energy levels the risk for suicide may increase (Keltner & Warren 2003). Hence, ongoing thorough nursing assessment of clients in this situation both in inpatient settings and in the community is very important.

Mood stabilisers

Mood stabilisers are prescribed for people with bipolar disorder. Three agents are effective: lithium carbonate, divalproex sodium and carbamazepine. Because of its widespread and long-term use, lithium is focused on here. Research shows that between 59 per cent and 91 per cent of people with acute mania have a moderate to marked positive response to lithium (Bailey et al. 2002). For one-third of long-term clients, lithium is not therapeutic. The initial side-effects usually disappear after a month, and lithium is non-sedating and non-addictive.

Lithium is the psychotropic medication where therapeutic levels are closest to its toxicity range: the lowest possible therapeutic dose should be used and serum lithium levels should be between 0.6 and 1.2 mEq/L. As lithium is a salt, fluid balance issues are crucial for its safe use. In the body, lithium substitutes for sodium, calcium, potassium and magnesium, and therefore the higher the sodium levels, for example, the lower the lithium levels and vice versa (Fontaine 2003). Hence, clients must be very careful when they have a fever, diarrhoea or vomiting. At serum levels above 2.5 mEq/L lithium is toxic and between 1.5 and 2.5 mEq/L, side-effects are very significant indicators of incipient toxicity. These side-effects include the following:

- increased tremor
- diarrhoea
- nausea and vomiting

- coordination difficulties and ataxia
- slurred speech (Bailey et al. 2002).

Misinformation and lack of information about medication contributes to non-adherence. In summary, teaching clients about medications as well as observing those in acute inpatient units for side-effects is an integral part of nursing assessment, interventions, psychoeducation and discharge planning.

CONCLUSION

This chapter has drawn on international mental health nursing literature and interviews with four Australian registered nurses with expertise in working with clients with mood disorders. Key issues addressed are the knowledge, understanding and skills required for students and graduates to appreciate the complexity of depression and mania. Clients with depression and mania commonly reveal altered feelings, thoughts and behaviours as well as bodily changes such as impaired sleeping and diminished appetite. With good nursing interventions using the principles outlined in this chapter—usually in association with prescribed antidepressant medication—mood disorders respond to treatment and the person often regains their former level of abilities.

EXERCISES FOR CLASS ENGAGEMENT

- According to Boyd (2002), many people from China, Japan, Korea, the Philippines and Vietnam consider mental illness to be caused by character weakness, emotional strain, lack of self-discipline, physical exhaustion, unrequited love or Yin-Yang imbalance. Mental illness may be viewed as shameful among immigrants from these countries. It is not surprising, therefore, that mentally ill family members are often hidden, and assistance from health professionals is only sought when behaviours become extreme or unmanageable (Boyd 2002).

Working in groups, discuss the following questions.
  - What consequences would arise for a depressed person from family shame and the fear of cultural insensitivity from health-care providers?
  - Define stereotyping. How might cultural stereotyping affect a depressed person in an inpatient unit?
  - European or Westernised cultures value autonomy, independence and individualism, but many Aboriginal Australian, African, Asian and Pacific Island cultures value the collective over the individual, and family obligation and commitment to the community are central precepts for living. The aim of most psychological treatments for depression is to enhance personal autonomy: what difficulties may then arise for a depressed person from a culture that prizes the group as a whole? (See Donnelly 2002 for further discussion.)

- Chronic low self-esteem is a nursing diagnosis associated with depression and some other mental illnesses. The evidence for low self-esteem includes expression of inappropriate guilt, self-negating statements, and passivity in relation to others (Bailey, Sauer & Herrell 2002).

In a group, develop at least six detailed nursing interventions and rationales to improve a depressed person's self-esteem over twelve months.

- Blame can be understood as under-responsibility for self; and guilt may be defined as over-responsibility for others.

During the next week, listen to conversations within your family and friends for expressions of inappropriate blame and guilt. Share your findings with your group and discuss how such cognitions impede recovery from depression, and what strategies can be used to ameliorate them.

REFERENCES

American Psychiatric Association (APA) 2000, *Diagnostic and Statistical Manual of Mental Disorders* (4th edn, text rev.), APA, Washington.

Australian Bureau of Statistics 1998, Mental health and wellbeing profile of adults, Australia, AGPS, Canberra.

Bailey KP, Sauer CD & Herrell C 2002, Mood disorders. In: Boyd MA (ed.), *Psychiatric Nursing. Contemporary Practice* (2nd edn), Lippincott, Philadelphia, pp 410–51.

Baker JA 2001, Bipolar disorders: an overview of current literature, *Journal of Psychiatric and Mental Health Nursing*, 8(5), pp 437–41.

Barker P 2001, The tidal model: developing a person-centred approach to psychiatric and mental health nursing, *Perspectives in Psychiatric Care*, 37(3), pp 79–87.

Boyd MA 2002, Cultural issues related to mental health care. In: Boyd MA (ed.), *Psychiatric Nursing. Contemporary Practice* (2nd edn), Lippincott, Philadelphia, pp 16–28.

Brugman T 2002, Physical exercise and improvements in mental health, *Journal of Psychosocial Nursing*, 40(8), pp 25–31.

Buckley NA & McManus PR 2002, Fatal toxicity of serotoninergic and other antidepressant drugs: analysis of UK mortality data, *British Medical Journal*, 325(7376), pp 1332–3.

Choi H, Stafford L, Meininger JC, Roberts RE & Smith D 2002, Psychometric properties of the DSM scale for depression with Korean–American youths, *Issues in Mental Health Nursing*, 23(8), pp 735–56.

Cleary M, Jordan R, Horsfall J, Mazoudier P & Delaney J 1999, Suicidal patients and special observation, *Journal of Psychiatric and Mental Health Nursing*, 6(6), pp 461–7.

Coker AL, Smith PH, Thompson MP, McKeown RE, Bethea L & Davis K 2001, Social support protects against the negative effects of partner violence on mental health, *Journal of Women's Health and Gender-based Medicine*, 11(5), pp 465–76.

Cutcliffe JR & Barker P 2002, Considering the care of the suicidal client and the case for 'engagement and inspiring hope' or 'observations', *Journal of Psychiatric and Mental Health Nursing*, 9(5), pp 611–21.

Cutler CG 2001, Self-care agency and symptom management in clients treated for mood disorder, *Archives of Psychiatric Nursing*, XV(1), pp 24–31.

Donnelly TT 2002, Contextual analysis of coping: implications for immigrants' mental health care, *Issues in Mental Health Nursing*, 23(7), pp 715–32.

Drew BL 2001, Self-harm behavior and no-suicide contracting in psychiatric inpatient settings, *Archives of Psychiatric Nursing*, XV(3), pp 99–106.

Fontaine KL 2003, *Mental Health Nursing* (5th edn), Pearson, Upper Saddle River, USA.

Horsfall J 1994, *Social Constructions in Women's Mental Health*, University of New England Press, Armidale, NSW.

Horsfall J 2001, Gender and mental illness: an Australian overview, *Issues in Mental Health Nursing*, 22(4), pp 421–38.

Horsfall J, Stuhlmiller C & Champ S 2000, *Interpersonal Nursing for Mental Health*, McLennan & Petty, Sydney.

Jacik M 1996, Loss along the journey. In: Carson VB & Arnold EN (eds), *Mental Health Nursing: The Nurse Patient Journey*, WB Saunders, Philadelphia, pp 661–88.

Keltner NL 2003, Bipolar disorders. In: Keltner NL, Schwecke LH & Bostrom CE (eds), *Psychiatric Nursing*, Mosby, St Louis, pp 366–80.

Keltner NL & Warren BJ 2003, Depression. In: Keltner NK, Schwecke LH & Bostrom CE (eds), *Psychiatric Nursing*, Mosby, St Louis, pp 340–65.

Kirchner JE, Curran GM, Thrush CR, Owen RR, Fortney JC & Booth BM 2002, Depressive disorders and alcohol dependence in a community population, *Community Mental Health Journal*, 38(5), pp 361–73.

Latorre MA 2002, Spirituality and psychotherapy: an important combination, *Perspectives in Psychiatric Care*, 38(3), pp 108–10.

Puotiniemi TA, Kyngas HA & Nikkonen MJ 2002, The resources of parents with a child in psychiatric inpatient care, *Journal of Psychiatric and Mental Health Nursing*, 9(1), pp 15–22.

Resnick WM & Carson VB 1996, The journey colored by mood disorders. In: Carson VB & Arnold EN (eds), *Mental Health Nursing: The Nurse Patient Journey*, WB Saunders, Philadelphia, pp 759–92.

Seligman MEP 1975, *Helplessness: On Depression, Development and Death*, Freeman, San Francisco.

Skärsäter I, Agren H & Dencker K 2001, Subjective lack of social support and presence of dependent stressful life events characterize patients suffering from major depression compared with healthy volunteers, *Journal of Psychiatric and Mental Health Nursing*, 8(2), pp 107–14.

Stuart GW 2001a, Therapeutic nurse–patient relationship. In: Stuart GW & Laraia MT (eds), *Principles and Practice of Psychiatric Nursing* (7th edn), Mosby, St Louis, pp 15–48.

Stuart GW 2001b, Emotional responses and mood disorders. In: Stuart GW & Laraia MT (eds), *Principles and Practice of Psychiatric Nursing* (7th edn), Mosby, St Louis, pp 345–80.

Talseth AG, Lindseth A, Jacobson L & Norberg A 1999, The meaning of suicidal in-patients' experiences of being cared for by mental health nurses, *Journal of Advanced Nursing*, 29(5), pp 1034–41.

Valente S 2002, Overcoming barriers to suicide risk management, *Journal of Psychosocial Nursing*, 40(7), pp 22–33.

Varcarolis EM 2002, Mood disorders: depression. In: Varcarolis EM (ed.), *Foundations of Psychiatric Mental Health Nursing. A Clinical Approach*, WB Saunders, Philadelphia, pp 452–91.

Yonge O 2002, Psychiatric patients' perceptions of constant care, *Journal of Psychosocial Nursing*, 40(6), pp 23–9.

Acknowledgments

We wish to thank the senior nurse who suggested the four mental health nurse contributors and made the initial contact with them. Thanks especially to each expert for sharing their excellent insights into nursing people with major depression with focus, clarity and conciseness. One nurse requested anonymity; a second nurse did not show a clear interest in being acknowledged; the third wished to be acknowledged at the end of the chapter; and the fourth nurse was happy to have her name attached to her vignette. Hence, all nurse and client names have been changed except Philippa's. Thanks to Heather Keens and Philippa Mazoudier.

CHAPTER

16

Personality Disorders

Gerry Farrell and
Christina Bobrowski

KEY POINTS

- The DSM-IV-TR categorises personality disorders into three behavioural clusters: (A) odd or eccentric; (B) dramatic, emotional or erratic; and (C) anxious or fearful.
- People with personality disorders are considered by nurses and others to be among the most challenging clients to care for.
- Although personality characteristics are formed early in life and evolve over time, once established they are resistant to change.
- People with personality disorder have problems relating to others at home, work, school, and in the community.
- Personality disorders are longstanding, pervasive and maladaptive behaviours that are resistant to treatment and are not caused by another psychiatric disorder, but may coexist with another psychiatric disorder.
- There are several theories of personality disorder with varying degrees of explanatory power.
- Evolution-based theory provides a broad base for understanding personality disorder by addressing fundamental developmental processes.
- People with personality disorders may exhibit self-destructive behaviours such as self-mutilation, eating disorders, alcohol or substance abuse or even shoplifting.
- Improvement can only be achieved when the person with the disorder commits to exploring and re-evaluating their behaviour and relationships and then formulates realistic expectations, although, given the symptoms of personality disorder, this may be a very lengthy process.
- People diagnosed with personality disorder fall into psychiatry's grey area: they are often complained about for exhibiting the behaviours that led to their hospitalisation in the first place.
- There is an urgent need for nursing practice in this field to be based on evidence that demonstrates and validates the contribution that nurses make to the management of these clients.

KEY TERMS

- agenda setting
- antisocial
- avoidant
- borderline
- collusion
- dependency
- dependent
- histrionic
- limit-setting
- narcissistic
- obsessive-compulsive
- paranoid
- personality
- personality disorder
- personality traits
- schizoid personality disorder
- schizotypal personality disorder
- self-harm
- splitting

LEARNING OUTCOMES

The material in this chapter will assist you to:
- differentiate between a personality trait and a personality disorder
- identify the main characteristics of each of the three clusters of personality disorders
- develop an awareness of the feelings that may be experienced by nurses and other health-care workers when working with people who have a personality disorder
- understand the importance of maintaining clear professional boundaries when working with people who have a personality disorder
- identify appropriate nursing interventions and treatments for the care of people with personality disorder
- comprehend the evolutionary theory of personality disorder
- appreciate the need for research into the study and treatment of personality disorder.

INTRODUCTION

People with personality disorders suffer from maladaptive and self-destructive behaviour that can be difficult to change and may coexist with another psychiatric disorder. These people tread an uneasy path between being seen as deserving treatment and being seen as not having a 'real' psychiatric disorder. Nurses managing such patients need appropriate education and training to be able to engage therapeutically with them. This chapter explains the main categories of personality disorders and their diagnosis. Nursing interventions are described, and challenges in working with people who have a personality disorder are discussed. Limitations in our understanding of personality disorders, and problems in categorisation, diagnosis and treatment are also discussed.

'TRAIT' VERSUS 'DISORDER'

Each of us has a personality and a commonsense understanding of what that means. We describe ourselves and others as 'outgoing' or 'assertive', or maybe 'withdrawn' or 'shy'. Sometimes the terms we might choose to describe ourselves are not those that would be chosen by those who know us. Some individuals have personalities that seem to draw people to them. They may be described as charismatic, extroverted, friendly, good team players, helpful or kind. Others seem to have difficulty attracting others or maintaining relationships. They may appear to be unreceptive, cold, aloof, isolative or eccentric, or perhaps they are moody, aggressive or reckless. Our personality may be thought of as the expression of our feelings, thoughts and patterns of behaviour that evolve over time. Our genetics, life experiences and the environment we are exposed to all serve to shape our personality. Our personality manifests in our moods, attitudes and opinions and is clearly expressed when we interact with others.

Enduring aspects or features of our personality are referred to as *personality traits*. These traits are what make us unique and interesting and they differentiate us from each other. Social mores provide unwritten boundaries for what constitutes a 'normal' personality trait. For example, if a student expresses concern at having to present their work to the class because they are shy, and public speaking makes them anxious, we regard that as being within the bounds of normal behaviour. It is very common for people to feel uncomfortable at the prospect of standing up in front of an audience, even one composed of their peers. With encouragement and support, most people are able to jump this particular hurdle. However, some individuals feel so strongly about appearing in public that they avoid all social situations where this may be required of them, to the point where they will withdraw from an enjoyable course of study or well-paid employment or even contact with their family. This behaviour is beyond what is socially regarded as shyness. The personality trait has moved beyond normal boundaries to a point where it may be understood in terms of psychopathology. Some individuals display personality traits that seem to be beyond the scope of what is considered reasonable as observed by their behaviour and attitudes to others, and, as in the foregoing example, will do almost anything to avoid feeling ridiculed, rejected or embarrassed.

When these manifestations of personality start to interfere negatively with a person's life or with the lives of those close to them, the person is diagnosed as suffering from a *personality disorder*. The challenge for nurses, and indeed for anyone involved with such an individual, lies in determining appropriate behaviour, given that norms relating to behaviour are socially and culturally

---

CASE STUDY: Jodie

Jodie is 28 years old. She is an only child and still lives at home with her parents. She is particularly close to her mother. Jodie works as an administrative assistant for a small law firm where she is considered to be very good at her job. She is highly productive and has always been reliable. However, her colleagues state that they don't know 'what to do with her'. She has a fixation on her boss John, the senior partner in the firm. She believes, despite her feelings not being reciprocated, despite the considerable difference in their ages and despite their working together, that there are no barriers to their having a relationship. She is in love with him and believes they are meant to be together. She talks at length about him to her work mates. She becomes tearful and despondent and has been sent home 'sick' on a number of occasions by Laura, the office manager. Jodie blames her boss's inability to see how perfect they are for each other for her inability to function at work on these occasions.

The situation reached crisis point at the firm's Christmas party. Everyone from the office was treated to a dinner cruise with food, wine and music. Initially, Jodie appeared to be having a great time, laughing, flirting and expending a lot of energy on trying to get John to dance with her. After a while, however, Laura noticed that Jodie was missing. Laura found Jodie sitting apart from the main group, crying and sobbing, 'Why won't he come to his senses? How can he do this to me?'. Jodie was clutching a handful of tablets. She told Laura that she had already swallowed a handful and she refused to say what they were. The boat had to return prematurely to port and an ambulance was called. The guests felt uncomfortable about eating the beautiful food that had been hurriedly presented to them and fell silent. Some were angry, while others were also confused. The party was ruined. In Jodie's opinion it was all John's fault.

constructed. When is the expression of someone's personality to be considered disordered? Let us set the scene for our contemplation of this question by considering the case study of Jodie.

Clearly, Jodie has some problems. In particular, she seems to have trouble with her relationships and with discerning appropriate ways of dealing with disappointment. It is one thing to have unrequited feelings for someone and to feel sad. It is quite another to deal with the situation as Jodie did. Jodie may be exhibiting the features of a personality disorder. In order to determine whether Jodie does have such a disorder, an assessment would need to be conducted that considered more than the events that triggered her attempted overdose and ensuing admission. A full psychosocial history would be obtained to enable clinicians to detect patterns in Jodie's behaviour over time. Without a comprehensive assessment, Jodie's behaviour may be interpreted as resulting from a fixed delusion on her boss. The problem is compounded by the fact that we believe that these behaviours are usually enacted unconsciously—that is, sufferers have little or no conscious awareness of their disorder.

However, it is rare for a person who has a personality disorder to present to a clinical setting because of the disorder. Rather, people tend to present to their medical practitioner for secondary mental health issues such as depression, feeling unable to cope or because of the effects of a situational crisis they may find themselves in.

CLASSIFICATION OF PERSONALITY DISORDERS

While each of the personality disorders described in the *Diagnostic and Statistical Manual of Mental Disorders*, fourth edition, DSM-IV-TR (American Psychiatric Association 2000) has particular characteristics, they also have certain features in common. Personality disorders are recognised by persistent and enduring patterns of behaviour that are often destructive and nearly always characterised by maladaptive and inflexible ways of coping with stress (such as Jodie's response to John's rejection). As a result, those affected experience significant impairment in their ability to relate satisfactorily to others at work or socially. People with personality disorder also seem to have an outsized capacity to evoke interpersonal conflict and therefore have an intense, often negative, impact on those around them.

One of the difficulties of caring for these people is that they tend to have very little or no insight into their condition. Clinicians often comment that the trouble with working with people with personality disorder is that as far as they are concerned, the problem is yours, not theirs! This lack of insight stems from an inability to empathise with others, which can be seen to be related to impaired cognition, affect, interpersonal functioning and impulse control (APA 1994). Of course we have to acknowledge that this view is the orthodox one and it may simply be that clients are unwilling to share with us how they feel and what they believe.

The DSM-IV-TR groups personality disorders into three clusters: A, B and C. Cluster A is composed of the disorders of an odd or eccentric nature; cluster B includes dramatic, erratic and emotional disorders and cluster C the anxious and fearful group. Table 16.1 summarises the disorders covered by each cluster along with the diagnostic criteria used in clinical settings. It should be noted that the DSM-IV also provides a category to accommodate the diagnosis of people whose personality disorders do not fit the criteria for any specific disorder, which is referred to as 'personality disorder: not otherwise specified'.

PROBLEMS OF DIAGNOSIS

The rise of evidence-based practice cautions health professionals to acknowledge the individual determinants of disease. Health professionals are urged to look at clients holistically and not reduce them to a label based purely on a collection of signs and symptoms. Individual client predicaments and concerns should be given equal weight alongside the research and diagnostic evidence, so that together, clinicians and clients can make informed choices about what might be the optimum care in a given situation (Farrell 1997, p 1). Psychologists remind us also of the interplay between psychological and physical determinants of illness and treatment outcomes. Yet it appears that psychiatry is moving ever more towards a reductionist approach to illness, whereby mental disorders are categorised into discreet entities based on the presence of specific symptoms or signs. One only has to review the DSM-IV-TR and compare its present size to earlier editions. Each later edition of this manual increases in size as the diagnostic categories expand to include disorders such as caffeine addiction.

While the layperson may be forgiven for thinking that psychiatric diagnoses are reliable and valid, the mental health nurse should be aware that psychiatric diagnosis is problematic at best and flawed at worst. The DSM-IV (APA 1994) issues a cautionary statement to clinicians regarding the interpretation of its diagnostic categories. It acknowledges that:

> there is no assumption that each category of mental disorder is a completely discrete entity with absolute boundaries dividing it from other mental disorders or from no mental disorder. There is also no assumption that all individuals described as having the same mental disorder are alike in all important ways. The clinician using DSM-IV should therefore consider that individuals sharing a diagnosis are likely to be heterogeneous even in regard to the defining features of the diagnosis and that boundary cases will be difficult to diagnose in any but a probabilistic fashion.

(APA 1994, DSM-IV, p xxii)

Table 16.1 Criteria for classification of the personality disorders

Cluster A: *Odd or eccentric*	*Criteria*
Paranoid personality disorder	■ The person has expectations of being harmed or exploited without sufficient reason ■ There is a preoccupation with unjustified doubts ■ There is an unwillingness to confide in others ■ Perceive hidden, demeaning or threatening messages in innocent remarks or comments by others ■ There is a tendency to bear grudges ■ Perceive attacks upon their character or reputation that are not apparent to others ■ Suspicion regarding the fidelity of their spouse or partner
Schizoid personality disorder	■ The person neither enjoys nor desires close relationships ■ There is a preference for solitary activities ■ There is little interest in sexual activity ■ There is indifference to either praise or criticism ■ Emotional frigidity is apparent
Schizotypal personality disorder	■ The person exhibits evidence that they are experiencing ideas of reference ■ The person expresses odd beliefs and thinking in their speech and is odd in their appearance ■ There is evidence of some paranoid ideation ■ There is social anxiety ■ They lack a social network/friends
Cluster B: *Dramatic, erratic & emotional*	*Criteria*
Antisocial personality disorder	■ The person is at least 18 years old ■ They may have expressed a conduct disorder before age 15 years ■ Exhibit a disregard for the law ■ Exhibit reckless, aggressive, deceitful and impulsive behaviour ■ Do not exhibit remorse ■ There is an inability to sustain employment/study
Borderline personality disorder	■ The person is terrified of abandonment and actively attempts to avoid it ■ Experience intense and unstable moods ■ Form intense and unstable relationships ■ Experience disturbances of identity ■ Engage in impulsive self-destructive behaviours ■ Exhibit recurrent suicidal behaviour ■ Experience chronic feelings of emptiness and transient paranoia
Histrionic personality disorder	■ The person craves being the centre of attention and engages in self-dramatisation/physical appearance to attain this ■ Displays inappropriately sexually seductive behaviour ■ Speech is used to impress others but is lacking in depth ■ Prone to exaggeration and dramatic expression of emotion ■ There is a tendency to exaggerate the degree of intimacy that they share with others ■ Tendency to be easily led by others
Narcissistic personality disorder	■ The person brims with self-importance and grandiosity ■ There is a preoccupation with fantasies of success, power, genius and/or beauty ■ There is a profound belief that one is special ■ It follows that the person exudes a sense of entitlement, i.e. is deserving of special treatment and favours ■ They display arrogance ■ There is a need to be admired ■ There is a lack of empathy ■ There is a tendency to exploit others for their own benefit
Cluster C: *Anxious and fearful*	*Criteria*
Avoidant personality disorder	■ The person fears disapproval, rejection and ridicule and so avoids occupations and social situations where this may occur *. . . continues*

INTERVENTIONS

Despite the prevalence of personality disorders, they are notoriously frustrating to treat. However, effective interventions do exist to alleviate symptoms and reduce the problematic behaviours that accompany personality disorders. Although people usually improve in terms of clinical and statistical significance, they might not reach 'normalcy' (Sanislow & McGlashan 1998). From the client's perspective this may mean dealing with their personality disorder to some degree for the rest of their lives. Therefore, long-term management plans need to be instituted for these people in order to promote the quality of their life, including their relationships.

When planning care for a person with a personality disorder there are some factors that require consideration regardless of which disorder the person may have. These factors relate to culture, insight, co-morbidity and self-destructive behaviours. Cultural factors, including religion and ethnicity, must always be recognised, as a failure to do so could undermine any therapeutic intention the treatment team or therapist may have.

Given the intrinsic nature of personality, it is difficult to effect change if the client does not acknowledge the need for it. Given that many of these clients will exhibit very low levels of insight, and are prone to noncompliance due to their inability to appreciate the need for intervention, the challenge is obvious for both client and clinician. Altering aspects of personality takes place over extended periods of time and, though gains may be very limited, they should be celebrated. So while the coexisting disorder may respond to the standard treatments for that condition, the underlying personality disorder may remain resistant to change. The principles of caring for the client with a personality disorder are listed in Box 16.2.

Box 16.2 Principles of care

- Monitor for signs of self-harm and suicidality
- Ensure consistency of care among treatment team members
- Communicate frequently and clearly with the treatment team
- Enact firm, fair and consistent limit-setting on client
- Involve client in setting limits and determining consequences

---

The nurse must monitor the client for signs of self-harm and suicidality. Although such behaviours may on occasion be dismissed by members of the treatment team as attention seeking or non-lethal manipulation, they are nonetheless an aspect of the client's disorder and may well have been the motivating factor in admission. There must be consensus among team members as to how these behaviours are to be managed. Clear and frequent communication among team members will assist in this regard. Firm, fair and consistent limit-setting enacted with a non-judgmental attitude should be continually strived for. Limit-setting aims to offer clients a degree of control over their behaviour. Whenever limit-setting is employed the client should know in advance the behaviours expected (for example, attend group therapy daily), as well as the consequences for breaches (for example, forfeit attendance at the late-night cinema). As far as practicable, the client should be involved in setting the limits and determining the consequences. The use of contracts (where the client and staff both sign a written agreement that sets out acceptable standards of behaviour), time-out (where the client is offered monitored time in a quiet, private, slow stimulus environment until the urge to self-harm passes) have both been found to be useful tools in practice. The first gives the client boundaries within which to operate and concrete consequences for behaviour. The second encourages the client to attempt to deal with maladaptive behaviours in a more positive and acceptable way. Carried out consistently by a team that communicates well, the behaviours (see Box 16.3) of seduction, dependency, rejection, agenda setting, collusion and staff splitting (Tredget 2001) may be avoided.

Box 16.3 Definition of terms

- *Seduction*—the client engages in behaviours that can range from simple flattery to sexual seduction.
- *Dependency*—the nurse experiences gratification from the client's perceived dependency on them.
- *Rejection*—the client rejects the nurse/s because they feel it is inevitable that the nurse/s will reject them.
- *Agenda setting*—the client is allowed to control the therapeutic relationship and the treatment regimen.
- *Collusion*—the client attempts to persuade individual staff members to endorse their way of behaving.
- *Staff splitting*—the client attempts to split the treatment team by appealing to individual members by sharing 'secrets' and suggesting that the staff member is the 'only one' who understands or is approachable.

Such manipulative behaviour is analogous to the client's propensity for dividing the world into 'good' and 'bad' with no individual or thing having both qualities at the same time. In an attempt to overcome some of these difficulties it is worth remembering that as a nurse, your task is to accept that your role is to establish a relationship with a person who needs relief from feelings, has no reason to trust you, has experienced a lifetime of betrayal, lives in a state of chronic arousal, and cannot comfort or soothe themselves (Gallop 2002). Gallop (2002) suggests that nurses need to set modest, client-centred, short-term goals so that success can be easily recognised and experienced.

Interactive therapies

Increasingly, mental health nurses have been trained in cognitive behavioural therapy (CBT). Cognitive behavioural therapy uses aspects of both cognitive therapy, which primarily seeks to identify and alter unhelpful patterns of belief, and behaviour therapy, which seeks to identify unhelpful patterns of behaviour and to implement strategies to break these patterns. Cognitive behavioural therapy aims to help people to develop more efficient coping mechanisms by equipping them with strategies that promote logical ways of thinking about and responding to everyday situations.

Dialectical behaviour therapy (DBT) is similar to CBT, but it also actively incorporates social skills training. The focus of this therapy is: first, the attenuation of parasuicidal and life-threatening behaviours; second, the attenuation of behaviours that hinder therapy; and third, the attenuation of behaviours that frustrate the client's ability to improve their quality of life. Essentially, this therapy, developed by Linehan (1998, 2000) moves between validation and acceptance of the person. Therapeutic procedures include attention to the present moment, being non-judgmental and focusing on effectiveness. Change strategies include behavioural analysis of maladaptive behaviours and problem-solving techniques, such as skills training, contingency management (using reinforcers and punishment), cognitive modification, and exposure-based strategies (assisting clients to confront difficult situations) (Linehan 1998, 2000).

In a meta-analysis of the effects of the two most frequently applied forms of psychotherapy in the treatment of personality disorders, psychodynamic therapy and CBT, it was found that both these therapies can be effective treatments for personality disorder. However, these results should be regarded as preliminary due to the limited number of studies that were included in the meta-analysis (Leichsenring & Leibing 2003). Both these therapies are discussed in Chapter 23.

Pharmacological intervention

Medication has been of limited use in the treatment of personality disorder. However, there is some indication that antipsychotic medications may alleviate paranoid, schizoid and schizotypal symptoms (Sadock & Sadock 2003, p 804). Mood stabilisers such as lithium, and anticonvulsants such as carbamazepine and sodium valproate, and selective serotonin reuptake inhibitors such as sertraline hydrochloride or fluoxetine, may help to control the compulsive element of the dramatic disorders. Although antidepressant and anti-anxiety medications may have little effect on something as fundamental as personality, medical practitioners and psychiatrists find that if they prescribe medication that relieves the stress that comes with living such disordered lives, then some clients may be motivated or enabled to undertake the therapies described above.

Therapeutic community

Tredget (2001) defines a therapeutic community as a setting where a conscious effort is made to ensure that the potential of all clients and staff is used to create a social environment that is conducive to personal development. This style of care seeks to minimise hierarchical power relationships so that there is equality between clients and staff in relation to decisions concerning treatment and the running of the community. In Australia and New Zealand, the most prominent exponent of this style of care is The Richmond Fellowship. Originally founded by a social worker in England, the Fellowship maintains many residences offering the opportunity for personal growth and development to young people with a range of mental disorders. Chapter 21 offers further discussion about therapeutic community.

Team or triumvirate nursing interventions

Given the propensity for people with personality disorder to staff split, this form of care delivery might be useful, particularly in the inpatient setting, although empirical evidence to substantiate its degree of efficacy is lacking. It involves nurses working in teams of three, each with equal responsibility for the provision of care to the clients assigned to them. Two nurses of the team of three conduct sessions with the client. A debriefing session is conducted with the third nurse after each occasion. Tredget (2001) describes this role as the clinical coordinator role, as this person attempts to constructively challenge what has transpired in the therapy sessions with the client. This provides an appropriate, professional forum for dealing with any issues that may have arisen and facilitates reflective practice. The nurses' roles are interchangeable, so that no one nurse is always the clinical coordinator. For this system to work well, staffing and rostering issues must be taken into account to maintain viable teams. The point of this exercise is to ensure that all staff involved in the client's care, regardless of whether they are full-time or part-time workers, are privy to the same information in relation to the client's management while at work.

WORKING WITH PEOPLE WITH PERSONALITY DISORDER

Given the discussion thus far, it will not surprise you to learn that working with people who have a personality disorder can be very challenging for all concerned. This particular diagnosis is especially prone to having a loaded label. By 'loaded label' we mean that the very term itself carries negative connotations. Listen to the way people say 'PDs' and in what context and ask yourself what images it conjures up for you. The nurse and indeed all those involved with such clients must resist the temptation to respond to these clients in a way that may negatively affect their care.

One of the behaviours that is particularly difficult to work with is that of self-harm/self-mutilation. Self-harming behaviours may be regarded as occurring along

CHAPTER

17

Anxiety Disorders

*Sue Henderson and
Stephen Elsom*

KEY POINTS

- Anxiety disorders are the most common mental disorder in the community.
- People with an anxiety disorder are less likely to seek treatment than people with a mood disorder.
- Every nurse should be able to recognise the different presentations of the various anxiety disorders and refer clients to appropriate services.
- All nurses should possess the skills to manage a panic attack in any setting.
- Mobilising appropriate coping skills and implementing stress-management techniques is a core nursing skill.
- The major psychotherapeutic methods of treating anxiety disorders include stress-management techniques such as progressive muscle relaxation.
- The major classes of drugs used in the treatment of anxiety disorders are antidepressants and anxiolytics.

LEARNING OUTCOMES

The material in this chapter will assist you to:
- define key terms related to anxiety disorders
- distinguish between normal anxiety and the anxiety experienced in anxiety disorders
- discuss the epidemiology, aetiology and treatment of anxiety disorders
- explain the different types of anxiety disorders
- describe the assessment of individuals with anxiety disorders
- discuss interventions appropriate to the care of individuals with anxiety disorders
- provide teaching to individuals and the community to facilitate early intervention for persons with anxiety disorders.

KEY TERMS

- acute stress disorder (ASD)
- adjustment-related disorders
- agoraphobia
- anxiety
- compulsions
- coping
- generalised anxiety disorder (GAD)
- obsessions
- obsessive-compulsive disorder (OCD)
- panic attack
- panic disorder
- phobic disorder
- post-traumatic stress disorder (PTSD)

INTRODUCTION

Nurses frequently interact with anxious clients who are facing threats to their health and wellbeing. Experienced nurses become adept at reassuring and supporting clients in coping with the threat and crisis posed by ill health and trauma. Anxiety is a normal emotion experienced in varying degrees by everyone. Carpenito (2002, p 113) defines anxiety as 'a state in which the individual/group experiences feelings of uneasiness (apprehension) and activation of the autonomic nervous system in response to a vague, non-specific threat'. Anxiety may manifest as:

- thought, e.g. excessive worry or an intrusive, unwanted idea
- feeling, e.g. feeling of impending doom
- behaviours, e.g. performing repetitive actions or avoiding objects or situations
- physical change, e.g. increased heart rate, trembling.

Fear manifests in exactly the same way as anxiety but is a response to a known threat. 'Fear is the knowledge that a threat exists; anxiety is the emotion generated by fear' (Videbeck 2001, p 261). However, the presence of anxiety does not signify that the client has an anxiety disorder. Anxiety disorders are specific diagnostic entities that are the primary problem.

Anxiety disorders are the most common mental disorders. They disrupt the individual's everyday life yet often go unrecognised by clients and health professionals alike. There is a tendency for clients, health professionals and others to dismiss the symptoms of anxiety disorders as nerves, worry or excessive shyness. As a result, anxiety disorders often go untreated, under-treated or inappropriately treated.

If this situation is to be reversed it is imperative that all nurses have an accurate understanding of anxiety and its relationship to anxiety disorders. A sound appreciation of the prevalence, causes, assessment, treatment and nursing management of anxiety disorders will enable the nurse to provide evidence-based nursing care. In addition, a sound knowledge base will facilitate the accurate dissemination of information about anxiety disorders to clients, families and communities. Increased mental health literacy about anxiety disorders may facilitate early intervention for people with anxiety disorders, which could, with appropriate treatment, reduce the incidence of anxiety disorders in the Australian and New Zealand populations.

CRITICAL THINKING CHALLENGE 17.1

Consider the following client scenarios and ask yourself:
- Is this anxiety normal or does it constitute a disorder?
- How long must anxiety persist before it is classified as a disorder?
- What level of anxiety constitutes a disorder?
- What more needs to be known, to be sure that the individual has met the diagnostic criteria for a specific anxiety disorder?

Scenarios:
- Sharon organises her clothes according to fabric type and colour.
- Michael continues to have nightmares five years after he was robbed at a petrol station.
- Seb has never liked spiders.
- Alicia stays at home all day every day.
- Glenda worries about everything and has done so for years.
- Nick avoids eating in public.

The common link in these presentations is excessive anxiety. In order to make this assessment we need to know how long the symptoms have been occurring. We also need to know how much time is devoted to the behaviours and to what degree they interfere with the individual's daily functioning.

For example, in examining Sharon's situation, if we found that Sharon organises her clothes after cleaning the wardrobe, then this would not be regarded as a disorder. If Sharon rigidly arranged her clothes after completing the laundry but spent no more than a few minutes on the task, this behaviour may indicate a personality *trait* but not a disorder. However, if Sharon spends considerable time each day rearranging her clothes, feels distressed if she cannot complete the ritual and cannot leave the house until she has repeatedly checked that the clothes are in order, her behaviour may be considered a *disorder*.

EPIDEMIOLOGY

Anxiety disorders are the most common mental disorder experienced by Australian adults, with a twelve-month prevalence of 9.7 per cent or 1,300,000 Australian adults (470,000 males and 830,000 females) (ABS 1998). An examination of the contemporary epidemiology of anxiety disorders reveals that they are highly prevalent, disabling, largely unrecognised and under-treated. In 1997 the Australian Bureau of Statistics (ABS) conducted the National Survey of Mental Health and Wellbeing (NSMHW) to determine the rate of mental disorders in the Australian community. The ABS interviewed a representative sample of the Australian population—comprising 10,641 community-dwelling Australians. The survey was the first national study to provide information on the prevalence and patterns of mental disorders in the Australian adult population. The twelve-month prevalence of mental disorders in Australian adults is provided in Table 17.1.

Among the major findings of this survey were that people who live alone have a higher rate of anxiety disorder than people who live with one or more persons. Women who live outside capital cities have a higher rate of anxiety disorder than females residing in cities (ABS

Nursing interventions

A panic attack can occur in any setting, and therefore nurses must be prepared for a range of situations, from delivering first aid for a panic attack in a shopping centre, to managing the panicked client in a fully equipped clinical environment.

The presenting symptoms of a panic attack may include palpitations, chest pain, sweating and shortness of breath. Consequently clients often present to the nearest accident and emergency department with their first panic attack. In this environment clients are assessed for physical problems and when none can be found they are frequently told that there is 'nothing' wrong and they are discharged from the department without follow-up. A valuable opportunity to teach the client about their condition and its management is missed. Early recognition and appropriate treatment can, at best, prevent the development of an anxiety disorder and, at the least, ensure that clients do not make continual visits to health professionals seeking a physical reason for their symptoms.

During a panic attack—Stay with the client during the panic attack, as the panic will escalate if they are left on their own (Schultz & Videbeck 2002). The presence of another individual has a calming effect on the panicking client. An unattended client in panic may try to escape their current situation, and in doing so put themselves in danger.

If the clinical environment in which the client has presented with a panic attack is a high-stimulus area, take the client to a calmer, more private setting. Avoid very small rooms or areas were the client might feel trapped. Avoid public areas where the vulnerable client can be observed by passers-by.

Some people lose control of their limbs or become dizzy during a panic attack and are unable to walk independently to another venue. In such a situation it is preferable to modify the environment (reduce noise, lighting, people moving and talking), rather than insist that the client relocate. The panic attack will pass with time, whereas attempting to move a dizzy, fainting client could result in injury to the client should they fall, or muscle-strain for the helper.

In a first-aid situation it may be beneficial to help the client overcome the panic attack in the environment that triggered it. The client's first response will be to flee the situation. In engaging in this behaviour they reinforce avoidance as a coping strategy.

The client experiencing a panic attack may present with apparent cardiac symptoms. In a first-aid situation the nurse will not have access to monitoring equipment that can help exclude a cardiac cause for the symptoms. However, if the chest pain eases when the client slows their breathing it is unlikely to be due to a heart attack. Nevertheless the nurse must be ready to activate an emergency plan, while at the same time remaining calm and presenting an image of confidence and control. An anxious client can make a nurse anxious and in turn an anxious nurse can make an anxious client more anxious. This ability to transmit anxiety from one person to another has been referred to as *infectious anxiety*. At its most extreme, infectious anxiety can cause mass hysteria.

Speak to the client in short, simple and audible sentences. A client at panic-level anxiety can only process one detail at a time and their sense of hearing can also be reduced (Fortinash & Holoday-Worret 2003). During the panic attack take a directive approach; instruct the client to 'Please sit down' rather than asking 'Would you like to sit down?'. The client experiencing panic will not be able to decide what to do when offered the choice of whether to sit or not and needs direction at this time. When the client has regained control they can resume responsibility for their own decisions.

Continue with a calm, reassuring tone: 'You are having a panic attack' and 'I will stay with you'.

Instruct the client to take a slow, medium breath (*not* a deep breath) through their nose and to hold it briefly before exhaling slowly through their nose. Aim to reduce the client's respiration rate to ten breaths per minute by using a six-second cycle per respiration—for example, say 'in-2-3, out-2-3' (Andrews & Garrity 2000). Instruct the client to breathe using their diaphragm, not their chest. Continue coaching the client until their anxiety subsides. Some clients are aware that they are hyperventilating and try to slow their breathing, whereas others are not aware and make no attempt to reduce their respiration rate. Shallow, increased breathing or deep breathing results in the client exhaling too much carbon dioxide, which will manifest as dizziness and tingling or pins and needles in the extremities. To correct this you can ask the client to breathe into a paper bag. They will then re-breathe the carbon dioxide and regain the correct balance. However, some people find the prospect of having a bag over their mouth and nose too smothering or embarrassing and will become more panicky. Also, your chances of obtaining a paper bag in a first-aid situation in this age of plastic will be slim. You must be prepared to modify any anxiety reduction intervention to the individual concerned.

Continue to coach the client in the slow-breathing technique because it is important for them to learn that the panic attack will pass and that reducing their breathing rate has helped them to regain control. As the client's panic subsides, try and encourage them to stay and further reduce their anxiety rather than fleeing as soon as they can. This is an important step in proving to the client that they can regain their composure, which is empowering, rather than reinforcing the idea that the current environment is a dangerous place. A client who experiences a panic attack in a specific setting may come to associate that setting with danger and thus avoid it in future. This is how panic attacks can lead to agoraphobia, as the client has another panic attack in another venue and adds this to the list of places to be avoided.

In a clinical setting, if the above techniques fail or the client is experiencing disorganised thoughts, perceptual disturbances or agitation that could escalate to aggression, consider administering a prescribed anti-anxiety medication that can be given as necessary. Even in a clinical situation, medication should only be used as a last resort because it communicates to the client that they are incapable of regaining control and sets up a future expectation that anxiety can be eliminated by medication. An oral dose from the benzodiazepine group (Therapeutic Guidelines Limited 2000), preferably in syrup form, followed by a glass of water will have a quicker onset of action than an intramuscular injection (Therapeutic Guidelines Limited 2000). Although benzodiazepines are very effective at reducing anxiety, they are associated with dependence and should only be used in the short term (preferably no longer than two weeks). Long-term use can result in withdrawal symptoms that mimic the anxiety symptoms that precipitated the client taking them in the first place, thus convincing the client that they cannot do without their 'pills' (National Prescribing Service 1999a).

A small minority of clients experiencing very severe symptoms may require intravenous administration of a benzodiazepine by a medical practitioner.

After a panic attack—Once the panic attack has abated, tell the client again that what they have just experienced was a panic attack. Be aware that most of the information given to the client during the panic attack will not have been retained. Continue to keep your explanations short and simple. Ask the client if they have previously experienced a panic attack and, if so, when was their last attack, how many previous attacks have they had and is there anything in particular that triggers them?

Give the client a list of the classic symptoms of a panic attack. Ask them to put a tick next to each symptom that they have experienced (Treatment Protocol Project 1997). Discuss the list with the client to determine whether they agree that what they have experienced was a panic attack. Some clients may continue to harbour a belief they have a physical problem that has yet to be diagnosed.

However, if this was the client's first panic attack, and it has occurred in a community environment, it is important to refer the client to a health professional for a thorough physical examination to exclude a physical cause for their symptoms. Once a physical cause for the client's symptoms has been excluded and the diagnosis of panic attack has been confirmed, no further follow-up is warranted, as one panic attack does not constitute an anxiety disorder. However, the client should be informed that if they have further panic attacks they should seek appropriate help early.

Panic disorder
Panic disorder is defined as 'the presence of recurrent, unexpected panic attacks followed by at least one month of persistent concern about having another panic attack, or a significant behavioural change related to the attacks' (American Psychiatric Association 2000, p 433). The individual must have experienced at least two unexpected panic attacks to be diagnosed with panic disorder. There are two types of panic disorder: panic disorder without agoraphobia and panic disorder with agoraphobia. The frequency and severity of panic disorder varies widely from one panic attack per week for months, to daily panic attacks, separated by weeks or months without an attack. The characteristics of panic disorder are:

- fear that attacks indicate the presence of an undiagnosed, life-threatening illness
- remaining unconvinced by repeated negative medical tests and positive reassurance
- fear that they are going crazy or have a weak character
- development of avoidance behaviours
- fear of having another attack.

The associated features of panic disorder include: a constant or intermittent anxiety that is not focused on anything specific; apprehension about routine activities; and anticipation of catastrophic consequences related to mild symptoms (for example, worrying that a headache is really an undiagnosed brain tumour). The client may also be hypersensitive to medication side-effects.

Panic disorder can lead to damage or loss of interpersonal relationships. The individual can be so disabled by the panic that they are no longer able to fulfil their usual roles.

Co-morbid disorders to panic disorder include depression, with rates varying from 10 to 65 per cent. In one-third of clients, depression precedes the panic disorder. In two-thirds of clients, depression coincides with panic disorder. Clients will often self-medicate with alcohol or other medication and are at high risk of developing a substance-use disorder. Other anxiety disorders and numerous general medical conditions are also common in panic disorder (APA 2000). The case study of Ian illustrates role impairment and co-morbidity associated with panic disorder.

The New South Wales Mental Health Service (ABS 1998) found that the prevalence of mental disorders is much higher in clinical populations. Panic disorder occurs in 10 per cent of clients in mental health settings; in 10–30 per cent of general medical clients (especially in vestibular, respiratory and neurology settings) and in up to 60 per cent of clients in cardiology settings (APA 2000).

Panic disorder has a peak onset in adolescence and a smaller peak in the mid-thirties. It is rare in children and people over 45 years of age. Panic disorder has a chronic, fluctuating course. Agoraphobia usually develops within the first year of panic attacks.

Panic disorder is more common in families. A client with a first-degree relative with panic disorder is eight times more likely to develop panic disorder than the

---

CASE STUDY

'Heather is a 48-year-old woman whose husband of eighteen years recently left her. Heather has always been shy and anxious, and recalls a particularly awkward adolescence. She remembers being eighteen, having few friends, and being painfully shy with boys. She never went to school dances, rarely went out at night, tried to avoid looking people in the eye, and hardly ever spoke to people unless she knew them well. Since these early days, Heather's confidence has grown a little as she matured, but she has always found it difficult to be in any social situation. Heather believes that she looks awkward and unattractive and whenever the conversation turns to her, she immediately feels that people will think she is stupid. She avoids parties and dinners whenever she can and rarely starts conversations. She always tries to fit in with others and even avoids walking around in crowded places because she thinks everyone is watching her.'

Source: Rapee RM 2001, *Overcoming Shyness and Social Phobia: A Step-By-Step Guide* (2nd edn), Lifestyle Press, Killara, NSW, p xiii.

Specific phobia

Specific phobia is defined as a 'marked and persistent fear that is excessive or unreasonable, cued by the presence or anticipation of a specific object or situation (e.g. flying, heights, animals, receiving an injection, seeing blood). Exposure to the phobic stimulus almost invariably provokes an immediate anxiety response . . . which may take the form of a panic attack' (APA 2000, p 449).

In specific phobia the person recognises that the fear is excessive. They avoid the phobic stimulus or endure it with intense anxiety. The avoidance, anxious anticipation or distress interferes significantly with the individual's daily functioning. Individuals under eighteen years of age must have symptoms for longer than six months to receive a diagnosis of specific phobia. This is in recognition that there are many fears related to a child's developmental level, such as fear of the dark or fear of strangers.

A useful mnemonic to remember the key elements necessary for a diagnosis of phobia is 'PHOBIA':
P—persistent
H—handicapping (restricted lifestyle)
O—object/situation
B—behaviour (avoidance)
I—irrational fears (recognised as such by client)
A—anxiety response.
For a diagnosis of specific phobia, the individual's fear must result in significant interference with their functioning. Significant distress alone is not sufficient for a diagnosis of phobia.

There are five different subtypes of specific phobia, depending on the type of trigger:
- animal—animals or insects
- natural environment—storms, heights, water etc (generally childhood onset)
- blood/injection/injury—seeing blood or injury or receiving an injection or other procedure (vasovagal fainting response)
- situational—bridges, elevators, flying etc
- other—choking, vomiting, contracting an illness.

Often more than one type will be present. Features associated with specific phobia include a restricted lifestyle. Co-morbid conditions include other anxiety disorders, mood disorders and substance-related disorders.

Specific phobias are common in clinical settings but, with the exception of the blood/injection/injury type, are rarely the focus of attention. In contrast to other specific phobias, clients with the blood/injection/injury type experience an initial brief increase in heart rate and blood pressure, followed by a decreased heart rate and blood pressure. Three-quarters of clients will faint when their blood pressure drops. There is a risk to the client's physical health if they avoid seeking treatment for a medical condition because of their phobia (APA 2000). Some clients would rather die than have a needle. The case study below illustrates that this type of phobia is not confined to the 'weakling' stereotype.

CASE STUDY

A 32-year-old healthy male farmer told his physician during an examination that he always faints when stuck with a needle. The physician did not listen and assumed the patient was exaggerating, because the patient was otherwise very healthy, strong and able to deal with all the physical demands of farming, including delivering animals and giving them shots. The patient fainted before the needle was inserted for a blood sample, fell backward off the examination table, and had to be lifted back onto the table while unconscious. Fortunately, except for some sore, stretched muscles, the patient was unhurt.

Source: Travis TA 1998, *Solving Patient Problems: Psychiatry*, Blackwell Science, Madison, p 57.

Less than a third of people with a specific phobia seek professional treatment. Clients with a high level of impairment and those who are phobic about commonly encountered objects and situations are more likely to seek help.

Females are twice as likely as males to have a specific phobia but rates vary with the different subtypes. Animal, natural and situational phobias are strongly associated with being female. In the blood/injection/injury type, 55–70 per cent are female. The prevalence of specific phobias was not measured in the ASMHW (ABS 1998).

Specific phobias develop in childhood and early adolescence. Females develop them at a younger age than males. Predisposing factors to the development of specific phobias include traumatic events such as being bitten by a dog, an unexpected panic attack in a specific situation, observation of others undergoing trauma, and repeated warnings of danger by, for example, parents or the media.

Phobia rates are higher in individuals with other family members with a phobia. Blood/injection/injury phobias have strong familial patterns. Remission occurs in only 20 per cent of clients with a phobia that persists into adulthood (APA 2000).

Nursing interventions for phobias

Carpenito (2002, p 380) defines fear as 'a state in which an individual or group experiences a feeling of physio-logical or emotional disruption related to an identifiable source that is perceived as dangerous'.

Exposure therapy is an effective non-drug therapy used in a range of anxiety disorders. Exposure therapy is defined as the gradual facing of feared situations to reduce associated anxiety and distress (Rogers & Gournay 2001). *Systematic desensitisation* is similar to exposure but pairs a conscious relaxation technique with exposure to decrease the anxiety response to an identified phobic trigger (Schultz & Videbeck 2002). Exposure therapy relies on naturally occurring 'habituation' rather than a conscious induction of relaxation. Before commencing a course of exposure therapy the nurse must fully explain the procedure and provide support to the client in the initial stages of therapy.

According to Rogers & Gournay (2001) there are several components of exposure:

- graded
- prolonged
- repeated
- focused
- practised.

Graded exposure

The client develops a hierarchy of fears from most feared to least feared. These fears are written down in point form and discussed with the nurse. For example, the client with social phobia may develop the following hierarchy:

- speaking to people in authority
- initiating a conversation with a stranger at a party
- eating in front of others.

The client with agoraphobia would generate a different list of phobic triggers:

- visiting the shopping plaza
- walking to the end of the street
- going to the letterbox
- leaving the house and standing on the front step.

As would the client with a specific phobia:

- patting a dog
- standing next to a dog
- standing within arm's reach of a dog
- looking at pictures of dogs.

After the list has been generated and committed to paper, start with the least-fearful trigger and negotiate the manner and duration of exposure. Assist the client to set goals for exposure. Ask the client: 'What would you most like to be able to do if you didn't have this phobia?'. Some examples elected by the client with social phobia may include:

- looking people in the eye
- speaking in a confident tone
- inviting a friend over for a coffee
- initiating a conversation with the boss.
- chatting up girls (or boys).

Prolonged exposure

The aim is for the client to remain exposed to the phobic trigger for as long as it takes their anxiety to subside. This will vary from one client to another. At least a fifty per cent reduction from beginning-level anxiety is required for the exposure therapy to be effective.

Repeated exposure

The clients must face the phobic trigger at least daily for exposure therapy to be successful.

Focused exposure

The client may revert to avoidance behaviours during the exposure. The client has been using these maladaptive coping mechanisms for some time and it is difficult to break the habit. Examples include distraction techniques. Keep the client focused on feeling the initial fear on exposure and then commenting on the natural reduction of anxiety that accompanies prolonged exposure.

Practised exposure

Practising exposure on a regular basis will maintain the gains. A family member can be enlisted to coach the client to maintain a daily schedule of exposure (Rogers & Gournay 2001).

CRITICAL THINKING CHALLENGE 17.4

Think of a person you know who has a phobia. What measures do they take to avoid coming in contact with the phobic stimulus? What effect does this avoidance behaviour have on their daily functioning?

STRESS-RELATED DISORDERS

Adjustment disorder

An adjustment disorder is an exaggerated emotional or behavioural response to a significant life change or stressor such as a relationship break-up, bereavement, divorce, business difficulties, illness, migration and so on. Adjustment disorders occupy a separate chapter from anxiety disorders in the *Diagnostic and Statistical*

Manual of Mental Disorders. However, they are discussed here because adjustment disorders such as acute stress disorder (ASD) and post-traumatic stress disorder (PTSD) are characterised by the presence of a stressor, although unlike ASD and PTSD, the stressor is not beyond the realm of everyday experiences.

The onset of adjustment disorder is within three months of exposure to the stressor. Acute adjustment disorder resolves within six months of the cessation of the stressor and its consequences. Chronic adjustment disorder occurs when a stressor, such as ill health, persists for longer than six months.

The symptoms experienced by the person are beyond what would normally be expected of a person in the given situation and significantly impair the individual's social, academic or occupational functioning. The decision of what is 'in excess of what would normally be expected' is subjective and thus prone to cultural and/or clinician bias.

People experiencing an adjustment disorder may have particular symptoms that dominate, such as depressed mood, anxiety or a disturbance of conduct (truancy, reckless driving, overspending, fighting). The diagnosis is only made when the person does not meet the diagnostic criteria for any other mental disorder. A normal grief reaction to the loss of a loved one would not be classified as an adjustment disorder; however, if the grief is excessive or prolonged, adjustment disorder may be diagnosed. Associated features include decreased performance at work, school, changed relationships, suicide attempts and suicide, substance abuse and somatic complaints.

Prevalence varies widely from two to eight per cent of community samples, to twelve per cent of general hospital clients, up to a third of mental health outpatients and up to half of clients in specialist settings such as post cardiac surgery (APA 2000).

Assessment consists of determining whether the person meets the criteria for another mental or personality disorder first, and exploring the nature of the stressor (duration, severity) and the individual's symptoms in relation to the stressor. Because the response is out of the norm, conducting a detailed assessment of the individual's personality traits and support structure would provide a sound base for a management plan.

As the disorder does not meet the diagnostic criteria of other DSM-IV-TR disorders, first-line management consists of removal or modification of the stressor if possible, allowing the individual to ventilate feelings, crisis intervention, instituting problem-solving and stress management. Anti-anxiety medication or antidepressants are not appropriate in the initial stages but may be indicated at a later date. People experiencing ongoing stressors will need ongoing support, whereas those experiencing a response to an acute stressor may not require treatment or support after the initial crisis intervention. Most people experiencing an adjustment disorder recover fully.

CASE STUDY

Emma, a 23-year-old employed female, presented to her GP after an argument with her work colleague. Emma complains of feeling 'nervy' and on edge. She describes it as a feeling of tension that stops her from being able to relax. She lies awake until the early hours of the morning going over the argument. The feeling of tension has dulled her appetite and she does not enjoy her meals. Two days after the argument she is still thinking about it most of the time.

Once the crisis has passed it can be helpful to teach clients a range of coping skills. Box 17.2 lists some common methods of coping with difficulties.

Box 17.2 Common coping methods

- Problem solving—weighing up the pros and cons
- Tension reduction—play, exercise, hobbies
- Social skills—negotiation, humour, good communication
- Self-disclosure—sharing feelings
- Structuring—organising coping resources, planning ahead
- Seeking information—friends, self-help groups, health professionals, literature
- Stress monitoring—awareness of our own tension and events that increase it
- Assertive response—being able to request our needs and wants clearly, without infringing on others' rights
- Avoidance/withdrawal—getting away from things for a while. Not facing up to things at all is not adaptive.
- Self-medication—in the short term a glass of alcohol can help you relax. Self-medication becomes maladaptive when you rely on substances to relax.
- Social support network—friends can provide a great deal of support. The absence of friends and family or loneliness can be a precursor to mental illness.
- Belief/values—many clients say it is their belief in God or reliance on their values that has helped them through a crisis
- Wellness—keeping fit, eating nutritious meals and getting enough rest and sleep
- Self-esteem/confidence—prizing oneself

Stress-management techniques include progressive muscle relaxation, guided imagery and meditation.

CRITICAL THINKING CHALLENGE 17.5

Think of a time when you had a crisis in you life. How did you cope with the problem?

Acute stress disorder

Acute stress disorder (ASD) is a transient response to a severe trauma such as an accident, natural disaster, crime or combat. The characteristic symptoms of anxiety, dissociation and other intense autonomic arousal occur within one month after exposure to the stressor. The characteristic symptoms of ASD occur either while experiencing the trauma or within one month of the traumatic event. The diagnostic criteria require three or more of the following characteristic symptoms:

- numbing, detachment or no emotional response
- being in a daze
- derealisation (feeling that the world is unreal or distorted)
- depersonalisation (feeling of unreality, detachment or being outside one's body or mind, like an observer)
- dissociative amnesia (inability to recall significant aspects of the trauma).

The person persistently re-experiences the traumatic event in at least one of the following ways:

- recurrent images
- recurrent thoughts or dreams
- illusions
- flashbacks
- distress on reminders of the event.

The symptoms of ASD must last for at least two days and may persist for up to four weeks after the trauma. If the symptoms persist beyond one month after the trauma, ASD is reclassified as post-traumatic stress disorder (APA 2000).

Nursing interventions

Debriefing—Debriefing is an interpersonal technique that assists people to mobilise adaptive coping strategies in order to overcome the effects of exposure to traumatic events. Debriefing helps the individual gain a clear understanding of the trauma, come to terms with their thoughts and reactions to the trauma and identify any stress-related symptoms they may be experiencing. The debriefer provides information about the normal stress response to abnormal stressors, promotes problem solving and supports the individual as they come to terms with the trauma (Department of Human Services 1997).

Progressive muscle relaxation—Progressive muscle relaxation is a useful technique to practise regularly in order to manage the stresses and strains of everyday life. It is not useful as a strategy to control panic in a person who has not previously mastered the technique, but it can be used in the early stages of anxiety. This is why it is so important for the client to learn his or her own early warning signs of increased anxiety and institute anxiety-reduction techniques as soon as they emerge.

Progressive muscle relaxation follows a logical sequence, starting with the hands, then the arms, upward to the shoulders and neck, down the back and so on to the toes.

Start by instructing the client to adopt a comfortable position in a chair with arm rests. Prepare the room so that there will be no interruptions for the duration of the session. Ask the client to make a hard fist and hold it until you tell them to let their hands fall into their lap. Encourage the client to notice the tension and then the feeling of relaxation. Continue throughout the body from the head to the toes.

All trainee health professionals have to start somewhere in developing their helping skills. The best way to master the technique of progressive muscle relaxation is to enrol in a class at the local community health centre and then practise the techniques on a regular basis. Written scripts, setting out the exact wording in the correct sequence, can be used until you are skilled in the format (see Stern 1995). It is important to practise speaking in a calm, unhurried tone, which aids in relaxation. Relaxation tapes are available from retail outlets and can be useful, but it is advisable that the client starts with a personal instructor before moving to the audiotape method. Working with a health professional will increase motivation and adherence to the program, whereas a tape can easily be put off or ignored.

Guided imagery—Guided imagery can be used to deepen the relaxation response obtained during progressive muscle relaxation. After achieving a state of relaxation the client is asked to imagine a place that they find beautiful and relaxing (Fortinash & Holoday-Worret 2003). Ask them to conjure up an image of the scenery and focus on specific aspects such as the feeling of wind on their face, or the sound of waves, or the smell of gum leaves.

Meditation—Ask the client to adopt a comfortable position in a quiet place. Every time they exhale they should say the word 'calm'. While guided imagery encourages the client to use their imagination to conjure up pleasant images, meditation aims to still the mind. People who lead busy lives find this very difficult to do. The moment they have five minutes to spare they start thinking about the next three things they have to do. Tell the client that as a thought comes into their head they should concentrate on their breathing and saying the word 'calm' as they exhale. They should practise meditation regularly.

Post-traumatic stress disorder

Post-traumatic stress disorder (PTSD) is defined as the *development of characteristic symptoms following exposure to an extreme traumatic stressor involving direct personal experience of an event that involves actual or threatened death or serious injury, or other threat to one's integrity; or witnessing an event that involves death, injury, or a threat to the physical integrity of another person; or learning about unexpected or violent death, serious harm, or threat of death or injury experienced by a family member or other close associate.*

(APA 2000, p 463)

Traumatic events that may trigger PTSD include military combat, violent personal assault, disasters, a severe car accident, being diagnosed with a life-threatening illness, and child sexual abuse. All of these events are outside the realm of normal human experience.

The characteristic symptoms of PTSD include: recurrent, intrusive recollections of the event; recurrent distressing dreams of the event; acting or feeling as if the traumatic event were recurring (flashbacks); intense distress at exposure to cues that resemble an aspect of the trauma; and physiological hyper-arousal on exposure to the cues.

The client adopts avoidance behaviours such as a persistent avoidance of the stimuli associated with the trauma, avoiding talking or thinking about the trauma, avoiding activities and places or people that remind the client of the trauma. The client may be unable to recall important aspects of the trauma, display decreased interest and participation in important activities, feel detached from others and have a restricted range of feelings towards loved ones. Clients no longer expect to live a long life or have a career; they suffer from increased arousal, difficulty falling asleep, irritability or outbursts of anger, difficulty concentrating, hyper-vigilance and an exaggerated startle reflex.

Post-traumatic stress disorder may be acute, with symptoms resolving within three months, or chronic, whereby symptoms persist for longer than three months. Some clients experience a delayed onset, with symptoms occurring at least six months after the trauma. Features associated with PTSD include survivor guilt, marital conflict, loss of employment and co-morbid major depression, substance-related disorders or other anxiety disorders. The prevalence of PTSD varies with the group studied. Groups exposed to trauma, such as refugees or military personnel, can have rates from a third to half of those exposed.

Post-traumatic stress disorder can occur at any age. Predisposing factors include the client's premorbid personality, family background and the presence of a pre-existing mental disorder; however, PTSD can develop in individuals without any predisposing factors. Intriguingly, there is an increased vulnerability in clients with a first-degree relative with a history of PTSD or depression (APA 2000).

Generalised anxiety disorder

Generalised anxiety disorder (GAD) is defined as 'excessive anxiety and worry (apprehensive expectation), occurring more days than not for a period of at least six months, about a number of events or activities. The individual finds it difficult to control the worry' (APA 2000, p 472). For a diagnosis of GAD to be made, the anxiety and worry must be accompanied by at least three of the following symptoms: restlessness, being easily fatigued, difficulty concentrating, irritability, muscle tension and disturbed sleep. The typical worries of the client with generalised anxiety disorder are about everyday routine events like job responsibilities, finances, health of family members and household tasks. The client may shift from one worry to another.

Features not part of the diagnostic criteria but associated with GAD include muscle tension, trembling, twitching, feeling shaky, muscle aches and soreness. The client may raise somatic complaints of sweating, nausea and diarrhoea. People with GAD are on edge and may have an exaggerated startle response. Hyper-arousal, characterised by increased heart rate, shortness of breath and dizziness, is less prominent in GAD than in other anxiety disorders.

People with GAD are more likely to also have a mood disorder, other anxiety disorder, substance-related disorder, irritable bowel syndrome or headaches.

Generalised anxiety disorder is more common in females than males, in families with relatives with the disorder, and it runs a chronic, fluctuating course exacerbated by stress. Half of clients with GAD state that they have had the symptoms since childhood or adolescence (APA 2000).

CASE STUDY

Tamara, a 25-year-old woman, presented with worries about her health, her career and her relationships. She said that she had always worried easily, but over the past several months she had felt more tense and agitated. The current increase in anxiety began following a dispute with a colleague who she believed had taken advantage of her, but since then she had been unable to assert herself with this colleague. She frequently worried about the quality of her work and worried that making a mistake would ultimately cause her to lose her job. Over this time she had developed a pattern of waking frequently during the night and being unable to get back to sleep for two to three hours while thinking about all her worries. She had also come to see her GP for various somatic complaints over the years, which she worried were signs of a serious physical illness.

Source: Andrews G & Hunt C 1998, Treatments that work in anxiety disorders, *Medical Journal of Australia*, 168(12), pp 26–32, p 28.

Nursing interventions

Problem solving—The problem-solving technique should be familiar to nurses because the nursing process is based on a problem-solving framework. The first step is to describe the problem clearly and accurately. This is not as easy as it sounds, as people do not always identify the exact problem. For example, Tamara states: 'I am worried that I will make a mistake and lose my job.' Further probing reveals that Tamara had a dispute with a colleague and did not assert herself. Tamara's real problem is a lack of assertion skills.

The second step is to generate a list of possible solutions to the problem. Brainstorming, a process whereby any solution, no matter how far-fetched, is recorded. Tamara could ask her assertive cousin how she would deal with the situation, or she could watch other assertive people at her workplace to see how they go about asserting themselves, or she could hire an actor to take her place at the office to 'deal' with her colleague. While the third solution sounds outlandish, all solutions are listed because they may contain an element of usefulness in solving the problem. The last solution may indicate to Tamara that acting a part until she feels more confident may be more helpful than waiting until she feels confident to act.

Step three involves weighing the pros and cons of each generated solution and choosing the best or most practical solution.

The next step is to plan the best way to implement the chosen solution. What resources are needed and are they available? What does Tamara need to learn to implement the solution? A list is made in point form, detailing each step.

The plan is then implemented and evaluated. Did the solution work? What else needs to be done to solve the problem?

Although the problem-solving method looks incredibly easy, people with an anxiety disorder often have difficulty understanding their problems clearly and tend to choose solutions that reinforce their problem. Tamara may insist that she is in danger of losing her job and choose not to assert herself with her work colleague (avoidance behaviour) as a solution to her problem. It is for this reason that clients often need assistance in applying the problem-solving method in the early stages of therapy.

Obsessive-compulsive disorder

Obsessive-compulsive disorder (OCD) consists of 'recurrent obsessions or compulsions that are severe enough to be time consuming (i.e. they take more than one hour a day) or cause marked distress or significant impairment' (APA 2000, p 456). To put it simplistically, *obsessions* are mental processes and *compulsions* are actions. There are some nuances, however, as the following definitions illustrate:

- Obsessions are 'recurrent persistent thoughts, impulses, or images that are experienced as intrusive and inappropriate and that cause marked anxiety or distress' (APA 2000, p 457). The most common obsessions are thoughts about contamination, repeated doubts (e.g. 'Did I turn the iron off?'), a need to have things in a particular order, aggressive or horrific impulses, and sexual imagery.
- Compulsions are 'repetitive behaviours (e.g. handwashing, ordering, checking) or mental acts (e.g. praying, counting, repeating words silently), the goal of which is to prevent or reduce anxiety or distress, not to provide pleasure or gratification' (APA 2000, p 457). The most common compulsions are washing and cleaning, counting, checking, requesting or demanding assurances, repeating actions and arranging objects in order.

The next case study illustrates the link between obsessions and compulsions and how the client does not gain any enjoyment from the ritual but relents in an effort to ward off uncomfortable anxiety.

CASE STUDY

A 26-year-old man is very concerned about cleanliness and hygiene. He spends a significant amount of time each day washing his hands and showering, especially after touching a toilet seat, doorknob or any other item he thinks may be dirty or contaminated. The client explains that he is concerned about becoming infected or sick from touching these objects. He periodically acknowledges that the washing is excessive but explains that he becomes very anxious when he tries to avoid washing and eventually feels compelled to wash even more to make up for the omission.

Source: Fauman MA 2002, *Study Guide to DSM-IV-TR*, American Psychiatric Publications, Washington DC, p 223.

Features associated with OCD include avoidance of situations that involve the content of the obsession, and hypochondriasis, with repeated visits to doctors for reassurance. The client may feel guilty about the content of their thoughts or the time devoted to rituals; they may experience insomnia and abuse alcohol or drugs in an effort to cope. Engaging in the 'rituals' is time-consuming and thus detracts from relationships, work and social activities.

Clients with OCD have higher rates of major depression, experience other anxiety disorders and may also have an obsessive-compulsive personality disorder. Children with OCD have an increased incidence of learning disorders and disruptive behaviours. One-third to half of people with Tourette's disorder also have OCD. Twenty to thirty per cent of clients with OCD display tics. Clients who engage in excessive washing may have concurrent dermatitis (APA 2000).

19 Substance-related Disorders and Dual Diagnosis

Janette Curtis

KEY POINTS

- It is estimated that ten per cent of the population consume alcohol or other drugs at levels that are hazardous or harmful.
- Alcohol consumption at harmful levels accounts for nearly five per cent of the total disease burden in Australia, and illicit drug use for two per cent.
- Approximately two per cent of the total burden of disease in Australia can be attributed to illicit drug use.
- Excessive alcohol use is estimated to cost $4.5 billion in Australia and $1.4–4.6 billion in New Zealand. Alcohol is also associated with liver disease, pancreatitis, some cancers, diabetes, epilepsy, motor vehicle accidents and a range of injuries and social problems such as neglect and abuse.
- There is a considerable degree of coexistence between substance use disorder (particularly alcohol) and other mental health disorders.
- Hazardous use is a repetitive pattern of use that poses a risk of harmful physical and psychological problems.
- Psychoactive drugs can cause harm through intoxication or through dependence. They are classified as depressants, stimulants or hallucinogens.
- Specific assessment tools and criteria are used for a client who presents with a substance disorder or who has a dual diagnosis.
- Interventions include harm reduction, management of the intoxicated client, detoxification and early and brief interventions.
- Accurate assessment and appropriate management of clients with a dual diagnosis is essential.
- Treatment for dual diagnosis clients can include pharmacological treatment and psychological interventions to reduce substance use.

KEY TERMS

- abstinence
- affective disorders
- alcohol use disorders
- anxiety disorders
- AOD use
- assessment
- coexisting disorder
- co-morbidity
- dependence
- detoxification
- drug use disorders
- dual diagnosis
- harm reduction
- harmful use
- hazardous use
- illicit
- injecting drug use
- intoxication
- pharmacodynamics
- pharmacokinetics
- physical dependence
- problematic substance use
- psychoactive drugs
- psychological dependence
- psychosis
- risk
- substance misuse
- substance-related disorders
- therapeutic use
- tolerance
- toxicity
- withdrawal

LEARNING OUTCOMES

The material in this chapter will assist you to:
- discuss the incidence and significance of substance-related disorders and dual diagnosis in Australia and New Zealand
- differentiate between and describe the pharmacokinetics and pharmacodynamics of psychoactive drugs
- identify the importance of undertaking an alcohol and other drug assessment for all mental health clients
- describe a range of interventions that can be used for clients with a coexisting substance-use disorder and a mental illness
- apply your knowledge of the nursing process to the client who is dependent on alcohol and/or other drugs
- critically analyse the range of treatment services available for clients with a dual diagnosis.

INTRODUCTION

This chapter explores issues of substance use, substance-related disorders and dual diagnosis. It begins by outlining the use of alcohol and other drugs (AOD) in Australia and New Zealand and highlights the costs of AOD use to the individual, family and community. The pharmacological dimension of psychoactive drugs is explored, terms are defined and the diagnostic criteria for substance abuse are presented. How to elicit information and undertake a comprehensive AOD assessment are detailed and specific interventions such as early and brief interventions and harm reduction are explored. Interventions for assessing and treating clients who are intoxicated or withdrawing from substances are described.

The final section of the chapter discusses dual diagnosis (mental illness and substance use disorder), including the clinical significance of dual diagnosis, an exploration of why people with a mental illness use alcohol and other drugs, and treatment models and interventions. The emphasis throughout this chapter is on the problematic use of alcohol and other drugs. You will find additional information and specific nursing interventions for dual diagnosis in other relevant chapters. The interventions described are applicable to any client with a substance-use disorder, including the client who is dually diagnosed.

SUBSTANCE USE AND MISUSE IN AUSTRALIA AND NEW ZEALAND

Tobacco and alcohol account for 83 per cent of the cost of drug abuse in Australia. By measuring hospital bed days and other health costs and deaths in 1998–99 it has been estimated that involuntary (passive) smoking costs the country $47 million (Intergovernmental Committee on Drugs 2001). Tobacco use is included as one of the 'other drugs'. The principles of alcohol and other drug (AOD) assessment, interventions and harm-reduction strategies are used with a person who wants to reduce or cease their use of tobacco as with any other substance.

Excluding tobacco, alcohol is the most used drug in Australia and New Zealand. It is present on most social and celebratory occasions, from diplomatic banquets to informal meetings with friends. Social drinking is a rule-laden activity. Drunkenness may be considered appropriate during certain rites of passage such as stag nights, but there is a clear line between this form of social interaction and continuous, excessive drinking, which has a strong impact on the individual, the community and the economy. Negative effects can follow heavy or excessive regular (chronic) alcohol consumption or single (acute) episodes of alcohol misuse.

Illicit drug use (illegal drugs and the illicit use of drugs and volatile substances, including the non-medical use of prescription drugs) can also be acute or chronic, and have negative effects on individuals, their families and the community. People with a mental illness have been identified as being at particular risk of alcohol and other drug related problems (Intergovernmental Committee on Drugs 2001).

Epidemiology

Australia and New Zealand have two of the highest rates of alcohol consumption in the English-speaking world; only the United Kingdom has a higher consumption. Excessive alcohol use is estimated to cost Australia $4.5 billion, and New Zealand between $1.4 and $4.6 billion per year (Lopatko et al. 2002). It has been estimated that the harm caused by alcohol consumption accounts for 4.9 per cent of the total disease burden in Australia (Australian Institute of Health and Welfare 2000). Conditions associated with hazardous and harmful alcohol use include some cancers, liver disease, pancreatitis, diabetes and epilepsy. Alcohol is also a significant factor in motor vehicle fatalities and injuries, falls, drowning, burns, suicide and occupational injuries. In addition, social costs associated with the excessive use of alcohol include such factors as neglect, and physical and verbal abuse (AIHW 2000).

Chronic, excessive alcohol consumption can result in thiamine deficiency, which affects the central nervous system and can lead to what is termed Wernicke-Korsakoff syndrome (Lopatko et al. 2002; Anderson et al. 2002). Wernicke's disease is the acute phase of the syndrome, which results in damage to the sixth nerve, causing nystagmus (involuntary, rhythmic movement of the eyes), ataxia (staggering gait) and confusion. This is reversible with thiamine therapy. Korsakoff's psychosis is the chronic phase of the syndrome, resulting in short-term memory loss and confabulation (Homewood & Bond 1999). Recovery from this syndrome is usually incomplete. Irreversible alcoholic dementia may also occur (Ambrose, Bowden & Whelan 2001; Jacques 2000).

Approximately two per cent of the total burden of disease in Australia can be attributed to illicit drug use. Data from the 1998 National Drug Strategy Household Survey show that an estimated 3.3 million Australians aged fourteen years or over had used an illicit drug in the previous twelve months. Around 2.7 million people, the greatest proportion, had used cannabis within the past twelve months (AIHW 2000; White 2000). Studies over the past decade suggest that 40–50 per cent of Australians and New Zealanders have tried cannabis at least once and most people who use cannabis do so only occasionally. Approximately 10–20 per cent of New Zealanders use cannabis regularly (Fergussen & Holmwood 2000). According to Todd et al. (2002), rates of cannabis use and dependence appear higher in New Zealand Maori than in New Zealand non-Maori, with rates of dependence approximately 1.8 times higher (Todd et al. 2002).

It is estimated that approximately 100,000 Australians inject drugs regularly and an additional 175,000 inject drugs occasionally. New Zealand has approximately

30,000 drug injectors. In Australasia the number of injecting drug users is estimated to have doubled every ten years since the 1960s, with heroin or amphetamine being the most frequently injected drugs in Australia, and opioids such as morphine and home bake (extracted from codeine tablets) the most frequently used in New Zealand (Australasian Society for HIV Medicine 2001). Injection of illicit drugs and non-prescribed pharmaceuticals can have adverse health effects including drug overdose and acquiring of blood-borne infections (such as hepatitis C virus (HCV) or HIV).

Substance use and misuse among indigenous Australians

Although there is considerable regional variation, the percentages of indigenous Australians who have never drunk alcohol or who drink occasionally are roughly the same as non-indigenous Australians. However, among regular drinkers the percentage who drink at hazardous levels is higher than in the non-indigenous population (Hunter, Brady & Hall 2000). Moreover, as a consequence of the relatively higher frequency of hazardous consumption, indigenous Australians account for a higher number of hospital bed-days per person. Tobacco use is approximately twice as high among indigenous than non-indigenous people and accounts for approximately 13 per cent of deaths among indigenous people (Gray et al. 2002).

Fifty per cent of indigenous Australians have reported using cannabis, compared to forty per cent of non-indigenous Australians. Overall, illicit drugs account for less than one per cent of deaths. However, there has been an increase in the number of indigenous Australians being admitted for problems such as cannabis misuse, amphetamine misuse and drug-induced psychosis (Gray et al. 2002). In some small rural communities in central and northern Australia, the inhalation of petrol fumes is a serious problem. Prior to the introduction of unleaded petrol and aviation fuel in remote communities, lead poisoning was a major health problem for petrol sniffers. Although this problem has been alleviated, the inhalation of other solvents such as aerosols remains a significant issue for some communities (Gray et al. 1995, 1998, 2002; Hunter, Brady & Hall 2000).

Substance use and misuse among New Zealand Maori

In common with indigenous Australians, alcohol use among New Zealand Maori indicates that compared to the general population, fewer Maori than non-Maori drink. Those who do drink, drink less frequently but consume more on each occasion (Adamson et al. 2000). After alcohol, nicotine is the most commonly used drug, with percentages of smokers estimated to be as high as 50 per cent of women and 35 per cent of men (Robertson et al. 2002). Cannabis use is viewed by some as being more problematic for Maori due to the favourable cultivation climate and the socioeconomic status of some Maori. A recent survey indicated that 60 per cent of Maori used cannabis at some time, that 18 per cent were regular users (Dacey & Moewaka Barnes 2000) and that Maori cannabis users are over-represented in AOD services. Benzodiazepine use is also increasing among Maori, and solvents continue to be used among some young, usually male, sections of the population (Dacey & Moewaka Barnes 2000).

PHARMACOLOGY OF PSYCHOACTIVE DRUGS

The World Health Organization (WHO) uses the term 'drug' to describe a chemical entity used non-medically and self-administered for its psychoactive effect. The psychoactive effect is an essential component of the description and usually includes a change in mood, arousal and/or perception, cognition (thinking) and/or behaviour (WHO 1993).

All psychoactive drugs have the capacity to produce drug dependence. These drugs may be produced in a laboratory (e.g. amphetamines or ecstasy) or extracted from plants (e.g. heroin or cocaine). They can also be legal (such as alcohol) or illicit (e.g. cannabis). Psychoactive drugs can cause harm either through intoxication or through dependence (Whelan 1999). They can be classified in many ways. One of the most common methods is to classify them as depressants, stimulants or hallucinogens. Some drugs have multiple actions and therefore can be placed in more than one category (Teesson & Hall 2001).

Depressants are drugs that slow down the activity of the brain. When used in small doses they produce relaxation or drowsiness; in larger doses they produce a loss of consciousness similar to a deep sleep. Some can produce impaired coordination, depression and, in large quantities, coma and death. Depressant drugs include ethanol (alcohol), benzodiazepines (e.g. diazepam), sleeping tablets (e.g. Normison), opioids and painkillers (e.g. codeine, morphine, heroin), and solvents and inhalants (e.g. petrol, nitrous oxide, amyl nitrate) (Teesson & Hall 2001; Whelan 1999).

Stimulant drugs accelerate activity in the nervous system and increase the body's sense of arousal. In small doses they increase awareness and concentration and decrease fatigue. Irritability, activity, nervousness and insomnia increase as the amount taken increases, and some individuals experience delusions and hallucinations. Excessive doses can lead to convulsions and death. Stimulants include amphetamines (commonly known as speed), methamphetamines (commonly known as crystal meth, ice), *d*-amphetamine (dexamphetamine) and methylphenidate (Ritalin). Other stimulant drugs include cocaine, nicotine, caffeine and 3,4 methylenedioxymethamphetamine (MDMA, commonly known as ecstasy) (Teesson & Hall 2001; Whelan 1999).

Hallucinogens (also called psychedelics or psychotomimetics) share properties with both of the previous categories. However, their specific function is to distort perception and consequently induce hallucinations (auditory, tactile and/or visual). In small doses, some hallucinogens such as cannabis reduce inhibitions and cause the user to become more relaxed and feel more sociable. Hallucinogens include lysergic acid diethylamind (LSD), psilocybin (magic mushrooms) and mescaline (part of the Mexican cactus, peyote). Some amphetamine derivatives such as MDMA (ecstasy) are chemically related to mescaline and have both stimulant and hallucinatory properties and may be placed in both categories for classification purposes (Teesson & Hall 2001; Whelan 1999).

Although cannabis is commonly placed with the hallucinogenic group of drugs, it is often difficult to classify in pharmacological terms as it has a mixture of mood, cognitive, motor and perceptual effects and does not clearly belong with any one drug class (Ashton 2001).

HOW DO DRUGS WORK?

The effects of drugs on the body can be understood through two concepts: pharmacokinetics and pharmacodynamics.

Pharmacokinetics is the study of the action of the drugs within the body, including the mechanisms of absorption, distribution, metabolism and excretion (Anderson et al. 2002). The pharmacokinetics of each drug differs; for example, the oral administration of amphetamines produces peak cardiovascular effects after approximately one hour, while central nervous system (CNS) effects peak about two hours after administration. The effects last between four and six hours. However, if the drug is administered intranasally (snorting), the effects are felt within a few minutes. Intravenous injection produces even faster results. Amphetamines are eliminated by metabolism in the liver and excreted by the kidneys, and much is excreted as unchanged amphetamine (Latt et al. 2002).

In comparison, smoking cannabis delivers the active ingredient tetrahydrocannabinol (THC) rapidly to the blood and brain. Plasma THC peaks at the end of smoking (approximately 14 minutes) and falls to low values within two hours. If cannabis is consumed orally, its absorption is lower and its effects are more variable and also often less pronounced. THC is fat-soluble, which results in a slow elimination of metabolites and can be detected in the urine several days after administration and well after the acute effects of THC have disappeared (Todd et al. 2002).

Pharmacodynamics is the study of how a drug acts on a living organism, including the pharmacological response and the duration and magnitude of response observed relative to the concentration of the drug at an active site in the organism (Anderson et al. 2002). As with pharmacokinetics, each drug action is different; for example, amphetamines activate the CNS and have peripheral sympathomimetic actions. The CNS stimulation results in euphoria, an increased feeling of well-being, increased energy and confidence, improved cognitive and psychomotor performance, insomnia and suppression of appetite. Sympathomimetic effects include elevated blood pressure and tachycardia (Latt et al. 2002).

In contrast, the effects of cannabis are mediated by the actions of THC at CB1 receptors in the brain and peripheral tissues (e.g. endothelial cells and testes). Cannabis taken in low doses produces a mixture of stimulatory and depressant effects; at high doses the effects are mainly depressant. The effects of cannabis include euphoria, relaxation and a feeling of wellbeing. In addition, there are perceptual distortions such as altered time sense. Memory, cognition and skilled task-performance are impaired, although many users may feel confident and highly creative. Peripheral effects include tachycardia, vasodilatation and hypotension. Cannabis stimulates the appetite and is also an anti-emetic, and people who have taken cannabis often experience 'the munchies' when they feel hungry and crave certain foods (Todd et al. 2002). As with all psychoactive drugs, the effects vary between individuals depending on the amount taken, the manner of administration, the frequency of use, concurrent use with other drugs, past exposure and the environment in which the drug is used.

CORE DIAGNOSES FOR SUBSTANCE USE

Substance use exists on a continuum that extends from abstinence through intermittent non-hazardous (and sometimes beneficial) use, risky or hazardous use, and harmful use, to dependence (Saunders & Young 2002). In general, the greater the frequency of use and the greater the amount of AOD consumed per occasion, the more severe the consequences for the user's health, the psychosocial consequences and the risk of dependence. However, problems may occur due to occasional, high-level (binge) use, and/or repeated harmful but not dependent use. The terms 'substance abuse' and 'dependence' can be difficult to define precisely, as there are extraneous factors that must be taken into account, such as culture and ideology. For example, in some cultures the use of psychoactive drugs for religious or spiritual ceremonies is accepted but in other cultures is prohibited.

The descriptive terms that are most often used are:

- intoxication
- hazardous use
- harmful use
- substance abuse
- dependence.

These are discussed on the following pages.

The evidence for levels of alcohol consumption are based on a systematic review of international literature commissioned by the National Health and Medical Research Council (NHMRC) (NHMRC 1999).

Intoxication

Intoxication occurs when a person's intake of a substance exceeds their tolerance and produces behavioural and/or physical changes. There is no formally agreed definition, although it is usually taken to refer to an elevated blood alcohol concentration such that a person cannot function within their normal range of physical/cognitive abilities. The DSM-IV-TR criteria for intoxication (see Box 19.1) are used for diagnosis. Women become intoxicated after drinking smaller amounts of alcohol than men, because of their smaller body weight, smaller liver size and smaller blood volume than men, so that the concentration of alcohol in their vital organs is higher for a given dose. It is important for nurses to manage intoxication correctly because it complicates assessment and client management, even when it is not life-threatening. Intoxication can be dangerous because it can mimic or mask serious illness or injury (infections, hypoxia, head injury, hypoglycaemia, temporal lobe epilepsy, drug toxicity (Dilantin, Digoxin), meningitis, cerebral vascular accidents, transient ischaemic accidents).

Box 19.1 DSM-IV-TR criteria for substance intoxication

A The development of a reversible substance-specific syndrome due to recent ingestion of (or exposure to) a substance. **Note**: Different substances may produce similar or identical syndromes.

B Clinically significant maladaptive behavioural or psychological changes that are due to the effect of the substance on the central nervous system (e.g. belligerence, mood lability, cognitive impairment, impaired judgment, impaired social or occupational functioning) and develop during or shortly after use of the substance.

C The symptoms are not due to a general medical condition and are not better accounted for by another mental disorder.

Source: American Psychiatric Association (APA) 2000, *Diagnostic and Statistical Manual of Mental Disorders* (4th edn, text rev.), APA, Washington, DC.

Psychoactive drugs affect mood, cognition, behaviour and physiological functioning. Intoxication can be life-threatening because it can cause altered physical functioning (for example, depressed respiration, alterations in temperature regulation and altered mental function such as panic or paranoia, which can result in accidental injuries).

The essential feature of substance intoxication is that it is reversible and is due to the recent ingestion of, or exposure to, a substance. The maladaptive behavioural or psychological changes associated with intoxication are due to the direct physiological effects of the substance on the central nervous system and develop during or shortly after the use of the substance. The symptoms are not due to a general medical condition or are not better accounted for by another mental disorder. Intoxication is often associated with substance abuse or dependence, but this category does not apply to nicotine (APA 2000).

Box 19.2 Indications of intoxication

- *Alcohol*: loss of control of voluntary movements, slurred speech, disinhibition, low blood pressure, smells of alcohol
- *Benzodiazepines*: slurred speech, loss of control of voluntary movements, sedation, nystagmus (repetitive eye movement), low blood pressure, drooling, disinhibition
- *Opioids*: pinpoint pupils (pupillary constriction), sedation, low blood pressure, slowed pulse, itching and scratching

Source: Hulse G, White J & Cape G 2002, *Management of Alcohol and Drug Problems*, Oxford University Press, Melbourne.

Hazardous use

Hazardous use is defined as a repetitive pattern of use that poses a risk of harmful physical and psychological consequences (potential problem). Hazardous substance use is defined in terms of at-risk behaviours such as sharing intravenous needles, bingeing and using substances in unsafe settings such as when using machinery (Saunders & Young 2002). The NHMRC in Australia defines hazardous consumption of alcohol as a regular daily intake of more than forty grams for men or more than twenty grams for women.

There is evidence that high levels of alcohol consumption during pregnancy can contribute to a variety of adverse outcomes in the newborn child. However, the evidence of the effects on the fetus of drinking lower levels is less clear. Overall, the most consistent evidence to date identifies an average of one standard drink per day as the level below which no discernible evidence has been found for harm to the unborn child (Single et al. 1999).

Harmful use

The term 'harmful use' is used when the pattern of substance use is actually causing harm. Both the Australian NHMRC and the New Zealand definition of harmful alcohol use emphasise high-risk levels of alcohol consumption rather than specific consequences. In Australia this level is over sixty grams per day for men and over forty grams per day for women. In New Zealand the same quantity is used but is applied to 'per session' (Saunders & Young 2002).

Substance abuse

The term 'substance abuse' is often associated with addiction and dependence. It is considered value laden, and has limited use in contemporary addiction literature in the United Kingdom (Hussein Rassool 2002). In Australia and New Zealand the *Diagnostic and Statistical Manual of Mental Disorders* DSM-IV-TR (APA 2000) is used to diagnose substance dependence. It focuses on social and interpersonal consequences of substance abuse such as failure in role obligations, and recurrent legal, social or interpersonal problems. Thus, substance abuse can be defined as the use of drugs or alcohol in a way that disrupts prevailing social norms, remembering that these norms vary with culture, gender and generation (Saunders & Young 2002).

Box 19.3 DSM-IV-TR diagnostic criteria for substance abuse

A A maladaptive pattern of substance use leading to clinically significant impairment or distress, as manifested by one (or more) of the following occurring within a 12-month period:

- recurrent substance use resulting in a failure to fulfil major role obligations at work, school or home (e.g. repeated absences or poor work performance related to substance use; substance-related absences, suspensions, or expulsions from school; neglect of children or household)
- recurrent substance use in situations in which it is physically hazardous (e.g. driving an automobile or operating a machine when impaired by substance use)
- recurrent substance-related legal problems (e.g. arrests for substance-related disorderly conduct)
- continued substance use despite having persistent or recurrent social or interpersonal problems caused or exacerbated by the effects of the substance (e.g. arguments with spouse about consequences of intoxication, physical fights)

B The symptoms have never met the criteria for this class of substance.

Source: American Psychiatric Association (APA) 2000, *Diagnostic and Statistical Manual of Mental Disorders* (4th edn, text rev.), APA, Washington, DC.

Dependence

Saunders & Young (2002) describe one paradox of substance use, which is the persistent use of a substance despite negative consequences. Often these negative consequences contradict the original motive for substance use in the early stages. For example, a person who is alcohol dependent may have initially used alcohol as a way of coping with anxiety, yet now maintains dependent use despite increased financial, relationship, physical and employment worries. The individual may consider that the reinforcing effects of alcohol use outweigh the negative consequences of its use. Dependence can be both physical and psychological. It is often referred to as a

psychobiological syndrome (Saunders, Young & Dore 2001), which exists along a continuum. It consists of a number of behavioural, cognitive and physiological disturbances that cluster together at the same time. The DSM-IV-TR criteria for dependence are presented in Box 19.4.

Box 19.4 DSM-IV-TR diagnostic criteria for substance dependence

A maladaptive pattern of substance use, leading to clinically significant impairment or distress, as manifested by three (or more) of the following, occurring at any time in the same 12-month period:

1 Tolerance, as defined by either of the following:
- a need for markedly increased amounts of the substance to achieve intoxication or desired effect
- markedly diminished effect with continued use of the same amount of the substance

2 Withdrawal, as manifested by either of the following:
- the characteristic withdrawal syndrome for the substance
- the same or a closely related substance is taken to relieve or avoid withdrawal symptoms

3 The substance is often taken in larger amounts or over a longer period than was intended.

4 There is a persistent desire or unsuccessful efforts to cut down or control substance use.

5 A great deal of time is spent in activities necessary to obtain the substance (e.g. visiting multiple doctors or driving long distances), use of the substance (e.g. chain smoking), or recovering from its effects.

6 Important social, occupational or recreational activities are given up or reduced because of substance use.

7 The substance use is continued despite knowledge of having a persistent or recurrent physical or psychological problem that it is likely to have been caused or exacerbated by the substance (e.g. current cocaine use despite recognition of cocaine-induced depression, or continued drinking despite recognition that an ulcer was made worse by alcohol consumption).

Specify if:
- **With physiological dependence**: evidence of tolerance or withdrawal (i.e. either item 1 or 2 is present)
- **Without physiological dependence**: no evidence of tolerance or withdrawal (i.e. neither 1 nor 2 is present)

Source: American Psychiatric Association (APA) 2000, *Diagnostic and Statistical Manual of Mental Disorders* (4th edn, text rev.), APA, Washington, DC.

ASSESSMENT AND DIAGNOSIS

The use of alcohol and other drugs is very common in Australia and New Zealand (as well as other countries) and AOD use must be considered as a possibility with every client that a nurse sees in any setting. Specific

regular basis will need to be withdrawn more slowly; however, the use of these drugs for short periods of time in a controlled unit such as an inpatient unit is probably safe and warranted for most clients (Todd 2002).

Less than five per cent of people with chronic alcohol use who withdraw from alcohol may experience a major withdrawal syndrome known as *delirium tremens* (Saunders & Young 2000). This syndrome occurs three to ten days after the person has had their last drink. The client may present with agitation, disorientation, high fever, paranoia and visual hallucinations (Townsend 2002). A medical practitioner must see clients who present with a major withdrawal syndrome.

Nursing attention for a client experiencing delirium tremens must be vigilant. The client must be nursed in a separate room. Intravenous fluid replacement may be required if there is severe dehydration and excessive sweating. In addition, specific electrolyte replacement (calcium, phosphate, magnesium and/or potassium) may be required. It is essential to reduce any agitation and the client must be kept calm to reduce exhaustion. Intravenous diazepam may be prescribed to relieve withdrawal symptoms, and antipsychotic medication such as haloperidol may also be prescribed (Garbutt et al. 1999).

There are some factors that predict the likely severity of the alcohol withdrawal syndrome. One factor is whether the client has a long history of regular heavy alcohol use that meets the criteria of hazardous or dependent as detailed earlier in this chapter (Saunders & Young 2002). Another factor is the use of other psychotropic drugs, particularly CNS depressants (Dale & Marsh 2000a). Furthermore, if the person has a past history of withdrawal syndrome, particularly delirium tremens, this places them at greater risk of withdrawal (NSW Health Department 2000a).

The Index for Suspicion of Alcohol Withdrawal is a useful tool for nurses to use as a guide to questions to ask a client regarding their alcohol use and to alert them to the possibility of withdrawal.

Other interventions

Evidence supports the need to offer a wide spectrum of treatment approaches. Non-residential rehabilitation services include self-help groups, of which the most common are Alcoholics Anonymous (AA) and Narcotics Anonymous (NA) (AA 2000), which are self-help groups based on an abstinence philosophy. Community drug and alcohol services provide a range of interventions including individual and group counselling, pharmacotherapies such as methadone maintenance for opiate-dependent clients, cognitive behavioural therapy (CBT), which teaches clients to moderate their responses to their environment by improving social coping and problem solving skills, and motivational interviewing (Cochrane Library http://www.cochrane.org/cochrane/revabstr/g360index.htm; Hulse, White & Conigrave 2002; Ritter & Lintzeris 1998).

Box 19.8 Index of suspicion of alcohol withdrawal

Questions to ask:

- Has the client had a regular intake of 80 grams of alcohol (eight standard drinks) or more per day?
- Has the client taken even small amounts of alcohol in conjunction with other CNS depressants?
- Has the client had previous episodes of alcohol withdrawal?
- Is the client's current admission for an alcohol-related reason?
- Does the client have a previous history of alcohol-related disease (e.g. alcoholic hepatitis, pancreatitis)?
- Does the client's physical condition indicate chronic alcohol use (e.g. parotid swelling, cushingoid face, reddened eyes or signs of liver disease—ascites, jaundice, limb muscle wasting)?
- Do the client's pathology results show raised serum GGT and/or raised mean cell volume (MCV)?
- Does the client display symptoms such as anxiety, agitation, tremor, sweatiness or early morning retching which might be due to an alcohol withdrawal syndrome?

Source: NSW Health Department 2000, Alcohol and Other Drugs Policy for Nursing Practice in NSW: Clinical Guidelines 2000–2003, NSW Health Department, Sydney, pp 41–2.

CRITICAL THINKING CHALLENGE 19.3

- A 36-year-old man is admitted to the unit on which you are working, with the following symptoms: T 38.1, P 106, R 28, BP 189/93, profuse perspiration and tremulousness. He appears highly agitated. A mental status examination reveals confusion, disorientation and visual and tactile hallucinations. His partner informs you that he had been a heavy drinker of alcohol, but he stopped two days ago. What substance-induced disorder would the client be experiencing?

  A substance-induced psychosis

  B alcohol withdrawal syndrome

  C delirium tremens

  D substance-induced anxiety disorder

- When the nurse does an initial admission interview on a client being admitted for detoxification, which of the following areas is it critical to assess?

  A type(s) of drug used

  B family history

  C reason for admission

  D physical history

(All these therapeutic interventions are described more fully in Ch 23.) The goal of motivational interviewing is to encourage the client to recognise both the problems and benefits associated with drug use and to determine whether the consequences outweigh the benefits (Blume & Marlatt 2000; McMahon & Jones 1992; Martino et al. 2000; Miller & Rollnick 1991). Other approaches include residential treatment services such as Odyssey House (a therapeutic community), which offers rehabilitation to a person after they have completed their detoxification program (Mattick & Jarvis 1993).

The integration of different treatment philosophies that meet the needs of clients has been shown to be problematic (Gomez et al. 2000; Torrey et al. 2002), but the most important aspect of treatment interventions is to match the client to the counsellor and to the treatment (Dale & Marsh 2000b; Capelhorn, Hartel & Irwig 1997).

DUAL DIAGNOSIS

Several terms are used to describe someone who has more than one disorder at the same time. Mental health and AOD clinicians use the terms 'dual diagnosis', 'co-morbidity' or 'coexisting disorder' interchangeably. There is no universal acceptance of any one term.

There is a considerable degree of coexistence between substance use disorders and other mental health disorders. Alcohol-use disorders coexisting with a mental illness are approximately three times more common than other drug disorders coexisting with a mental illness (AIHW 2000; Intergovernmental Committee on Drugs 2001). Alcohol and other drugs, even at low levels of consumption, can interact adversely with most of the medications commonly prescribed for the treatment of mental health problems. The prevalence rates of dual diagnosis vary significantly, depending on the definitions used and the populations studied. Most studies exclude tobacco use from their data; however, McEvoy & Allen (2003) estimate that between 70 and 80 per cent of people with schizophrenia and 65 and 78 per cent of people with a mood disorder smoke, while Ziedonis & Williams (2003) state that people with mental illness smoke nearly half of all cigarettes consumed in the United States, and that their risk of developing tobacco-related medical illnesses is two to three times that of the rest of the population.

Studies indicate that substance-use disorder is the most common co-morbidity for individuals with severe mental illness, with approximately 50 per cent of individuals with severe mental illness having a dual diagnosis (Alverson, Alverson & Drake 2000; Brunette et al. 2001). Laudet et al. (2000) report that the rate of co-occurring substance abuse and mental health disorders in the United States ranges between 29 and 59 per cent. Silver (1999) reports similar statistics, indicating that 25–27 per cent of individuals who have a mental illness also misuse substances such as illicit drugs and alcohol. Drake et al. (2001) state that substance abuse is the most common

and clinically significant dual diagnosis among individuals with mental illness.

Patterns of dual diagnosis are dependent on the drug and the type of psychiatric disorder (Kandel, Huang & Davies 2001). For example, the highest rates of substance abuse were seen in antisocial personality disorders, and greater dependence on substance use was seen in individuals who used illicit drugs. Patterns of co-morbidity also appear to be age dependent (Prigerson, Desai & Rosenheck 2001). Younger persons with dual diagnosis were more likely to use illicit substances; older persons were more likely to use legal substances such as alcohol (Kandel et al. 2001). Data from the National Survey of Mental Health and Wellbeing (AIHW 2000), which was a cross-sectional survey of 10,641 Australian adults conducted in 1997, found that approximately one-third of respondents with an alcohol-use disorder (abuse or dependence using DSM-IV and ICD-10 criteria) also met criteria for at least one concurrent mental disorder in the previous twelve months (Burns & Teesson 2002). Although the studies vary a little in their results, they all demonstrate that the prevalence rates for clients with a dual diagnosis are considerable and that nurses and other health professionals must find ways to address the problem.

Clinical significance of dual diagnosis

There is considerable evidence to suggest that clients with a dual diagnosis do less well than those with either a mental health problem or a substance use problem. They are more difficult to manage due to their complex health and social needs, have higher rates of noncompliance with treatment, and are more likely to be violent and to be exposed to violence (Drake et al. 2001; Teesson & Hall 2001). Clients with a dual diagnosis are more likely to have a chronic disability and consequently result in more service utilisation (Primm et al. 2000). They have less access to treatment services (Sitharthan et al. 1999) and have a greater chance of experiencing 'marriage breakdown, social isolation, poor educational attainment, unemployment and chronic financial difficulties' (Hall 1996, p 168). These clients often have a number of surrounding issues that combine and add to the complexity of treatment goals and outcomes. 'Such issues may include impending legal action from illegal activity, having a child placed in care due to parental alcohol and/or other drug abuse, lack of accommodation and psychological problems' (Dale & Marsh 2000b, p 45).

Why do people with a mental illness use non-prescribed drugs?

A number of reasons have been proposed for the increase in numbers of people with a mental illness using non-prescribed drugs. Since deinstitutionalisation, the number of people with a mental illness living in the community has increased and this exposes them to a substance-using culture that they may not have been exposed to when separated from mainstream society and living in institutions. Furthermore, an increase in the social acceptability and prevalence of substance use may contribute to higher levels of disorders (NSW Health Department 2000b). There may also be increased awareness of and interest in dual diagnosis, with more clinicians actively assessing their clients; or it may be that substance abuse can precipitate or perpetuate a psychiatric illness.

In a frequently cited work, Smith & Hucker (1994) suggest that people with a mental illness use psychoactive drugs for the following reasons:

- to self-medicate symptoms of psychiatric illness
- to reduce the side-effects of prescribed medication
- to facilitate social interaction
- to participate in certain subcultures
- to develop an identity more acceptable than that of a person with a mental illness
- to help cope with the disabilities of mental illness such as isolation, poverty, lack of affordable housing and social drift.

Williams & Cohen (2000) suggest that the availability of illicit drugs in psychiatric institutions may be a contributory factor, and that some individuals are introduced to drug use when they are inpatients for treatment of their mental illness.

It has been identified that nicotine may improve the poor attention to and processing of sensory stimulation of individuals with schizophrenia. Nicotine improves eye acceleration and integration of visual information into motor commands for people with schizophrenia (McEvoy & Allen 2003). Management of the side-effects of medication may be another reason for tobacco dependence—medications are metabolised more quickly and blood levels are lower in people who smoke. Smokers with mental illness report that smoking reduces their symptoms and improves their cognitive functioning. Cigarettes were rated as a core need by all subjects in the study and rated as more important than food (Ziedonis & Williams 2003). However, evidence from recent clinical trials shows that continued smoking adversely affects treatment for marijuana dependence and that smoking cessation is recommended for substance-dependent people. Cessation could actually protect against relapse in the illicit drug user (Cantwell 2003).

Assessing for AOD in a mental health unit

For people presenting to a mental health unit it is important to undertake an AOD assessment, as the percentage of people presenting with a dual diagnosis is estimated at between 30 and 80 per cent (Alverson et al. 2000; Drake et al. 2001; Prigerson et al. 2001; Silver 1999). For example, psychiatric disorders (particularly schizophrenia and depression) are commonly associated with alcohol use or dependence (Lopatko et al. 2002). In addition, anxiety disorders and substance use are also commonly dually

diagnosed (McKeehan & Martin 2002). It may sometimes be difficult to discern whether depression is the result or the cause of an alcohol-use disorder (Garbutt et al. 1999). With repeated use of large doses of stimulants a psychotic state resembling acute schizophrenia can develop and is characterised by agitation, paranoid delusions and visual hallucinations. It is sometimes difficult to differentiate stimulant-induced psychosis from acute paranoid schizophrenia, although psychotic symptoms usually subside as the drug concentration declines (Latt et al. 2002). Drug use can mask a mental illness, exacerbate the symptoms and prolong the episode (McKeehan & Martin 2002; White 2001). Depression, anxiety disorders and bulimia are all more common in women with alcohol problems than in men with alcohol problems (Dore 1998).

Guidelines for differentiating between a primary psychotic disorder and a substance-abuse disorder are provided in Box 19.9.

Box 19.9 Guidelines for differentiating between a primary psychotic and a substance-induced disorder

Substance-induced psychotic symptoms can result from intoxication, chronic use or withdrawal.

- Intoxication with cannabis can induce a transient, self-limiting psychotic disorder characterised by hallucinations and agitation.
- Prolonged heavy use of psychostimulants (e.g. amphetamines) can produce a psychotic picture similar to schizophrenia.
- Hallucinogen-induced psychosis is usually transient, but may persist if use is sustained.
- Heavy alcohol use has been associated with alcoholic hallucinosis and morbid jealousy.
- Psychotic symptoms can also occur during withdrawal (e.g. delirium tremens) and delirious states.

A non-substance-induced psychotic disorder should be considered when:

- psychosis preceded the onset of substance use
- psychosis persists for longer than one month after acute withdrawal or severe intoxication
- psychotic symptoms are not consistent with the substance used
- there is a history of psychotic symptoms during periods (> one month) of abstinence
- there is a personal or family history of a non-substance-induced psychotic disorder.

Source: Lubman D & Sundram S 2003, Substance misuse in patients with schizophrenia: a primary care guide, *Medical Journal of Australia*, 178(9), pp 571–5.

Management of clients with a dual diagnosis

Clients with dual diagnoses can be very complex and difficult to treat. Nursing staff are usually not trained or educated in both areas (AOD and mental health) and, as noted earlier in this chapter, nurses often hold negative attitudes towards clients who use alcohol and other drugs. Dually diagnosed clients often evoke powerful, unpleasant feelings in health professionals, and nurses may feel unskilled in working with them and overwhelmed by the multiplicity of their problems (Lubman & Sundram 2003). Many nurses are pessimistic regarding outcomes and believe that intensive time spent with these clients will produce minimal gains. In addition, dually diagnosed clients may feel stigmatised by mental health nurses' attitudes when these are related to an abstinence model that is in direct contrast to the harm-minimisation model supported by the AOD sector.

This group of clients offers many challenges to nursing staff, as most dually diagnosed clients have a range of personal and social problems and have difficulty maintaining a concurrent level of wellness in both areas. Continued drug use (e.g. of cannabis) may exacerbate positive symptoms of schizophrenia and lead to decompensation and admission or readmission to hospital.

The key principles of AOD history taking and assessment have been detailed under the section on assessment in this chapter. Developing a collaborative therapeutic alliance is essential and the nurse needs to adopt an empathetic and non-judgmental approach. It is important to accurately assess clients and to screen them for substance use, as many clients with schizophrenia or other mental illness will often deny or under-state their substance use. Once a diagnosis has been made, appropriate management combines pharmacological treatment of the psychotic episode and psychosocial interventions to reduce substance abuse. Ideally, a client's mental state should be relatively stable before attempting detoxification, although this is not always possible. Early and brief interventions can be used in both outpatient and inpatient settings.

Management principles for clients with schizophrenia and substance abuse are outlined in Box 19.10.

As with all aspects of nursing care, safety is the main concern. If a client has been admitted to a mental health facility in a psychotic state, it is essential that the psychosis be managed, and when the client's mental state is more settled the nurse can engage in psychosocial interventions to assist the client with their problematic substance use. These interventions will need to be continued once the client has been discharged from hospital. If the client is at risk of withdrawal from one or more substances, detoxification strategies as outlined earlier in this chapter need to be implemented immediately. The client will need to be monitored closely and examined by the medical officer/psychiatrist and appropriate medication prescribed. When the client is more settled, the nurse can begin to explore reasons for the client's substance use, including the relationship of the substance to the client's psychiatric symptoms, treatment for their mental illness and feelings of social isolation related to their negative symptoms.

Box 19.10 **Management principles for clients with schizophrenia and substance abuse**

Assessment
- Screen clients with psychosis for substance misuse.
- Determine severity of use and associated risk-taking behaviours (e.g. injecting practices, unsafe sex).
- Exclude organic illness or physical complications of substance misuse.
- Seek collateral history—families or close supports should be involved where possible.

Treatment
- First engage the client using a non-judgmental attitude.
- Educate the client:
  - Give general advice about harmful effects of substance misuse.
  - Advise about safe and responsible levels of substance use (NH&MRC guidelines).
  - Make individual links between substance misuse and client's problems (e.g. cannabis use and worsening paranoia).
  - Inform the patient about safer practices (e.g. safe sexual practices).
- Treat psychotic illness and monitor the client for side-effects.
- Help the client establish advantages and disadvantages of current use and motivate client to change.
- With medical staff, evaluate the need for concurrent substance-use medications (e.g. methadone, acamprosate, nicotine replacement therapy).
- Refer the client to appropriate community services as appropriate.
- Devise relapse-prevention strategies that address both psychosis and substance misuse.
- Identify triggers for relapse (e.g. meeting other drug users, family conflict) and explore alternative coping strategies.

Source: adapted from Lubman D & Sundram S 2003, Substance misuse in patients with schizophrenia: a primary care guide, *Medical Journal of Australia*, 178(9), pp 571–5.

The client's readiness to change and their degree of commitment to treatment of both their mental illness and their substance use need to be explored (Lubman & Sundram 2003). (Refer to Ch 23 for motivational interviewing and other interventions.) Remember: clients may be at different stages of readiness in their problematic drug use and their mental illness, and interventions need to reflect this. For example, a client may be at a precontemplation stage for their substance use and at an action stage for their mental illness.

Adopt a concrete problem-solving approach with the client whenever possible. For example, set tasks that are readily achievable, such as keeping a daily diary of

20

Somatoform and Dissociative Disorders

Ruth Elder

KEY POINTS

- The somatoform disorders are psychiatric illnesses that present as physical disorders.
- The somatoform disorders are not to be confused with malingering, which is the intentional production of symptoms to avoid some responsibility or duty.
- Somatisation is a method of expressing anxiety and distress and is found in all cultural groups.
- The distress and suffering experienced by clients with a somatoform disorder are real, although the medical basis for their symptoms is not.
- Clients with a somatoform disorder are most frequently encountered in general health settings.
- The dissociative disorders are marked by an abrupt, temporary change in consciousness, cognition, memory, identity or behaviour.

LEARNING OUTCOMES

The material in this chapter will assist you to:
- define somatoform and dissociative disorders
- define key terms related to somatoform and dissociative disorders
- distinguish disorders that present as physical disorders from malingering
- describe the major conditions categorised as somatoform or dissociative disorders
- describe the assessment of people with somatoform and dissociative disorders
- discuss interventions appropriate to persons with somatoform and dissociative disorders.

KEY TERMS

- amnesia
- conversion
- depersonalisation
- derealisation
- dissociation
- fugue
- hypochondriasis
- hysteria
- *la belle indifference*
- malingering
- neurosis
- primary gain
- reassurance
- secondary gain
- somatisation

INTRODUCTION

The disorders discussed in this chapter are the somatoform disorders and dissociative disorders. In both groups of disorders, sufferers present complaining of physical symptoms, although no medical condition is found to exist. All these disorders as well as the anxiety disorders, phobias, compulsions and obsessions (see Ch 17) and disorders of sexual functioning were once classified as 'neurotic reactions' or 'neurotic disorders'. The term 'neurosis' is not used in the *Diagnostic and Statistical Manual of Mental Disorders* DSM-IV and later editions, but is of mainly historical interest and can be found in a number of seminal texts on psychiatry. The concept of neurosis was developed in 1769 by William Cullen from Edinburgh University, who believed that madness was the result of excessive irritation of the nerves (Porter 2002) and used the term to refer to nervous system disease. Since the time of Freud its meaning has changed to refer to a non-psychotic disorder characterised mainly by anxiety. The disorders that fall under the label of neurosis are *ego-dystonic*—that is, the symptoms are experienced as distressing to the individual.

SOMATOFORM DISORDERS

The somatoform disorders (see Box 20.1) are a heterogeneous group of disorders whose distinguishing characteristic is the presence of physical symptoms in the absence of a readily apparent medical condition. In order for the patient to be diagnosed as suffering from a somatoform disorder, the symptoms cannot be fully accounted for by a physical disease or another psychiatric disorder, or the effects of drugs or medication. There is usually no evidence of injury. However, these disorders are often confused with actual physical disorders and the client suffering from them truly believes they are physically ill. The symptoms cause the afflicted person significant distress and can interfere with their normal functioning. Although no medical condition exists, hospitalisation can occur, and numerous diagnostic tests and even surgery are performed (Clarke & Smith 2001). These disorders well illustrate how 'suffering and illness are only indirectly related to the presence or absence of disease' (Epstein, Quill & McWhinney 1999, p 221).

The somatoform disorders should be distinguished from *malingering*. The physical symptoms are not fabricated intentionally, whereas in malingering there is the intentional production of symptoms in order to avoid some specific duty or responsibility. In malingering, the incentive for the person to become sick is clearly identifiable. For example, the person might be required to stand trial, or wants to evade the police, or is simply looking for a bed for the night.

The symptoms that accompany the disorders are referred to as either somatisation or, more commonly

---

Box 20.1 The somatoform disorders

- The symptoms or deficits cannot, after appropriate investigation, be fully explained by a general medical condition, or by the direct effects of a substance, or as a culturally sanctioned behaviour or experience.
- The symptoms are not intentionally produced or feigned (as in factitious disorder or malingering).

Somatisation disorder
- History of multiple symptoms before age thirty occurring over several years and results in treatment being sought or significant impairment in social, occupational or other important areas of functioning.
- All of the following symptoms must have occurred during the course of the disturbance:
  - four pain symptoms e.g. head, back, joints, rectum, during menstruation
  - two gastrointestinal symptoms e.g. bloating, nausea, vomiting, diarrhoea
  - one sexual symptom e.g. sexual indifference, erectile dysfunction
  - one pseudoneurologic symptom e.g. paralysis, weakness, aphonia.

Conversion disorder
- Symptoms or deficits affecting voluntary motor or sensory function that suggest a neurological or general medical condition, and are associated with psychological factors.

Pain disorder
- Pain in one or more sites of significant focus or severity, causing significant distress or impairment and associated with psychological factors.

Hypochondriasis
- Preoccupation with fears of having, or the idea that one has, a serious disease based on the person's misinterpretation of bodily symptoms or normal functions.

Body dysmorphic disorder
- Preoccupation with an imagined defect in appearance. If a slight physical anomaly is present, the person's concern is markedly excessive.

Undifferentiated somatoform disorder
- One or more physical symptoms (e.g. fatigue, loss of appetite) that cause clinically significant impairments in social, occupational or other functioning lasting at least six months.

Somatoform disorder not otherwise specified
- Somatoform symptoms that do not meet the criteria for other somatoform disorders.

Source: adapted from DSM-IV-TR, American Psychiatric Association (APA) 2000, *Diagnostic and Statistical Manual of Mental Disorders* (4th edn, text rev.), APA, Washington DC.

Aetiology

The causes of the somatoform disorders are unknown. However, somatisation has been recognised since the ancient Egyptians (Sadock & Sadock 2003), and BDD has been recognised for centuries. References to it can be found in Greek mythology, European, Russian and Japanese literature (Biby 1998). Theories about their possible origins can roughly be divided into two: those that consider the disorders to originate in organic structures and processes (*neurogenesis*) and those that believe they originate in mental phenomena (*psychogenesis*) (Shorter 1994). The latter position reached its apotheosis in psychoanalytic doctrine in the first half of the twentieth century, but can be traced to the seventeenth-century physician Thomas Sydenham, who believed somatisation to be a disease of the mind (Sharpe & Carson 2001). The former position is much older, but was out of favour while psychoanalytic doctrine was dominant. The term 'hysteria' itself, by focusing on a particular bodily function, namely the uterus, suggested a belief in its organic basis. However, Thomas Willis, a seventeenth-century neurologist, believed the symptoms derived from the head (Sharpe & Carson 2001). Briquet, a nineteenth-century French physician, was convinced that hysteria had a genetic component (Shorter 1994). He was among the first to believe that patients inherited psychosomatic illnesses. Pierre Janet (1903) also thought that the condition he termed 'psychasthenia' was biological in origin (Shorter 1994).

Psychoanalysis

Psychodynamic theory explains somatisation as an outcome of early life experiences and as a defence against psychological conflict (see Ch 7). Emotions are expressed physically when they cannot be expressed verbally through either guilt or fear (Hardy et al. 2001).

Used as a defence mechanism, the client stands to accrue a number of short-term advantages, which are referred to as primary and secondary gains. The *primary gain* is the decrease in anxiety which results from psychological pain and conflict. A physical symptom gives legitimacy to 'feeling bad'. Rather than changing the 'self', the problem is a body part. The *secondary gain* is the attention and support provided by others for a physical illness. Through physical conditions and symptoms the person might be able to avoid their obligations such as going to work or doing the housework. For example, in conversion disorder the person who witnesses a fatal accident might develop blindness, as might a person who feels guilty about looking at erotic material. Keeping the upsetting material out of consciousness and thus helping reduce anxiety is the primary gain. Secondary gain is achieved when the symptom helps the person avoid a particular duty, for example in the case of a soldier who develops a paralysis of the hand and therefore cannot fire a gun.

The concepts of primary and secondary gains are not intended to imply that the symptoms are simulated or figments of the imagination; the symptoms are not 'all in the mind'. Clients really do experience the symptoms in the body.

Amplification

Amplification theory proposes that in some people, normal bodily sensations are amplified or heightened. Some people simply may be hypersensitive to normal bodily stimuli and attribute pathological meaning to normal somatic sensations and functions (Hardy et al. 2001). Others, however, may become susceptible to media influence, public health campaigns or simple word of mouth, so symptoms that were previously ignored or dismissed are brought into awareness and assume new meaning (Barsky & Borus 1999).

Interpersonal theory

Interpersonal theory has been used as an explanation for hypochondriasis. This theory suggests that children with hypochondriasis model their behaviour on the responses to pain and illness they have observed in another family member or other adults who are ill. From an interpersonal perspective, the antecedents of hypochondriasis are believed to be found in childhood adversity where early attachments have been marked by insecurity, which, in turn, produces persistent separation anxiety (Noyes Jr et al. 2002).

Developmental theory

Developmental theory suggests that translating psychological distress into physical symptoms is a learned response. The child may not have learnt adequate verbal and cognitive skills to express their psychological distress. Parents may also model somatic behaviour, thus teaching it to their children.

Personality

Personality factors appear to be important in the genesis of the somatoform disorders. For example, the personality characteristics of anxiousness and fearfulness are commonly associated with these disorders (Bass & Tyrer 2000). Furthermore, high numbers of clients with anxiety disorders or major depression suffer from the somatoform disorders.

Biological theories

There is as yet no strong evidence for any biological basis for the somatoform disorders, although a number of interesting hypotheses are being pursued. Sharpe & Carson (2001) suggest that new evidence supports the idea that the functional disorders are disturbances of the nervous system.

Familial factors

Body dysmorphic disorder has been found to be four times as prevalent in those who have first-degree relatives with the condition. For hypochondriasis, studies have indicated high rates of concordance for twins (Hardy, Warmbrodt & Chrisman 2001).

Culture

According to Shorter (1994), culture is important in shaping illness. In this theory, culture shapes illness behaviour by conferring legitimacy and, hence, respectability, to certain forms of behaviour. In Western cultures greater legitimacy is accorded somatic complaints and both patients and doctors act to interpret symptoms as indicative of bodily, rather than psychological, processes.

Assessment

The first step in assessment is taking a comprehensive history. The point to keep in mind here is that it is the client's concerns that are paramount, rather than the health professional's need to diagnose. Fischhoff & Wessely (2003, pp 595–6) provide some questions that can help focus on the areas of concern to the client, rather than the health professional:

- What decisions face them?
- What concerns weigh on them, including non-medical issues (e.g. insurance, family)?
- What conflicting claims, beliefs and observations confuse them?
- What information, and misinformation, do they have already?
- Which knowledge gaps and misconceptions provide the greatest barrier to understanding?

It is useful to enquire as to any stresses in the client's life at the time the symptom(s) first appeared.

Somatisation disorder

Somatisation disorder is characterised predominantly by multiple physical complaints, and usually runs a chronic course (Bass & Tyrer 2000; Escobar, Hoyos-Nervi & Gara 2002). Persons with unexplained somatic symptoms have usually sought medical treatment many times over many years (Maynard 2003). The symptoms they present with tend to be multiple and recurring. They will often present in a dramatic way, providing vivid descriptions of the effect of the symptoms on their lives, but are vague about the details of the symptoms themselves. The most common symptoms clients complain about are listed in Box 20.4.

Clients are often described as appearing anxious and/or angry. The distress clients experience should be treated as real, as should the experience of the symptoms. They are not lying or imagining their symptoms. The client should be asked what they think has caused the symptoms, how the symptoms interfere with their everyday activities and how they handle them. Examples of helpful questions the nurse could ask the client are listed in Box 20.5.

Box 20.4 Common symptoms of somatisation disorder

Headaches
Abdominal distress
Other aches and pains
Dizziness
Palpitations
Other symptoms of anxiety
Constipation or diarrhoea (irritable bowel syndrome)
Depression or anxiety

Source: Treatment Protocol Project 2000, *Management of Mental Disorders*, World Health Organization Collaborating Centre for Mental Health and Substance Abuse, Sydney.

Box 20.5 Helpful questions

- Why do you think you are having this problem?
- At what age did you start having this problem?
- How do you feel about it?
- How many health-care providers have you seen over the past five years?
- What do you consider to be the major stressors in your life now?
- How does your body usually respond to stress?
- Is there something that you fear is wrong with you?
- What do you think would help your problem most right now?
- How is this problem affecting your life?
- If the problem cannot be cured, what would you consider to be reasonable goals?

Source: adapted from Maynard CK 2003, Assess and manage somatization, *The Nurse Practitioner*, 28(4), pp 20–9.

Communication is often impaired because there are sometimes gaps in the client's history, and they are often inclined to over-dramatise, to make false generalisations about what is happening to them from limited evidence, and to oversimplify. They are also said to be very demanding of health professionals' time and attention, because, despite the numerous negative tests, they will not be reassured that there is nothing physically wrong with them. They may also express feelings of helplessness in the face of perceived failures on the part of health professionals to cure them and at the same time will usually refuse to see a psychiatrist or will simply ignore the referral. In contrast to clients with other chronic disorders such as rheumatoid arthritis or diabetes, Holloway & Zerbe (2000) report that the clients with somatisation disorder tend to be passive with respect to finding a cure.

Most physicians (see, for example, Singh 1998 and Barsky & Borus 1999) advocate ruling out a physical cause for the client's complaints before contemplating the possibility of a psychological cause for the symptoms.

given an explanation that fits their frame of reference. Empowering explanations are marked by 'a tangible, usually physical, causal mechanism [chemicals or neurones in the brain]; they exculpate the patient by attributing symptoms to causes for which the patient could not be blamed; and they involve the patient by invoking internal adjustment or suggesting external factor(s) that the patient could influence' (Salmon, Peters & Stanley 1999, p 375).

Relief of symptoms

There is little agreement among authors about whether to focus on symptoms. Some argue that to focus on symptoms leads to their amplification and perpetuation (Barsky & Borus 1999) or reinforcement (Servan-Schreiber et al. 2000). Others believe that such a focus shows compassion (Fischhoff & Wessely 2003). Overall, it seems a balance needs to be achieved and a distinction made between people with a somatoform disorder and those who have somatic symptoms. The reality of the symptoms for the client needs to be acknowledged—they can be told that they are not 'all in their head'. The focus, over the long term, should be on the client, their beliefs and expectations, their everyday functioning, and how the symptoms interfere with their functioning rather than the symptoms themselves (Epstein et al. 1999; Escobar 1996; Maynard 2003; Servan-Schreiber et al. 2000). In this way, unwittingly reinforcing the symptoms by challenging them and thus making them the centre of the therapeutic encounter can be avoided.

However, it is important to focus on relieving the symptoms as much as possible. Such relief may be provided through carefully listening to the client's history and acknowledging uncertainty. Naming the condition (Fischhoff & Wessely 2003; Starcevic 2002) has also proved helpful. Clients generally do not want to be told, 'There is nothing wrong with you' or 'You have no illness'. These statements serve only to heighten the client's concerns. Instead, a concrete rendering of their symptoms is needed, which might involve saying, 'You have a depression which is the result of a chemical imbalance in the brain' or 'Your headaches are a result of the stress you've been experiencing at work leading you to tense your muscles'.

Cognitive behavioural therapies

For clients who attend mental health professionals, cognitive behavioural therapy (CBT) has proved effective (Sharpe & Carson 2001). Cognitive behavioural interventions have been found to reduce the intensity and frequency of somatic complaints (Servan-Schreiber et al. 2000). Cognitive behavioural therapy aims to help the client modify the thoughts that reinforce their symptoms (see Ch 23 for a discussion of CBT). A basic premise is that the client's beliefs are false. There are numerous techniques that aim to overcome false beliefs. For example, the client can be taught about the relationship between cognitive beliefs and physiological responses. For example, simply believing in danger can stimulate the sympathetic responses that raise blood pressure and heart rate (Hardy et al. 2001). Clients also can be encouraged to formulate alternative explanations for their experience of bodily symptoms. They can be encouraged to write a list for and against the chances of having a particular disease (Hardy et al. 2001). There is often a physiological explanation for a client's symptoms that the client can be educated about. For example, the client may be unaware of how stress can lead to muscular tension in their neck and shoulders that, in turn, can give rise to headaches. These types of explanations can also be used to help overcome client beliefs that the mind and body are separate—for example, a preoccupation with bodily functions can lead to anxiety, which can lead to hyperventilation, which can produce a tingling in the fingers.

Some hypochondriacal clients are helped by insight therapy or explanatory therapy (Hardy et al. 2001). This therapy seeks to help clients understand the origin of their symptoms, which might be an earlier traumatic event that led to an intense focus on bodily symptoms.

Therapies that focus on the body, such as relaxation, exercise, physiotherapy and massage, are often well accepted by clients (Epstein et al. 1999). These therapies are also useful in helping reduce anxiety. Sometimes training the client in assertiveness and general social skills, so they learn to ask for what they want clearly and directly, can help the client cope better. The clients' new abilities with these skills also provide opportunities to reward them with praise and support, helping undermine their previous dependence on gaining support from physical symptoms.

Behaviour therapy has a place especially in the treatment of those clients who achieve secondary gains from their symptoms. However, it is also useful when the client agrees that whatever they have been doing about the symptoms has not been successful so far. The client's beliefs can gently be challenged.

Cognitive behavioural therapy is also useful in helping BDD clients develop a more realistic picture of themselves. It can also help the client resist the urge to engage in compulsive behaviours such as checking their appearance in the mirror, and face social situations that were previously avoided (Patterson et al. 2001).

Psychopharmacology

Medications have a place in the treatment of coexisting illnesses such as depression and anxiety. Careful education about side-effects is necessary so that the client does not discontinue the medication through misattribution of symptoms to side-effects of the medication (Holloway & Zerbe 2000). They also have a role in the treatment of real physical illnesses, but care needs to be taken with those medications that somatising clients are apt to over-use, such as anti-anxiety agents, analgesics and hypnotics (Clarke & Smith 2001), which also have the potential to be addictive. If they are prescribed, then they are administered for a specific time over a specific period; for example, an analgesic might be prescribed for the first two days of the menstrual period. In pain disorder, the medications used for pain tend to be limited to aspirin and non-steroidal anti-inflammatory agents.

Antidepressants have been shown to be beneficial in the MUS syndromes, even in the absence of a depressive disorder (Kroenke & Swindle 2000). They have also proved efficacious in the treatment of the various functional pain syndromes (Singh 1998).

Successful treatment of BDD with the tricyclic antidepressant imipramine has been reported (Fontenelle et al. 2002). The selective serotonin reuptake inhibitor (SSRI) antidepressants are also used. Clomipramine (approx. 175 mg/day), fluoxetine (approx. 50 mg/day) and fluvoxamine (approx. 260 mg/day) have all been used effectively (Phillips 1995). These medications appear to help by reducing the distressing preoccupation with the body and its associated depression and anxiety. They are especially helpful in those cases where the person has attempted suicide. Patterson et al. (2001) suggest that BDD clients can be helped to accept medication by telling them that it will help with their feelings of distress and demoralisation about their appearance.

Support

Many of the somatoform disorders are chronic; therefore it is unlikely that the client will be cured. In these cases a number of psychiatrists suggest that care, rather than cure, is the appropriate intervention model (Holloway & Zerbe 2000; Singh 1998). Kroenke & Swindle (2000, p 206) have termed this the 'hand-holding' approach—that is, 'regularly scheduled visits with a primary care provider, limited subspecialty referrals or diagnostic testing, legitimation of the patient's complaints and sustained reassurance'. Nurses especially can play an important role by visiting or phoning clients regularly and spending time listening to the client's concerns. This routine can help minimise the client's need to develop new symptoms in order to get the support and attention they crave. The goal is to help the client express their emotional conflicts verbally and to reduce, if not eliminate entirely, their reliance on expressing them in physical complaints.

Supportive therapies are usually the treatment of choice for people with hypochondriasis. Communication needs to be simple, straightforward and clear. The results of all laboratory tests and screening procedures need to be told to the client. The condition needs to be fully explained. The client should be told they have a fear of disease, and what this means should be discussed with them. Clients will often vacillate between accepting and rejecting the diagnosis. This vacillation means they will need to be seen supportively for some time. Some clients may never fully accept the diagnosis, so long-term education will be in order.

Family involvement

It is also useful to involve the family in treatment if possible. The family can be educated about the disorder, especially with a view to helping them understand what their contribution to the realisation of secondary gains might be. They can also be enlisted in helping the client avoid unnecessary treatments and surgery, and to respond supportively without recourse to talk about disease. They can be taught to help get the client to exercise and avoid inactivity. They can learn to respond supportively without encouraging 'pain' or 'disease' (Katon 1993, cited in Meyer 1999, pp 81–2).

Validation

Validation has been found to be a useful strategy with hypochondriacal clients. There is no point telling clients that their symptoms are imaginary and that they must give them up. As Starcevic (2002) argues, hypochondriacal clients need to feel accepted. He suggests that we can convey acceptance by validating the client's experience. He provides the following examples of validating statements:

- 'It is reasonable to concentrate so much on your body when it keeps sending you signals.'
- 'I understand why you're listening to your body, as the body seems to be trying to tell you something, and perhaps only you can make some sense of it, despite what the doctors tell you.'
- 'You seem to be expressing something through symptoms that are difficult to understand, but the language of symptoms is yours and the one with which you are now trying to communicate as best as you can' (Starcevic 2002, p 172).

Rather than telling the client, 'You are a hypochondriac', it can be helpful to reframe the diagnosis as 'excessive worry about health' or 'fear of illness' (Hardy et al. 2001). This re-framing can also help overcome potential client resistance to understanding their behaviour as hypochondriacal. If an alternative rational explanation is available for a client's symptoms, then it should be given. For example, a 'pounding heart' is a normal response to exertion, not a sign of heart disease.

Reality therapy

Reality therapy or confrontation–insight therapy has had some limited success with clients with pain disorder. The therapy involves confronting the client with the fact that there is no plausible reason for their pain, but there are 'rewards'. This type of confrontation is not intended to be conflictual, or to drive the client away from therapy.

Lifestyle interventions

Servan-Schreiber et al. (2000) recommend physical exercise for twenty minutes three times a week for clients who believe themselves to be physically impaired. The client should be encouraged to get moving psychologically and physically (Katon 1993, cited in Meyer 1999, pp 81–2). Inactivity and rest tend to be counterproductive in that the client might then ruminate on their symptoms.

Box 20.8 Principles for intervening in somatisation

Develop a strong therapeutic alliance
Treat the client's distress as real
Focus on activities of daily living
Focus on the client, not the symptoms
Tell the client they do not have a life-threatening illness
Reassure the client about their health
Encourage physical activity
Educate the client about physiological processes
Set up routine visits

CRITICAL THINKING CHALLENGE 20.1

How do you think you might react to clients who seem to be always complaining about physical symptoms that you know are not real? If you think you might feel angry or frustrated, can you identify why you might feel that way?

DISSOCIATIVE DISORDERS

The dissociative disorders are rare. Before DSM-III-R they were known as hysterical neuroses of the dissociative type. They are marked by an abrupt, temporary change in consciousness, cognition, memory, identity or behaviour. Clients suffering from one of these disorders frequently report that they suddenly cannot remember important events or aspects of their own identity such as who they are or how old they are. Many studies demonstrate a relationship between traumatic childhood events, such as physical and sexual abuse and dissociative phenomena. Dissociation as a response to abuse is considered a coping mechanism; that is, it provides a means for the person to physically, emotionally or cognitively absent themselves from the traumatic situation.

The DSM-IV-TR diagnostic criteria for dissociative disorders are listed in Box 20.9.

Pierre Janet (1889, cited in Witztum & van der Hart 1998), in the early part of the twentieth century, first conceptualised the dissociative disorders as forms of 'splitting off' or dissociating parts of consciousness. Certain parts of the personality were considered to separate from the habitual personality and slip outside the control of conscious awareness. These personality parts could then assume a life of their own. However, it was Freud who developed the idea of a dynamic unconscious where emotions and ideas unacceptable to the person were kept out of awareness or repressed. The person is thus protected from the anxiety and emotional pain associated with psychological conflicts or other disturbing circumstances by compartmentalising and 'forgetting' the unpleasant material.

Amnesia is a feature of dissociative amnesia, dissociative fugue and dissociative identity disorder. To the outside observer, who is not aware of the presence of a

---

Box 20.9 Diagnostic criteria for the dissociative disorders

Dissociative amnesia
- The predominant disturbance is one or more episodes of inability to recall important personal information, usually of a traumatic or stressful nature, that is too extensive to be explained by ordinary forgetfulness.
- The symptoms cause clinically significant distress or impairment in social, occupational or other important areas of functioning.

Dissociative fugue
- The predominant disturbance is sudden, unexpected travel away from home or one's customary place of work, with inability to recall one's past.
- Confusion about personal identity or assumption of a new identity (partial or complete).
- The symptoms cause clinically significant distress or impairment in social, occupational or other important areas of functioning.

Dissociative identity disorder (previously known as multiple personality disorder)
- The presence of two or more distinct identities or personality states (each with its own relatively enduring pattern of perceiving, relating to, and thinking about the environment and self).
- At least two of these identities recurrently take control of the person's behaviour.
- Inability to recall important personal information that is too extensive to be explained by ordinary forgetfulness.

Depersonalisation disorder
- Persistent or recurrent experiences of feeling detached from, and as if one is an outside observer of, one's mental processes or body (e.g. feeling like one is in a dream).
- During the depersonalisation experience, reality testing remains intact.
- The depersonalisation causes clinically significant distress or impairment in social, occupational or other important areas of functioning.

Dissociative disorder not otherwise specified
- This category is included for disorders in which the predominant feature is a dissociative symptom that does not meet the criteria for any specific dissociative disorder.

Source: adapted from DSM-IV-TR, American Psychiatric Association (APA) 2000, *Diagnostic and Statistical Manual of Mental Disorders* (4th edn, text rev.), APA, Washington DC.

disorder, the person might appear to be functioning entirely normally. Unlike clients with amnesia related to dementia or other organic processes, there is rarely confusion or disorganised behaviour.

Similarly to the somatoform disorders and the process of somatisation, the dissociative disorders and the process of dissociation need to be distinguished. The experience of mild dissociation is very common, occurring in more than 95 per cent of the world's cultures, and is most often considered normal (Kleinman 1996, p 23). Nearly everyone experiences dissociation at some time or another. For example, a person might be driving somewhere and, while focused on their own internal thoughts, they might be unaware of what is happening around them. They then suddenly realise that they can't remember driving during the previous few minutes, or they might find themselves driving to work instead of to a friend's house. Daydreaming is a very mild form of dissociation. Another form of dissociation is when we are surprised at how quickly time has gone by when we 'get lost' in a book or other enjoyable activity. Hypnosis is an example of a dissociative state produced in normal people.

Dissociative amnesia

This disorder is sometimes referred to as psychogenic amnesia. Clients with dissociative amnesia are suddenly aware that they are unable to remember events, which are usually of a particularly stressful or traumatic nature, during a particular period. It has been extensively documented among soldiers who have been in combat (Witztum & Maragalit 2002). The most common form is *localised amnesia*, where the person forgets events of a few hours to a few days. This type of amnesia can occur in people who might have survived a car crash in which another family member has been killed (APA 2000). *Selective amnesia* is the failure to recall some, but not all, events during a short period of time; for example, an abused child might remember only some of the events connected to abusive episodes. *Generalised amnesia* is the loss of a whole lifetime's memories. *Systematised amnesia* is the loss of memory for a specific category of information—for example, all memories relating to a particular person.

Primary and secondary gains can also be associated with amnesia. The soldier who forgets the horrors witnessed during combat protects himself from painful emotions, as does the mother who forgets the car accident in which her children were killed.

Dissociative fugue

Dissociative fugue is a very rare disorder and is most likely to occur after a critical event. A client with this disorder suddenly and unexpectedly travels far away, often thousands of kilometres from home. The journey can last from a few hours to many days, and sometimes several months, at a time. The dissociated part of the personality appears to take control of the person's life. The person is unable to remember their past. The person may also be confused about their identity, unable to remember their name or their occupation. A very small number adopt a new identity.

Other types of trauma might also be seen, such as war experiences. Families may also report there have been times when the client has mysteriously disappeared for varying periods of time and/or been found in places some distance from their homes. Families may also be able to provide information about trauma or stressful situations previously experienced by the client. Family and friendship relations in general may have become highly disrupted because of the client's apparent abrupt withdrawal.

Dissociative identity disorder

Dissociative identity disorder (DID), a rare disorder that is often severe and chronic, is most popularly known by its former name of multiple personality disorder. It has sometimes been confused in the popular imagination with schizophrenia, to which it is not related. Clients with this disorder have at least two distinct personalities. Neither or none of the personalities should be confused with having imaginary playmates. The development of autonomous personalities appears to resolve deep-seated conflicting beliefs and desires, because the alternate personalities often have characteristics quite different to those of the core or host personality. The transition or switching from one personality to another is rapid and the core personality usually forgets or is unaware of the existence of the others, although the host is often aware that they have lost time or that there are periods of blackout. The alternate personalities, however, are usually aware of the core personality. The alternate personalities are relatively self-contained, having their own set of roles and relationships distinct from those of the core personality, and are in control at different times or situations. The alternate

CASE STUDY

Marla was a 23-year-old doctor's receptionist who failed to return to work from lunch one day. She had been working for the doctor for six months and there had been no indication that anything was wrong. Ten days later, she was found in a small country town 600 kilometres away. She had been taken in by a woman who had been unable to find out her name, but was concerned because 'she seemed so confused'. Marla's true identity became known when she suddenly 'came to'. She was unable to account for how she had come to the town. In therapy it emerged that Marla had suffered physical abuse by her stepfather from the age of eight until fourteen, when he died.

personalities allow the person to cope in situations or with events that the core personality finds overwhelming.

The classic story of split personality is Robert Louis Stevenson's *Dr Jekyll and Mr Hyde* (Stevenson 1925). *Sybil* (Schreiber 1975) and *The Three Faces of Eve* (Thigpen 1960) were two best-selling books about this disorder that were also made into films, which helped further popularise this condition. Despite this popularity, however, little is known about the incidence of this disorder. It is overwhelmingly a disorder of females, with 90 per cent of cases occurring in women and most of these in the United States (Meyer 1999). People with this disorder rarely seek treatment. If they become known to mental health professionals, it is usually because they may have attempted suicide or are suffering from another disorder, usually major depression or schizophrenia.

This condition is also most likely the one that clients suffer from when they are believed to be 'possessed' or in some cultures such as India, where there is an expectation of possession. In some other cultures, such as Indonesia, Malaysia and Latin America, as well as India, dissociative disorders are associated with trance states, which are usually induced and which are not usually associated with distress or dysfunction.

A history of childhood physical or sexual abuse or neglect is common in DID clients' backgrounds. Common symptoms of dissociation include headaches, switching, mood swings, time lapses, auditory hallucinations, intrusive memories and anxiety (McAllister 2000). Seemingly innocuous triggers such as certain fruits, sounds or colours can start the dissociative process. The person will usually have experienced a loss of time and be unable to recall events from when the alternate personality dominated. Some clients with DID also suffer from an eating disorder or are dependent on substances.

Depersonalisation disorder

In depersonalisation disorder, a client experiences one or more episodes of feelings of unreality. The client's sense of their personal reality is lost or altered, such that they feel estranged from themselves, as if they are in a dream, or feel 'spaced out', or that their actions are mechanical, or that they are otherwise detached from their body or mind. Persons with this disorder often report that they feel they are 'going crazy' and are often highly anxious. Time and space can feel distorted. In order to be diagnosed with this disorder the feelings must not have been induced by drugs.

Derealisation is another, related, phenomenon where the person's sense of the object world is altered. The person might perceive objects to be bigger or smaller than they really are, or that once-familiar objects now seem strange.

Depersonalisation is often a symptom in numerous other mental and physical illnesses, such as panic attacks and schizophrenia. Many normal persons also experience depersonalisation during periods of anxiety or stress (Clarke & Smith 2001), and sometimes when intoxicated, but usually continue to function and not feel overwhelmed by them.

Assessment

As with the somatoform disorders, underlying organic pathology, such as brain tumour or temporal lobe epilepsy, must be ruled out. The focus of assessment will be identity, memory and consciousness. Although the symptoms appear abruptly, sometimes a history of emotional and/or physical abuse and trauma can be uncovered. These disorders have the potential to interfere with social and occupational functioning, so these aspects are worth exploring. Like the somatoform disorders, the dissociative disorders need to be distinguished from malingering.

Interventions

The dissociative disorders are difficult to manage and interventions tend to be targeted to troublesome symptoms. The interventions in this section will be usually applicable to all of the dissociative disorders, although exceptions and particular cases will be identified. First and foremost among the interventions is the development of a sound therapeutic relationship. Such a relationship is crucial, as progress is often slow and long-term. In some cases, psychodynamically oriented psychotherapy might be offered (see Ch 23). However, this form of treatment is usually outside the expertise of most nurses. Hypnotic techniques are still used with DID and are most likely to be provided by psychologists and psychiatrists (see below). Drugs will be used to treat any coexisting disorders, especially depression and anxiety, but there are none specific to the dissociative disorders. Nursing interventions will be psychotherapeutically oriented and will target social and environmental supports, advocating and teaching stress-reduction strategies and skill-acquisition strategies where necessary (see Ch 23).

If there is a history of childhood abuse, then the client can benefit from being able to disclose the abuse and their feelings about the abuse in a non-judgmental, safe environment. Sometimes their lost memories can be recovered through hypnosis (Degun-Mather 2002), deep relaxation techniques (see Ch 23) or free association (McAllister 2000). Hypnosis involves inducing a trance in the client. In the trance, clients can recall to consciousness memories that were once lost and some can regress to earlier stages of development (Sadock & Sadock 2003). Free association was a technique developed by Freud. The fundamental rule guiding the technique is that the client tells the analyst whatever comes into their mind. Inevitably, however, the client censors the material, usually unconsciously through the defence mechanism of repression, sometimes consciously as when the client feels embarrassed. This censoring is known as 'resistance' and becomes the focus of the therapeutic encounter.

Some clients are receptive to explanations that their dissociative disorder is psychogenic in origin. For example, a client can be told that they have blocked out events that would be too stressful or traumatic to bear consciously (Degun-Mather 2002). They can also be told that this is a natural defence against pain.

The family is often included in therapy where possible. Such therapy can help the family learn new ways of interacting with the client, so they no longer reinforce any secondary gains the client is achieving.

CRITICAL THINKING CHALLENGE 20.2

- Do you believe that simply listening to a client with one of the somatoform or dissociative disorders can be helpful to the client? Why or why not?
- In what way can dissociation serve to protect a client from overwhelming anxiety?

CONCLUSION

In this chapter the somatoform and dissociative disorders have been discussed. The somatoform disorders are psychiatric illnesses that present as physical disorders. Clients with these disorders often prove difficult to treat because they perceive their problems as physical, not psychological. Somatisation is an extremely common means of communicating anxiety and some members of all cultural groups express their distress in this way. The dissociative disorders are marked by an abrupt, temporary change in consciousness, cognition, memory, identity or behaviour.

EXERCISES FOR CLASS ENGAGEMENT

- In a group, discuss how you might respond to a client who insists that the dyspepsia she experiences is cancer and not related to the problems she is experiencing in her marriage and at work.

- Discuss the advantages and disadvantages of excluding physical causes for a client's symptoms before considering possible psychological reasons.

REFERENCES

American Psychiatric Association (APA) 2000, *Diagnostic and Statistical Manual of Mental Disorders* (4th edn, text rev.), APA, Washington.

Barsky AJ & Borus JF 1999, Functional somatic syndromes, *Annals of Internal Medicine*, 130(11), pp 910–21.

Bass C & Tyrer P 2000, The somatoform conundrum: a question of nosological values, *General Hospital Psychiatry*, 22(1), pp 49–50.

Biby EL 1998, The relationship between body dysmorphic disorder and depression, self-esteem, somatisation, and obsessive-compulsive disorder, *Journal of Clinical Psychology*, 54(4), pp 489–99.

Cansever A, Uzun O, Dönmez E & Ozsahin A 2003, The prevalence and clinical features of body dysmorphic disorder in college students: a study in a Turkish sample, *Comprehensive Psychiatry*, 44(1), pp 60–4.

Castillo RJ 1997, *Culture and Mental Illness: A Client-centered Approach*, Brooks/Cole, Pacific Grove, California.

Castillo RJ (ed.) 1998, *Meanings of Madness*, Brooks/Cole, Pacific Grove, California.

Clarke D & Smith G 2001, Somatoform disorders. In: Meadows G & Singh B (eds), *Mental Health in Australia: Collaborative Community Practice*, Oxford University Press, Melbourne, pp 375–86.

Degun-Mather M 2002, Hypnosis in the treatment of a case of dissociative amnesia for a 12-year period, *Contemporary Hypnosis*, 19(1), pp 33–41.

Epstein RM, Quill TE & McWhinney IR 1999, Somatization reconsidered: incorporating the patient's experiences of illness, *Archives of Internal Medicine*, 159(3), pp 215–22.

Escobar J 1996, Overview of somatisation: diagnosis, epidemiology, and management, *Psychopharmacology Bulletin*, 32(4), pp 589–96.

Escobar JI, Hoyos-Nervi I & Gara M 2002, Medically unexplained physical symptoms in medical practice: a psychiatric perspective, *Environmental Health Perspectives*, 110(suppl. 4), pp 631–6.

Fischhoff B & Wessely S 2003, Managing patients with inexplicable health problems, *British Medical Journal*, 326(7389), pp 595–7.

Fontenelle LF, Mendlowicz MV, Mussi TC, Marques C & Versiani M 2002, The man with the purple nostrils: a case of rhinotrichotillomania secondary to body dysmorphic disorder, *Acta Psychiatrica Scandinavica*, 106(6), pp 464–7.

Halligan PW, Bass C & Wade DT 2000, New approaches to conversion hysteria, *British Medical Journal*, 320(7248), pp 1488–90.

Hardy ER, Warmbrodt L & Chrisman SK 2001, Recognizing hypochondria in primary care, *Nurse Practitioner*, 26(6), pp 26–35.

Holloway KL & Zerbe KJ 2000, Simplified approach to somatisation disorder: when less may prove to be more, *Postgraduate Medicine*, 108(6), p 89.

Janet P 1889, *L'Automatisme Psychologique*, Félix Alcan, Paris.

Janet P 1903, *Les Obsessions et la Psychasthénie*, vols 1 & 2, Félix Alcan, Paris.

Kihlstrom JF & Kihlstrom LC 2001, Somatisation as illness behavior, *Advances in Mind–Body Medicine*, 17(4), pp 240–3.

Kipen HM & Fiedler N 2002, Environmental factors in medically unexplained symptoms and related syndromes: the evidence and the challenge. *Environmental Health Perspectives*, 110(suppl. 4), pp 597–9.

Kirmayer LJ 1996, Cultural notes and somatoform and dissociative disorders 1. In: Mezzich JE, Kleinman A, Fabrega Jr H & Parron DL (eds), *Culture and Psychiatric Diagnosis: A DSM-IV Perspective*, American Psychiatric Press, Washington, pp 151–8.

Kleinman 1996, How is culture important for DSM-IV?. In: Mezzich JE, Kleinman A, Fabrega Jr H & Parron DL (eds), *Culture and Psychiatric Diagnosis: A DSM-IV Perspective*, American Psychiatric Press, Washington, pp 15–26.

Kroenke K & Swindle R 2000, Cognitive-behavioral therapy for somatisation and symptom syndromes: a critical review of controlled clinical trials, *Psychotherapy and Psychosomatics*, 69(4), 205–15.

Lipsitt DR 2001, The time has come to speak of many things, *Advances in Mind-Body Medicine*, 17(4), pp 249–56.

Lyles JS, Hodges A, Collins C, Lein C, Given W, Given B et al. 2003, Using nurse practitioners to implement an intervention in primary care for high-utilizing patients with medically unexplained symptoms, *General Hospital Psychiatry*, 25(2), pp 63–73.

Maynard CK 2003, Assess and manage somatization, *The Nurse Practitioner*, 28(4), pp 20–9.

McAllister MM 2000, Dissociative identity disorder: a literature review, *Journal of Psychiatric and Mental Health Nursing*, 7(1), pp 25–33.

McWhinney IR, Epstein RM & Freeman TR 1997, Rethinking somatization, *Annals of Internal Medicine*, 126(9), pp 747–50.

Merskey H 2000, Pain, psychogenesis, and psychiatric diagnosis, *International Review of Psychiatry*, 12(2), pp 99–102.

Meyer RG 1999, *Case Studies in Abnormal Behaviour*, Allyn & Bacon, Boston.

Morrison J 1995, *DSM-IV Made Easy: The Clinician's Guide to Diagnosis*, Guilford Press, New York.

Noyes Jr R, Stuart S, Langbehn DR & Happel RL 2002, Childhood antecedents of hypochondriasis, *Psychosomatics*, 43(4), pp 282–9.

Olivardia R 2001, Mirror, mirror on the wall, who's the largest of them all? The features and phenomenology of muscle dysmorphia, *Harvard Review of Psychiatry*, 9(5), pp 254–9.

Otto MW, Wilhelm S, Cohen LS & Harlow BL 2001, Prevalence of body dysmorphic disorder in a community sample of women, *American Journal of Psychiatry*, 158(12), pp 2061–3.

Page LA & Wessely S 2003 Medically unexplained symptoms: exacerbating factors in the doctor–patient encounter, *Journal of the Royal Society of Medicine*, 96(5), pp 223–7.

Patterson WM, Bienvenu OJ, Chodynicki MP, Janniger CK & Schwartz RA 2001 Body dysmorphic disorder. *International Journal of Dermatology*, 40, pp 688–90.

Phillips KA 1995, Body dysmorphic disorder: clinical features and drug treatment, *CNS Drugs*, 3, pp 30–40.

Phillips KA & Castle DJ 2001, Body dysmorphic disorder in men, *British Medical Journal*, 323(7320), pp 1015–17.

Phillips KA, Grant J, Siniscalchi & Albertini RS 2001, Surgical and non-psychiatric treatment of patients with body dysmorphic disorder, *Psychosomatics*, 42(6), pp 504–10.

Porter R 2002, *Madness: A Brief History*, Oxford University Press, Oxford.

Punamaki R-L, Kanninen K, Qouta S & El-Sarraj E 2002 The role of psychological defences in moderating trauma and post-traumatic symptoms among Palestinian men, *International Journal of Psychology*, 37(5), pp 286–97.

Ramsay S 2000, Controversy over UK surgeon who amputated healthy limbs, *Lancet*, 355(9202), p 476.

Ringel Y & Drossman DA 1999, From gut to brain and back—a new perspective into functional gastrointestinal disorders, *Journal of Psychosomatic Research*, 47(3), pp. 20–10.

Sadock BJ & Sadock VA 2003, Somatoform disorders. In: Sadock BJ & Sadock VA (eds), *Kaplan & Sadock's Synopsis of Psychiatry: Behavioral Sciences/Clinical Psychiatry* (9th edn), Lippincott Williams & Wilkins, Philadelphia, pp 643–60.

Salmon P, Peters S & Stanley I 1999, Patients' perceptions of medical explanations for somatisation disorders: qualitative analysis, *British Medical Journal*, 318(7180), pp 372–6.

Schreiber FR 1975, *Sybil: The True Story of a Woman Possessed by Sixteen Different Personalities*, Harmondsworth, Penguin.

Servan-Schreiber D, Tabas G & Kolb N 2000, Somatizing patients: part II, practical management, *American Family Physician*, 61, pp 1423–8, 1431–2.

Sharpe M & Carson A 2001 'Unexplained' somatic symptoms, functional syndromes, and somatization: do we need a paradigm shift?, *Annals of Internal Medicine*, 134(9 part 2), pp 926–30.

Shorter E 1994 *From the Mind into the Body: The Cultural Origins of Psychosomatic Symptoms*, Free Press, New York.

Showalter E 1997, *Hystories: Hysterical Epidemics and Modern Culture*, Columbia University Press, New York.

Singh B 1998, Managing somatoform disorders, *Medical Journal of Australia*, 168, pp 572–7.

Starcevic V 2002, Overcoming therapeutic pessimism in hypochondriasis, *American Journal of Psychotherapy*, 56(2), pp 167–78.

Stevenson RL 1925, *Dr Jekyll and Mr Hyde*, Dent, London.

Thigpen CH 1960, *The Three Faces of Eve*, Pan, London.

Treatment Protocol Project 2000, *Management of Mental Disorders*, World Health Organization Collaborating Centre for Mental Health and Substance Abuse, Sydney.

Veale D, Boocock A, Gourna, K, Dryden W, Shah F, Willson R et al. 1996, Body dysmorphic disorder, a survey of fifty cases, *British Journal of Psychiatry*, 169(2), pp 196–201.

Waitzkin H & Magaña H 1997, The black box in somatisation: unexplained physical symptoms, culture, and narratives of trauma, *Social Science and Medicine*, 45(6), pp 811–25.

Wessely S, Nimnuan C & Sharpe M 1999 Functional somatic syndromes: one or many? *Lancet*, 354(9182), pp 936–9.

Witztum E & Maragalit H 2002, Combat-induced dissociative amnesia: review and case example of generalized dissociative amnesia, *Journal of Trauma & Dissociation*, 32(2), pp 35–55.

Witztum E & van der Hart O 1998, Possession and persecution by demons: Janet's use of hypnotic techniques in treating hysterical psychosis. In: Castillo RJ (ed.), *Meanings of Madness*, Brooks/Cole, Pacific Grove, California.

PART

4

Developing Skills for Mental Health Nursing

21

Settings for Mental Health Care

Ruth Elder

KEY POINTS

- The quality of the environment is important to client recovery and rehabilitation.
- The preferred environment for the care of the mentally ill over time has been the home.
- Environmental strategies in the care of the mentally ill became more important in the eighteenth century, when it was noticed that patients were more manageable in a pleasant environment.
- Confinement of the mentally ill in large public asylums was largely an innovation of the nineteenth century.
- The therapeutic milieu is a consciously organised environment.
- Maxwell Jones in the United States and Thomas Main in the United Kingdom pioneered the concept of the hospital and environment as treatment tools.
- The goals of the therapeutic milieu are containment, structure, support, involvement, validation, symptom management, and maintaining links with family and the community.
- The principles on which the therapeutic milieu is based include: open communication, democratisation, reality confrontation, permissiveness, group cohesion and the multidisciplinary team.
- The principle guiding the care of clients in the community is that of the least-restrictive alternative.
- The therapeutic community residence is an environment that encourages the development of the client as a person in interaction with others, rather than as someone suffering from a health problem or disability.
- The preferred contemporary setting for the provision of mental health care is the community.
- The predominant form of service delivery in the community is case management, which has been found to be most effective for people with severe mental illnesses.
- The principles of caring in the community are self-determination, normalisation, a focus on client strengths, and the community as a resource.

KEY TERMS

- case management
- community care
- community integration
- community meeting
- continuity of care
- custodial care
- deinstitutionalisation
- democratisation
- empowerment
- group cohesion
- least restrictive alternative
- milieu
- milieu therapy
- moral treatment
- multidisciplinary team
- normalisation
- observation
- open communication
- partnership
- permissiveness
- reality confrontation
- revolving door
- therapeutic community

LEARNING OUTCOMES

The material in this chapter will assist you to:
- define and describe the therapeutic milieu
- discuss the historical antecedents of the therapeutic milieu
- appraise the characteristics and goals of the therapeutic milieu
- discuss the role of the nurse in the therapeutic milieu
- describe the components and functions of the multidisciplinary team
- identify forms of community accommodation for mentally ill clients
- compare six types of case management
- examine principles of caring in the community.

INTRODUCTION

The medical model, which underpins the management of mental illness in the contemporary Australian and New Zealand health-care systems and is focused on alleviating symptoms through the use of biological treatments such as psychotropic drugs and electroconvulsive therapy, has tended to underplay the usefulness of the environment as an aid to the care of the mentally ill. However, far from being an outmoded concept or form of treatment, the setting in which care takes place is an important and necessary component of client recovery and is a means of assessing and rehabilitating people with mental illnesses. Persons who are psychotic, profoundly depressed, suicidal or dangerous will all need the protection afforded by a well-structured inpatient ward. On discharge, many will also need ongoing assistance in the form of halfway houses in order to regain lost functioning, and will need assistance with integration into the community in order to ensure their continued wellbeing.

This chapter is concerned with the environment as a therapeutic tool. 'Milieu', 'therapeutic milieu', 'milieu therapy' and 'therapeutic community' are terms that have been used in psychiatry to refer to the qualities of the environment believed to be beneficial to people with mental illnesses. These terms can refer to a wide variety of programs and contexts, from whole institutions, to psychiatric wards located in general hospitals, to community residences. Despite a number of attempts to differentiate them, the terms lack precise definition and are often used interchangeably. For the purposes of this chapter, however, the terms 'milieu' and 'milieu therapy' will be used to refer to inpatient psychiatric settings, while 'therapeutic community' will be used to refer to environments where the emphasis is on normal functioning rather than a psychiatric illness or disability. In the inpatient setting, the people who are being treated are usually referred to as 'patients' or 'clients', while in therapeutic community environments they are known as 'residents' or 'consumers'.

This chapter begins by providing the historical context and development of ideas about the therapeutic potential of the environment in which care occurs. A discussion of the history of the terms should aid clarity and understanding and the appraisal of their usefulness in modern mental health care. The brief history will then be followed by an examination of the application of the concepts in a variety of settings.

HISTORICAL OVERVIEW

Ideas about what is considered a suitable environment for the care of the mentally ill have varied little over time or across cultures. On the whole, the mentally ill have been considered a domestic responsibility (Porter 2002), irrespective of beliefs about the nature of mental disorder. However, these beliefs have at times been highly influential, even if the conclusions drawn from them have been contradictory. For example, throughout most of history it has been believed that the mentally ill were possessed by supernatural forces. This belief usually led to their being feared and avoided. However, one exception to this rule is the Belgian colony of Gheel (sometimes spelt Geel), whose role as a haven for the mentally ill was founded on familial/community support and has existed since the thirteenth century. At Gheel is the church of St Dymphna, the patron saint of the mentally ill, to which the mentally ill seeking to exorcise their affliction have made pilgrimages (Sedgwick 1982). Many of them settled there. The inhabitants of this farming town made, and still make, available their homes for shelter and care, and their fields for work to severely disturbed, mentally ill patients. This township thus became one of the precursors to the idea of a community-based, therapeutic environment.

However, the acceptance shown the mentally ill by the townspeople of Gheel has proved exceptional during much of the period it has been in existence. In the seventeenth century, when it was more generally believed that the mentally ill were insane—that is, they were believed to be without reason and akin to wild beasts rather than possessed—small, private and public asylums were developed, wherein they could be segregated from the sane. The asylums varied markedly in terms of the quality of care they provided, and many meted out brutal treatments. Two infamous madhouses of the time were St Mary of Bethlehem in London, from whence the word *bedlam* is derived and the Hôpital Générale in Paris. The inmates at both were chained and tortured, and at Bedlam the inmates were put on display for the amusement and edification of Sunday visitors.

The eighteenth-century Enlightenment brought a general reforming zeal as well as new ideas about madness as a mental condition which could be best treated by mental means. Furthermore, greater experience with managing the mentally ill gave rise to the idea that the asylum could be used as a therapeutic tool as opposed to a means only of confinement. One of the foremost advocates of this progressive thinking was Philippe Pinel (1745–1826). Pinel, who is considered the founder of modern psychiatry, freed the inmates of the Bicêtre and Salpêtrière asylums in Paris from their chains (Shorter 1997). He also provided them with nourishing food, warm baths and useful activity, abolished whips and other instruments of torture, and treated them with kindness. An important outcome of these acts was that many inmates improved dramatically, while others were less violent when allowed to move around. Pinel coined the term 'le traitement moral' which translated as 'moral treatment', a phrase later popularised by the Englishman and Quaker tea merchant, William Tuke (1732–1822) (Shorter 1997). Tuke's humanitarian philosophy, which was in stark contrast to the bleedings, purges, chains and denial of basic necessities for life that had marked other treatment approaches, was that mental illness was best

---

Box 21.9 Core functions of case management

Assessment
Planning
Linking
Monitoring
Evaluation

Source: Intagliata J 1982, cited in Mueser KT, Bond GR, Drake RE & Resnick SG 1998, Models of community care for severe mental illness: a review of research on case management, *Schizophrenia Bulletin*, 24(1), pp 37–74.

The tasks involved in the implementation of each of these vary according to the client. Examples of what might be involved in the assessment of medication management and linking a client to community services are provided in Box 21.10.

Box 21.10 Examples of case management functions

Assessment of medication management
Questions to ask the client directly:
- What type of medication are you on?
- What dose?
- How often is the medication supposed to be taken?
- When do you take it?
- What does it do?
- What side-effects are there?
- Do you alter the times or do you follow the prescription exactly?
- Where do you get your medication from?

Observe the client for their ability to:
- read the directions on the medicine container
- see the pills
- discriminate between pills of different colour
- manipulate the pills
- count out pills or measure liquids
- remember the regimen.

Linking a client who enjoys reading:
- Where is the closest public library?
- What is the best means of transportation to the library?
- Does the client need to be accompanied? If so, does the case manager do this or is there someone else in the community who can?
- Can the client use this form of transport?
- Does the client need help to join the library?
- Can the client use a computerised retrieval system?
- Does the client have suitable clothing to wear?

There is no standard definition of case management. However, Mueser et al. (1998) have delineated six types (see Box 21.11).

Box 21.11 Typology of case management

Broker
Clinical
Assertive community treatment
Intensive case management
Strengths
Rehabilitation

The broker model

In the broker model, an individual case manager assesses clients and provides a linking and coordinating function with various needed services. The case manager may also monitor but does not provide a direct clinical service. This model was one of the first designed to assist clients to navigate the community mental health system. Its major flaw was that the relationship with the client was under-rated. Staff in the community need to be able to assess risk and to respond quickly. In order to provide this care, staff must know the client well, monitor the client regularly and be attuned to signs of relapse. Practitioners also need to monitor clients who refuse to engage with services. Education of clients regarding their illness, and their medication and its effects also needs to be ongoing. Furthermore, it has been found that clients place a very high value on their relationship with their caregiver (O'Brien et al. 2001; Wolf, Parkman & Gawith 2000). Clinical case management was then developed and was designed to overcome the fault in the brokerage model of the clinician not providing a clinical service.

Neither of these models proved sufficient to meet the needs of the severely mentally ill. This group of clients were often characterised by frequent, numerous hospital admissions, an unstable psychotic illness, resistance to treatment, and homelessness. This was the group who, in the early days of deinstitutionalisation, became part of the phenomenon of the revolving door, where they would be discharged from hospital only to return in a very short time. Eventually the problem was identified as one of service delivery and the idea of a team of professionals assuming responsibility for providing the necessary mix of services was born. The team, like the hospital, made services available 24 hours a day, seven days a week.

Assertive community treatment

Assertive community treatment (ACT) most closely 'mirrors the medical model of care in which psychiatrists and nurses have critical roles' (Schaedle et al. 2002, p 210). However, clinicians share a caseload rather than assuming individual responsibility for clients. Another feature of ACT is a low client-to-staff ratio (for example, 10:1). The low caseload allows for the development of close relationships with clients, which has been found helpful in increasing client tenure in the community (Rapp 1998). The size of the ACT team is usually ten to twelve staff, which is large enough to provide the necessary mix of services but small enough for all team members to know all clients.

An important feature of this model, and from where it derives its description as assertive, is case finding or *outreach*. The goal of outreach is to identify those individuals in greatest need. These are often the clients who have had multiple hospital admissions. The objective of outreach is to try to find ways to interrupt the process that leads to hospitalisation (Witheridge 1989). In some cases this approach might involve relapse-prevention techniques, or supported accommodation could be required. Outreach involves developing and maintaining working relationships with hospitals and other community agencies that might come into contact with this clientele.

Other features include: 24-hour coverage; services provided directly, not brokered out; services provided in the community, not an office; and no time limit on services (Mueser et al. 1998). This model has been found most effective in reducing hospitalisation for clients with schizophrenia whose illness is unstable, who are treatment resistant and have nowhere to live (Drake et al. 2001).

Intensive case management

Intensive case management developed from the clinical case management model (Issakidis et al. 1999). It shares many of the features of the ACT model but caseloads are not always shared. When implemented, its practitioners also often have a strengths focus and are concerned with linking clients and coordinating services (Schaedle et al. 2002). This model was designed for those clients who are defined as high service users—that is, the severely mentally ill—and has been found effective in engaging clients in treatment.

The strengths model

The strengths model (Rapp 1998) was developed in response to a perceived emphasis in other models on the problems and handicaps associated with psychiatric disability and illness, rather than the client's strengths and talents. In this model individual professionals work closely with individual clients. The relationship between case manager and client, which is the first linking activity, is considered paramount and also provides a vehicle for the monitoring function. In this model the community is conceptualised as a resource, and as being full of resources capable of meeting the diverse needs of a wide variety of clients.

The rehabilitation model

The rehabilitation model (Anthony, Forbess & Cohen 1993), similarly to the strengths model, emphasises the need to deliver services that clients want, rather than the goals of the mental health delivery system. However, the focus of this model is on assessing and developing the skills clients require to lead a normal, satisfying life. Through the

development of skills the client is helped to create a meaningful identity that fosters hope (McQuistion, Goisman & Tennison Jr 2000). This focus is in keeping with a philosophy that is centred on client wellbeing and quality of life, not just keeping the client out of hospital. It is rehabilitative in that it focuses on wellness and competence rather than illness and disability. The type of training offered is usually training in daily living tasks. These tasks might include such things as how to work the washing machine or where to go to pay the rent. This training is best provided *in vivo*—that is, at the client's place and with the client's materials and tools. In vivo training overcomes problems with the transfer of skills from one setting to another and ensures that the client can function in their particular environment.

The type of case management offered should be determined by client needs and goals. Too often the focus is on what the mental health delivery system is able to provide. When clients are asked about the goals they seek for themselves, they indicate that these are, in order of priority: money, availability of health care, a decent place to live, transportation, socialisation, and help if needed (Rapp 1998). These goals contrast with those of the mental health service delivery system, which seeks reduced hospital bed-days, integration, mainstreaming and continuity of care. They also contrast with those of many service providers, who often simply want the client to adhere to their medication regimen.

Clients in the community require a wide range of support services according to their varying needs at any one time. Care in the community seeks to encourage the development of the client as a person in interaction with others, rather than as someone suffering from a health problem or disability. The focus of care is more on day-to-day functioning and less on illness management. The major goals of community care are to assist people toward independent living, and to help them fit into the community and develop a sense of belonging. In the community, the client needs functional skills such as being able to budget, plan meals and manage their medication. He or she also needs social competencies, such as being able to establish and use relationships with family and peers, and to express feelings without losing control (Yurkovich & Smyer 1998).

Some of the principles of caring for people in the community are self-determination, normalisation, a focus on client strengths and recruiting environmental agencies (Box 21.12). These principles are the topic of the next section.

> **Box 21.12 Principles of caring in the community**
>
> Self-determination
> Normalisation
> Focus on client strengths
> Recruiting environmental agencies

Principles of caring in the community

The relationships developed with individual clients in the community are often long-lasting, unlike the short relationships developed in the hospital setting. It is not sufficient to simply empathise with the client. These relationships are more like partnerships—clients are empowered by being helped to find their own solutions to problems, and given hope through recognition of their abilities. Some of the principles that can assist in achieving this are: self-determination, normalisation, a focus on client strengths, and recruiting environmental agencies and forces (Cnaan et al. 1990). Implementing these principles might involve a great variety in interventions, some of which may seem alien to those trained in professional disciplines.

Self-determination

One of the major aims of the shift to community care was to foster client self-determination. In the community, clients are not treated like hospitalised patients. Clients have consistently demonstrated their desire to be informed about their treatment and to make decisions about it. This independence can be supported by helping clients to identify and pursue their own goals, and to take responsibility for their actions and behaviour, and respecting their decisions about medication. However, there is still progress to be made in improving consumer participation in treatment and recovery plans (SCESNNHP 2002). Client self-determination is the key to developing a partnership with clients because the client's goals and aspirations become the centre of the relationship. Self-determination can best be catered for by engaging in activities such as: ensuring that the client's consent to involve their family or others in the treatment plan is obtained; getting the client to help plan the activities they want to engage in; encouraging the client to set their own goals; and ensuring that the client can refuse, if they wish, to participate in activities. Success is gauged by the pursuit of the client's goals, not by the extent to which the client has conformed to the expectations of the mental health system or service providers. From this perspective, the emphasis is on *trying* to achieve the goal, rather than on whether or not the client succeeds.

Normalisation

Another principle of community care is normalisation. Normalisation can be achieved by: encouraging clients to set the rules for behaviour; engaging in trips and excursions with clients; setting expectations for appropriate behaviour and expressing disapproval of deviant behaviour; and encouraging a normal routine in matters such as hygiene, housework and dressing. Clients can be helped to integrate into the community by helping them develop social networks, for example by introducing them to community groups. Some services provide a mini-van whereby clients can be transported to various community venues such as local social, cultural and sporting clubs and participate alongside other community members. However, care must be taken that this strategy does not increase social isolation by identifying the clients as a homogeneous group (Evans & Moltzen 2000). Integration into the community can also be assisted by encouraging clients to use mainstream health services such as the local general practitioner for their medication rather than specialist mental health services (see Box 21.13 for an overview of primary mental health care). Clients may also need help in developing work and leisure skills. For example, a client may demonstrate artistic aptitude and skills, and wish to use their leisure time more meaningfully. The system response to this desire might be to provide a professional in a day hospital setting to teach the client a craft such as leatherwork. An alternative would be to find a group of clients with similar wants and then advertise for volunteers to teach the clients particular skills for a limited period. Volunteers could be drawn from art schools and colleges, or they might be practising or retired artists, who could be asked to teach specific skills to the clients for half a day weekly, for ten weeks. One of the great advantages of this method is that clients would be helped to better integrate into the community, rather than being marginalised and identified as a 'special' group.

Box 21.13 **Primary mental health care**

Primary care is the local, accessible, universal, front-line health services available to a community. GPs, pharmacists, podiatrists, physiotherapists, dentists, optometrists, community health centres, and primary care clinics in general hospitals are all among the major providers of primary care services.

In Australia, the National Primary Mental Health Care Initiative was established in 1999 under the National Mental Health Strategy. This initiative was a response, in part, to the finding from the National Survey of Health and Wellbeing (Australian Bureau of Statistics 1998) that mental illnesses are far more prevalent in the community than previously thought. Many illnesses, such as depression and anxiety, entailed significant disability and were treatable, but the people suffering from them were often unable to access public mental health services. This failure of public mental health services has been attributed to their restricting the definition of a 'serious' mental disorder to psychosis.

The National Primary Mental Health Care Initiative seeks to further the integration of services by emphasising the role of primary care in delivering mental health services to the community through the development of partnerships between primary health care providers and specialist mental health services.

Focus on client strengths

A focus on clients' strengths rather than their problems and weaknesses can enhance motivation. When considering strengths, the nurse, in collaboration with the consumer, assesses what the client *wants* rather than their needs (Rapp 1998). For example, if the client wants to live independently of their family, then what they need to do to achieve this goal—such as adhering to their medication regimen or learning to budget—can be placed in a context relevant to the client.

Recruiting environmental agencies

Recruiting environmental agencies involves working effectively with community services. In the community, very little of the environment, unlike that in a hospital, is under the control of mental health professionals. One of the major goals of working in the community setting is to modify the environment in which the client lives, works, plays and interacts so that it is better aligned with their abilities. These modifications will demand collaboration with community agencies. Mentally ill clients will often need assistance in procuring housing and work or education. They might need help in using public transport, shopping and budgeting. It is therefore useful for the mental health professional to get to know and meet regularly with local doctors, shopkeepers, employers and the police.

Recruiting community forces also means taking account of the families of the mentally ill. In the community, family and significant others are often expected to shoulder a large burden of care for their mentally ill relative. It is not uncommon for families to feel they are being blamed for their relative's illness, and they have often been ignored when it comes to being informed about diagnoses and treatment. They have not been able to participate fully and meaningfully in treatment and recovery planning (SCESNNHP 2002). However, carers are usually keen to be involved. They want up-to-date information and need to be confident that support will be prompt and available when needed. Nurses provide families and caregivers with advice and education about mental illness and its treatment, and offer support to them in the management of any problems. Family education has been found to be one of the core interventions that help clients achieve quality of life (Drake et al. 2001). Families may also require information about the government services they are entitled to, and the voluntary services that might assist them.

CONCLUSION

In this chapter it has been argued that the quality of the environment in which client care takes place is important to their recovery and rehabilitation. Environmental strategies in the care of the mentally ill have a long history, but their application over time has been patchy. These strategies reached their peak in the eighteenth century, when it was noticed that patients were more manageable in a pleasant environment. In the twentieth century, Thomas Main and Maxwell Jones pioneered the concept of the hospital and environment as treatment tools. The principles on which the therapeutic milieu is based include open communication, democratisation, reality confrontation, permissiveness, group cohesion and the multidisciplinary team. The goals of the inpatient therapeutic milieu are containment, structure, support, involvement, validation, symptom management and maintaining links with family and the community.

The preferred contemporary setting for the provision of mental health care is the community, which accords best with the principle of caring for people in the least-restrictive environment. The predominant form of service delivery in the community is case management, which has been found to be most effective for people with severe mental illnesses. The principles of caring in the community are self-determination, normalisation, a focus on client strengths and the community as a resource.

EXERCISES FOR CLASS ENGAGEMENT

Discuss the following questions with your tutorial group.
- How can an emphasis on safety in the inpatient setting promote or detract from the development of therapeutic relationships?
- How can nurses in an inpatient setting provide support to families?
- Is it possible and/or desirable to maintain a nursing identity when working in a community setting?
- What services are available in your community to assist mentally ill clients?

REFERENCES

Anthony WA, Forbess R & Cohen MR 1993, Rehabilitation oriented case management. In: Harris M & Bergman H (eds), *Case Management for Mentally Ill Patients: Theory and Practice*, Harwood Academic, Chur, Switzerland.

Australian Bureau of Statistics 1998, *Mental Health and Wellbeing: Profile of Adults, Australia, 1997*, ABS, Canberra.

Barker PJ & Walker L 2000, Nurses' perceptions of multidisciplinary teamwork in acute psychiatric settings, *Journal of Psychiatric and Mental Health Nursing*, 7(6), pp 539–46.

Benbow R & Bowers L 1998, Rehabilitation using therapeutic community principles, *Nursing Times*, 94(1), pp 56–7.

Bland R 2001, The social worker. In: Meadows G & Singh B (eds), *Mental Health in Australia: Collaborative Community Practice*, Oxford University Press, London.

Cleary M, Edwards C & Meehan T 1999, Factors influencing nurse–patient interaction in the acute psychiatric setting: an exploratory investigation, *Australian and New Zealand Journal of Mental Health Nursing*, 8(3), pp 109–16.

Cnaan RA, Blankertz L, Messinger KW & Gardner JR 1990, Experts' assessment of psychosocial rehabilitation principles, *Psychosocial Rehabilitation Journal*, 13(3), pp 59–73.

Cooper D 1967, *Psychiatry and Anti-psychiatry*, Tavistock, London.

Creedy D & Crowe M 1996, Establishing a therapeutic milieu with adolescents, *Australian and New Zealand Journal of Mental Health Nursing*, 5(2), pp 84–9.

Delaney KR 1992, Nursing in child psychiatric milieus. Part 1: What nurses do, *Journal of Child Psychiatric Nursing*, 5(1), pp 15–19.

Delaney KR, Pitula CR & Perraud S 2000, Psychiatric hospitalization and process description: what will nursing add?, *Journal of Psychosocial Nursing and Mental Health Services*, 38(3), pp 7–13.

Dowling R-M, Fossey E, Meadows G & Purtell C 2001, Case management. In: Meadows G & Singh B (eds), *Mental Health in Australia: Collaborative Community Practice*, Oxford University Press, London.

Drake RE, Goldman HH, Leff HS, Lehman AF, Dixon L, Mueser KT & Torrey WC 2001, Implementing evidence-based practices in routine mental health service settings, *Psychiatric Services*, 52(2), pp 179–82.

Duffy D 1995, Out of the shadows: a study of the special observation of suicidal psychiatric in-patients, *Journal of Advanced Nursing*, 21(5), pp 944–50.

Elsom S 2001, The mental health nurse. In: Meadows G & Singh B (eds), *Mental Health in Australia: Collaborative Community Practice*, Oxford University Press, London.

Evans IM & Moltzen NL 2000, Defining effective community support for long-term psychiatric patients according to behavioural principles, *Australian and New Zealand Journal of Psychiatry*, 34, pp 637–44.

Farhall J 2001, Clinical psychologists. In: Meadows G & Singh B (eds), *Mental Health in Australia: Collaborative Community Practice*, Oxford University Press, London.

Foucault M 1967, *Madness and Civilisation: A History of Insanity in the Age of Reason*, Routledge, Tavistock, London.

Greene JA 1997, Milieu therapy. In: Johnson BS (ed.), *Psychiatric-mental Health Nursing: Adaptation and Growth*, Lippincott-Raven, Philadelphia, pp 221–31.

Hummelvoll JK & Severinsson E 2001, Coping with everyday reality: mental health professionals' reflections on the care provided in an acute psychiatric ward, *Australian and New Zealand Journal of Mental Health Nursing*, 10(3), pp 156–66.

Intagliata J 1982, Improving the quality of community care for the chronically mentally disabled: the role of case management, *Schizophrenia Bulletin*, 8(4), pp 655–74.

Issakidis C, Sanderson K, Teesson M, Johnston S & Buhrich N 1999, Intensive case management in Australia: a randomised controlled trial, *Acta Psychiatrica Scandinavica*, 99, pp 360–7.

Jansen E 1980, Editor's discussion. In: Jansen E (ed.), *The Therapeutic Community: Outside the Hospital*, Croom Helm, London, pp 19–51.

Jones J, Ward M, Wellman N & Lowe T 2000, Psychiatric inpatients' experience of nursing observation: a United Kingdom perspective, *Journal of Psychosocial Nursing*, 28(12), pp 10–20.

Jones M 1953, *The Therapeutic Community*, Basic Books, New York.

Kahn EM 1994, The patient–staff community meeting: old tools, new rules, *Journal of Psychosocial Nursing*, 32(8), pp 23–6.

Krauss JB & Slavinsky AT 1982, *The Chronically Ill Psychiatric Patient and the Community*, Blackwell Scientific Publications, Boston.

LeCuyer EA 1992, Milieu therapy for short stay units: a transformed practice theory, *Archives of Psychiatric Nursing*, VI(2), pp 108–16.

Main T 1946, The hospital as a therapeutic community, *Bulletin of the Menninger Clinic*, 10, pp 66–70.

Main T 1980, Some basic concepts in therapeutic community work. In: Jansen E (ed.), *The Therapeutic Community: Outside the Hospital*, Croom Helm, London, pp 52–63.

McQuistion HL, Goisman RM & Tennison Jr CR 2000, Psychosocial rehabilitation: issues and answers for psychiatry, *Community Mental Health Journal*, 36(6), pp 605–16.

Morrison P, Lehane M, Palmer C & Meehan T 1997, The use of behavioural mapping in a study of seclusion, *Australian and New Zealand Journal of Mental Health Nursing*, 6(1), pp 11–18.

Mueser, KT, Bond GR, Drake RE & Resnick SG 1998, Models of community care for severe mental illness: a review of research on case management, *Schizophrenia Bulletin*, 24(1), pp 37–74.

Munich RL 2000, Leadership and restructured roles: the evolving inpatient treatment team, *Bulletin of the Menninger Clinic*, 64(4), pp 482–94.

Munich RL 2002, Efforts to preserve the mind in contemporary hospital treatment, *Bulletin of the Menninger Clinic*, 67(3), pp 167–86.

Murray RB & Baier M 1993, Use of therapeutic milieu in a community setting, *Journal of Psychosocial Nursing*, 31(10), pp 11–16.

O'Brien AP, Woods M & Palmer C 2001, The emancipation of nursing practice: applying anti-psychiatry to the therapeutic community, *Australian and New Zealand Journal of Mental Health Nursing*, 10(1), pp 3–9.

Onyett S 1999, Community mental health team working as a socially valued enterprise, *Journal of Mental Health*, 8(3), pp 245–51.

Onyett S & Ford R 1996, Multidisciplinary community teams: where is the wreckage?, *Journal of Mental Health*, 5(1), pp 47–55.

Porter R 2002, *Madness: A Brief History*, Oxford University Press, Oxford.

Prebble K & McDonald B 1997, Adaptation to the mental health setting: the lived experience of comprehensive nurse graduates, *Australian New Zealand Journal of Mental Health Nursing*, 6(1), pp 30–36.

Pyke J 1999, Community services and supports. In: Clinton M & Nelson S (eds), *Advanced Practice in Mental Health Nursing*, Blackwell Science, Oxford.

Rapp C 1998, *The Strengths Model: Case Management with People Suffering from Severe and Persistent Mental Illness*, Oxford University Press, New York.

Renouf N & Meadows G 2001, Teamwork. In: Meadows G & Singh B (eds), *Mental Health in Australia: Collaborative Community Practice*, Oxford University Press, London.

Schaedle R, McGrew JH, Bond GR & Epstein I 2002, A comparison of experts' perspectives on assertive community treatment and intensive case management, *Psychiatric Services*, 53(2), pp 207–10.

Sedgwick P 1982, *Psychopolitics*, Pluto Press, London.

Shorter E 1997, *A History of Psychiatry: From the Era of the Asylum to the Age of Prozac*, John Wiley & Sons, New York.

Steering Committee for the Evaluation of the Second National Mental Health Plan 2002, *Evaluation of the Second National Mental Health Plan*, Canberra.

Thomas SP, Shattell M & Martin T 2002, What's therapeutic about the therapeutic milieu?, *Archives of Psychiatric Nursing*, XVI(3), pp 99–107.

Tobias G & Haslam-Hopwood G 2003, The role of the primary clinician in the multidisciplinary team, *Bulletin of the Menninger Clinic*, 67(1), pp 5–17.

Tuck I & Keels MC 1992, Milieu therapy: a review of development of this concept and its implications for psychiatric nursing, *Issues in Mental Health Nursing*, 13, pp 51–8.

Watson J 1992, Maintenance of therapeutic community principles in an age of biopharmacology and economic restraints, *Archives of Psychiatric Nursing*, VI(3), pp 183–8.

Witheridge TF 1989, The assertive community treatment worker: an emerging role and its implications for professional training, *Hospital & Community Psychiatry*, 40, pp 620–4.

Wolf J, Parkman S & Gawith L 2000, Professionals' performance in community mental health settings: a conceptual exploration, *Journal of Mental Health*, 9(1), pp 63–76.

Yalom ID 1983, *Inpatient Group Therapy*, Basic Books, New York.

Yurkovich E 1989, Patient and nurse roles in the therapeutic community, *Perspectives in Psychiatric Care*, XXV(3/4), pp 18–22.

Yurkovich E & Smyer T 1998, Strategies for maintaining optimal wellness in the chronic mentally ill, *Perspectives in Psychiatric Care*, 34(3), pp 17–24.

The **Patient** as **Person**

*Kim Usher, Lauretta Luck
and Kim Foster*

22

KEY POINTS

- Communication is a skill that underpins all mental health nursing interventions.
- Self-harm and suicidal behaviour need to be differentiated.
- Assessment of client risk behaviours is an essential part of assessment.
- Effective interventions can be implemented when working with people who exhibit aggressive, violent, self-harming and suicidal behaviour.
- Patient choice and informed consent underlie care considerations in regard to patients who exhibit challenging behaviour.
- The individual strengths and limitations of the nurse and client must be recognised and considered in care planning and delivery.

KEY TERMS

- aggression
- anger
- communication skills
- competency
- counter-transference
- empathy
- ethico-legal issues
- informed choice
- informed consent

- limit-setting
- professional boundaries
- seclusion
- self-harm
- suicide
- therapeutic relationship
- transference
- violence

LEARNING OUTCOMES

The material in this chapter will assist you to:
- define the key terms related to communicating with individuals
- describe the key communication skills necessary to establish and maintain a therapeutic nurse–patient relationship
- understand nursing assessment and management of distressed patients who may be aggressive
- understand the principles of teaching anger management/impulse control
- understand nursing strategies for patients who are suicidal and patients who self-harm
- outline the skills nurses use to work with patients who demonstrate risk behaviours such as aggression, violence, self-harm and suicide
- distinguish between the terms used in regard to suicide and self-harm
- outline the relevant ethico-legal issues related to informed consent and seclusion.

INTRODUCTION

This chapter outlines interpersonal skills related to mental health nursing. It is based on a perspective that values the strengths and skills of both the mental health nurse and the person who is the patient, while recognising that both can have vulnerabilities (Hem & Heggen 2003). The chapter is divided into three sections. It begins with an overview of the communication skills that underpin the therapeutic nurse–patient relationship. These are the underlying skills that the mental health nurse needs when working with patients in special situations. Issues related to nurse vulnerabilities are discussed in this section, particularly in relation to use of self. The second section of the chapter discusses risk. In this section the management of patients at risk of self-harm, suicide, aggression and violence is addressed. Special attention is given to risk assessment. Tools to aid assessment, and subsequent nursing interventions, are included. Section three introduces the ethico-legal issues of patient choice and consent, which are important when planning and implementing nursing skills.

COMMUNICATION SKILLS

Arguably, mental health nurses use 'self' as their most essential therapeutic tool, and the nurse–patient relationship is one of the most vital clinical components of nursing practice (Lauder et al. 2002; Stein-Parbury 2000). 'Self' in this context relates to the need for the mental health nurse to understand and be aware of his or her own subjective and experiential world while using specialist skills. This use of self includes professional detachment, self-awareness, and understanding of personal emotions, beliefs and values. This personal understanding is used to facilitate the therapeutic relationship, where the outcome is a focus on the patient's needs (Fontaine 2003; Horsfall, Stuhmiller & Champ 2000). The therapeutic relationship is a balance between the personal self, offering human closeness, and professional distance (Hem & Heggen 2003). What does this mean for nurses practising in this specialty? It challenges nurses to review who they are in ways that may not be as rigorously required in other nursing specialties. In addition, there is an increased emphasis on interpersonal communication skills. It is understandable that some undergraduate and novice nurses have difficulty with the notion that communication is a 'skill' and that these skills require theory, understanding, practice and personal reflection. One of the activities we all engage in throughout our lives is communication—we communicate with others individually, in groups, via the telephone, via electronic means, in writing, and in a variety of social, informal and formal situations. It could therefore be claimed that this amount of understanding, practice and personal involvement in communication would mean that we already have a degree of expertise when it comes to communication. Although this argument seems reasonable, there are many indicators to suggest that we are not always good at communicating.

> ### CRITICAL THINKING CHALLENGE 22.1
>
> Take a minute to think about communication situations that you find difficult.
>
> Think of a recent conversation you have had with someone significant or important to you. Think of how you felt about this interaction and reflect on what was said during your conversation. What went well and why? What was difficult and why?
>
> For many of us, tutorial presentations may spring to mind!

Communication as it applies to mental health nursing has other attributes in addition to those with which we are most familiar. Mental health nurses use communication skills in developing the therapeutic relationship. Additional focused communication skills are required with respect to communication theory, skills and practice, and these are discussed below.

Therapeutic relationship

A cornerstone skill for initiation, development and maintenance of a therapeutic relationship between nurse and patient is interpersonal communication (Kunyk & Olson 2001; Lauder et al. 2002). A therapeutic relationship is an enabling relationship that supports the needs of the patient. The nurse is entrusted to understand what the patient needs, in order to enable the patient to understand their own needs and therefore become empowered in their life (Lauder et al. 2002). Mutually agreed goals for nursing practice are enhanced as a function of the therapeutic relationship. A therapeutic relationship is based on *rapport*—establishing a connection with the person and developing trust—and is distinct from interviewing, counselling and education. Therapeutic relationship differs from other interactions in its structure, purpose and intent. The value of the relationship is exhibited by improvement in the patient's wellbeing and capacity to take control of their life (Lauder et al. 2002). Therapeutic relationships also differ from social relationships and intimate relationships (Horsfall et al. 2000). Whilst establishing and engaging in a therapeutic relationship, the mental health nurse focuses his or her skills on the patient and judiciously uses self-disclosure.

Empathy

Empathy is not sympathy. *Sympathy* is about pity, compassion, commiseration and condolence, and while there are social situations where the offering of sympathy may be culturally and socially relevant, still it is not empathy. Nor is sympathy appropriate for the therapeutic relationship. Five conceptualisations of *empathy* have been proposed: empathy as a human trait, a professional state, a communication process, caring and a special relationship (Kunyk & Olson 2001). Empathy as a communication process and professional state can offer us a clear understanding of what we mean by 'empathy' and a theoretical basis for our understanding.

Empathy is about observing, listening, understanding and attending. It is 'being' with the person physically, cognitively and emotionally, and understanding their story, thoughts, feelings, beliefs and emotions. It is an ability to understand the person as fully as we can, and from their subjectively expressed view. It means not making judgments and not giving advice, but genuinely and honestly striving to understand the client's subjective experience and communicating this understanding to the person. Here empathy is conceptualised as both a communication process and a professional process (Kunyk & Olson 2001).

Empathy involves perceptiveness, listening to meaning, listening to feelings, and listening in context, attending, responding appropriately and maintaining presence with the person (Motyka, Motyka & Wsolek 1997). In this sense, empathy is linked to the therapeutic use of self. The mental health nurse is able to actively listen to both the cognitive content of the patient's story and the subjective meaning this has for the patient. Nurses need to be honest about their own experiences and subjective responses, such that they are able to clearly hear, respect and understand the experience of the patient. This means that the patient's experience is acknowledged (Collins & Cutcliffe 2003). It is one of the important building blocks of a constructive therapeutic alliance between nurse and patient.

Earlier research suggested that rather than the five conceptualisations of empathy listed above, there are two types of empathy (Alligood 1992, cited in Evans et al. 1998). The first is *basic empathy*. This is essentially our trait capacity to understand and feel for others. 'Trait capacity' refers to our subjective capacity to feel for other people. These personal characteristics are shaped by our family, social environment and culture, and are contextually and culturally expressed. The second type of empathy suggested is *trained empathy* (Evans et al. 1998). Trained empathy is a professional skill that is taught, learned and developed. Trained empathy enables the nurse to create a trusting relationship in which the patient feels able to discuss their feelings and thoughts, thus facilitating the nurse's understanding of the patient, the patient's responses and health needs (Reynolds & Scott 2000). These two types of empathy are in fact reflected in the five conceptualisations and can be aligned with 'empathy as a human trait' and 'empathy as a professional state' (Kunyk & Olson 2001, p 319).

Two personal characteristics of the nurse that contribute to the skill of empathy are the capacity for immediacy and the ability to be open-minded. The skill of *immediacy* refers to the capacity of the mental health nurse to respond to the patient and their feelings, in the 'here and now' with warmth and genuineness (Kneisl Wilson & Trigoboff 2004; Reynolds & Scott 2000). It is a combination of both an appropriate physical presence and the clinical use of communications skills, such as the ones discussed in this chapter. *Open-minded* people tend to have a dynamic or fluid (rather than static) world view. Open-mindedness can convey an attitude of acceptance to the person and an ability on the nurse's part to 'take the person as they are'.

Active listening

Active listening requires attention, genuineness and an ability to 'hear' what the patient has to say and validate the meaning of the patient's perceptions. This does not mean that the nurse overtly or inadvertently agrees with (or, for that matter, disagrees with) delusions or hallucinations, but that the patient's perception and experience are heard and acknowledged. The skilful use of active listening requires practice and reflection on the part of the mental health nurse and contributes to the capacity of the nurse to maintain presence with the patient. Again, the examined self affects many such 'micro' skills that are valuable in the therapeutic relationship.

Listening to patients is improved by being available in the best environment for communication—one with reduced distractions and noise. The ideal may not always be possible, but consideration of the safety and privacy of the environment demonstrates good communication skills on behalf of the nurse. Often when we first start working with people in the mental health context, we are overly worried about what we will say next rather than what the patient is saying. A good way to increase your skills and be more effective is to concentrate on what the patient is saying and become an effective and active listener.

Mental health nurses' communication skills are a combination, and purposeful extension, of a number of personal and professional communication strategies. While the skills discussed here are not exhaustive, they offer some explanation and description of communication strategies, including closed and open-ended questions, reflective listening, paraphrasing, summarising, body language, touch, transference and counter-transference.

Closed and open-ended questions

Closed and open-ended questions elicit different types of responses from the patient, and both are useful in mental health nursing. A *closed question* is one that elicits a brief answer, often a single word. Asking many closed questions in a row can seem like an interrogation, but there is value in asking closed questions in order to gather specific information. An *open-ended question* allows the respondent to answer more fully. Open-ended questions have the advantage of not narrowing down or directing the response, and so the answer can give you information that you may not have expected. This style of questioning also allows the patient to tell their subjective experiences, an important communication strategy that enhances the nurse–patient therapeutic relationship. Individuals will nevertheless share information at the level they feel comfortable or safe with, so you may find that a closed question elicits a detailed response or an open-ended question is answered with a single word. Ordinarily, however, these questioning styles are a good guide for communication.

Table 22.1 Examples of closed and open-ended questions

Closed	Open-ended
Are you feeling good today?	How are you feeling today?
Are you still getting side-effects from your medication?	How are your medications affecting you now?
Do you want to come to group?	What would you like to do today?
Does feeling stressed still make you feel like harming yourself?	How does your stress affect you now?

Reflective listening

Reflective listening means literally echoing the patient's communication. Reflective listening can include reflecting the content of the communication or reflecting the patient's feelings (Stein-Parbury 2000). Reflection of feelings, however, requires a good therapeutic relationship as well as prudent, skilful use. Over-use of reflective listening can seem contrived and stilted. This skill redirects the content or feelings back to the patient.

Patient: I feel really sad about my family.
Nurse: You feel really sad about your family?
Patient: I want to go home.
Nurse: You want to go home?

Paraphrasing

Essentially, paraphrasing is confirming the main points made by the patient—either the content of the communication or the feelings—by re-stating them (Stein-Parbury 2000). Re-stating these main points can be a combination of your own words or the same phrases that the patient has used. Paraphrasing is a useful communication skill that is different to, but can overlap with, other skills. Paraphrasing can be used to clarify that you have heard and understood the patient's subjective experience or perception. Any misunderstandings can also be clarified with the use of paraphrasing (Stein-Parbury 2000). It indicates that you have been actively listening to both content and feelings.

Patient: I am sorry for the mess I am in. It's just that some days I can't find the energy to tidy up or do anything.

Nurse: I see. You're feeling distressed about your lack of energy.
Patient: If they do that to me one more time I am just going to have to tell them, that's all.
Nurse: It sounds like you're feeling angry about this issue and think it is time to let people know.

Summarising

Summarising means putting together the main issues and ensuring that you have understood them from the patient's perspective. The main issues could be focused on the content, perceptions or feelings of the patient. This communication strategy can be useful for clarifying what you have shared, or for gaining some new perspectives or insights, or it can be used to conclude your current communication with the patient (Stein-Parbury 2000).

Nurse: So, the important issues for you are finding suitable accommodation, repaying your car loan and getting organised so you can return to your university studies.

The use of 'rote' learned responses ('tell me about that') or reflective paraphrasing ('so you say you feel down') might impede the development of the nurse–patient relationship, as the nurse may not convey empathy (Evans et al. 1998). Clearly there are times when active listening is indeed the best response and minimal verbal responses and silence enable the patient to better express their perceptions and feelings. The point here is that when the emphasis of communication is restricted to 'rote' and learned responses, the nurse is unable to express genuine concern and empathy, and this in turn impedes the development of the therapeutic relationship. Development of skilful communication requires practice and self-awareness so that the nurse can use a variety of responses that are congruent with who she or he is as a person.

Body language and touch

Communication, of course, is not only verbal exchanges. Body language is an integral part of how we send and receive messages. Both verbal messages and messages sent via our body language can be misunderstood or misinterpreted. Body language, or non-verbal signals, include all the cues we send with our body; how we stand, our facial expressions, how close to other people we position ourselves, what we wear, how much we move our hands, if we cross our arms and any other physical movement that can be interpreted (or misinterpreted) by the recipient of our communication (Stein-Parbury 2000). There may be times when we communicate one message verbally but give a conflicting or different message with our body language. The importance of body language can be clearly demonstrated in everyday ways. Nurses need to consider both the impact of their body language alone (a raised eyebrow or hands on hips) and the congruence between their body language and their verbal communication.

Congruence between verbal messages and body language is important.

Body language and the issue of touch have particular significance in the mental health setting. Regard for the patient's perceptions includes understanding the possible impact of 'touch'. The nurse touching the patient may have significance for the patient beyond, or other than, that intended by the nurse. In some circumstances touch may be perceived fearfully, as a threat, or as seduction. It may also be culturally inappropriate. Remaining sensitive to patient feedback about the level of eye contact is also important in therapeutic nurse–patient communications. Inappropriate eye contact, in particular a fixed gaze or stare, may also be misinterpreted or culturally inappropriate. Touch and eye contact are two significant considerations when communicating with patients with mental illness and are clear examples of the necessity of competently and skilfully understanding the particular health problems and needs of the client.

Influence

We influence other people by what we say, what we do not say, what we focus on (feelings, content, context), our body language and our attitude to the other person's communication. That is, we have interpersonal and mutual influence. This is particularly so when we are in a professional role caring for patients who have perceptual, emotional, language or cognitive impairment as a result of their mental illness. Patients will feel more able to trust a nurse who demonstrates that he or she understands the patient's needs and feelings (Reynolds & Scott 2000). In addition to the many micro skills that we can learn and practise to improve our communication skills, attitudes and values are important elements of therapeutic communication. Treating patients with respect, dignity, genuineness and honesty are among the characteristics that interweave with trained empathy to enhance the therapeutic relationship and build trust. Talking and approaching situations in a calm manner is also an important feature of effective and therapeutic communication in the mental health setting (Street & Walsh 1998). These skills require nurses to recognise their own strengths and limitations and seek appropriate resources and/or mentors.

Transference and counter-transference

So far we have looked at the impact of our communications on the patient, their perceptions and feelings. What of the impact of the patient on our perceptions and feelings? In order to understand the issues of transference and counter-transference, it is important to gain some insights into where these concepts originated. Sigmund Freud (1856–1939) was the founder of the psychoanalytic model and it is from Freud's work that these concepts emerged (see Ch 7). Without detailing his work, it is important to grasp Freud's notion of the 'unconscious'. Unlike the way

we might use this idea in everyday language, the 'unconscious' in psychoanalytic terms means that the person is not aware, or not conscious, of the motivation for their thoughts, feelings or actions. This is pivotal to the idea of transference and counter-transference.

The process of *transference* occurs when a person transfers beliefs, feelings, thoughts or behaviours that occurred in one situation, usually in their past, to a situation that is happening in the present. Traditionally it was meant to refer to the patient with unconscious feelings or beliefs about someone in their past, transferring these feelings or beliefs onto the psychoanalyst. Past issues and conflicts experienced by the patient are carried into the therapeutic relationship (Pearson 2001). These can include issues with authority, sibling rivalry, anxiety and dependence. The patient brings these unresolved issues from the past into the present one-to-one relationship with the nurse. These feelings in the therapeutic relationship may be triggered by the nurse's manner, look, position or speech. The transference may be displayed by covert or overt hostility, contempt for the nurse, lack of cooperation, or deference and submissiveness.

The patient's self-awareness is reduced as a result of transference. Helping the patient to identify the past issues, deal with the feelings and emotions, and to examine their meaning in the present, is an effective way to support the patient to work through the transference. This supportive strategy develops the patient's capacity to make choices. Dealing with transference in an empathic and honest manner, through judicious and skilful reality-based self-disclosure, can effectively disengage the transference (Pearson 2001).

Counter-transference is regarded as the response of the analyst to the patient. It is also referred to as the response of the analyst to the patient's transference (O'Kelly 1998). Generally the nursing perspective is that counter-transference is the response of the nurse to the patient (whether this is due to unconscious or conscious reasons). One cue that you might be experiencing counter-transference is having strong feelings towards a patient—either negative or positive. For instance, the patient may have similarities to you in their age, gender, family relationships, life situation or personal issues that generate strong positive feelings for you. Alternatively, you may experience a strong feeling of dislike or avoidance of a particular patient related to their behaviours, such as aggressive or self-harming behaviours, or you may feel a lack of understanding of their behaviours and communications due to their mental illness, particularly patients with personality disorders (Ens 1999).

Boundaries

Finally, one salient feature of a working therapeutic relationship involves respecting the needs of the patient while remaining professional, and that includes the setting of boundaries (Horsfall, Cleary & Jordan 1999). The core

important that such outcomes do occur in the event of the unwanted behaviour. It is therefore imperative that all staff are aware of the plan and that everyone agrees to follow through with the action in the event of the unwanted behaviour. However, remember that some inpatient environments are perceived as coercive and controlling and, because of limited space, may make the patient more likely to become violent (Quintal 2002).

Box 22.2 Nursing skills for use with the aggressive patient

- Approach the patient calmly.
- Speak softly and slowly.
- Avoid prolonged eye contact.
- Keep space between you and the patient.
- Demonstrate control over the situation.
- Always use a non-threatening manner of speech and action.
- Provide the patient with choices if appropriate.
- Listen to the patient.
- Use other staff wisely—for example, have other staff nearby before intervening with the patient; nominate one staff member to speak with the patient; call for back-up staff if necessary.
- Follow local protocols if available.
- Use medication and seclusion if necessary.

An Australian study (Wynaden et al. 2002) found that when managing difficult behaviours, nurses used a management hierarchy that had seclusion at the bottom. The hierarchy included things like distraction, the use of outdoor areas to separate patients, encouraging the patient to regain control of their behaviour, and communication techniques. They also found that the nurses used intuitive judgments when deciding whether or not to seclude a patient, and would use seclusion if it had been successful in a similar situation in the past.

Seclusion

Why use seclusion?

Seclusion is usually instigated when other methods, such as medication and talking, have failed to manage a difficult behaviour (Muir-Cochrane et al. 2002). Its use is based on the therapeutic principles of containment, isolation and decrease in sensory input (Guthiel 1978). A recent study found that the most common reason nurses gave for using seclusion was the immediate control of violent behaviour. Other reasons given were to protect the safety of staff and other patients (Terpstra et al. 2001). Even though aggression and violence are the most common reasons for seclusion in the inpatient setting (Meehan 1997; Muir-Cochrane 1995), patients have reported being secluded for inappropriate reasons, such as refusing to attend an activity or refusing to take medications (Heyman 1987).

Seclusion is the practice of placing a person in a locked, purpose-built area for a set period of time (Baradell 1985). Muir-Cochrane et al. (2002) explain that this practice, although long considered an important practice in the treatment and control of the mentally ill, is controversial. The controversy is said to focus on legal, ethical, professional, attitudinal and safety issues (Wynaden et al. 2002). Seclusion raises issues of nursing 'control' and there are questions regarding how these issues are ethically balanced with patients' rights. Differences in staff level of experience, nurses' perception of seclusion and individual nurses' perceptions of the seriousness of patients' behaviours also affect the practice of seclusion (Lowe, Wellman & Taylor 2003; Muir-Cochrane 1996). The implementation of and preference for seclusion in a consistent and appropriate manner is also of concern to mental health nurses. Issues of staff–patient ratio are also reported to have a statistical relationship with the use of seclusion (Donat 2002). A decreased use of patient seclusion followed a focused effort to increase staffing numbers. This strategy was concurrent with supportive patient behavioural treatment plans and staff training. Because of the controversy, the use of seclusion continues to be varied, with some facilities using it routinely, some sparingly, and others not at all. The practice continues to be recognised by clinicians in Australia and New Zealand as an acceptable tool for the management of certain behaviours (Muir-Cochrane et al. 2002), even though current practice in psychiatry is based on use of the least-restrictive environment wherever possible (Australian Health Ministers 1998).

Holmes (1998) explains how the term 'seclusion' refers to different things, such as time out, open seclusion, isolation, quiet room and so on. However, whichever way it is conceived, seclusion still tends to be perceived in a negative way by patients (Farrell & Dares 1996; Griffith 2001).

Patient perspectives on seclusion

Some patients have actually reported that they felt seclusion aided their recovery (Heyman 1987; Plutchik et al. 1978; Soliday 1985). However, others have reported the opposite. These patients reported that seclusion made them feel helpless, punished, depressed, disgusted, afraid, vulnerable and worthless (Binder & McCoy 1983; Heyman 1987; Martinez et al. 1999; Norris & Kennedy 1992; Plutchik et al. 1978; Soliday 1985). In a study by Meehan (1997), patients supported the use of seclusion in the inpatient unit but claimed it was over-used. They also reported that rather than helping a patient feel safe, seclusion can actually make a person feel vulnerable, neglected and punished. An Australian qualitative study of patients' perspectives on the experience of seclusion found that most patients perceived the experience in a negative way. The patients reported similar feelings to those reported in earlier studies, such as abandonment, fear and isolation; however, they also reported feeling under-informed about the seclusion process (Meehan, Vermeer & Windsor 2000).

Nurse perspectives on seclusion

Staff attitudes to seclusion have been the focus of a number of studies (Terpstra et al. 2001). Some mental health staff defend the use of seclusion as an acceptable way to manage the destructive or violent behaviour of severely disturbed patients. Not all health-care professionals, however, believe seclusion to be desirable or efficacious. Some say its use is a violation of freedom and dignity and that it may in fact be counter-therapeutic and lead to dependency on staff, cause hallucinations due to sensory deprivation, and cause feelings of abandonment (Tooke & Brown 1992). One study found that 85 per cent of nurses prefer to use medication rather than seclusion as they consider it to be less restrictive (Terpstra et al. 2001).

Legal perspectives on seclusion

The Australian State and Territory Mental Health Acts, the New Zealand Mental Health Act and local institutional policies govern the use of seclusion. Clinicians must be aware of the relevant Act and local policy related to their place of work. The relevant Acts should be referred to, to determine such aspects as when seclusion can be used, who can instigate seclusion and under what conditions, the timing of observations of the patient in seclusion, how long seclusion can be used, and when seclusion should be terminated. There is variation across Australia in the policies prescribing monitoring, review and observation practices for seclusion episodes (Muir-Cochrane & Holmes 2001). In addition, the legal issues related to seclusion remain complex and unclear: 'the Australian and New Zealand Mental Health Acts appear to adopt an uneasy mix of ideology, legal projections and the need to provide practical approaches to difficult situations. There is still a lack of consensus about what constitutes seclusion, under what circumstances it may be applied, how it ought to be managed and when it should be terminated' (Muir-Cochrane et al. 2002, p 143). Therefore, it is important for the clinician to be aware of the relevant Mental Health Act (see the website link in the box below) and local policy on seclusion.

Links to the Mental Health Acts

The website below provides links to all Australian State and Territory Mental Health Acts and to the New Zealand sites. Select your country, State or Territory and follow the links to the appropriate legislation.
http://www.austlii.edu.au

CASE STUDY: Maria (part A)

Maria, a 23-year-old female, was brought to the emergency department on an emergency examination order by the police after threatening to stab her boyfriend with a knife, and acting 'quite bizarrely' when the police attended. At the time of the Crisis Assessment and Treatment Team's arrival she was in the isolation room, pacing up and down and yelling in a threatening manner at all staff who passed. The police were still in attendance.

The staff initially approached Maria from outside the room by introducing themselves and explaining their role in being present. (Only one person spoke to Maria.) The staff ensured that in interacting with Maria they maintained an open posture. Direct eye contact was maintained as was appropriate to the situation. Staff explained the situation to Maria. During this time a constant assessment was made of Maria's response to the assessors, and her level of arousal. As Maria stopped pacing and appeared to be engaging with the staff, she was asked if she would like to sit down and talk about what had occurred. Maria agreed to this.

CASE STUDY: Maria (part B)

By being open and honest with Maria, and acting in an assertive, but non-aggressive manner, staff were able to reduce Maria's hostility enough to engage in an assessment process. After the interview, Maria expressed her appreciation that someone wanted to listen and hear her side of the story. Maria does have a mental illness, which is currently well controlled with the medication she takes. Unfortunately her relationship is volatile, due partly to her boyfriend's overprotectiveness. He is always checking on what she has been up to, and whether she has taken her medication. Today they had been arguing about housework, when he started to blame her anger with him on her not taking her medication.

At this point Maria became extremely frustrated and picked up a knife from the kitchen bench. Maria denies any intention to use the knife, stating that she was just frustrated and wanted to get her point across. Maria agreed that this was not the best response to the situation.

Following discussion with Maria's case manager it was agreed that her case manager would help her to develop more effective communication strategies, and would provide support and psychoeducation for Maria's boyfriend. Maria was discharged home.

The authors would like to acknowledge Kym Park, CN Community Assessment and Treatment Team, Cairns Mental Health Service for this case study.

CRITICAL THINKING CHALLENGE 22.2

■ In part A, what are the immediate management priorities for Maria? Consider the context of her presentation, the current setting and the available staff.

■ From the information provided in the case study, identify the strategies the staff used to defuse Maria's aggression. In your opinion, do they seem to have been effective? How do you know this?

CRITICAL THINKING CHALLENGE 22.3

■ Does the situation in part B seem to have ended successfully? Provide rationales for your responses

■ Applying the principles of developing a therapeutic rapport with clients, identify the strategies staff used in this situation that enhanced rapport and trust.

■ In this situation, there was a precipitating factor and psychosocial issues surrounding the event. What were they? Does the management plan developed by the staff adequately address them?

■ This situation may have been handled differently based on staff responses to Maria's aggression. What other strategies may have been used to manage Maria's behaviour? Consider the viability of the use of psychotropic medication and restraint.

Working with the patient who self-harms or is suicidal

Self-harming behaviours and suicide risk

A number of terms are used to describe behaviour that may be damaging to the self. Note that suicidal behaviour can be seen to exist on a continuum. For instance, there is a clear risk that the person who deliberately self-harms may eventually go on to commit suicide (Holdsworth, Belshaw & Murray 2001; Slaven & Kisely 2002). Some of the terms are used interchangeably, although there are distinctions to be made between them. The terms listed in Box 22.3 are in order of increasing level of harm or risk.

The issues of suicide and deliberate self-harm or injury will almost certainly be encountered by nurses in their practice, whether in a community mental health setting, inpatient mental health unit, emergency department or other health setting. In a recent Australian study, for example, 96.3 per cent of nurse respondents had had experience with people who deliberately self-harm (McAllister et al. 2002a). Suicide and/or self-harm may engender concern and anxiety in the nurse due to personal attitudes, and the moral, ethical, legal and practical requirements of care. The care of patients who are suicidal or self-harming may necessitate the provision of support and clinical supervision to the mental health nurse by experienced staff, to enable them to continue working with these patients and to develop the necessary attitudes, knowledge and skills needed to care for them (Cutcliffe & Barker 2002).

Working with the person who self-harms

Self-harm may be distinguished from suicidal behaviour in that self-harm is a non-lethal, sometimes impulsive, method of alleviating emotional distress where the person deliberately inflicts injury on himself or herself. The person may self-harm without having suicidal intent (Holdsworth et al. 2001). It is estimated that between one and four per cent of the population self-harm in order to deal with their feelings and/or situation (Martinson 2002; McAllister et al. 2002b). A recent Australian study on nurses' attitudes toward patients who self-harmed found that nurses who saw themselves as skilled in working with these patients were more likely to feel positive towards them and less likely to demonstrate negative attitudes. This highlights the importance of nurses having relevant intervention and therapeutic skills in this area (McAllister et al. 2002b).

Reasons for self-harming behaviour—There are complex reasons why patients self-harm. Self-harm is generally considered to be a negative or self-destructive act, yet it can be viewed from another perspective. It may be empowering or affirming of the person's individuality and strength in expressing themselves and/or dealing with

---

Box 22.3 Terms used to describe self-harm and suicide

■ *Self-harm or injury/deliberate self-harm*: any intentional damage to the person's body, without a conscious intention to die. Includes the use of cutting, burning, carving, branding, head-banging, scratching, biting, bruising, abrasions and pulling skin and hair. This is distinct from suicidality and self-harm that results from psychosis.

■ *Parasuicidal behaviour*: actions that are intended to cause self-injury but not intended to be lethal (eg cutting wrists or taking an overdose of a drug in low doses and/or drugs that will not cause death)

■ *Self-poisoning*: intentionally ingesting a substance in more than the recommended dose, either through accident or to deliberately self-harm

■ *Suicidal ideation*: thoughts or ideas about suicide

■ *Lethality of suicide threat*: the seriousness of the threat or attempt to suicide and the degree to which the action is likely to result in death

■ *Suicide*: the deliberate and conscious attempt to kill oneself. May be either completed (results in death) or attempted.

strong emotions. The use of self-harm can therefore be interpreted as an act of power rather than the more common perception of it as an act of emotional pain and/or the inability to cope with feelings or experiences.

It may be that self-harm actually reveals the person's will to live or survive, as the patient's use of self-harm can be seen as a way of maintaining psychological integrity through releasing unbearable feelings and therefore easing an urge toward suicide. It may be a rite of passage for some young people—for instance, where body scars from cutting reveal a sense of 'tribal belonging' (Martin 2002). Some people use physical self-injury to deal with overwhelming emotions or situations, and to relieve tension.

It is common for people who self-harm to have a history of abuse, and to be anxious and/or depressed, and/or diagnosed with borderline personality disorder or dissociative identity disorder. Episodes of self-harm have also been associated with recreational substance use (Holdsworth et al. 2001). The self-harm behaviour of the person can be a way to express and 'release' psychic pain through the flow of blood. It can represent a destructive way of dealing with perceived uncontrollable negative feelings such as intense anger or desperation. The perception that self-harm is used as a way of attention-seeking has not been found to be accurate. People who self-harm often do so in private as a secret and shameful practice (McAllister et al. 2002b) as they may feel that there is no other option available to them. It can be seen as a method of expressing deep needs that require skilful help (Hopkins 2002).

Providing care and communicating with the person who self-harms—Research has found that nurses generally hold more negative than positive attitudes towards patients who are self-harming. The reasons for this include their own feelings of anxiety about the act of self-injury, and frustration that other care priorities prevent them from giving these patients the time and space needed to explore their use of self-harm. Nurses can find it stressful and can feel helpless to prevent repetitive self-harm attempts (Holdsworth et al. 2001; Hopkins 2002; McAllister et al. 2002b; McKinlay, Coustan & Cowan 2001; Smith 2002). The clinician may end up being ambivalent towards the person, and resent the demands placed upon them (Hopkins 2002). This can interfere with the development of therapeutic rapport, so the ability to empathise is compromised and engagement becomes more difficult. The health-care context that can lead to a more transient connection between nurse and patient may also make it difficult for nurses to find the time or energy to subjectively engage with patients, so their hearing of patient stories remains incomplete. There is a need for nurses to work with this ambiguity through reflective practice and to navigate between the positions of neutrality, distance and empathy (Holdsworth et al. 2001; Hopkins 2002; McAllister 2001).

CRITICAL THINKING CHALLENGE 22.4

- How do you think you would feel if you were working with a patient who had deliberately self-harmed?
- What factors in your life may have led to your opinions and feelings about this issue? Consider your own background in terms of religion, family beliefs about the value of life, etc.
- What measures could you take to protect the therapeutic relationship if you found you were experiencing either very negative or overly positive countertransference feelings toward a patient who self-harmed?

Comprehensive assessment of the person who self-harms—The lack of structure to guide assessment, management and discharge planning for the patient who is self-harming is a significant issue raised by nurses working with these patients (Slaven & Kisely 2002). The five-dimensional nursing assessments model (Rawlins, Williams & Beck 1993) covers physical, intellectual, emotional, social and spiritual aspects of the patient and is a comprehensive tool for use in assessment of patients who self-harm. This model goes beyond the more traditional biopsychosocial model as it considers all dimensions of the person, including the spiritual.

It is important that assessment also focuses on the person's strengths as well as problems or needs. As the previous discussion has highlighted, this approach provides a more accurate and comprehensive overview of the patient than simply viewing them and their behaviour from a pathogenic or illness perspective (McAllister & Estefan 2002).

Interventions for self-harming behaviour—Patients report that it is helpful for a nurse to sit down and talk with them. One complaint patients have is that nurses do not necessarily understand the reasons for the self-harm, and that they offer medication rather than making themselves available to talk (Smith 2002). These are important messages to consider when working with patients who self-harm. Box 22.4 outlines some useful skills for dealing with a patient who has self-harmed.

Working with the person who is suicidal

Many people experience temporary or fleeting thoughts of suicide at some point in their lives, but most of us do not go on to try it (Pirkis et al. 2002; Treatment Protocol Project 2000). In Australia in 1998, two per cent of all deaths were attributed to suicide (ABS 2000b). The overall rate of suicide has remained fairly static since 1921 at 14 suicides per 100,000 persons, with a total of 2683 suicides in 1998, although rates within the various demographic groups have fluctuated over time (ABS 2000a). This is relatively consistent with the statistics for New Zealand, where the suicide rate in 2000 for the total population was 11.2 per 100,000,

---

Box 22.4 Nursing skills used with the person who is self-harming

- Approach the person with an open mind and a supportive attitude.
- Encourage the person to share their thoughts and feelings regarding the self-harm.
- Remove potentially harmful objects such as razors, glass, pins, scissors, knives, lighter.
- Assess for any precipitating factors prior to self-harm and remove/reduce them if possible.
- Assess for risk of suicide.
- Convey a sense of calm, control and safety to the person.
- If the person is distressed, reassure them of their safety.
- Remain available to the person for emotional support.
- Explore alternative coping methods for expressing negative feelings.

- Follow the setting's protocol with regard to level of observation.
- Use seclusion and/or medication only if absolutely necessary and according to the setting's policy.
- Review the episode with the person afterwards and develop with them a mutually agreed plan for managing possible future episodes, e.g. note what factors precipitate self-harm and try to reduce or eliminate them.
- Gain the patient's agreement that they will contact a staff member if they feel overwhelming negative feelings that may lead to self-harm behaviours.
- Agree to spend time with the person and support them when they require emotional support.

Sources: Whitehead L & Royles M 2002, Deliberate self-harm: assessment and treatment interventions. In: Regel S & Roberts D (eds), *Mental Health Liaison: A Handbook for Nurses and Health Professionals*, Bailliere Tindall, London; Horsfall J, Stuhlmiller C & Champ S 2000, *Interpersonal Nursing for Mental Health*, McLennan & Petty, Sydney.

---

compared to 12.1 per 100,000 in 1990 (New Zealand Health Information Service 2003).

People aged 25 to 44 years had the highest rate of suicide in 1998, at 23 suicides per 100,000 persons, followed by people in the 15–24 year age group, at 17 per 100,000 persons, whose rate of suicide has continued to increase. The male suicide rate is consistently higher than the female rate; however, women are twice as likely to attempt suicide as men. The most common method of suicide in 1998 for both males and females was hanging. In 1998, 15 per cent of males and 18 per cent of females who suicided had a diagnosis of a mental health disorder. In general, marriage appears to be protective against suicide, with married people (at 9 per 100,000) being less likely to commit suicide than never-married people

(22 per 100,000), widowed people (13 per 100,000) or divorced people (26 per 100,000). This is consistent for both genders (ABS 2000a,b).

The largest increase in deaths from suicide between 1921 and 1998 has been in males in the 15–24 year age group. Concern over rising rates of suicide for young people has resulted in its emergence as a major public health issue, with a number of national programs and strategies instituted such as the National Youth Suicide Prevention Strategy and the National Action Plan on Youth Suicide Prevention (ABS 2000b).

Reasons for suicidal behaviours—Although the reasons for attempting suicide vary, it is commonly related to an effort to deal with relationship difficulties (Queensland

---

NURSE'S STORY: Self-harm

I was working in the emergency department one day when Sally arrived for assessment. Sally is pretty. When she is wearing long sleeves you wouldn't think she had a care in the world. In short sleeves, however, the picture isn't so pretty. There are about fifty self-inflicted scars running laterally across both inner arms from each radial pulse up to the biceps. We can't use her left arm for taking a blood pressure—the drum of the stethoscope won't sit flat on all the lumpy scar tissue.

Sally is wearing a tank-top; the scars are reminders that our work as mental health nurses is important. Using the language of a mental health professional, I said that talking through things is a safe alternative to cutting herself, but now that she's talking I feel afraid . . . I have no idea what she, or I, will say. How can I relate to her experiences? How can I understand her life? What if I mess things up?

Sally is doubtful too. She speaks of the release that cutting offers: 'When I slash-up I'm not trying to kill myself. I just

want to feel something—anything's better than nothing.' It doesn't hurt to slash-up; the blood-letting takes some of the pain and the anger away, she says. Sally feels embarrassed and sore afterwards. That's why she's running an 'experiment' with me to see if talking helps.

Months later I realise something that I probably should have known. Not knowing and not experiencing self-harm, I start to realise that Sally's life isn't a disadvantage to her. She needs to tell her story, without somebody interrupting with their story or with clichés. She needs somebody who knows what counter-transference is, and tries not to let it get in the way. She needs somebody to challenge her unrealistic beliefs, but still believe in her. She needs support and being listened to without judging, not rescuing.

Paul McNamara, CNC Community Liaison Team, Cairns Base Hospital

Health 2000). It is also commonly related to the presence of mental health disorders such as schizophrenia, depression, and dual diagnosis of both severe mental illness and substance abuse (Gournay & Bowers 2000; Pirkis et al. 2000). An attempt to suicide is often reported by patients as reflecting their feelings of powerlessness or the experience of loss and disappointment, where they want freedom from the psychic pain they feel rather than actually wanting to die (Talseth, Jacobsson & Norberg 2001). It is this ambivalence, where the person wants to escape from their feelings yet retain an underlying desire to live, that nurses can try to understand and access when they work with the person who is suicidal.

Box 22.5 Risk factors for suicidal behaviour

Risk factors associated with suicide include:
- being male and aged between 15 and 30 years
- being an indigenous Australian or Maori youth
- previous deliberate self-harm
- previous history of suicide attempts
- psychiatric disorder: primarily depression and schizophrenia
- substance/alcohol abuse
- dual diagnosis of mental illness and substance abuse
- recent stressful events such as divorce, loss of job, breakdown of relationship, death of a loved one
- anniversaries of previous losses.

Assessing for risk of suicide—If the nurse is concerned about a person they think may be suicidal, it is important that they talk directly with them about suicide. Prevention of suicide is far better than having to treat the consequences of a suicidal act. However, the nurse may be concerned about directly asking the person about suicide, for fear of unintentionally causing the person to become suicidal. Discussing suicide will not make the person more likely to attempt suicide. Talking openly about the possibility of it and giving the patient a chance to talk about it may lead to the person realising that it is not the best solution for their problem (Treatment Protocol Project 2000).

As well as conducting a comprehensive mental state and psychosocial assessment, the nurse can specifically structure their questioning of suicide risk according to the five broad areas shown in Box 22.6, which each reveal an escalating level of risk.

Therefore, if a person has thoughts about committing suicide, has a plan to take pills, and has the pills in their home with the immediate intention of acting out their plan, they are at an acute and high level of suicide risk. A person who has thoughts about committing suicide and a vague plan of taking some pills, but is not sure what pills they might take and does not have any pills

available, is not at as high a risk of suicide. There is obviously a need for regular re-assessment of risk for suicide as the person's risk level may change at any time.

Box 22.6 Assessment of suicidality: questions

Examples of questions for assessing risk for suicide:
- Has the person been having thoughts about killing themselves?
- Is there a plan about how they would go about killing themselves? (eg taking pills, hanging, etc)
- Is there a means to carry out the plan? (e.g. does the person have access to these pills, do they have a rope or other device?)
- What is the timeframe for their plan? (e.g. is it immediate, or is it something they have thought about for the future?)
- Has the person ever tried to kill themselves before?

Box 22.7 Assessment of suicidality: direct questions

Examples of direct questions that may be used for assessing suicidal ideation:
- Have you been feeling 'down' or depressed for a few days at a time?
- Do you ever feel that life is not worth living?
- When you feel like this, have you ever had thoughts of killing yourself?
- What did you think you might do to kill yourself?
- Have you taken steps towards doing this (i.e. buying pills)?
- Have you thought about when you might kill yourself?
- What has stopped you from doing this so far?
- What could help make it easier for you to deal with your problems?

Source: adapted from Treatment Protocol Project 2000, *Management of Mental Disorders* (3rd edn), World Health Organization Collaborating Centre for Mental Health and Substance Abuse, Sydney.

Suicide risk assessment tool

For a comprehensive tool for assessment of suicide risk, see the following website:
http://www.dao.wa.gov.au/wadaso/html/contents/publications/best-practice/questionnaires/suicide-risk/pdf

---

Caring for and communicating with the person who is suicidal—As highlighted throughout this chapter, the nurse–patient relationship is pivotal in the provision of care in a mental health setting, and particularly in providing care for the person who is suicidal. The key aspects of providing interpersonal care for the person who is suicidal may be seen as inspiring hope, communication and engagement (Cutcliffe & Barker 2002; Samuelsson et al. 2000).

However, nurses can struggle to understand why a person should want to try and kill themselves or to injure themselves through self-harm. It may be seen as irrational and/or be mystifying to them (Hopkins 2002). Some nurses may feel distressed and find that they either avoid working with these people, or become overly involved in their care and extremely upset if the person eventually commits suicide (McLaughlin 1999). It is understandable that when the nurse has cared for a patient and worked closely with them over time, their personal sense of loss can be significant if the patient suicides. It is important that nurses are able to respect the individual's particular situation, beliefs and right to self-determination. Although the provision of hope is crucial and the vast majority of patients will eventually overcome their suicidal feelings, the realistic understanding that not all patients will survive is a difficult but ultimately essential realisation for the nurse.

The nurse can use a number of support strategies when working with suicidal patients. These include receiving ongoing professional clinical supervision in order to increase their professional skills and coping skills. Clinical supervision may also provide a safe avenue for nurses to express their feelings. Nurses can ensure that they attend in-service and/or regularly update their knowledge of suicidality and management through professional journals and/or texts. Use of collaborative care planning with the patient, which results in individualised care (Samuelsson et al. 2000), can also improve the nurse's sense of self-efficacy and the patient's experience of receiving comprehensive and relevant care.

Patient perspectives on being cared for while suicidal

Patients who are suicidal report that the most distressing aspects of their experience are the loneliness, suffering and despair they feel, and the need to feel respected as people and given responsibility for their own lives. They ask to be cared for as human beings. Nurses need to have an understanding of the meaning of this experience for the person as well as a deeper understanding of their own experiences in taking care of the person, rather than simply understanding suicide in terms of theories or models (Samuelsson et al. 2000; Talseth et al. 2001). Patients can feel ashamed of being a psychiatric patient and embarrassed that they require treatment. They may sense a lack of respect from staff and feel that staff do not trust them. However, they have also reported positive experiences of care received. Feeling cared for and secure with staff who were friendly, welcoming, accepting of them and allowed them to talk about their problems contributed to positive experiences (McLaughlin 1999; Samuelsson et al. 2000). The skills and attitudes that the nurse holds clearly play an important role when working with patients who are suicidal.

Nursing interventions for the person who is suicidal

Nurses themselves consider that the most important skill a mental health nurse must have when working with patients who are suicidal, is effective communication (McLaughlin 1999). Throughout this chapter the need for effective communication has been highlighted as the basis from which the nurse can be therapeutic when working with the patient. Nevertheless, the major focus of care for suicidal patients in the inpatient setting seems to be that of *observation*, albeit often linked with therapeutic communication and engagement (Cutcliffe & Barker 2002; Horsfall & Cleary 2000). Observation includes terms such as 'one-to-one' care, 'specialling' or 'close observation'. Observation usually ranges from intensive 24-hour care where the nurse is never more than an arm's length away from the patient, through to lower-level 'category' observations where there are periodic and regular 'checks' of the patient's whereabouts and well-being. Observation has the aim of preventing the patient attempting suicide by reducing risk (Bowers, Gourney & Duffy 2000; Cutcliffe & Barker 2002; Horsfall & Cleary 2000). Although observation may be commonly used as a strategy it also needs to be consistently and appropriately implemented (Bowers et al. 2000). The issue of patient rights and the use of power by staff need to be considered (Horsfall & Cleary 2000). It is imperative that nurses have an awareness that nursing *engagement* could replace observation as a more effective way to inspire hope in the person through use of the interpersonal relationship. The engagement approach advocates the use of the nurse–patient therapeutic relationship where the nurse attempts to explore with the patient the issues that led to their suicidal behaviour. An understanding of these issues by another person may help to address the patient's need for physical and emotional security (Cutcliffe & Barker 2002).

The use of the *no-suicide contract* is also a frequently used strategy by nurses working in crisis assessment teams, inpatient mental health settings, and community mental health settings. It is used for both assessment of risk and as a management strategy (Farrow 2002). The contract addresses the prevention of a suicide attempt by the patient and may be a written contract, although it is more often a verbal agreement between the nurse and patient. It usually includes an agreement that when the patient feels they may attempt suicide, they agree instead to contact the nurse (or other agreed person) and discuss their feelings rather than acting on them. If the patient does not comply with the agreed contract the consequence may be that they face a more restrictive level of care, such as involuntary admission under the Mental Health Act.

NURSE'S STORY: Managing the person who is at risk

I have been a mental health nurse since 1988 and have worked mainly in acute settings. One of the most difficult clinical situations I have encountered is known as an 'A' special. This means being no further than an arm's length away from the client at all times, including bathroom activities. The fact that it is done to prevent the person from coming to harm, either by their own hand or due to their altered judgment, makes it no less difficult. The client gets cross at times because they feel that their space is being invaded and that the nurse is stopping them from doing what they want to do. If the client is responding to hallucinations or delusional beliefs, you can become a part of these thoughts, and the patient can become paranoid about you.

I remember looking after a young man (eighteen years old) who was transferred to our inpatient unit for reasons of safety. It was late in the evening (2200 hours) and at this time he was not an 'A' special client. He had presented with suicidal ideation, delusions and auditory hallucinations, and this was his first admission to a mental health unit. On arrival on our unit, he was hyper-vigilant and restless. He was given some PRN medication (valium) to help reduce his agitation, and then settled into his room. I found it difficult to relax about this young man, chose to observe him closely, and discussed my feelings and observations with my colleague. I couldn't voice my exact concerns, but he just didn't 'feel right' to me. He wasn't expressing any suicidal ideation to us, but he remained restless. I observed

him looking perplexed and walking up to the exits. My colleague agreed with my observations and we decided between us to observe him closely overnight. We decided to continue to observe him at ten-minute intervals while he was asleep, and constantly when he was awake. Throughout the next day he became increasingly distressed and at greater risk of self-harm. He was placed on an 'A' special.

Once his pharmacotherapy levels were established, his symptoms decreased. The degree of observation lessened and supportive therapy was commenced. He was later discharged home into the care of his family, with community case management.

As a mental health nurse, I think the important thing about close observation is that it requires the use of personal qualities such as empathy, patience, warmth, and being able to understand and tolerate anxiety and anger.

Close observation is also one situation where the nurse really needs, and uses, interpersonal skills such as listening, reflecting, observing and building rapport. This can be a tense and uncomfortable situation, but it can also provide a unique opportunity to work closely with a client, supporting them through this time so they can stay safe and eventually get well. I think it is one of the most important things we can do for our clients.

Donna-Maree Bates, CN Alcohol Tobacco and Other Drugs Service,
Cairns Base Hospital

Box 22.8 **Nursing strategies for use with the patient who is suicidal**

- Approach the person calmly and maintain a non-judgmental attitude.
- Provide reassurance of safety.
- Develop rapport and genuine regard for the person.
- Enable regular time and space to allow the person to talk freely about their thoughts and feelings.
- Maintain a safe environment through removal of potentially injurious objects including knives, glass, razor blades.
- Follow local protocol concerning regular observation of person's safety and location.
- Judiciously use self-control options (such as no-suicide contracts) that the person can use when they are feeling on the verge of attempting suicide, e.g. contact the nurse or other staff member.
- Involuntary admission may need to be considered for the person who is in the community.
- Ensure the person has 24-hour access to help.

CASE STUDY: Ben (part A)

Ben is a 47-year-old man who is transported by ambulance to the emergency department of the local hospital accompanied by the police. He has been unwillingly brought in to hospital and presents as combative and uncooperative, and seems confused. The ambulance officer reports that they were called out by Ben's ex-wife Amelia, after she received a call from him, where he sounded intoxicated, was crying and expressing remorse about their relationship breakdown. Ben told her he had taken an overdose of paracetamol, sertraline and diazepam and wanted to die. This is the second time in the last month that Ben has presented at the emergency department with a suicide attempt.

Therefore, there are significant ethical and legal implications for their use. Although they are commonly used, recent research has indicated that no-suicide contracts may be more a protective strategy for nurses or a result of a lack of available alternatives or resources such as inpatient facilities or nursing skills, rather than necessarily being the best decision regarding care (Farrow 2002). In summary, the commonly accepted use of observation and no-suicide contracts by nurses working with the person who is suicidal needs to be thoughtfully considered before implementation.

CRITICAL THINKING CHALLENGE 22.5

- What right do the police and ambulance officers have to take Ben to hospital against his will?
- What are the immediate nursing priorities for Ben? Consider issues such as the drugs taken, his repeat suicide attempt, and his aggression and confusion.
- Ben is combative, confused, uncooperative and non-compliant, but the medical officer won't prescribe sedation. What likely reason(s) are there for this decision?
- How would you feel about nursing a person who had made repeated suicide attempts? Consider factors such as your own beliefs and background.

CASE STUDY: Ben (part B)

Ben is nursed overnight in the critical care bay of the emergency department and is administered activated charcoal via nasogastric tube and intravenous acetylcysteine, with regular observations including Glasgow Coma Scores and vital signs. A nurse 'specials' Ben during this time. Ben is angry and uncooperative with the nurse. Towards the end of the shift, Ben says to the nurse, 'What the f . . . is wrong with you? You haven't saved my life. You've just delayed the inevitable. I'll top myself the moment I get out of here.'

The nurse from the Mental Health Consultation Liaison service later interviews Ben and conducts a full assessment. The findings include that Ben is employed full time but has some current financial stressors, has a large network of friends, and no significant medical history. He shows signs of depression and is overweight, with poor self-care and diet. He has been drinking large amounts of alcohol lately, and appears to have low self-esteem. However, he has good communication skills and a good rapport is developed during the interview. Ben agrees to be transferred as a voluntary patient to the mental health inpatient unit 'for a night or two'.

The authors would like to acknowledge Paul McNamara, CNC Community Liaison Team, Cairns Base Hospital for this case study.

CRITICAL THINKING CHALLENGE 22.6

- If you were the nurse specialling Ben, how would you feel about him swearing at you and saying he would kill himself? How could you best respond to his statements?
- What are the aims of specialling the person who is suicidal? Explore the benefits and disadvantages of specialling for both the patient and the nurse.
- Explore the skills and strategies the nurse could use to develop rapport with Ben.
- Based on the information provided, identify Ben's likely strengths and vulnerabilities. How could these be addressed in terms of risk management?

- If Ben had not agreed to transfer to the unit as a voluntary patient, should he be made an involuntary patient under mental health legislation? Consider issues such as patient rights, dignity, empowerment, duty of care and risk assessment.
- When planning is made for Ben to be discharged from hospital, what issues need to be considered? How might these be best addressed?

ETHICO-LEGAL ISSUES
Patient choice in the therapeutic setting

People are often called upon to make decisions or choices about their health care. Being involved in choices about treatment is part of the right to self-determination. People in any type of hospital or health-care setting can be called upon to make or be involved in decisions about their care, and mental health and psychiatric facilities are no different. Mental health patients make frequent choices related to their care and treatment. The nurse is often the person the patient will turn to for advice when such choices need to be made. There is ever-increasing pressure from consumer groups, the profession and government policy for nurses to encourage patient participation in decision-making related to their care (Usher & Arthur 1998). Participation in decision-making by the patient promotes autonomy and indicates respect for the rights of the patient. Involving the patient in choices about their care and assisting them to make choices in the role of advocate has additional therapeutic advantages. The respect shown the patient when involving them in decisions about their care may result in enhanced self-esteem and a reduction in helplessness (Brabbins, Butler & Bentall 1996). It may also lead to mutual respect and regard between the nurse and the patient (Munhall 1991). It is also necessary for the person to have sufficient information about the proposed treatment strategy in order for them to make a reasonable decision about their care. We must remember that it is the person/patient rather than a third party who can determine what information is needed to make a meaningful decision (Aveyard 2002).

Informed consent

Everyone has the right to be informed about and to give consent to any form of treatment. Unfortunately, it is often assumed that consent is only required when major clinical interventions are to be undertaken or where the proposed intervention presents a significant risk to the person. However, consent should be obtained for all procedures, including nursing procedures, wherever patient autonomy is at stake (Aveyard 2002). Procedures where a recognised risk of side-effects or adverse effects exists, as is the case with many medications used in psychiatric treatment, is cited as an area where consent is required (Wallace 2001).

In psychiatric facilities there are times when consent may not be necessary—for example, when a patient is involuntarily detained and prescribed a course of treatment against his or her will according to the relevant Act. However, because a person has a mental illness or is detained in a psychiatric facility does not mean they cannot consent to treatment. In fact, even patients who are involuntarily detained may be considered capable of consenting to some things, some of the time. However, the culture in psychiatric hospitals has encouraged patients to be passive recipients of expertise. As a result, little consultation with or participation by patients in treatment decisions has occurred in the past (Brabbins et al. 1996).

The administration of interventions or procedures without the consent of the patient can result in a legal action against the health-care provider and/or the health-care facility. Therefore, obtaining informed consent prior to nursing interventions is an important practice. Nurses need to be aware of the patient's consent status, of any orders that have been made, and of the need to inform the patient about the treatment they are to receive and to encourage the patient's cooperation in decision-making (Wallace 2001).

Informed consent assumes that the following requirements have been satisfied:

- A fair description of the procedure to be followed has been supplied.
- Description of the possible risks and discomforts has been explained.
- Description of the benefits to be expected has been supplied.
- Disclosure of any alternative procedures that might be advantageous has been made.
- An offer to answer any queries has been made.
- Instruction that the person is free to refuse or withdraw consent at any time has been clearly explained (Usher & Arthur 1998; Wallace 2001).

For consent to be informed it must be voluntary, specific and come from a competent person. The last of these is often the problematic area for mental health nurses. We will examine each aspect in detail.

Consent must be voluntary

For consent to be voluntary it must be given freely without any form of duress. Care must be taken when dealing with mental health patients as persistent persuasion, often considered to be a reasonable part of psychiatric practice, may be perceived by the patient as duress. For example, if the nurse uses persuasion to ensure a patient takes their medication and if the patient understands or believes that he or she has no other choice but to follow the advice of the prescriber, this does not constitute informed consent (Brabbins et al. 1996). In other words, if the patient is of the opinion that she or he has no other choice but to take the medication, then informed consent is not achieved.

Consent must be specific

For consent to be specific the patient must be aware of what it is he or she is consenting to. In other words, patients must be given sufficient information to make decisions about the proposed treatments.

Competency to give consent

Competency is a key issue in any health-care context where judgments of competency are critical to deciding: whether a patient can or should decide and/or be permitted to decide for themselves; and the point at which another or others will need to, or should, decide for the patient. This issue becomes even more complicated when it is realised that a patient deemed to be 'rationally incompetent' can still be capable of making self-interested choices and, further, that even if these choices are deemed irrational, they may not necessarily be harmful (Wallace 2001).

From a legal perspective, a voluntary patient in a psychiatric unit must be considered to be like any other adult of sound mind (Wallace 2001). Neither the existence of a mental illness nor hospitalisation is sufficient grounds to deny an individual's right to make informed choices about their care. It is only when a patient is involuntary that their refusal to consent to treatment can be overridden. However, whether a person can give consent should be determined individually, regardless of whether the person has a mental illness (Brabbins et al. 1996). The hospitalised mental health patient may have been considered (at least temporarily) incompetent to care for themselves outside the inpatient setting. However, it does not automatically follow that the patient is generally incompetent to make any treatment or other decisions related to their care (Schafer 1985). Competence to make decisions may vary for one person across time and across tasks; that is, a person may be held competent to make one decision but not another. This recognition of limited competence creates a problem for those who work with people who experience mental illness, for it means that someone must judge which of these categories a person may reasonably belong to (Usher & Holmes 1997). Therefore, the mental health nurse must have a means by which competency is determined. Five tests of competency proposed by Roth et al. (1983, p 173) are:

- evidencing a choice
- 'reasonable' outcome of choice
- choice based on 'rational' reasons
- ability to understand
- actual understanding.

A sixth test of competency was proposed by Gunn (1994). This test is that of appreciation—that is, the patient is able not only to understand the information supplied but also to appreciate its implications and relevance to their situation.

Ongoing consent

A further process has been considered necessary to ensure that informed consent is current and that it involves the patient in a mutual decision-making process (Usher & Arthur 1998). The authors argue that consent should not

ETHICAL DILEMMA

If a voluntary patient is prescribed medication but refuses to take it, what should the nurse do? If the nurse uses persuasion or coercion to get the patient to take the medication, this could be said to rest on the principle of paternalism—that is, the nurse believes they know the best for the patient. Does this persuasion make the consent invalid? What do you think is the right thing to do in this situation?

What if the patient had an involuntary treatment order according to the Act? Do they have the right to refuse to take medications? This has already been addressed in the American cases of *Rennie vs Klein* (1983) and *Rogers vs Orkin* (1980), where it was held that involuntarily committed patients have a right to refuse medication under certain circumstances (Oriol & Oriol 1986). This situation may present an ethical dilemma for the nurse who, while believing the patient will benefit from the medication, realises that any form of coercion could make the consent invalid (Gallagher & Usher 1993).

be seen as static, but rather as an ongoing dynamic process in which the patient has a vital role. An ongoing consensual process keeps the patient involved at each step of the therapeutic process. It also keeps them up to date and informed about treatment decisions and, further, it requires that the patient's competency to make decisions and choices is not considered static.

CONCLUSION

This chapter has focused on the nursing skills that underpin the provision of therapeutic care for patients in the specialty of mental health nursing. In particular, the chapter has discussed selected communication and nursing skills surrounding patients at risk, issues of violence, aggression and seclusion, and ethico-legal considerations including consent. These are important skills for the nurse to develop when working with people who have a mental health problem, as each nurse–patient encounter is a unique interaction with the potential to heal and support. As stated, these nursing issues have acknowledged both the nurse and patient as people with strengths, vulnerabilities and opportunities. In other words, the interaction between nurse and patient is an opportunity for both to learn and grow.

EXERCISES FOR CLASS ENGAGEMENT

- The personal qualities of the nurse are a significant factor in determining the nature of the therapeutic relationship they form with their patients. Describe your own qualities and explain how they might assist or impede the development of therapeutic rapport. In a small group, outline ways you could develop therapeutic qualities.

- Identify the specific communication skills you will need in order to develop and maintain an effective therapeutic nurse–patient relationship. As a group, choose the three skills you believe are critical.

- Describe the elements of risk assessment. How can a comprehensive risk assessment assist in the management of persons identified as being at risk?

- Management of aggressive behaviour can be challenging for the nurse. Describe some effective verbal strategies that may be used to defuse the person's aggression before it escalates.

- Differentiate between the terms 'self-harm' and 'suicidal'. Outline the major nursing issues and strategies for the person who is self-harming, and the person who is suicidal. What beliefs do you hold concerning people who self-harm and people who are suicidal? How can you manage these in order to provide effective nursing care?

- Describe your understanding of the term 'informed consent'. What aspect(s) of informed consent may be affected when the person is mentally ill, and how can this/these be addressed ethically and legally? How might the issue of choice be relevant to informed consent?

REFERENCES

ABS 2000a, ABS Finds Suicide Highest in 25–44 Age Group. Commonwealth of Australia. Online: http://www.abs.gov.au.austats/abs@nsf/0/040B5B63A136A2B2CA2568B7001B06C, accessed 20 January 2003.

ABS 2000b, Australian Social Trends 2000: Health—Mortality and Morbidity: Suicide. Commonwealth of Australia. Online: http://www.abs.gov.au/ausstats/abs@nsf/94713ad445ff1425ca25682000192af2/2d9cecf2, accessed 20 January 2003.

Aquilina C 1991, Violence by psychiatric inpatients, *Medicine, Science and Law*, 31, pp 441–7.

Australian Health Ministers 1998, *Second National Mental Health Plan*, Mental Health Branch, Commonwealth Department of Health and Family Services, AGPS, Canberra.

Aveyard H 2002, Implied consent prior to nursing care procedures, *Journal of Advanced Nursing*, 39(2), pp 201–7.

Baradell JG 1985, Humanistic care of the patient in seclusion, *Journal of Psychosocial Nursing*, 23(2), pp 9–14.

Binder R & McCoy S 1983, A study of patients' attitudes towards placement in seclusion, *Hospital and Community Psychiatry*, 34, pp 1052–4.

Blair T 1991, Assaultive behaviour: does provocation begin in the front office?, *Journal of Psychosocial Nursing and Mental Health Services*, 29(5), pp 21–6.

Bowers L, Gournay K & Duffy D 2000, Suicide and self-harm in inpatient psychiatric units: a national survey of observation policies, *Journal of Advanced Nursing*, 32(2), pp 437–44.

Brabbins C, Butler J & Bentall R 1996, Consent to neuroleptic medication for schizophrenia: clinical, ethical and legal issues, *British Journal of Psychiatry*, 168, pp 540–4.

Cleary M, Jordan R & Horsfall J 2002, Ethical mental health nursing practice. In: Horsfall J (ed.), *Mental Health Nursing: Shaping Practice*, Central Sydney Area Health Service, Nursing Division.

Collins S & Cutcliffe JR 2003, Addressing hopelessness in people with suicidal ideation: building upon the therapeutic relationship utilizing a cognitive behavioural approach, *Journal of Psychiatric and Mental Health Nursing*, 10(2), pp 175–85.

Cutcliffe JR & Barker P 2002, Considering the care of the suicidal client and the case for 'engagement and inspiring hope' or 'observations', *Journal of Psychiatric and Mental Health Nursing*, 9, pp 611–21.

Delaney J, Cleary M, Jordan R & Horsfall J 2001, An exploratory investigation into the nursing management of aggression in acute psychiatric settings, *Journal of Psychiatric and Mental Health Nursing*, 8, pp 77–84.

Distasio CA 2002, Protecting yourself from violence in the workplace, *Nursing*, 32(6), pp 58–64.

Donat DC 2002, Impact of improved staffing on seclusion/restraint reliance in a public psychiatric hospital, *Psychiatric Rehabilitation Journal*, 25(4), pp 413–16.

Doyle M & Dolan M 2002, Violence risk assessment: combining actuarial and clinical information to structure clinical judgements for the formulation and management of risk, *Journal of Psychiatric and Mental Health Nursing*, 9, pp 649–57.

Duxbury J 2002, An evaluation of staff and patient views of and strategies employed to manage inpatient aggression and violence on one mental health unit: a pluralistic design, *Journal of Psychiatric and Mental Health Nursing*, 9, pp 325–37.

Ens IJ 1999, The lived experience of countertransference in psychiatric/ mental health nursing, *Archives of Psychiatric Nursing*, 6, pp 321–9.

Evans GW, Wil DL, Alligood MR & O'Neil M 1998, Empathy: a study of two types, *Issues in Mental Health Nursing*, 19(5), pp 453–61.

Farrell G & Dares G 1996, Seclusion or solitary confinement: therapeutic or punitive treatment?, *Australian and New Zealand Journal of Mental Health Nursing*, 5(4), pp 171–9.

Farrow T 2002, Owning their expertise: why nurses use 'no suicide contracts' rather than their own assessments, *International Journal of Mental Health Nursing*, 11(4), pp 214–19.

Fontaine KL 2003, *Mental Health Nursing* (2nd edn), Pearson Education, New Jersey.

Fry AJ, O'Riordan D, Turner M & Mills KL 2002, Survey of aggressive incidents experienced by community mental health staff, *International Journal of Mental Health Nursing*, 11(2), pp 112–20.

Gallagher F & Usher K 1993, Informed consent in mental health nursing, *Proceedings of the 20th Annual Convention of the Australian College of Mental Health Nurses*, Sydney.

Garnham P 2001, Understanding and dealing with anger, aggression and violence, *Nursing Standard*, 16(6), pp 37–42.

Gournay K & Bowers L 2000, Suicide and self-harm in inpatient psychiatric units: a study of nursing issues in 31 cases, *Journal of Advanced Nursing*, 32(1), pp 124–31.

Griffith L 2001, Does seclusion have a role to play in modern mental health nursing?, *British Journal of Nursing*, 10(10), pp 656–61.

Gunn M 1994, The meaning of incapacity, *Medical Law Review*, 2(1), pp 8–29.

Gutheil T 1978, Observations on the theoretical bases for seclusion of the psychiatric inpatient, *American Journal of Psychiatry*, 135(3), pp 325–8.

Hem MH & Heggen K 2003, Being professional and being human: one nurse's relationship with a psychiatric patient, *Journal of Advanced Nursing*, 43(1), pp 101–8.

Heyman E 1987, Seclusion, *Journal of Psychosocial Nursing*, 25(11), pp 9–12.

Holdsworth N, Belshaw D & Murray S 2001, Developing A&E nursing responses to people who deliberately self-harm: the provision and evaluation of a series of reflective workshops, *Journal of Psychiatric and Mental Health Nursing*, 8(5), pp 449–58.

Holmes CA 1998, *The Policies and Practices of Seclusion: An Advisory Report for the Western Sydney Area Mental Health Service*, Western Sydney Area Health Service, Parramatta, NSW.

Hopkins C 2002, 'But what about the really ill, poorly people?'. An ethnographic study into what it means to nurses on medical admissions units to have people who have harmed themselves as their patients, *Journal of Psychiatric and Mental Health Nursing*, 9(2), pp 147–54.

Horsfall J & Cleary M 2000, Discourse analysis of an 'observation levels' nursing policy, *Journal of Advanced Nursing*, 32(5), pp 1291–7.

Horsfall J, Cleary M & Jordan R 1999, *Towards Ethical Mental Health Nursing Practice*, Australian & New Zealand College of Mental Health Nurses Inc., South Australia.

Horsfall J, Stuhlmiller C & Champ S 2000, *Interpersonal Nursing for Mental Health*, McLennan & Petty, Sydney.

Hurlebaus AE & Link S 1997, The effects of an aggressive behaviour management program on nurses' levels of knowledge, confidence, and safety, *Journal of Nursing Staff Development*, 13(5), pp 260–5.

Kelly T, Simmons W & Gregory E 2002, Risk assessment and management: a community forensic mental health practice, *International Journal of Mental Health Nursing*, 11(4), pp 206–13.

Kneisl CR, Wilson HS & Trigoboff E 2004, *Contemporary Psychiatric–Mental Health Nursing*, Pearson Education, New Jersey.

Kunyk D & Olson JK 2001, Clarification of conceptualizations of empathy, *Journal of Advanced Nursing*, 35(3), pp 317–25.

Lanza ML 1988, Factors relevant to patient assault, *Issues in Mental Health Nursing*, 9(3), pp 239–57.

Lauder W, Reynolds W, Smith A & Sharkey S 2002, A comparison of therapeutic commitment, role support, role competency and empathy in three cohorts of nursing students, *Journal of Psychiatric and Mental Health Nursing*, 9(4), pp 483–91.

Linaker OM & Busch-Iversen H 1995, Predictors of imminent violence in psychiatric inpatients, *Acta Psychiatrica Scandinavica*, 92(4), pp 250–4.

Littrell P & Littrell S 1998, Current understanding of violence and aggression: assessment and treatment, *Journal of Advanced Nursing*, 41(2), pp 154–61.

Martin G 2002, Self-injury in context, *Ausinetter*, 16(3), p 9.

Martinez RJ, Grimm M & Adamson M 1999, From the other side of the door: patient views on seclusion, *Journal of Psychosocial and Mental Health Nursing*, 37(3), pp 13–22.

Martinson D 2002, What is self-injury?, *Ausinetter*, 16(3), p 8.

McAllister MM 2001, In harm's way: a postmodern narrative inquiry, *Journal of Psychiatric and Mental Health Nursing*, 8(5), pp 391–7.

McAllister MM & Estefan A 2002, Principles and strategies for teaching therapeutic responses to self-harm, *Journal of Psychiatric and Mental Health Nursing*, 9(5), pp 573–83.

McAllister MM, Creedy D, Moyle W & Farrugia C 2002a, Nurses' attitudes towards clients who self-harm, *Journal of Advanced Nursing*, 40(5), pp 578–86.

McAllister MM, Creedy D, Moyle W & Farrugia C 2002b, Study of Queensland emergency department nurses' actions and formal and informal procedures for clients who self-harm, *International Journal of Mental Health Nursing*, 8(4), pp 184–90.

McKinlay A, Couston M & Cowan S 2001, Nurses' behavioural intentions towards self-poisoning patients: a theory of reasoned action, comparison of attitudes and subjective norms as predictive variables, *Journal of Advanced Nursing*, 34(1), pp 107–16.

McLaughlin C 1999, An exploration of psychiatric nurses' and patients' opinions regarding inpatient care for suicidal patients, *Journal of Advanced Nursing*, 29(5), pp 1042–51.

Meehan T 1997, Nurse researchers investigate effect of seclusion on mentally ill, *Nursing Review*, February, Royal College of Nursing.

Meehan T, Vermeer C & Windsor C 2000, Patients' perceptions of seclusion: a qualitative investigation, *Journal of Advanced Nursing*, 31(2), pp 370–7.

Morrison EF 1998, The culture of caregiving and aggression in psychiatric settings, *Archives of Psychiatric Nursing*, XII, pp 21–31.

Motyka M, Motyka H & Wsolek R 1997, Elements of psychological support in nursing care, *Journal of Advanced Nursing*, 26(5), 909–12.

Muir-Cochrane E 1995, An exploration of ethical issues associated with the seclusion of psychiatric patients, *Collegian*, 2(3), pp 14–20.

Muir-Cochrane E 1996, An investigation into nurses' perceptions of secluding patients on closed psychiatric wards, *Journal of Advanced Nursing*, 23(3), pp 555–63.

Muir-Cochrane E & Holmes CA 2001, Legal and ethical aspects of seclusion: an Australian perspective, *Journal of Psychiatric and Mental Health Nursing*, 8(6), pp 501–6.

Muir-Cochrane E, Holmes C & Walton J 2002, Law and policy in relation to the use of seclusion in psychiatric hospitals in Australia and New Zealand, *Contemporary Nurse*, 13(2/3), pp 136–45.

Munhall PL 1991, Institutional review of qualitative research proposals: a task of no small consequence. In: Morse JM (ed.), *Qualitative Nursing Research: A Contemporary Dialogue*, Sage, Mewbury Park, California, pp 258–71.

New Zealand Health Information Service 2003, Health Statistics: Suicide—all ages. Online: http://www.nzhis.govt.nz/stats/suicidefacts1.html, accessed 18 August 2003, last updated 14 May 2003.

Nijman HL, Camp JMLG, Ravelli DP & Merckelbach HLGJ 1999, A tentative model of aggression on inpatient psychiatric wards, *Psychiatric Services*, 50(6), pp 832–4.

Norris M & Kennedy C 1992, The view from within: how patients perceive the seclusion process, *Journal of Psychosocial and Mental Health Nursing*, 30(3), pp 7–13.

O'Kelly G 1998, Countertransference in the nurse–patient relationship: a review of the literature, *Journal of Advanced Nursing*, 28(2), pp 391–7.

Oriol MD & Oriol RD 1986, Involuntary commitment and the right to refuse medication, *Journal of Psychosocial Nursing*, 24(11), pp 15–20.

Owen C, Tarantello C, Jones M & Tennant C 1998, Violence and aggression in psychiatric units, *Psychiatric Services*, 49(11), pp 1452–7.

Pearson L 2001, The clinician–patient experience: understanding transference and countertransference, *Nurse Practitioner*, 26(6), pp 8–11.

Pearson M, Wilmot E & Padi M 1986, A study of violent behaviour amongst inpatients in a psychiatric hospital, *British Journal of Psychiatry*, 149(2), pp 232–5.

Pirkis J, Francis C, Warwick Blood R, Burgess P, Morley B, Stewart A et al. 2002, Reporting of suicide in the Australian media, *Australian and New Zealand Journal of Psychiatry*, 36(2), pp 190–7.

Plutchik R, Karasu T, Conte H, Siegel B & Jerrett I 1978, Toward a rationale for the seclusion process, *Journal of Nervous and Mental Disease*, 166(8), pp 571–9.

Queensland Health 2000, Suicidality Assessment Policy: Logan-Beaudesert Health Service District Manual. Online: http://10.109.65.254/qheps/divisions/mental/policies/00062.pdf, accessed 21 January 2003.

Quintal SA 2002, Violence against psychiatric nurses: An untreated epidemic?, *Journal of Psychosocial and Mental Health Services*, 40(1), pp 46–55.

Rawlins RP, Williams SR & Beck CK (eds) 1993, *Mental Health–Psychiatric Nursing: A Holistic Life-Cycle Approach* (3rd edn), Mosby-Year Book, St Louis.

Reynolds WJ & Scott B 2000, Do nurses and other professional helpers normally display much empathy?, *Journal of Advanced Nursing*, 31(1), pp 226–34.

Roth LH, Meisel A & Lidz CW 1983, Tests of competency to consent to treatment. In: Gorovitz S, Macklin R, Jameton AL, O'Connor JM & Sherwin A (eds), *Moral Problems in Medicine* (2nd edn), Prentice Hall, Englewood Cliffs, New Jersey, pp 172–9 (reprinted from *American Journal of Psychiatry*, 134(4), pp 279–84).

Samuelsson M, Wiklander M, Asberg M & Saveman BI 2000, Psychiatric care as seen by the attempted suicide patient, *Journal of Advanced Nursing*, 32(3), pp 635–43.

Schafer A 1985, The right of institutionalized psychiatric patients to refuse treatment, *Canada's Mental Health*, 33(3), pp 12–16.

Shepherd M & Lavender T 1999, Putting aggression into context: an investigation into contextual factors influencing the rate of aggressive incidents in a psychiatric hospital, *Journal of Mental Health*, 8(2), pp 159–70.

Slaven J & Kisely S 2002, Staff perceptions of care for deliberate self-harm patients in rural Western Australia: a qualitative study, *Australian Journal of Rural Health*, 10(5), pp 233–8.

Smith SE 2002, Perceptions of service provision for clients who self-injure in the absence of expressed suicidal intent, *Journal of Psychiatric and Mental Health Nursing*, 9(5), pp 595–601.

Soliday SM 1985, A comparison of patient and staff attitudes toward seclusion, *Journal of Nervous and Mental Disease*, 173(5), pp 282–6.

Stein-Parbury J 2000, *Patient and Person: Developing Interpersonal Skills in Nursing* (2nd edn), Harcourt, Sydney.

Street A & Walsh C 1998, Nursing assessments in New Zealand mental health, *Journal of Advanced Nursing*, 27(3), pp 553–9.

Talseth A-G, Jacobsson L & Norberg A 2001, The meaning of suicidal psychiatric inpatients' experiences of being treated by physicians, *Journal of Advanced Nursing*, 34(1), pp 96–106

Tardiff K 1998, Prediction of violence in patients, *Journal of Practical Psychiatry and Behavioural Health*, 4(1), p 12.

Terpstra Tammy L, Terpstra Terry L, Pettee EJ & Hunter M 2001, Nursing staff's attitudes toward seclusions and restraint, *Journal of Psychosocial Nursing and Mental Health Services*, 39(5), pp 20–8.

Tooke SK & Brown JS 1992, Perceptions of seclusion: comparing patient and staff reactions, *Journal of Psychosocial Nursing and Mental Health Services*, 30(8), pp 23–6.

Treatment Protocol Project 2000, *Management of Mental Disorders* (3rd edn), World Health Organization Collaborating Centre for Mental Health and Substance Abuse, Sydney.

Turnbull J & Patterson B 1999, *Aggression and Violence*, Macmillan, London.

Usher K & Arthur D 1998, Process consent: a model for enhancing informed consent in mental health nursing, *Journal of Advanced Nursing*, 27(4), pp 692–7.

Usher K & Holmes C 1997, Ethical aspects of phenomenological research with mentally ill people, *Nursing Ethics*, 4(1), pp 49–56.

Vanderslott J 1998, A study of violence towards staff by patients in an NHS Trust hospital, *Journal of Psychiatric and Mental Health Nursing*, 5(4), pp 291–8.

Wallace M 2001, *Health Care and the Law: A Guide for Nurses* (3rd edn), Law Book, Sydney.

Whitehead L & Royles M 2002, Deliberate self-harm: assessment and treatment interventions. In: Regel S & Roberts D (eds), *Mental Health Liaison: A Handbook for Nurses and Health Professionals*, Bailliere Tindall, London.

Whittington R & Wykes T 1994, An observation of associations between nurse behaviour and violence in psychiatric hospitals, *Journal of Psychiatric and Mental Health Nursing*, 1, pp 85–92.

Wynaden D, Chapman R, McGowan S, Holmes C, Ash P & Boschman A 2002, Through the eye of the beholder: to seclude or not to seclude, *International Journal of Mental Health Nursing*, 11, pp 260–8.

Yegdich T 1999, On the phenomenology of empathy in nursing: empathy or sympathy?, *Journal of Advanced Nursing*, 30(1), pp 83–93.

Yudofsky S, Silver J, Jackson W, Endicott J & Williams D 1986, The overt aggression scale for the objective rating of verbal and physical aggression, *American Journal of Psychiatry*, 143(1), pp 35–9.

Therapeutic Interventions

Christine Palmer

23

KEY POINTS

- Mental health nurses use a range of therapeutic interventions when they work with people who have mental health problems and/or serious mental illnesses.
- You will be more therapeutic in a mental health context if you understand yourself.
- Being able to identify the stressors in your life will enable you to help others with their stress.
- Relaxation skills and assertiveness skills can be learned and are useful for all nurses.
- Risk assessment and crisis intervention strategies are used in a range of environments or settings.
- Psychotherapies include individual psychotherapy, planned short-term psychotherapy, motivational interviewing, cognitive behavioural therapy and dialectical behaviour therapy.
- Behaviour is learned, and so it can be unlearned through behaviour therapy.
- Group therapy is a cost-effective and therapeutic way to treat larger numbers of people at the same time.
- Family therapy is an intervention that works to effect change in the family system.
- Psychoeducation is a family-oriented intervention designed to empower and engage families in the care of the mentally ill.
- Client-centred ideas of recovery indicate that people will not engage with rehabilitation programs unless they have hope for a better life.
- Social skills training helps people to learn or re-learn social skills.
- Case management is a client-centred approach to working with people in the community in which the key worker assists the client to live in the community as independently as possible.
- Electroconvulsive therapy is an intervention with attendant nursing responsibilities.

KEY TERMS

- activity groups
- assertiveness skills
- behaviour therapy
- case management
- cognitive behavioural therapy
- crisis intervention
- dialectical behaviour therapy
- electroconvulsive therapy
- family therapy
- group therapy
- individual psychotherapy
- instillation of hope
- interviewing
- motivational interviewing
- planned short-term psychotherapy
- psychoeducation
- psychosocial rehabilitation
- psychotherapy
- relaxation skills
- risk assessment
- social skills training
- stress management
- telephone counselling

LEARNING OUTCOMES

The material in this chapter will assist you to:
- identify stressors and learn strategies for managing stress
- understand the implications of accurate risk assessment and crisis intervention
- differentiate between aggressive, passive and assertive response styles
- recognise fundamental concepts related to a range of psychotherapeutic intervention strategies such as individual psychotherapy, planned short-term psychotherapy, motivational interviewing, cognitive behavioural therapy and dialectical behaviour therapy
- describe how behaviour is learned, maintained and extinguished
- recognise the therapeutic factors as they occur within therapy and activity groups
- understand family-centred approaches to treatment
- realise how psychosocial rehabilitation contributes to recovery from mental illness
- consider how nurses can influence the recovery of people with enduring mental health problems
- understand how working alongside or with the client contributes to better outcomes for the client
- consider the ethical issues related to electroconvulsive therapy.

client. Changing destructive patterns of substance abuse and dependence does not happen all at once. Motivated by relevant and meaningful goals, the change occurs progressively (Finnell 2003). As relapse is viewed as part of the process of change, a return to earlier stages in the process is considered normal.

In addition to the spirit of MI, five principles underpin the model, as outlined by Miller et al. (1992).

- *Avoid argumentation*—there should not be any confrontation or arguing with the client. This will only result in the client returning with argumentation and withdrawing from the therapy. If the client were to deny having a problem with alcohol, despite the overwhelming evidence, the therapist would not argue the evidence with the client.
- *Express empathy*—this is considered critical to the approach. Expression of empathy gives clients the message that they are heard and understood. This is important because it is unlikely to have occurred within the family or the community. This leads to clients being more open to therapy and to sharing their stories. Clients are also more likely to be open to the gentle challenges that the therapist will make about their beliefs about substance use. Change occurs because clients are more comfortable in working with their ambivalence.
- *Support self-efficacy*—supporting a person's sense of self-efficacy contributes to the client's belief that change is possible. Self-efficacy is supported through acknowledging the person's past ability to change and by supporting the person to choose his or her own plan for change. Observing others who have made changes in their lives is also a powerful motivator for change.
- *Roll with resistance*—resistance from the client is considered normal and not to be contested. The counsellor rolls with the resistance by encouraging the client to find his or her own solutions to problems. Because there is no differentiation between the therapist and client, there is nothing for the client to fight against. The counsellor might offer new perspectives, but they are not imposed on the client.
- *Develop discrepancy*—this involves helping clients to see the discrepancies between what they hope to achieve (their goals) and how they are currently behaving. Recognising that their actions are leading them away from rather than toward the achievement of their important goals provides the motivation for change.

Motivational interviewing has been found to be very effective, particularly where a person's suffering from the effects of the addiction has increased, as it does over time. People have changed their patterns of substance dependence after as little as one to two hours of MI. And a single session of MI prior to embarking on a rehabilitation program has been found to double the chances of a person's abstinence continuing three months later (Miller 1998). And this is possible because someone has

actively listened to the client's problems, helped the client to acknowledge and resolve ambivalence and supported them in achieving the goal of a changed life.

Cognitive behavioural therapy

Cognitive behavioural therapy (CBT) grew out of behavioural therapy but is considered a planned short-term psychotherapeutic technique. It is usually conducted over around 16–20 sessions. Its premise is that there is an interrelationship between thoughts, feelings, behaviour, biology and the environment. That is, each factor influences the others. This has been understood for centuries. The Roman emperor Marcus Aurelius wrote:

If some external object distresses you, it is not the object itself but your judgement of it which causes pain. It is up to you to change your judgement. If it is your behaviour which troubles you, who stops you from changing it?

(Blackburn & Davidson 1990, p 16)

In the cognitive model, our thoughts are classified into three layers. The outer layer holds our automatic thoughts, the middle layer contains the intermediate beliefs or underlying assumptions, and the inner layer stores our core beliefs. The core beliefs develop during childhood as a result of experience and the influence of significant others. Cognitive behavioural therapy aims to cause change at each of these levels. The goal of treatment is to bring into conscious awareness the client's negative automatic thoughts, which are specific to certain situations, and the person's underlying assumptions, and to challenge them.

We all have negative automatic thoughts that are present when we are awake. They are responsible for many of our behaviours. An example of a negative automatic thought is: 'I can't cope'. This leads to the person behaving in a helpless way. The underlying assumption might be: 'If I can't work this out, then I'm no good'. The core belief for this person might be: 'I'm a failure'. The negative automatic thoughts are the most superficial and are more likely to be acknowledged. Once challenged, the client learns to develop new or revised beliefs. These are considered during therapy and practised in vivo (in real life).

Assessment for suitability to engage with the CBT model is carried out initially. This assessment will determine whether the client has the motivation to change and whether he or she has the ability to engage and to problem-solve. The model is prescriptive—that is, there is a distinct process for engaging in therapy with the client. Regardless of the person's difficulties, the same specific techniques and strategies central to the model are used. These include Socratic questioning (Calvert & Palmer 2003) and homework, such as charting behaviours and mood using a visual analogue scale, and keeping automatic thought records. Keeping an automatic thought record alerts the client to the negative automatic thoughts that continue to affect their feelings and behaviours, ultimately maintaining mental health problems. Homework is set after each session to ensure that the client remains motivated and learns the skills to take over his or her own therapy.

Initially, clients are given an overview of CBT and shown how the five-part model (illustrated in Figure 23.1) will be used to identify the more serious problems. Clients are asked to identify a situation that caused a strong negative emotional response. Then clients identify their specific emotional responses for that situation as well as their cognitions, physical responses and behaviours. The fifth aspect of the model, the environment, provides the context within which these responses occurred, including culture and personal history. Organising the person's experiences into the categories of thoughts, feelings, behaviour and physical responses is fundamental to CBT (Dattilio & Padesky 1990).

An example of this might be if an employee, 'Jane', received negative feedback about her work performance from her employer and had a strong emotional response. Figure 23.1 shows a description of the emotions, thoughts, actions and physical responses that occurred within the work environment for Jane during this scenario.

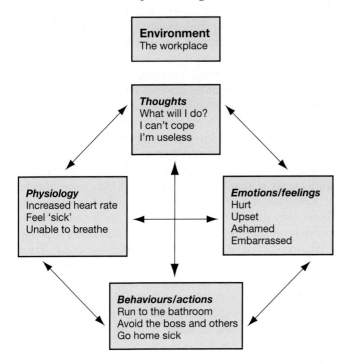

Figure 23.1 The five-part model for problem identification using cognitive behavioural therapy (adapted from Padesky CA & Mooney KA 1990, Presenting the cognitive model to clients, *International Cognitive Therapy Newsletter*, 6, pp 6–7)

The therapeutic relationship in CBT is collaborative. The client is an active participant in the process and is responsible for learning new ways of responding. There is also an emphasis on empiricism, which is the gathering of data to provide evidence to challenge current beliefs.

Clients are taught to identify their dysfunctional thoughts and the therapist then tests the validity of those beliefs. For example, in the situation described above and in Figure 23.1, Jane believes that everyone thinks she is stupid. The therapist would ask Jane for evidence of this. It is most unlikely that Jane would have any evidence. Ultimately clients learn to evaluate their own thoughts and manage their own responses (Dattilio & Padesky 1990).

Dialectical behaviour therapy

Dialectical behaviour therapy (DBT) was developed by Marsha Linehan and first published in 1993. It is a therapeutic technique designed specifically to treat people with borderline personality disorder, particularly those with chronic parasuicidal behaviours (self-harming without the intention to kill oneself). It is highly structured, goal-oriented and time-limited and is based on a cognitive behavioural approach.

The client's involvement in DBT is voluntary. Indeed, the client needs to be committed to work towards the behaviour change that is necessary to alter her or his lifestyle and subsequent difficulties. This is known as the pre-treatment phase of DBT. Without commitment from the client, DBT will not proceed. In particular, 'the client must agree to work on decreasing parasuicidal behaviours and interpersonal styles that interfere with therapy and on increasing behavioural skills' (Swales, Heard & Williams 2000, p 10). The core intervention strategies involved are 'validation' and 'problem solving'. The main work is carried out in weekly individual therapy sessions that focus on targeted behaviours. The therapist accepts the client as a valid human being while at the same time expecting change. The most important behaviour to be addressed is the parasuicidal behaviour. Once this is brought under control, other issues are addressed.

The group therapy aspect of DBT occurs concurrently with individual therapy and involves skills training. The person with borderline personality disorder has not developed effective coping skills, so learning how to solve problems effectively is very important. There are four groups of skills, or modules (Linehan 1993):

1 core mindfulness skills (derived from Buddhist meditation)

2 interpersonal effectiveness skills

3 emotion modulation skills

4 distress tolerance skills.

As skills are learned in the group sessions they are applied in the real world and also addressed in individual counselling sessions. The therapist acts as coach to support the use of these new skills as they are learned, both within sessions and over the telephone as problems arise (Wolpow 2000). It is the combination of acceptance or validation and active change or problem solving that brings about the alteration in personality style that enables these clients to lead more fulfilling lives.

Before considering DBT, it is important to consider what borderline personality disorder means (see also Ch 16), especially in the context of DBT. People with borderline personality disorder are very difficult to work with because of their personality style, which often develops as the result of a very challenging childhood. According to Linehan (1993), the experiences and responses of the child who develops borderline personality disorder were 'invalidated' or disqualified by the significant others around the child. This means that the child's experiences were not acknowledged or accepted as real. Sexual abuse is considered the ultimate form of invalidation and is frequently an aspect of the history of the person with borderline personality disorder. At the same time, Linehan argues that there exists a biological predisposition within the autonomic nervous system to react poorly to stress. It is important to note that the majority of people who are given the diagnosis of borderline personality disorder are women.

The person with borderline personality disorder classically has a dysfunctional lifestyle and staggers from one crisis to the next. Linehan points out that these clients are unable to regulate their emotions (have extreme emotional reactions to situations), have chaotic interpersonal relationships, have a disturbed sense of self, and are unable to regulate their thoughts and behaviours. They lack problem-solving skills and so respond to life haphazardly. They frequently engage in self-damaging behaviours such as substance abuse, promiscuity and overeating, but the most common behaviour is self-mutilation. According to the DBT approach, the diagnosis relates to a certain pattern of behaviours and so, once these behaviours cease, the diagnosis also no longer exists (Swales et al. 2000).

Originally DBT was designed as an individual therapy approach combined with group skills training, telephone contact between sessions and a strong emphasis on therapists also receiving DBT from each other. Therapist consultation is fundamental due to the risk of therapist burnout when working so intensively with clients with such challenging patterns of behaviour. Aspects of DBT can now be applied in a range of settings using the principles of treatment rather than these specific modes (Wolpow 2000), and for a range of conditions (Linehan et al. 1999). However, success is determined by the quality of the client–therapist relationship. In particular, the client learns that the needs of both the therapist and self are important.

BEHAVIOUR THERAPY

The behavioural model developed from the early work of Pavlov at the turn of the nineteenth century and Skinner during the early twentieth century. Pavlov's early experiments involving dogs showed that involuntary behaviours can be conditioned to occur (classical conditioning) and that, ultimately, this learned response can be unlearned (extinguished). It is normal for salivation to occur in response to the presentation of food, but it is not normal for salivation to occur at the sound of a tuning fork. Pavlov paired the presentation of food with the sound of a tuning fork until eventually salivation occurred at the sound of the tuning fork without the presence of food. The dogs had been conditioned to salivate at the sound of the tuning fork. Persistent sounding of the tuning fork without the presentation of food eventually led to extinction of this learned response—that is, the dogs no longer salivated at the sound of the tuning fork.

CRITICAL THINKING CHALLENGE 23.4

What are some of your conditioned responses? For example, consider how the sound of the school bell at the end of the day results in a lightening in mood for both students and teachers!

Skinner later developed the early work of Thorndike (1911, cited in Barker & Fraser 1985). He called this *operant conditioning* and showed that behaviours can be learned and unlearned through processes of positive and negative reinforcement. That is, behaviours can be strengthened through positive reinforcement or the presentation of rewards, and weakened through negative reinforcement involving the removal of rewards. Removing a reinforcer to a behaviour, such as walking away from the child having a temper tantrum, results in extinction of the temper tantrum behaviour. Be aware, though, that initially ignoring a behaviour will result in an increase in that behaviour before it begins to subside.

Punishment can also be used to change behaviour. When defined in behavioural terms, punishment refers to procedures designed to suppress behaviours, not the infliction of physical or psychological pain or harm. Punishment decreases the strength of certain behaviours rather than eliminating them (Sundel & Sundel 1993). Punishment can involve applying a punishing stimulus immediately after the unwanted behaviour is performed. An example of this is when the teacher humiliates a student verbally for arriving late to class. Alternatively, punishment might involve the removal of a positive reinforcer. Examples of this include a child being placed in time out following a temper tantrum, or a client with anorexia who loses weight or doesn't gain weight according to a prescribed schedule, losing the privilege of calling their friends for 48 hours. To be effective, the punisher needs to be applied consistently; that is, each time the behaviour presents, the punisher is applied. Punishment is most effective when applied immediately after the undesirable behaviour. It is also important to specify alternative behaviours that are more appropriate (Sundel & Sundel 1993).

Behaviour therapy has been found to be particularly useful in explaining the development of anxieties and fears and the ways in which these are generalised to a range of stimuli. For example, a person who has a fear of spiders may well find that the fear generalises to a range of crawling insects as well as toys and pictures of spiders. The events that occur prior to or after behaviours determine whether those behaviours will be learned, maintained or changed. For example, the presence of a spider will result in heightened anxiety. Moving away from the spider causes the anxiety to subside. Therefore, the person learns that spiders are to be feared and to avoid spiders. Unfortunately, this will result in avoidance of environments that have the potential to contain spiders, causing constriction of the person's social world.

It is important to point out that in the case study below, George is not aware that his avoidance of anxiety-provoking situations actually increases his anxiety. He would not accept that staying within an anxiety-provoking situation is helpful in managing his anxiety and in preventing future panic attacks. George believes that he will 'freak out' and that this would be the most awful outcome for him. He would feel vulnerable and that he might never get back home. Combined with education, staying with George and verbally supporting him to stay within the anxiety-provoking situation will show him that his most feared outcome will not be realised. Once he recognises that avoidance only worsens the situation and that he *can* cope with his anxiety and that terrible things won't happen to him, he can begin to make changes to his behaviour.

The target behaviour, the behaviour we wish to change, is the social isolation that George suffers as a result of his avoidance of anxiety-provoking situations. It is important to point out that 'the target behaviour is the behaviour to be observed and measured; it is the focus of modification' (Sundel & Sundel 1993, p 4). It can be the behaviour we want to increase (e.g. acceptable or appropriate social behaviour), or the behaviour we want to minimise (e.g. lying on the bed all day). George has hopes and goals that include working and living in a small beachside community. In order to achieve these goals, George needs to be able to cope with driving a vehicle or using public transport, meeting new people, and widening his social world without fear of losing control.

Prior to working with George and his problems, the nurse would need to carry out a behavioural assessment. This requires George to record the triggers, both internal and external to his anxiety, and to identify his physical, cognitive, emotional and behavioural responses. The frequency and duration of anxiety responses would also need to be recorded. This helps to identify specific cues to certain behaviours and also to determine improvement or deterioration. Treatment should address both his behavioural (e.g. social avoidance) and cognitive responses (e.g. believing that he will lose control and perhaps his life). This is because his beliefs continue to limit his ability to act.

After determining what causes and maintains certain behaviours, it is possible to develop a treatment plan together that specifies goals, what will need to be done to achieve those goals, how goal achievement will be measured, and a timeline for goal achievement. For example, George may set as his goal: being able to travel into the city in a car. A plan involving systematically working from sitting in a stationary car to driving short distances in the car, to travelling into the city, will need to be laid out. The plan will also need to indicate how many weeks or months this process will take.

CASE STUDY

George suffers from schizophrenia but is more disadvantaged by his social and panic anxiety (see Ch 17). Using Truax's (2002) model for behavioural case conceptualisation, the reinforcers and punishments that cause his anxieties to occur and persist, resulting in increasing social isolation, are:

- *Positive reinforcement*—an increase in a consequence leads to an increased probability that panic attacks will happen in the future. For example, George's family members carry out his weekly grocery shopping and manage his finances and bill paying for him. This reinforcement increases the likelihood of George not engaging in these behaviours and increases the probability of panic attacks occurring should he engage in these behaviours.
- *Negative reinforcement*—a decrease in an uncomfortable or aversive consequence or outcome leads to increased avoidance of anxiety-provoking situations in the future. When George stays at home rather than engaging in social situations or the use of public transport, it reduces his anxiety, thereby increasing his avoidance of these anxiety-provoking situations.
- *Positive punishment*—an increase in a negative consequence leads to decreased engagement in anxiety-provoking situations in the future. For example, when George goes for long walks far from his home but within his suburb, his anxiety increases because he fears 'freaking out'. He has now limited his walks to a small radius from his home, and so his social world is shrinking even further.
- *Negative punishment*—a decrease in a consequence leads to a decreased probability that he will stay in anxiety-provoking situations in the future. For example, George is unable to use positive self-talk to manage his anxiety and is therefore unable to stay in anxiety-provoking situations. He is so certain that he will 'freak out' that he no longer puts himself at risk.

GROUP THERAPY

Group therapy involves the engagement of two or more people in therapy at the same time. This mode of therapy is more cost effective than individual therapies because more people can be treated at once. Group counselling is also more efficient if the group is composed of people with similar problems (the homogeneous group)—for example, a psychoeducational group for families of people with schizophrenia. However, efficiency and cost effectiveness are not the most important reasons for engaging people in group therapy. There are immense benefits for clients who come together with others who experience the same or similar difficulties. Often the benefits are derived from interactions with others in the group rather than through the therapeutic efforts of the counsellor (Byrne & Byrne 1996).

There are as many approaches that can be taken in group therapy as there are for individual therapy (for example, see Cowan & Brunero (1997) for a nurse-led group in Australia). Group therapy provides an opportunity for people to explore their thoughts, feelings and behaviours and the impact they have on others. This is achieved through facilitation by the therapist/nurse therapist and through feedback from the other group members. Ultimately, learning occurs about relating to others. One thing that is certain is that almost everyone benefits from healthy interpersonal relationships. We are all social beings and we thrive on relating to others. An important outcome of any type of group is the relationships developed with others and the opportunity to learn better or more effective ways of relating.

Therapeutic groups can be divided into two main categories: general-purpose groups and problem-focused groups (Earley 2000). Addressing specific issues such as grief, sexual abuse or alcohol abuse is the goal of problem-focused groups. They aim to impart information and provide support to people in crisis and are consequently time-limited. General-purpose groups attempt to facilitate deeper character change by addressing problems that arise from the interpersonal processes that occur in groups (Earley 2000). This involves the expression of transference and counter-transference as early relationships and customary interpersonal difficulties are re-enacted in the group with other group members. These processes occur unconsciously and interactions within the group provide opportunities for other group members or the therapist to gently bring to the person's awareness what has been happening.

Yalom (1995) determined that there are eleven curative or therapeutic factors that occur in psychotherapy groups. When a psychotherapeutic group is working effectively, these curative factors are operating and group members are benefiting from them. The factors work interdependently—that is, they don't occur or function separately but interrelate with each other. The same factors operate in every type of group but their interplay and importance can vary widely from group to group. In addition, people from within the same group can benefit from differing clusters of therapeutic factors. These factors are:

- *Instillation of hope*: people are inspired by the improvements that others have made and the group provides opportunity for the therapist to point out the improvements people have made.
- *Universality*: entering a group enables people to see that they are not alone in their struggles. Hearing that others have the same difficulties is reassuring because people realise that their problems are not beyond solving.
- *Imparting information*: this might include learning about their illness or how to cope. Education might be an explicit or implicit part of the group.
- *Altruism*: group members get back from giving to and supporting others. Finding that they are valuable to others boosts self-esteem.
- *Corrective recapitulation of the family group*: the therapy group represents the family in many ways. This provides the opportunity to act out old family relationships and to recognise how earlier relationships continue to be acted out in current relationships.
- *Development of socialising techniques*: learning social skills might be an explicit part of the group or it may be more indirect, as people observe the behaviour of others.
- *Imitative behaviour*: group therapists influence the communication patterns in members by modelling certain behaviours such as self-disclosure or support.
- *Interpersonal learning*: the group becomes a social microcosm so that members are able to re-enact interpersonal behaviours typical of their lives outside the group. Feedback from others enables a person to see that their behaviours are responsible for interpersonal difficulties.
- *Group cohesiveness*: cohesiveness is essential for the other curative factors to operate. It involves members feeling warmth and comfort in the group and feeling that they belong and are accepted and supported by others.
- *Catharsis*: this is the expression and mutual working through of strong emotions that have not been previously expressed. The group provides a safe environment for this to happen. Therefore, catharsis will only occur once group cohesiveness develops.
- *Existential factors*: these are the elements in the group process that help members to develop an understanding of their individual existences. This is more likely to occur in groups where there is a focus on thinking, talking and feeling.

Some of these factors are self-evident, while others are more subtle and take an understanding of psychotherapy to enable their facilitation and expression. Nevertheless, when setting up a group therapy program, it is important to plan it well (Sharry 2001) and to consider the expectations or goals you have for the group. If you are the therapist you will need to decide whether it will be a closed group—that is, one that has a set number of members for a set period of time—or an open group. An open group allows different membership each time the group meets and the group membership at each session will determine to some extent the direction the group takes. Whichever type of group you facilitate, there will be a specific process of coming together or initial engagement, reaction and resistance to working, developing trust, working through issues, and termination or closure (Fehr 1999). In an open group, trust may take longer to develop as membership fluctuates.

Activity groups
Activity groups grew out of the perceived need to occupy people during the long hospital stays of the past. Ultimately, activity groups became a part of psychosocial rehabilitation programs and are also often part of an organised therapy program in psychiatric inpatient units today. While the task of organising an activity program has been taken on largely by occupational therapists, this role was historically a nursing responsibility. Given the amount of time that nurses spend with clients, nurses need to once again embrace this responsibility. Activity groups involve gathering together a group of people interested in a particular activity or those who need to develop skills in a particular area.

Examples of activity groups include cooking skills, gardening, art, walking, newspaper discussion, reminiscence and games and sporting groups. Many inpatient psychiatric units hold daily 'community meetings' that are designed to engage clients in daily planning and organisation. Originally developed to help construct a therapeutic milieu—that is, a physical and emotional ward environment that is therapeutic and empowering for clients—these community groups might also be viewed as activity groups in some respects. Despite the perception

that activity groups are not particularly challenging and that they only serve the purpose of keeping people occupied, many of Yalom's curative factors outlined above can operate. Not least of these are the development of socialising techniques and imitative behaviour.

FAMILY THERAPY
Family therapy developed in the 1950s out of the belief that the family was responsible for causing schizophrenia. In particular it was believed that certain communication styles within families were responsible for causing the illness (the skewed and schismatic families). A further belief centred on the communication style of the mother, the so-called schizophrenogenic mother. Although these ideas have long since been rejected, a group of interventions known as family therapy had been born (Goldenberg & Goldenberg 2000). Family therapy shifted the focus on therapy directed at unconscious material (psychotherapy) 'to a focus on the interpersonal process—that is, how family members interact with each other' (Kadis & McClendon 1998, p 6).

Family therapy is an approach to treatment that is based on the fundamental premise that when a person has a problem, it usually involves the whole family (Mellor, Storer & Firth 2000). Family interactions might be causing the problem or prolonging the problem for the identified client, or perhaps the problem or behaviours of the client are affecting other members of the family. Family therapists aim to effect change in the entire family system. While family therapy usually involves multiple family members, they need not be the same family members each time, or therapy might involve a single family member (Meech & Wood 2000).

Even when therapy involves a single individual, its impact will be experienced by the wider family. This might be demonstrated through an improvement in family functioning and/or through the alleviation of symptoms (Mellor et al. 2000). Unlike individual therapists who

NURSE'S STORY

I facilitate a discharge planning group in an acute inpatient setting. This is an open group due to the nature of the rapid turnover of clients in this setting. While I might plan for a reasonably structured group with specific goals, the members inevitably determine the direction of the group. I always begin with introductions and give each person an opportunity to identify short- and long-term goals. I also attempt to discuss any concerns about medications, accommodation, family relationships, employment and money management. The acuity of the mental health problems of the group members will dictate the issues addressed, however. For example, a group member who has a bipolar mood disorder and who is somewhat elevated in mood will inevitably find it difficult to

stay 'on track'. As the group facilitator, it's important to allow everyone to participate in the group. It may be necessary to gently point out the domination by a group member or to encourage others to have some say. Despite this challenge to the group process, it enables several of the curative factors to operate. These include and are probably not limited to universality, instillation of hope, altruism, interpersonal learning and the development of socialising techniques. So, despite the concerns of nurses that group therapy might not be effective or appropriate in an acute inpatient setting, coupled with the challenges that these groups will pose, group therapy is valuable at a range of levels, not least of which is having the opportunity to relate more effectively with others.

believe that problems reside within the person, family therapists believe that 'the dominant forces within our lives are located externally, within the family' (Nichols & Schwartz 2001, p 6). Therapy concentrates on the family and the way it is organised. Ultimately this affects the lives of each family member in some way. That is, the whole system is affected.

Nichols & Schwartz (2001) maintain that family therapy is particularly useful in working with children who are having problems. This is because they are strongly influenced by the family and must remain within its influence. Marital problems, family feuds and difficulties that develop in people when there has been a major family transition, are also particularly amenable to family therapy. The role of the family therapist is to understand the dynamics that occur within families and then to help the family members to reconsider the ways in which they interact with each other. The family therapist then motivates the family members to change.

When working with families, the problem is viewed as dysfunction in the relationship between family members. The relationship therefore becomes the focus of attention. Sometimes the person identified to be 'the problem' behaves in that way in order to hold the family together. For example, consider the child who misbehaves when his or her parents begin fighting. The misbehaviour distracts the parents from their conflict and so further fighting is averted. The parents then work together to manage the child's problem behaviour. Ultimately the problem is not with the child but with the marital relationship.

The two-way mirror is a useful tool in family therapy. While there is a therapist in the room with the family, behind the mirror sit a number of other members of the team observing the therapy in progress. This allows immediate feedback as the observers call in to the therapy room by telephone to give feedback or direction to the therapist and/or family. Observers may see things (communication styles, body language) that the therapist does not, so these can be communicated *during* the session rather than following it.

Another tool used in family therapy is the genogram, which is a graphic representation of the family and its patterns across generations. The genogram is drawn up with the involvement of the family, helping to engage all family members as the mapping process seeks input from everyone. Enduring and broken relationships, illegitimate and legitimate children, blended and nuclear family relationships are all depicted on the same page, revealing the emotional processes of the family to both the therapist and the family members (McGoldrick, Gerson & Shellenberger 1999).

Psychoeducation

Initially designed to help families develop skills to understand and cope with a family member with schizophrenia, psychoeducation is now used with families with any type of problem, including families with relationship problems (Goldenberg & Goldenberg 2000). In the mental health field, psychoeducation refers to the provision of information about a person's mental illness to that person and/or his or her family. Psychoeducation grew out of the belief that people with mental illness, particularly those with schizophrenia, are vulnerable to stress and that excessive stress in the person's life is likely to cause an exacerbation of the illness. That is, too much stress will cause the person to become unwell or relapse. Therefore psychoeducation is considered an intervention designed to reduce the impact of the illness on the client. For example, it has been found to be effective in reducing the number and duration of relapses for clients with bipolar affective disorders (Colom et al. 2003).

The early work of Brown (1958, cited in Bland 1986) claimed that some families contribute to stress through the ways they communicate and behave. These families were deemed to have high levels of expressed emotion (EE) and high EE was considered detrimental to the wellbeing of the client. Expressed emotion was originally defined as consisting of five constructs, including critical comments, hostility, emotional over-involvement, warmth and positive remarks (Jenkins & Karno 1992). Today, however, EE in families tends to be assessed only in terms of the first three, negative constructs. The level of EE in families is determined through a face-to-face interview, known as the Camberwell Family Interview of family members. Once a family is deemed to indicate high EE, psychoeducation is considered the appropriate intervention.

CASE STUDY

Bill and Joan have been married for thirty years. Joan has a bipolar affective disorder and had been moderately depressed for around two years. Around the time that Joan became well, Bill was made redundant from his job after a very lengthy period of employment with the company. Bill had always been the breadwinner and the caregiver in the family. Now his wife was supporting him emotionally and was independent of him. This role transition resulted in a great deal of conflict in the family. Bill had difficulty adjusting to his new role and in accepting that his wife no longer relied on him. Their teenage daughter blamed her mother for causing the conflict. Although Joan was being held responsible for the problems, no doubt due to her history of mental health problems, essentially the expected roles of family members had been reversed and there was now confusion about how to function. The therapy concentrated on the patterns of communication within the family and on accepting that Joan was now well and functioning in different and unexpected ways.

Psychoeducation programs are usually run in multi-family groups over several weeks but may also be organised around the needs of individual families. The benefit of several families coming together in a group is the sharing of information, the support they provide each other and the experience of universality—that is, the recognition that they are not alone in having these problems. Supportive family education programs need to attempt to reinforce strengths and promote resilience. Psychoeducation will also enable families in particular to understand the medical jargon we use and to appreciate the experience from the perspective of others, including the consumer. A comprehensive psychoeducation program will provide not only information about the specific mental illness, but also information about the available resources in the community as well as information on and practice of problem-solving skills (Palmer 1996).

Families and consumers need to be provided with information about mental illness, just as they would if the diagnosis was a threatening physical health problem. Indeed, Mullen, Murray & Happell (2002) argue that family interventions need to be considered 'core business' for mental health services. When there is an emphasis on providing information to *support* consumers and their families, they are more likely to benefit from the intervention. A collaborative approach that recognises the experiences of families and consumers and their unique knowledge of the disorder will convey to them that they are not to blame and that they have something to contribute to the overall care plan. Family problems need to be viewed as normal responses to very difficult situations that tax the family's usual coping resources (Kavanagh 1992).

Providing psychoeducation to families is designed to alert them to the need to reduce stress at home and to change the ways in which they relate to the person with mental illness. This is thought to reduce relapse rates and this is argued to be a cost-effective way of managing mental illness. Ultimately, though, the psychoeducation approach designed to reduce EE in families maintains a philosophy that families are responsible for the illness, or at least, responsible for contributing to hospitalisation and subsequent health-care costs. While historically families were blamed for directly causing mental illness, the shift to assessing EE and providing psychoeducation is a more subtle form of blaming families. Families experience considerable burden in taking care of family members with mental illness in the community. This perception of responsibility for the client's illness has the potential to add to that burden.

PSYCHOSOCIAL REHABILITATION

Psychosocial rehabilitation is a treatment approach designed for people who are severely disabled by long-term mental illness. Most people with enduring mental health problems have a diagnosis of schizophrenia. However, many people with bipolar affective disorder and depression also have long-term needs (Ekdawi & Conning 1994). The cognitive and emotional problems experienced by people with enduring mental health problems result in social disability, which in turn results in their needing help and support to negotiate the social world (Perkins & Repper 1996). In line with the shift from inpatient to community mental health care, most psychosocial rehabilitation is now carried out in the community (see also Ch 2 for issues related to consumers, recovery and rehabilitation).

Psychosocial rehabilitation is the process of assisting people to tap into and learn the internal and external skills, supports and resources necessary to be successful. Success is measured by the individual's satisfaction in living, learning and working in the environment(s) of their choice. At its most basic level, psychosocial rehabilitation seeks to help people determine and prioritise their goals, identify the pathways for achieving these goals, and develop the necessary skills and supports to achieve these goals (Anthony, Cohen & Farkas 1991). The concept of recovery from physical illness and disability does not mean that the suffering has disappeared, all the symptoms removed, and/or functioning completely restored. For example, as Deegan (1988) points out, a person with paraplegia can recover even though the spinal cord cannot. Similarly, a person with mental illness can recover even though the illness is not cured. Recovery is what people with disabilities do. Treatment, case management, and rehabilitation are what helpers do to facilitate recovery (Anthony 1993).

Before a person actively engages the rehabilitation services offered, it is argued that the person will need to have embarked on his or her personal journey of recovery (Anthony 1993). Psychosocial rehabilitation efforts designed to have a positive impact on severe mental illness can do more than leave the person less impaired, less dysfunctional, less disabled and less disadvantaged. These interventions can result in more meaning, purpose, success and satisfaction with one's life. Recovery outcomes include more subjective outcomes such as self-esteem, empowerment and self-determination.

Curtis (1997, p 16) has identified a number of recovery principles that, she argues, need to be reflected in the rehabilitation programs we offer:

- Recovery is an active, ongoing and individual process.
- Recovery is not linear; it entails growth, plateau, setbacks, side tracks and fast tracks.
- Recovery relates not only to the experience of symptoms, but also to the secondary assaults of stigma, discrimination and abuse.
- Hope is the most fundamental factor in recovery.
- Recovery requires the presence of people who believe in and stand by the person.

- Recovery can occur without professional intervention.
- The establishment of a sense of control or free will is critical to recovery.
- 'Remembering your track record', or learning from observing your own mental and emotional behaviour, is critical for coping.
- Self-directed coping strategies are effective and can be learned.
- Maintaining or developing connections to valued activities and people is critical to the recovery process.
- Connecting with other people on a human level is important.
- Recovery is a process of 'finding meaning in your experience'.

There are a number of possible stimulants to recovery. These may include other consumers who are in recovery or recovering effectively. Books, films and therapy groups may cause unexpected insights to occur about possible life options. Visiting new places and talking to various people are other ways in which the recovery process might be triggered. Critical to recovery is regaining the belief that there are options from which to choose, a belief perhaps even more important to recovery than the particular option one initially chooses (Curtis 1997). Therefore, we need to structure our settings so that recovery 'triggers' are present. Boring day treatment programs and inactive inpatient programs are characterised by a dearth of recovery stimulants (Anthony 1993). We need more creative programming. The strongest recovery-oriented programs identified to date are those that arise from and are operated by skilled consumer providers (Curtis 1997).

We cannot presume to know what a person hopes to achieve in life. We are all individual and have different desires and needs. As nurses, we may think we know what is best for a person, but this is at best naive and at worst paternalistic. Before engaging someone in rehabilitation services, it is important to find out what the client hopes to achieve. Having a rehabilitation program designed to be completed by everyone is unlikely to suit the needs of all consumers.

Instilling hope

There has been a great deal of research into what helps people with long-term mental illness to recover in such a way that they can live relatively normal and productive lives despite the re-emergence of symptoms of illness from time to time. It has been found that hope is considered fundamental before a person can choose to embark on recovery. Curtis (1997) identified a number of factors considered critical to recovery reported by consumers. The factor that was ranked as the most important was having 'just one person who believed in me'. This is one of the ingredients thought to be important in promoting a sense of hope. Morse & Penrod (1999) offer a process model for the development of hope following a critical life experience, such as being told that you have breast cancer or that you have a mental illness. This model was developed out of qualitative enquiry exploring emotional responses to the experience of illness.

The Morse & Penrod (1999) model flows through a number of overlapping phases that begin with a critical life event. People inevitably experience uncertainty, suffering, hope and the challenge of despair, and ultimately, the achievement of a 'reformulated self'. At each of these phases, a different level of knowing or perceiving is experienced.

- *Enduring*: after a critical life experience we initially focus on cultivating our powers of endurance, which involves suspending or suppressing emotions and remaining in control. We do this because we worry that we will 'lose it' or disintegrate. The level of knowing here is *awareness*.
- *Uncertainty*: this is evident when we *recognise* what has happened and know what our goals are for the future, but we are unable to choose a course of action from a range of options. This state of uncertainty paralyses hope. At this time we simply exist in an emotional state and suffer as a result of not being able to act. When we are in a state of uncertainty, we have no other choice but to tolerate the present.
- *Suffering*: the level of knowing here is *acknowledgement*. We begin to grasp the situation and

NURSE'S STORY

I routinely invite into the classroom two people with bipolar affective disorder who live independently in the community. They talk about their experiences with mental health services to groups of postgraduate nursing students. While one of these values himself according to his ability to remain employed, the other accepts that work is too stressful for him. Self-worth is gained from his ability to be a good husband and a good father to his two young daughters. To help identify clients' goals I routinely start my inpatient pre-discharge group therapy sessions with introductions and a request for people

to identify their short-term and five-year goals. The goals are almost always quite different from each other. For some, at this stage of their illness, a five-year projection into the future is impossible. However, everyone has a dream and this should be tapped into as dreams provide the impetus for goals. Further, it is not our place to decide whether the goals are realistic or not. Should a goal seem potentially unachievable, it might be wise to break it down into smaller and more achievable sub-goals. I would usually say, 'That sounds like a great goal. What do you think you'll need to do to achieve that?'.

consequently suffer emotionally. Morse & Penrod (1999, p 148) comment that 'the depth of the state of suffering is despair, utter hopelessness'. Out of this overwhelming emotional experience, we begin to piece reality together and develop a perception of the future. 'This process of piecing together a new future begins in small incremental pieces, eventually building to … acceptance of the event and identification of both a goal and the means to attain it, which eventually leads to hope' (Morse & Penrod 1999, p 148). So, suffering is viewed as integral to moving on and ultimately to repair.

■ *Hope*: the level of knowing is now *acceptance* and we become future-oriented. We are able to develop an action plan designed to achieve desired goals. When we have hope, we understand the reality of the event while also understanding the real possibility of negative outcomes. Indeed, 'bracing for negative outcomes is a powerful motivating force for developing hope' (Morse & Penrod 1999, p 148). Supportive relationships are now sought and hope is bolstered.

■ *Reformulated self*: there is now a sense of becoming a 'better person' for having suffered. This state has been labelled the 'reformulated self', where the past is accepted and we also accept that the future has been irrevocably changed and a choice is made to 'make the most of life'.

Understanding the process involved in developing a sense of hope for one's future is fundamental to helping nurses know how to respond to people during the phases of enduring, uncertainty and suffering. If these phases are acknowledged as normal or expected, we won't make the mistake of attempting to force people to have hope when they are not ready to accept it. The trauma involved in dealing with a critical life experience such as the diagnosis of a mental illness, results in a range of responses. These responses are part of a process that is not linear. We move back and forth between these phases and an understanding of this may also explain the delays for some in developing hope. These are normal responses, and so should not be assessed as being part of an illness.

Deegan (1996, 1997) was diagnosed with schizophrenia at seventeen years of age and is very clear about the need for health professionals to treat people with mental illness as human beings. Although this may seem like a simple thing to do, the medically dominant model of disease reinforces the notion of person as illness. Deegan (1993, p 9) says: 'it is as if the whole world has put on a pair of warped glasses that blind them to the person you are and leaves them seeing you as an illness'. Stocks (1995, cited in Hayne & Yonge 1997, p 319) agrees, saying, 'once our personal identities are transformed into a psychiatric label, we are objects that are never allowed to be people again'.

It is clearly important to see the person as separate from the illness. However, there are many ways in which we maintain the view of the person as an illness. These include a tendency to focus predominantly upon problems, interpreting all behaviour as part of the illness, over-emphasising assessment, diagnosis and prognosis, and neglecting to consult the client (Palmer 1999). These are all things that are likely to stifle hope. If nurses can't accept people with mental illness as human and social beings, who else in society will? After all, we are all human beings with unique abilities, shortcomings and, often, disabilities. We are all a psychological 'work in progress' and having a mental illness does not make one 'weak' or imperfect.

Social skills training

There are many types of skills training designed to improve problem-solving skills, relaxation skills, assertion skills and coping skills. Similarly, social skills can be learned. We are not born with them. How do you know how to greet someone in a culturally appropriate way? How do you know how to behave when you walk into a university classroom? These are taken-for-granted behaviours that we tend to think little about before doing them. These are examples of social skills and we have learned how to carry them out as we were socialised into our culture. Much of this learning took place during childhood and adolescence. By adulthood we pretty much have these skills well developed.

However, if you develop a mental illness during childhood or adolescence, it is unlikely that you will develop sound social skills. Mental illness can distort communication with family members and peers, and the separations that ensue if a child or adolescent is hospitalised can disrupt family life, social life and schooling, where we learn many early social skills. If you develop a long-term mental disorder later in life, it is likely that you will have fewer opportunities to practise learned social skills, and if you don't use them, you will lose them. Social isolation often occurs for people with serious mental illness because of the stigma and discrimination that result and because it is harder to communicate with others when you have bizarre thoughts and experiences. These interfere with the ability to sustain relationships and develop new ones.

Much of the social skills training in mental health services focuses on working with people with schizophrenia. People with social phobia and depression are also often in need of social skills training (O'Donohue & Krasner 1995). Essentially, though, most client groups will have social and interpersonal problems as part of their overall picture.

Social skills training centres on teaching people the skills necessary to communicate effectively with others. There are some general approaches to teaching people social skills. As with most skills training packages, social skills training is usually carried out in groups. However, there are opportunities at almost every encounter to teach skills and to reinforce those skills already taught and being practised. When we role model appropriate social skills we provide opportunities for learning. However, O'Donohue & Krasner (1995) recommend using a model similar in presentation to the group members so that the behaviour has more relevance to them. That is, the role model for a group of adolescents learning how to present for a job interview should be an adolescent who has suffered similar life problems.

Most social skills training groups combine instruction, modelling, rehearsal or role playing as well as coaching, feedback and reinforcement. Rehearsal and role playing involve practising the skill once instruction has been provided. Coaching involves having an instructor or teacher helping the group members to practise the skill accurately by giving feedback on performance and praise (positive reinforcement) when the skill is performed well. Homework is an essential component of training packages because without practice in the real world, the goal of improved social skills will never be achieved. That is, social skills are not simply taught, they are developed through practice and the more practice, the more socially able the person will be.

INTERVIEWING

While the skill of interviewing might not strictly be considered an intervention, the nurse's interviewing style may have considerable impact on the therapeutic outcomes. When you meet with a client to carry out a clinical interview, you need to engage or connect with that person in the same way that you might when being therapeutic. That is, it is important to develop rapport by being open, thoughtful, caring and honest, both verbally and non-verbally. Interviewing a person to attempt to find out what is happening is likely to be viewed as threatening if the approach taken is to fire off a list of questions that seek to arrive at a medical diagnosis. As part of the process of empowering people with mental illness, the assessment process (usually undertaken via clinical interview) needs to be a collaborative and shared process (see Ch 10).

It is the client who has the knowledge or information that is required to move toward the identification of problems and subsequent planning of care. As nurses, we currently ask questions from a power base rather than a discovery base. However, the client is the expert in his or her experience of mental illness, so we can share in the discovery of an understanding of the person's experience through the way in which we ask questions. At the outset, set the scene by letting the client know that your goal is to work together to arrive at some conclusion of what is going on at the moment. You might say something like, 'Let's talk about what's happening for you. You'd probably like to get a clearer idea of what's going on and I need to hear your story so that we can better know what to do next.' Ask questions that help people to understand themselves and, through this, also arrive at some

understanding of what is happening. Asking questions that recognise the expertise of the client and summarising that information is a collaborative approach to guided discovery (Palmer 1999).

CASE MANAGEMENT

Case management describes a pattern of service delivery for clients based in the community that arose as a result of deinstitutionalisation, the term used to describe the return of people to live in the community rather than in psychiatric institutions. The key worker is often a nurse but can also be a social worker, an occupational therapist, psychologist or psychiatrist—that is, anyone from the multidisciplinary team. So the key worker is considered to have generic skills or a core group of skills that allow him or her to provide a particular service to clients with enduring mental health problems in the community. People with a long-term mental health problem, or whose mental illness causes them to require frequent admission to hospital, are usually assigned a key worker, sometimes without their consent. People who do not accept the need for this type of supervision in the community may require this to be enforced under a Mental Health Act order for community treatment. Most people, however, agree to and welcome additional support in the community.

Staff who act as key workers deliver a range of services to clients including counselling, assistance with social and financial needs and supervision of medication (Johnston et al. 1998). In Australia, the Medicare system of health care covers the cost of visits to GPs for the administration of intramuscular injections of antipsychotic medications so this is usually not a requirement of key workers, although there may well be times when it is necessary (e.g. when a client refuses to visit a GP). In New Zealand, however, no such system exists, so key workers are also responsible for the administration of these medications. In addition, key workers are responsible for ongoing mental state assessment as well as risk assessment to ensure the person's safety and the safety of the community. Because case management is often carried out in the person's own home, there is often greater contact with family members and, therefore, greater opportunity to work with families.

Early models of case management had the client working through the key worker to access other services in the community. While this seemed reasonable, it had the effect of making the client dependent on the key worker. Today, the client is considered central and the key worker is just one form of community support. The client is encouraged and supported to access other community services independently. If, for example, the client seeks support to access social security services, the key worker would certainly be supportive. However, unless this help was requested, the key worker would expect the client to negotiate the community without support. The responsibility of the key worker might be to teach the negotiation and social skills necessary to do this independently. This model of case management supports consumer empowerment through partnership (Howgego et al. 2003).

NURSE'S STORY

As a key worker, most of my time with people is spent talking through any current concerns, from weight gain to marital difficulties. These are the personal issues that contribute to difficulties in living and they are the mental health issues that we all experience and need an active listener for. However, most of us don't have the additional burden of a serious mental illness. The therapeutic encounter is designed to provide support and to enable people to solve their problems through exploring their difficulties in greater depth. When a person has a recurrence of symptoms, we attempt to manage them (the symptoms) together in the community with more frequent visits and telephone contact. Whenever someone requires hospitalisation, I liaise with staff working in the ward and visit the person there throughout the hospitalisation. I am also involved in discharge planning and family meetings.

Routine case management usually involves caseloads or numbers of clients of around thirty to forty per case manager. For the more seriously disabled, there are now teams that provide intensive case management. This involves low client numbers with ratios of around eight to ten people per key worker. A cost-effectiveness analysis carried out in Sydney (Johnston et al. 1998) comparing the cost of routine case management with intensive case management revealed that there were greater improvements in functioning and higher rates of engagement in treatment in the intensive case management group. However, it costs considerably more for this type of support and, for this study, there was no reduction in hospital use after twelve months of intensive case management. Importantly, though, the routine case management group required four times as many visits from the community crisis team. This means that clients who have limited key worker support inevitably require more support from the community crisis team. Therefore, this study suggests that people with enduring mental illness require more intensive support than we realise, so cost savings are not realised.

A word of caution: the term 'case management' carries with it certain messages. It reduces people to *cases* that require *managing*. These words are loaded towards paternalism at a time when we are encouraged to view consumers/clients/service users as active participants in their own care and in their recovery from mental illness. The term 'case management' was used here because it is a term used universally, but the term 'key worker' better describes the role of the 'case manager', and is less paternalistic.

Cultural note

Because of the bicultural nature of New Zealand, there are Kaupapa Maori mental health services designed to meet the specific needs of Maori consumers (tangata whaiora). In addition to being assigned a clinical key worker in these services, each client is usually also assigned a cultural worker. This ensures that cultural protocols are observed and cultural needs are addressed. This arrangement is also in place in designated mental health services for Pacific Island people.

ELECTROCONVULSIVE THERAPY

Invented in 1938 in Italy by two eminent psychiatrists (Ugo Cerletti and Lucio Bini), electroconvulsive therapy was investigated at a time when a number of physical treatments were developed, including insulin coma therapy, metrazole convulsive therapy and psychosurgery. Electroconvulsive therapy (ECT) is the only one of these treatments used routinely today. Much of the controversy around ECT grew out of its initial indiscriminate use and abuse. At first ECT was also used without anaesthetic or muscle relaxation. The outcome of this was many adverse effects such as fractures, pain and cardiovascular problems.

Today, however, once a person is considered a candidate for ECT—that is, the person has an illness that may respond well to ECT—a full psychological and physical assessment is carried out. Wherever possible, consent for treatment is sought from the client. If this is not possible, the Mental Health Acts in Australia and New Zealand allow for treatment to proceed, but only pending wider consultation in Australia. Section 62 of the *New Zealand Mental Health (Assessment and Treatment) Act 1992 (1993)* allows the administration of ECT without consent only if it is considered to be necessary to save the person's life or to prevent serious damage to the person's health.

Electroconvulsive therapy involves the application of two metal electrodes to the head, through which an electric current is delivered. The electrodes can be applied either bilaterally (one on each side of the head, usually in the frontotemporal region) or unilaterally (both on the same side of the head). Whether applied bilaterally or unilaterally, the treatment is almost equally effective. However, different adverse effects can be experienced. According to Endler & Persad (1988, p 26), 'unilateral ECT to the non-dominant hemisphere is less stressful for the patient than bilateral; it minimises confusion and memory loss; and it is almost as efficacious as bilateral in terms of alleviating the symptoms of depression'.

Indeed, in a more recent study, high-dosage right unilateral ECT showed an equivalent response rate (Sackeim et al. 2000). This study also supported other findings that bilateral ECT results in greater impairment in memory (both anterograde and retrograde amnesia). These authors concluded: 'right unilateral ECT at high dosage is as effective as a robust form of bilateral ECT, but produces less severe and persistent cognitive effects' (Sackeim et al. 2000, p 425). And, in response to concerns about the effects of ECT on cerebral function, a study by Ende et al. (2000, p 941) found evidence that ECT does not cause tissue damage and that 'there is no hippocampal atrophy, neuronal damage, or cell death induced by ECT'.

Electroconvulsive therapy is widely accepted as an effective intervention in the treatment of severe depression, although it remains controversial (Persad 2001). There is contention not only among the public regarding ECT, but also within the mental health professions, as many professionals question its efficacy (Barker 2003; Challiner & Griffiths 2000). However, recent publications support earlier conclusions that antidepressants and ECT are effective and safe treatments for depressed elderly patients (Salzman, Wong & Wright 2002) and for people who are suicidal (Persad 2001).

In the past, ECT has been used to treat a wide range of mental disorders, including schizophrenia. An examination of both older and more recent research has revealed that ECT is as effective as antipsychotic medications in the treatment of schizophrenia, particularly with people experiencing an acute episode. When used in combination with antipsychotic medications, it has been found to be more effective than ECT or medication used alone (Keuneman, Weerasundera & Castle 2002).

Whether conducted in a general theatre or a specialised ECT suite attached to the inpatient psychiatric unit, ECT remains a physically intrusive treatment that requires specialised nursing skills. Generally, though, the role of the nurse in working with a person preparing for ECT is to support the person and to prepare him or her for the procedure, both physically and psychologically, just as you would for any procedure requiring a general anaesthetic. Other responsibilities for the nurse are also the same as for any operative procedure conducted under general anaesthesia. For example, you may be required to provide close observation to ensure that the client doesn't eat or drink any food prior to the procedure. You would also need to make certain that make-up and jewellery have been removed. These are basic safety measures to prevent complications and to ensure an accurate assessment of skin colour during the anaesthetic.

Electroconvulsive therapy remains a controversial intervention in psychiatry today. Much of this controversy stems from the historical use of ECT and from movie representations, such as that in the movie, *One Flew Over the Cuckoo's Nest* (Vermeulen 1999). This is despite substantial research and descriptive evidence testifying to its effectiveness. Those who have not observed ECT and who base their understandings on historical and media representations of it are likely to be surprised at

how innocuous it is. A positive attitude to ECT has been found to be directly related to greater exposure to and knowledge about ECT (Endler & Persad 1988; Gass 1998). Nevertheless, concern persists because we are not entirely certain how ECT works and because of the cognitive side-effects experienced. Ultimately, clients and families still express fears about the long-term effects on brain function.

CASE STUDY

A woman in her mid-thirties with whom I worked many years ago left a lasting impression on me in terms of the efficacy of ECT. She was a very attractive woman with a supportive husband and two young children. However, she suffered from major depression. When depressed she experienced feelings of hopelessness and delusions of worthlessness. She believed that she was so worthless that her family would be better off without her and that we really shouldn't bother helping her. As with any delusion, her thoughts could not be countered.

She began treatment with ECT at the usually prescribed rate of three times each week. She had a very quick recovery and I recall her saying to us not long before she was discharged home, 'Thank you for keeping me alive until I got well'. She was also overheard recommending ECT to other depressed clients in the hospital.

CONCLUSION

This chapter has given you some fundamental information about a number of therapeutic intervention strategies that will assist you in being with and working with people with mental illness. Some of these intervention strategies apply to specific situations or client difficulties but there is always a way of working effectively with people experiencing challenging mental health problems. Some are more technical than others and require further education and practice to master. But many of the skills outlined briefly here can be learned and applied to the interactions you will experience now as a novice nurse and later, as your experience develops.

Novice nurses have frequently expressed their concern to me that they might 'say the wrong thing' and make the situation more challenging for the client. If you take a caring and thoughtful approach that avoids the generous delivery of advice, it is unlikely that you will cause harm. However, if you take with you some specific skills and models for your practice, you are likely to feel more confident and to understand the goals of your interaction. It is also hoped that, through reading this chapter, you have developed a sense of the importance of treating people with mental health problems as valid human beings who require your support and help through a particularly troubling time.

EXERCISES FOR CLASS ENGAGEMENT

A number of exercises are presented here to help you to engage with and consolidate what you have learned from this chapter. You should discuss the issues raised with your group or class members. Some of these activities also ask you to reflect on your personal values, beliefs and actions so that this greater insight into yourself will help you to be more effective in your interactions with others.

- What are the main stressors in your life? Consider relationship problems, difficulties with children, problems with parents, financial worries, physical conditions, environmental factors, study pressures, work factors, nutrition and exercise, in addition to chemical factors such as nicotine, alcohol, caffeine and other substances. Identify those that you can learn to manage and list the stressors in terms of their importance or greatest impact.
- Using the written text from a book or an audiotape, follow the instructions for carrying out progressive muscle relaxation. Were you able to relax? What effect did the exercise have on your respiratory and heart rates?
- Which of the assertion skills (making requests, refusing requests, accepting and giving compliments, expressing opinions, giving negative feedback or being confrontational, initiating conversations, sharing intimate feelings and experiences with others and expressing affection) do you find difficult to manage? Why do you think this is? Of the situations that you find difficult to manage, which one in particular presents the greatest challenge to you? How do you feel whenever you fail to manage these situations assertively?
- Consider the kinds of life events that might cause an individual to experience crisis, such as rape, loss of a job, unplanned pregnancy, or death of a loved one. How would you respond to being admitted to hospital for colorectal surgery? How would you respond to being admitted involuntarily to an acute psychiatric unit?

- Mark is a 25-year old single male. He has just been diagnosed with genital herpes and is extremely distressed. Although he is intelligent and has coped well with previous life crises and has good relationships with family and friends, he feels so ashamed that he can't discuss this with anyone he knows well. He believes that life is no longer worth living as he believes he will never have a normal sex life or a meaningful relationship again. What do you make of Mark's perception of his problem? Which interventions do you think are necessary according to Aguilera's model for crisis intervention?
- What are your short-term goals (that is, what do you hope to achieve over the next few weeks or months)? What is your main five-year goal? What will you need to do over the next five years to achieve that goal? What is likely to interfere with your achievement of that goal? What is likely to support your achievement of that goal?
- As a group, rent and watch the DVD/video of *One Flew Over the Cuckoo's Nest*. What stereotypes are portrayed in this movie? Which of these persist today? How does the portrayal of ECT in this movie make you feel about ECT? In addition, what are your thoughts about the nurse–patient and doctor–patient relationships as portrayed for that era? How do you think a movie made today would portray these things?
- Consider your values concerning health and wellness as well as self-determination. What issues might arise for you if you were responsible for preparing a client for ECT against that person's wishes? How would you deal with this situation?

REFERENCES

Aguilera D 1994, *Crisis Intervention: Theory and Methodology* (7th edn), Mosby, St Louis.
Anthony WA 1993, Recovery from mental illness: the guiding vision of the mental health service system in the 1990s, *Psychosocial Rehabilitation Journal*, 16(4), pp 11–23.
Anthony WA, Cohen M & Farkas M 1991, *Psychiatric Rehabilitation*, Centre for Psychiatric Rehabilitation, Boston.
Barker P 2003, Barker's beat, *Mental Health Practice*, 6(10), pp 38–9.
Barker PJ & Fraser D (eds) 1985, *The Nurse as Therapist: A Behavioural Model*, Croom Helm, London.
Battison T 1997, *Beating Stress*, Allen and Unwin, London.
Blackburn I & Davidson K 1990, *Cognitive Therapy for Depression and Anxiety*, Blackwell Scientific, New York.
Bland R 1986, *Family Support Program*, Occasional Paper Vol. 86, No. 1, The University of Queensland, Brisbane.
Bloom BL 1997, *Planned Short-Term Psychotherapy: A Clinical Handbook* (2nd edn), Allyn and Bacon, Boston.
Byrne J & Byrne DG 1996, *Counselling Skills for Health Professionals*, MacMillan Education, Melbourne.

Calvert P & Palmer C 2003, Application of the cognitive therapy model to initial crisis assessment, *International Journal of Mental Health Nursing*, 12(1), pp 30–8.
Challiner V & Griffiths L 2000, Electroconvulsive therapy: a review of the literature, *Journal of Psychiatric and Mental Health Nursing*, 7(3), pp 191–8.
Colom F, Vieta E, Martinez-Aran A, Reinares M, Goikolea JM, Benabarre A et al. 2003, A randomised trial on the efficacy of group psychoeducation in the prophylaxis of recurrences in bipolar patients whose disease is in remission, *Archives of General Psychiatry*, 60(4), pp 402–7.
Cowan D & Brunero S 1997, Group therapy for anxiety disorders using rational emotive behaviour therapy, *Australian and New Zealand Journal of Mental Health Nursing*, 6(4), pp 164–8.
Curtis L 1997, *New Directions: International Overview of Best Practices in Recovery and Rehabilitation Services for People with Serious Mental Illness*, New Zealand Mental Health Commission, Wellington.
Dattilio FM & Padesky CA 1990, *Cognitive Therapy with Couples*, Professional Resource Exchange Inc., Sarasota, Florida.
Davis CM 1989, *Patient–Practitioner Interaction*, Slack, Thorofare, New Jersey.

Davis M, Robbins Eshelman E & McKay M 2000, *The Relaxation and Stress Reduction Workbook* (5th edn), New Harbinger, Oakland, California.

Deegan P 1988, Recovery: the lived experience of rehabilitation, *Psychosocial Rehabilitation Journal*, 11(4), pp 11–19.

Deegan P 1993, Recovering our sense of value after being labelled mentally ill, *Journal of Psychosocial Nursing*, 31(4), pp 7–11.

Deegan P 1996, Recovery as a journey of the heart, *Psychiatric Rehabilitation Journal*, 19(3), pp 91–7.

Deegan PE 1997, Recovery and empowerment for people with psychiatric disabilities, *Social Work in Health Care*, 25(3), pp 11–24.

Doyle M & Dolan M 2002, Violence risk assessment: combining actuarial and clinical information to structure clinical judgements for the formulation and management of risk, *Journal of Psychiatric and Mental Health Nursing*, 9(6), pp 649–57.

Earley J 2000, *Interactive Group Therapy: Integrating Interpersonal, Action-Oriented, and Psychodynamic Approaches*, Brunner/Mazel, Philadelphia.

Edwards D, Hannigan B, Fothergill A & Burnard P 2002, Stress management for mental health professionals: a review of effective techniques, *Stress and Health*, 18(5), pp 203–15.

Egan G 1998, *The Skilled Helper: A Problem-Management Approach to Helping* (6th edn), Brooks/Cole, Pacific Grove, California.

Ekdawi MY & Conning AM 1994, *Psychiatric Rehabilitation: A Practical Guide*, Chapman & Hall, London.

Ende G, Braus DF, Walter S, Weber-Fahr W & Henn FA 2000, The hippocampus in patients treated with electroconvulsive therapy: a proton magnetic resonance spectroscopic imaging study, *Archives of General Psychiatry*, 57(10), pp 937–43.

Endler NS & Persad E 1988, *Electroconvulsive Therapy: The Myths and the Realities*, Hans Huber, Toronto.

Escot C, Artero S, Gandubert C, Boulenger JP & Ritchie K 2001, Stress levels in nursing staff working in oncology, *Stress and Health*, 17(5), pp 273–9.

Fehr SS 1999, *Introduction to Group Therapy: A Practical Guide*, Haworth Press, New York.

Finnell DS 2003, Use of the transtheoretical model for individuals with co-occurring disorders, *Community Mental Health Journal*, 39(1), pp 3–15.

Freud S 1938/1965, *The Basic Writing of Sigmund Freud*, Modern Library, New York.

Gallop R & O'Brien L 2003, Re-establishing psychodynamic theory as foundational knowledge for psychiatric/mental health nursing, *Issues in Mental Health Nursing*, 24(2), pp 213–27.

Gambril E 1995, Assertion skills training. In: O'Donohue W & Krasner L (eds), *Handbook of Psychological Skills Training: Clinical Techniques and Applications*, Allyn & Bacon, Boston.

Gass JP 1998, The knowledge and attitudes of mental health nurses to electroconvulsive therapy, *Journal of Advanced Nursing*, 27(1), pp 83–90.

Goldenberg I & Goldenberg H 2000, *Family therapy: An overview* (5th edn), Brooks/Cole, Belmont, California.

Greenstone JL & Leviton SC 2002, *Elements of Crisis Intervention: Crises and How to Respond to Them* (2nd edn), Brooks/Cole, Pacific Grove, California.

Hayne Y & Yonge O 1997, The lifeworld analysis of the chronically mentally ill: an analysis of 40 written personal accounts, *Archives of Psychiatric Nursing*, 11(6), pp 314–24.

Health & Disability Commissioner 2002, *Southland District Health Board Mental Health Services February–March, 2001: A report by the Health & Disability Commissioner*, Health & Disability Commissioner, Auckland, New Zealand.

Howgego IM, Yellowlees P, Owen C, Meldrum L & Dark F 2003, The therapeutic alliance: the key to effective patient outcome? A descriptive review of the evidence in community mental health case management, *Australian and New Zealand Journal of Psychiatry*, 37(2), pp 169–83.

Jenkins JH & Karno M 1992, The meaning of expressed emotion: theoretical issues raised by cross-cultural research, *American Journal of Psychiatry*, 149(1), pp 9–21.

Johnston S, Salkeld G, Sanderson K, Issakidis C, Teesson M & Buhrich N 1998, Intensive case management: a cost-effectiveness analysis, *Australian and New Zealand Journal of Psychiatry*, 32, pp 551–9.

Kadis LB & McClendon R 1998, *Concise Guide to Marital and Family Therapy*, American Psychiatric Press, Washington.

Kavanagh DJ 1992, Recent developments in expressed emotion and schizophrenia, *British Journal of Psychiatry*, 160, pp 601–20.

Kelly T, Simmons W & Gregory E 2002, Risk assessment and management: a community forensic mental health practice model, *International Journal of Mental Health Nursing*, 11(4), pp 206–13.

Keuneman R, Weerasundera R & Castle D 2002, The role of ECT in schizophrenia, *Australasian Psychiatry*, 10(4), pp 385–8.

Lester D 2002, *Crisis Intervention and Counselling by Telephone* (2nd edn), Charles C Thomas, Springfield, Illinois.

Linehan MM 1993, *Cognitive Behaviour Therapy of Borderline Personality Disorder*, Guilford Press, New York.

Linehan MM, Schmidt H, Dimeff LA, Craft JC, Kanter J & Comtois KA 1999, Dialectical behaviour therapy for patients with borderline personality disorder and drug-dependence, *The American Journal on Addictions*, 8, pp 279–92.

McGoldrick M, Gerson R & Shellenberger S 1999, *Genograms: Assessment and Intervention* (2nd edn), WW Norton, New York.

Meech C & Wood A 2000, Reconnecting past, present and future lives: therapy with a young person who experienced severe childhood privation, *Australian and New Zealand Journal of Family Therapy*, 21(2), pp 102–7.

Mellor D, Storer S & Firth L 2000, Family therapy into the 21st century: can we work our way out of the epistemological maze?, *Australian and New Zealand Journal of Family Therapy*, 21(3), pp 151–4.

Mental Health (Assessment and Treatment) Act (1992) 1993, New Zealand Government, Wellington.

Mental Health Commission 1998, Report on the Present State of Clinical Risk Management in Mental Health Services, documentation provided Crown Health Enterprises, Mental Health Commission, Wellington, New Zealand.

Miller W 1998, Toward a motivational definition and understanding of addiction, *Motivational Interviewing Newsletter*, 5(3), pp 2–6.

Miller WR, Zweben A, DiClemente CC & Rychtarik RG 1992, *Motivational Enhancement Therapy Manual: A Clinical Research Guide for Therapists Treating Individuals with Alcohol Abuse and Dependence*, National Institute on Alcohol Abuse and Alcoholism, Rockville.

Monahan J, Steadman HJ, Silver E, Appelbaum PS, Clark Robbins P, Mulvey EP et al. 2001, *Rethinking Risk Assessment: The MacArthur Study of Mental Disorder and Violence*, Oxford University Press, Oxford.

Morse J & Penrod J 1999, Linking concepts of enduring, uncertainty, suffering, and hope, *Image: Journal of Nursing Scholarship*, 31(1), pp 145–50.

Mullen A, Murray L & Happell B 2002, Multiple family group interventions in first episode psychosis: enhancing knowledge and understanding, *International Journal of Mental Health Nursing*, 11, pp 225–32.

Mullen P 2002, Marijuana and Mental Illness, paper presented at the Mental Health Services Conference Inc. of Australia and New Zealand (The MHS), Sydney, 21 August.

Myer RA 2001, *Assessment for Crisis Intervention: A Triage Assessment Model*, Wadsworth, Toronto.

Nichols MP & Schwartz RC 2001, *Family Therapy: Concepts and Methods* (5th edn), Allyn & Bacon, Boston.

O'Donohue W & Krasner L 1995, *Handbook of Psychological Skills Training: Clinical Techniques and Applications*, Allyn & Bacon, Boston.

Padesky CA & Mooney KA 1990, Presenting the cognitive model to clients, *International Cognitive Therapy Newsletter*, 6, pp 6–7.

Palmer CJ 1996, *Education and Support for Families and Friends of People with Schizophrenia*, Masters dissertation, Queensland University of Technology, Brisbane.

Palmer CJ 1999, Recovery-focused Mental Health Nursing: A Model for the Future?, paper presented at the scientific meeting of the Australian and New Zealand College of Mental Health Nurses (ANZCMHN), Tasmania, 9–12 September.

Patel C 1991, *The Complete Guide to Stress Management*, Plenum Press, New York.

Perkins RE & Repper JM 1996, *Working Alongside People with Long Term Mental Health Problems*, Chapman & Hall, London.

Persad E 2001, Electroconvulsive therapy: the controversy and the evidence, *Canadian Journal of Psychiatry*, 46(8), pp 702–3.

Petchkovsky L, Morris P & Rushton P 2002, Choosing a psychodynamic psychotherapy model for an Australian public sector mental health service, *Australasian Psychiatry*, 10(4), pp 330–4.

Prochaska JO 2001, Treating entire populations for behaviour risks for cancer, *The Cancer Journal*, 7(5), pp 360–8.

Prochaska JO & DiClemente CC 1983, Stages and processes of self-change of smoking: toward an integrative model of change, *Journal of Consulting and Clinical Psychology*, 51(3), pp 390–5.

Rollnick S & Miller WR 1995, What is motivational interviewing?, *Behavioural and Cognitive Psychotherapy*, 23, pp 325–34.

Romas, JA & Sharma, M 1995, *Practical stress management*, Allyn & Bacon, Boston.

Sackeim HA, Prudic J, Devanand DP, Nobler MS, Lisanby SH, Peyser S et al. 2000, A prospective, randomised, double-blind comparison of bilateral and right unilateral electroconvulsive therapy at different stimulus intensities, *Archives of General Psychiatry*, 57(5), pp 425–34.

Salzman C, Wong E & Wright BC 2002, Drug and ECT treatment of depression in the elderly, 1996–2001: a literature review, *Biological Psychiatry*, 52(3), pp 265–84.

Sanders P 1996, *An Incomplete Guide to Using Counselling Skills on the Telephone* (2nd edn), PCCS Books, Manchester.

Sharry J 2001, *Solution-focused Groupwork*, Sage, London.

Slaikeu KA 1990, *Crisis Intervention: A Handbook for Practice and Research* (2nd edn), Allyn & Bacon, Boston.

Sundel SS & Sundel M 1993, *Behaviour Modification in the Human Services: A Systematic Introduction to Concepts and Applications* (3rd edn), Sage, Newbury Park, California.

Swales M, Heard HL & Williams JMG 2000, Linehan's dialectical behaviour therapy (DBT) for borderline personality disorder: overview and adaptation, *Journal of Mental Health*, 9(1), pp 7–23.

Truax P 2002, Behavioural case conceptualisation for adults. In: Hersen M (ed.), *Clinical Behavioural Therapy: Adults and Children*, John Wiley & Sons, New York.

Varcarolis EM 1998, *Foundations of Psychiatric-Mental Health Nursing* (3rd edn), WB Saunders, Philadelphia.

Vermeulen J 1999, A Personal Reflection by a Psychiatric Nurse: Electroconvulsive Therapy: History, Perception, Knowledge and Attitudes, paper presented at the scientific meeting of the Australian and New Zealand College of Mental Health Nurses (ANZCMHN), Launceston Tasmania, 9–12 September.

Wolpow S 2000, Adapting a dialectical behaviour therapy (DBT) group for use in a residential program, *Psychiatric Rehabilitation Journal*, 24(2), pp 135–41.

Yalom ID 1995, *The Theory and Practice of Group Psychotherapy* (4th edn), Basic Books, New York.

24

Psychopharmacology

*Kim Usher, Lauretta Luck
and Kim Foster*

KEY POINTS

- Psychotropic medications play an important role in the treatment of mental illness. The nurse plays a pivotal role in medication administration and patient education. It is also important for the nurse to be aware of the potential side-effects and interactions of these drugs.
- Assisting the patient to understand the importance of taking psychotropic medication as prescribed and the issues surrounding compliance/adherence is an important skill for the mental health nurse.
- Polypharmacy is to be avoided where possible, especially the tendency to use drugs from different classes at the same time. Its use with older people is not advised.
- Issues related to as-needed (PRN) medication administration are of contemporary relevance.
- Nursing assessment and interventions related to psychopharmacological side-effects is important knowledge for the mental health nurse.

LEARNING OUTCOMES

The material in this chapter will assist you to:

- describe the role of the nurse in the administration of psychotropic medication and related interventions, including medication indications, interactions, side-effects and precautions
- identify the important classes of psychotropic medications and the disorders for which they are used
- understand the issues for patients requiring psychotropic medications
- understand the action, use and side-effects related to anti-anxiety/sedative-hypnotic, anti-depressant, mood-stabilising and antipsychotic drugs
- understand the issues related to the as-needed (PRN) administration of psychotropic medication and related interventions
- outline the relevant legal and ethical issues related to the administration of psychotropic medication.

KEY TERMS

- akathisia
- anti-anxiety medications
- anticholinergic
- antidepressant medications
- antiparkinsonian medication
- antipsychotic medication
- atypical antipsychotic medication
- extrapyramidal symptoms
- medication compliance/ adherence
- mood-stabilising medication
- neuroleptic malignant syndrome
- neuroleptic medication
- Parkinson's syndrome
- polypharmacy
- pro re nata (PRN) medications
- psychopharmacology
- psychotropic medication
- tardive dyskinesia
- traditional antipsychotic medication

INTRODUCTION
This chapter provides an overview of the principles of psychopharmacology, which is the study of drugs used to treat psychiatric disorders. The chapter provides important information related to drug indications, interactions, side-effects and precautions, and discusses patient education and the issues of adherence and as-needed (PRN) medication administration.

The use of drugs that have a demonstrated ability to relieve the symptoms of psychiatric disorders has become widespread since the mid-1950s (Baldessarini & Tarazi 2001). The pharmacological agents used in current psychiatric practice are the anti-anxiety sedatives, antidepressants, mood-stabilising, neuroleptic and antipsychotic drugs. Collectively, these drugs are referred to as *psychotropic medications* and are the focus of discussion in this chapter.

It is important to remember that psychotropic medications are just one part of the patient's treatment and on their own should not be considered a 'quick fix' or cure-all. In fact, psychotropic medications are not helpful to all people who experience the symptoms of mental illness, and have many untoward effects that can cause discomfort and distress. An important adjunct group of medications that are used to manage some of these side-effects are the antiparkinsonians

Skilful mental health nursing encompasses an understanding of the particular pharmacological actions of the psychotropic agents as well as an empathic understanding of the potential issues for the person taking these medications. Regardless of the treatment setting, which can range from inpatient to community, mental health nurses play a pivotal role in working with patients and their families as they grapple with the issues surrounding these medications. It is important that the nurse develops a comprehensive understanding of both the medications and their impact on an individual as well as developing an understanding of the supportive and therapeutic nursing interventions that promote medication compliance/adherence.

IMPORTANT PHARMACOLOGICAL PRINCIPLES
Use of supportive and therapeutic nursing interventions enables the person to develop and maintain medication compliance/adherence and fosters an understanding of their medications. As the mental health nurse plays an important role in the administration of psychotropic medications, especially within inpatient units, it is essential to have a sound working knowledge of psychotropic medications including the pharmacology and relevant neurochemistry. This knowledge is important for the nurse when offering medication education to the person and their family.

All drugs are prescribed for particular effects or target symptoms that the prescriber hopes to change. Therefore it is important for the nurse to be aware of the symptoms that particular drugs target as well as the symptoms experienced by individual patients. The correct identification of symptoms is a key component of a thorough nursing assessment. Side-effects, on the other hand, are the expression of effects for which the drug was not intended. Not all side-effects are harmful, but some can be, so the nurse needs a sound working knowledge of this area of practice. Nurses also need to be aware of polypharmacy. Polypharmacy implies the use of multiple psychotropic drugs at the same time. Essentially it is defined as the use of two or more psychotropic drugs, or two or more drugs from the same chemical class, or two or more drugs with the same or similar pharmacological action to treat different conditions (Kingsbury, Yi & Simpson 2001). Although it might be useful at some stage for the management of persons with serious psychiatric disorders, polypharmacy can increase the chance of adverse drug side-effects and interactions. It can also be extremely problematic with certain groups of vulnerable people, including older people (Shupikai Rinomhota & Marshall 2000).

An understanding of how psychotropic drugs work is important for mental health nurses so that they can better understand the issues surrounding the prescription and administration of these drugs. Neurons are the basic functional unit of the brain and central nervous system and all communication in the brain involves neurons communicating across synapses at receptors. Receptors are the targets for the neurotransmitters or chemical messengers necessary for communication between neurons. The neurotransmitters acetylcholine, noradrenaline, dopamine, serotonin (5HT) and GABA (gamma-aminobutryric acid) are implicated in the development of mental illness. The psychotropic drugs produce their therapeutic action by altering communication among the neurons in the central nervous system (CNS). In particular, they alter the way neurotransmitters work at the synapse by modifying the reuptake of a neurotransmitter into the presynaptic neuron, activating or inhibiting postsynaptic receptors, or inhibiting enzyme activity (Shupikai Rinomhota & Marshall 2000).

IMPORTANT PSYCHOTROPIC DRUGS
This section explores the most important groups of psychotropic drugs in current use: the anxiolytics (anti-anxiety), antidepressants, mood-stabilising and antipsychotics (neuroleptic). These groups of drugs are listed in Table 24.1 and common examples from a local perspective are included.

Anti-anxiety or anxiolytic medications
Anxiety is a common human experience that is a normal reaction to a threat of some kind. It leads to a flight-or-fight response in the individual. Anxiety is also the feature of many mental health problems. When anxiety becomes

Table 24.1 Classification of psychotropic drugs

Type	Drug group	Example
Antipsychotic		
Traditional	Phenothiazines	Thioridazine
	Thioxanthines	Flupenthixol
	Butyrophenones	Haloperidol
	Diphenylbutylpiperidines	Pimozide
Atypical		Clozapine
		Risperidone
		Olanzapine
		Quetiapine
Antidepressant	Tricyclic and related drugs	Amitriptyline
		Lofepramine
		Trazodon
	Selective serotonin reuptake inhibitors and related drugs	Venlafaxine
		Fluoxetine
		Paroxetine
	Mono-amine oxidase inhibitors	Isocarboxazid
		Phenelzine
		Tranylcypromine
Mood stabilising	Lithium	Lithium carbonate
	Anticonvulsants	Carbamazipine
		Valproate
		Topiramate
Anti-anxiety	Benzodiazepines	Chlordiazepoxide
		Diazepam
		Clonazepam
		Alprazolam
		Lorazepam
	Azapirones	Buspirone
	Beta-adrenergic blocker	Propanolol
Sedative-hypnotic	Benzodiazepines	Flurazepam
		Temazepam
	Cyclopyrrolones	Zopiclone
	Imidazopyrimidines	Zolpidem

disabling, anti-anxiety medications may be useful (Shupikai Rinomhota & Marshall 2000). Anti-anxiety drugs can be divided into benzodiazepines and non-benzodiazepines. The benzodiazepines are probably the most commonly prescribed drugs in the world today and are the drug of choice for the short-term treatment of anxiety states.

Indications for use

The benzodiazepines are thought to reduce anxiety because of their potentiation of the inhibitory neurotransmitter GABA, which results in a clinical decrease in the individual's anxiety by an inhibition of neurotransmission (Shupikai Rinomhota & Marshall 2000). Clinically they are used to treat anxiety, insomnia, alcohol withdrawal, skeletal muscle relaxation, seizure disorders, anxiety associated with medical disease, and psychotic agitation (Ballanger 2000; Battaglia et al. 1997; Garza-Trevino et al. 1989). Therefore, although the

discussion here is primarily related to the use of these drugs as anti-anxiety agents, they also have a sedative effect and are also often used for that purpose.

Side-effects

Side-effects from the benzodiazepine drugs (see Table 24.2) are common, dose related, usually short term, and almost always harmless. They include drowsiness, reduced mental acuity and impaired motor performance. However, other effects such as headache, dizziness, feelings of detachment, nausea, hypotension and restlessness may also be experienced. Therefore the patient should be warned of the risk of accidents and cautioned about driving a car or operating dangerous machinery. They generally do not live up to their reputation of being strongly addictive, especially if they have been used for appropriate purposes, if their use has not been complicated by other factors such as the addition of other medications, and if their withdrawal is planned

Table 24.2 Managing benzodiazepine side-effects

Side-effect	Intervention
Drowsiness	Encourage appropriate activity but warn against engaging in action such as driving or operating machinery
Dizziness	Observe and take steps to prevent falls
Feelings of detachment	Encourage socialisation
Dependency, rebound insomnia/anxiety	Encourage short-term use; educate to avoid other drugs such as alcohol; plan for withdrawal

Box 24.1 Benzodiazepine withdrawal syndrome

- Agitation
- Anorexia
- Anxiety
- Autonomic arousal
- Dizziness
- Hallucinations
- Insomnia
- Irritability
- Nausea and vomiting
- Seizures
- Sensitivity to light and sounds
- Tinnitus
- Tremulousness

and gradual. However, if addiction does occur with these medications, the resulting physical dependence can lead to development of tolerance and onset of a withdrawal syndrome (see Box 24.1) if they are abruptly ceased.

It is also important to remember that older patients are more vulnerable to side-effects because the ageing brain is more sensitive to the action of sedatives (Shupikai Rinomhota & Marshall 2000).

Contraindications/precautions
Benzodiazepines should not be taken in conjunction with any other CNS depressants including alcohol. Their use in pregnancy is not established.

Interactions
Interactions may occur with alcohol, mono-amine oxidase inhibitors, phenytoin, antacids and agents with anticholinergic activity.

Patient education
The patient should be educated about the following:
- Driving or operating machinery should be avoided until tolerance develops.

- Alcohol and other CNS depressants potentiate the effects of benzodiazepines, so they should be avoided.
- Benzodiazepine use should not be stopped suddenly.
- The use of benzodiazepines during pregnancy is not recommended.

Non-benzodiazepine anti-anxiety drugs
Buspirone is a potent non-benzodiazepine anxiolytic drug with no addictive or sedative properties. It is effective in the treatment of anxiety and it has no muscle relaxant or anticonvulsant properties. It is of no use in the management of alcohol or other drug abuse or panic disorder. Generally it takes about three to six weeks before maximum anxiolytic effects are achieved.

Propanolol is a beta blocker that is useful in the treatment of anxiety. It blocks beta-noradrenergic receptors centrally as well as in the peripheral cardiac and pulmonary systems. Beta blockers reduce certain physiological symptoms of anxiety, especially tachycardia, rather than working directly on the anxiety.

Antidepressant drugs
Depression is a disorder characterised by symptoms such as depressed mood, lack of pleasure or interest, appetite disturbance, sleep disturbance and fatigue. Depression is thought to be a result of dysregulation of neurochemicals, particularly serotonin and norepinephrine. The physiological understanding of antidepressant drug action supports this theory. Antidepressant drugs enhance the transmission of these neurochemicals in a number of ways: they block the reuptake of the neurotransmitters at the synapse, inhibit their metabolism and destruction, and/or enhance the activity of the receptors. The action of these drugs at the synapse is immediate but it takes several weeks for antidepressants to have an effect on mood.

Indications for use
Antidepressant medications are indicated in the treatment of dysthymic disorders, major depression, maintenance treatment of depression and prevention of relapse, and anxiety disorders such as panic disorder and obsessive-compulsive disorder. The drugs elevate mood and alleviate the other symptoms experienced as part of depression. Choice of a particular antidepressant medication will depend on its symptom profile, side-effects, co-morbid medical conditions, concurrent medications and risk of drug interactions, and the individual's drug history. If the patient responds to the course of treatment with a particular drug, they should continue taking the drug at the same dosage for up to nine months. If they remain symptom-free during this time then the drug will be gradually withdrawn. Patients who have return of depressive symptoms after withdrawal of medication may need long-term maintenance (Treatment Protocol Project 2000).

Side-effects

Tricyclic antidepressants—The tricyclic drugs, available on the market for many years now, are clinically similar, so their effects and side-effects tend to vary little between individual drugs. They work primarily by serotonin and norepinephrine reuptake inhibition. The blockade of reuptake leads to extra transmitters available for receptor binding. Side-effects include sedation, dry mouth, constipation, blurred vision, seizures and urinary retention. They may also cause postural hypotension and serious cardiac problems such as heart block and arrhythmias. Because of their serious side-effects these drugs can lead to life-threatening consequences if taken in large quantities, such as in suicide attempts, and if this is suspected, immediate action to support life must be instigated. In the case of severely depressed patients where a potential for suicide is predicted, close supervision is required and when the person is not an inpatient, the dispensing of small, sublethal quantities is recommended (Baldessarini 2001).

Box 24.2 Signs of tricyclic overdose

- Agitation
- Confusion, drowsiness, delirium
- Convulsion
- Bowel and bladder paralysis
- Disturbances with the regulation of blood pressure and temperature
- Dilated pupils

Source: Treatment Protocol Project 2000, *Management of Mental Disorders* (3rd edn), World Health Organization Collaborating Centre for Mental Health and Substance Abuse, Sydney.

Mono-amine oxidase inhibitors—Mono-amine oxidase inhibitors (MAOIs) were the first group of anti-depressant drugs discovered. They remain very effective antidepressants; however, due to their potentially serious side-effects their use has mostly been replaced by the newer antidepressant drugs. The MAOIs work by inhibiting both types of the enzyme (MAO A and B) that metabolise serotonin and norepinephrine. Patients taking these drugs must avoid norepinephrine agonists, which include its dietary precursor, tyramine. Adverse effects include drowsiness or insomnia, agitation, fatigue, gastrointestinal disturbances, weight gain, hypotension and dizziness, dry mouth and skin, sexual dysfunction, constipation and blurred vision. The major concern with the use of these drugs is the potential to interact with specific foods that contain tyramine, and other amine drugs such as those found in any cough preparation (see Box 24.3). Such an interaction can result in excessive and dangerous elevation in blood pressure, known as a hypertensive crisis.

Box 24.3 Food and drugs to be avoided by patients taking MAOIs

Avoid:
- cheeses, especially matured cheeses
- pickled herrings, cured meats and beef extracts such as marmite
- liver and chicken livers
- whole broad beans, avocados, especially if overripe, soybean paste
- figs, especially if overripe
- large numbers of bananas
- alcoholic drinks, especially chianti and red wine
- other antidepressant drugs, nasal and sinus decongestants, narcotics, epinephrine,
- stimulants, hayfever and asthma drugs.

Selective serotonin reuptake inhibitors (SSRIs)—The selective serotonin reuptake inhibitor (SSRI) group of antidepressant drugs inhibit the reuptake of serotonin at the presynaptic membrane. This leads to an increased availability of serotonin in the synapse and therefore at the receptors, thereby promoting serotonin transmission. These drugs are as effective as the tricyclic antidepressants but safer as they cause less serious side-effects and have decreased risk of death by overdose. While the actions and effectiveness of these drugs are similar, they are all structurally different from each other, resulting in differences in their side-effects. Side-effects are similar to those of the tricyclic group except that they do not have the cardiovascular, sedative and anticholinergic side-effects. Nausea, diarrhoea, anxiety and restlessness, insomnia, sexual disturbances, loss of appetite, weight loss and headache are the most common. They should not be stopped abruptly; the withdrawal syndrome includes symptoms such as dizziness, paraesthesia, anxiety, sleep disturbance, agitation and tremor. They should not be combined with MAOIs (Shupikai Rinomhota & Marshall 2000).

Contraindications/precautions

Caution is warranted in the use of all antidepressant drugs. Once the drugs start to take effect and the patient's mood lifts, the patient may become a risk for suicide.

Selective serotonin reuptake inhibitors should not be combined with MAOI therapy. MAOIs should not be started within one week of tricyclic therapy and, conversely, tricyclic drugs should not be commenced within two weeks of stopping a MAOI. The tricyclics are a special risk with depressed people because of their severe cardiac toxicity if taken in large doses. Caution is warranted in patients with cardiac disease and with older patients. Tricyclics may also impair reaction times, especially at the beginning of treatment. Alcohol may increase the sedative effects of tricyclics.

Interactions

Tricyclics—hyperpyretic crisis, seizures or serious cardiac events may occur if administered in conjunction with MAOIs. They may prevent therapeutic effect of some antihypertensives.

MAOIs—hypertensive crisis may occur if administered with many other drugs including epinephrine, norepinephrine, reserpine, narcotic analgesics and vasoconstrictors. May also experience hypertensive crisis if tyramine-rich foods are ingested.

SSRIs—alcohol may potentiate effect. Use with cimetidine may result in increased concentrations of SSRIs in the bloodstream. Hypertensive crisis may occur if taken within fourteen days of MAOIs.

Patient education

Inform the patient of the time it will take for a marked effect to be experienced from the medication and that it is important for them to keep taking the medication even though they have not noticed an initial improvement in their condition.

Other information:

- Warn of problems when driving or operating machinery if sedation is experienced.
- Tell the patient to discuss with their doctor if they become pregnant or intend to breastfeed.
- Warn about the effect that alcohol may have if combined with antidepressant medication.
- Inform about possible interactions with foods and other drugs if taking MAOIs.

Mood stabilisers

Lithium, a naturally occurring salt, is the drug of choice for the treatment of acute mania and for the ongoing maintenance of patients with a history of mania. An Australian, John Cade, discovered its effectiveness as a treatment for mania in 1949. Just how lithium works is not clear, but it is known to mimic the effects of sodium, thereby compromising the ability of neurons to release, activate or respond to neurotransmitters. It does appear to reduce the sodium content of the brain, and increase central serotonin synthesis and noradrenaline reuptake (Shupikai Rinomhota & Marshall 2000). A number of other drugs have also been used successfully, either alone or in combination with lithium, to control the symptoms of mania. The antidepressants and a number of anticonvulsant drugs have also been used very successfully to reduce mania.

Indications for use

Lithium—Lithium is the drug of choice for the treatment of acute mania and the ongoing maintenance of people with bipolar disorders (Baldessarini & Tarazi 2001). It is also useful in the treatment of unipolar depression, aggressive behaviour, conduct disorder and schizoaffective disorder.

Anticonvulsants—A number of anticonvulsant drugs have also been used to treat mania, especially when lithium is ineffective. These drugs are now rapidly becoming the drug of choice for many patients. Carbamazepine, valproate and topiramate are examples of commonly used anticonvulsants. These drugs have been found to have acute antimanic and mood-stabilising effects. Carbamazepine, valproate and topiramate are recommended treatments for mixed or bipolar states, secondary mania, rapid cyclers and lithium refractoriness (Nassir Ghaemi et al. 2001; Shupikai Rinomhota & Marshall 2000).

Side-effects

Lithium—Drowsiness, metallic taste in the mouth, difficulty concentrating, increased thirst, dizziness, headache, dry mouth, GIT upset, nausea/vomiting, fine hand tremor, hypotension, arrhythmias, polyuria, dehydration, weight gain.

Anticonvulsants

- *Carbamazepine:* blood dyscrasias, drowsiness, nausea, vomiting, constipation or diarrhoea, hives or skin rashes, hepatitis.
- *Valproate:* prolonged bleeding time, GIT upset, tremor, ataxia, weight gain, somnolence, dizziness, hepatic failure.
- *Topiramate:* cognitive impairment, sedation, nausea, weight loss, dizziness, vomiting, rash, agitation, paraesthesias.

Contraindications/precautions

Lithium—Contraindicated with cardiac or renal disease, dehydration, sodium depletion, brain damage, pregnancy and lactation.

Care should be taken with thyroid disorders, diabetes, urinary retention and history of seizures. The therapeutic range for lithium is between 0.6 and 1.2 mmol/L for acute mania and 0.6 and 0.8 mmol/L for maintenance, but increasingly more conservative levels are being used. Symptoms of lithium toxicity rarely appear at levels below 1.2 mmol/L but are common above 2.0 mmol/L (Treatment Protocol Project 2000). Therefore, as the therapeutic and toxic levels are so close, extreme care must be taken in monitoring the patient's blood level regularly, especially during early phases of the treatment. If the level exceeds 1.5 mmol/L the next dose should be withheld and the doctor notified. Usually levels are monitored weekly until stable and then monthly. The blood samples for testing should be taken twelve hours after the last dose when lithium has been taken for at least five to seven days.

Anticonvulsants—Contraindicated with MAOIs and during lactation. Caution in older patients, cardiac/renal disease and pregnancy.

Before commencing *carbamazepine* a range of tests should be performed including blood film examination, electrolytes, liver and kidney function, and an ECG. Carbamazepine may also interfere with the metabolism and blood concentrations of other drugs, so care is needed with oral contraceptives and other drugs. There is risk of fetal malformation, so it should not be taken during pregnancy.

Valproate should not be taken with aspirin and some antipsychotics. It may enhance the effects of alcohol and other CNS depressants. There is also the risk of fetal malformation, so it should be avoided during pregnancy.

Interactions

Lithium—Diuretics, ACE inhibitors, neuroleptics, non-steroidal anti-inflammatory drugs, alcohol and caffeine may interfere with lithium absorption.

Anticonvulsants

- *Carbamazepine*: erythromycin, isoniazid, oral contraceptives, theophylline, fluoxetine.
- *Valproate*: may potentiate alcohol, carbamazepine, barbiturates. Should not be taken with aspirin or antipsychotics.
- *Topiramate*: concomitant use with lithium and valproate can cause cognitive impairment.

Patient education

Lithium

- The patient must be educated about the side-effects and signs of toxicity (see Box 24.4 and nurse's story, below), and informed of the need for regular blood levels.
- Encourage a regular intake of about ten glasses of water every day.
- Take medication regularly even when feeling well.
- Do not operate machinery until initial drowsiness subsides.
- Discuss risks of pregnancy while taking lithium.

Anticonvulsants

- Inform patient about avoiding sudden cessation of the tablets.

- Encourage patient to report unusual symptoms, such as spontaneous bruising, unusual bleeding, sore throat, fever, malaise, yellow skin or eyes, to the doctor.
- Take medications with meals if GIT upset occurs.
- Avoid taking alcohol or non-prescription drugs without consulting the doctor.
- Pregnancy must be avoided while taking the medication.
- Alternative methods of contraception may be required if taking valproate, as oral contraception may not be effective.

Box 24.4 Signs of lithium toxicity

- *Early stages*: anorexia, nausea, vomiting, diarrhoea, coarse hand tremor, twitching, lethargy, dysarthria, hyperactive deep tendon reflexes, ataxia, tinnitus, vertigo, weakness, drowsiness
- *Later stages*: fever, decreased urinary output, decreased blood pressure, irregular pulse, ECG changes, impaired consciousness, seizures, coma, death

Note: lithium toxicity is a medical emergency.

Antipsychotic or neuroleptic drugs

The traditional neuroleptic or antipsychotic drugs (also known as the typical antipsychotics) have been an important treatment for psychotic disorders since their discovery in the 1950s. These drugs revolutionised the treatment of mental illness and soon became the mainstay of treatment for most psychotic disorders. Each group of the traditional antipsychotics appears to be equally effective for the reduction or elimination of 'positive symptoms' of psychosis (for example delusions, hallucinations, motor disturbances) (Treatment Protocol Project 2000). However, the side-effects profile of the traditional antipsychotics became cause for concern because of their effect on quality of life and their link with noncompliance. The newer antipsychotics, commonly referred to as the atypicals or novel antipsychotics, were introduced in the 1990s. These drugs are better tolerated and less likely to lead to problems with medication adherence (Davies et al. 1998). Apart from

---

NURSE'S STORY: Lithium intoxication

An elderly patient was admitted to an inpatient unit for an episode of manic behaviour. She had experienced mania before and was on continuous treatment with lithium. The lithium dose was increased during the admission. The nurse returned to the ward after two days' leave and noticed that the patient appeared unwell, had a coarse tremor, was confused, ataxic, and had myoclonic jerks. She called the doctor on call, expressed her concern and told him she would withhold the evening dose of lithium. She asked him to see the patient as soon as possible and to organise to have blood taken for a

lithium level. The doctor refused to come to the ward and disagreed with the nurse's concern about the patient. He insisted she give the evening dose of the medication and said he would see the patient the next morning. The nurse refused to accept his decision and called her immediate supervisor and explained her concern for the patient's wellbeing. The medication was withheld, and an urgent blood request determined that the patient's lithium level was 2.2 mEq/L. The nurse had correctly diagnosed lithium toxicity and taken the correct action to advocate best care for the patient.

clozapine, which has superior efficacy to the traditional antipsychotics, they appear to be of equal efficacy to the traditional antipsychotics (Therapeutic Guidelines: Psychotropic 2000), while being more effective in decreasing the negative symptoms of psychosis.

The term 'neuroleptic drug', used to indicate movement and posture disorder caused as part of the extrapyramidal side-effects of the drugs, is often used synonymously with the term 'antipsychotic'. However, the term 'antipsychotic' is preferable or even considered more correct, especially since the introduction of the atypical drugs, which have little extrapyramidal action (Baldessarini & Tarazi 2001).

The traditional antipsychotics are dopamine antagonists. They block the postsynaptic D_2 receptors primarily but also exert other synaptic effects. They reduce the 'positive' symptoms of schizophrenia. Atypicals, on the other hand, have dopamine receptor subtype 2 (D_2) and serotonin receptor subtype 2 ($5HT_2$) blocking action. They not only reduce the positive symptoms of schizophrenia but also have an effect on the negative symptoms (such as blunting of affect, avolition and anhedonia) without the serious extrapyramidal side-effects.

Indications

Antipsychotics are indicated for the treatment of acute and chronic psychoses, delusional disorder, and severe depression where psychotic symptoms are present. Schizophrenia and schizoaffective disorders are the most common indications for antipsychotic drugs. Some of the phenothiazine group have other uses such as anti-emetic in the case of prochlorperazine and the treatment of intractable hiccoughs in the case of chlorpromazine for example. Many of the antipsychotic drugs, especially the lower-potency ones such as chlorpromazine and haloperidol, have a prominent sedative effect. This effect is particularly conspicuous early in treatment, although tolerance usually develops quickly.

Side-effects: traditional antipsychotics

The side-effects of the traditional antipsychotic drugs are varied. They can affect every system of the body and range from effects on the CNS, including movement disorders, sedation and seizures, through to potentially life-threatening side-effects such as neuroleptic malignant syndrome (see Table 24.3 for an overview of the side-effects of typical antipsychotics). The most troubling of the side-effects are the extrapyramidal reactions. These result from the effects of the antipsychotic drugs on the extrapyramidal motor system. This is the same system responsible for the movement disorders of Parkinson's disease. Acute dystonia, parkinsonism and akathisia occur early and can be managed by a variety of medications including the antiparkinsonian and benzodiazepine drugs. Tardive dyskinesia generally occurs later and has no effective treatment. The Abnormal Involuntary Movement Scale is a useful tool for nurses to detect movement

disorders in their patients. Neuroleptic malignant syndrome, an idiosyncratic hypersensitivity to antipsychotic drugs, is a rare but serious reaction that is potentially life-threatening (see Box 24.5). More information on traditional antipsychotic side-effects can be found in the following articles: Usher (2001) (for particular emphasis on the patient's perspective); Usher & Happell (1996); Usher & Happell (1997) and Arana (2000).

Box 24.5 Neuroleptic malignant syndrome

Neuroleptic malignant syndrome is a rare disorder that resembles a severe form of parkinsonism with coarse tremor and catatonia, fluctuating in intensity, accompanied by signs of autonomic instability (labile pulse and blood pressure, hyperthermia), stupor, elevation of creatinine kinase in serum, and sometimes myoglobinaemia. In severe forms it may persist for more than a week after ceasing the medication. The risk of death from this syndrome is high (more than 10 per cent); therefore immediate medical intervention is required if suspected

Source: Baldessarini RJ & Tarazi F 2001, Drugs and the treatment of psychiatric disorders: psychosis and mania. In: Hardman JG, Limbard LE & Gilman AG (eds), *Goodman and Gillman's the Pharmacological Basis of Therapeutics* (10th edn), McGraw Hill, New York, pp 485–543.

Antiparkinsonian medications—Antiparkinsonian medications, also referred to as anticholinergics, are used to reduce the extrapyramidal side-effects primarily from the traditional antipsychotic medications. Those antiparkinsonians with a central anticholinergic action act to reduce the symptoms associated with parkinsonism, acute dystonia and akathisia. They inhibit the action of acetylcholine and are presumed to decrease cholinergic influence in basal ganglia and thereby help to balance the effects of antipsychotic medication reduction of dopaminergic influence (Therapeutic Guidelines: Psychotropic 2000). (See Table 24.4 for action and side-effects.)

However, antiparkinsonians are not routinely administered as many patients taking antipsychotic medication do not experience extrapyramidal effects. The antiparkinsonian medications also have their own set of unwanted effects and there is considerable intentional misuse of these drugs for euphoric and sometimes hallucinogenic effects.

Side-effects: atypical antipsychotics

The atypical antipsychotics may cause some annoying side-effects such as weight gain, constipation, dizziness and paradoxical hypersalivation, which occurs primarily during sleep. They may also cause extrapyramidal side-effects (EPS) at higher doses. Seizures may also occur with too rapid a titration associated with increase in dosage. In addition, cardiac problems such as atrial fibrillation, atrial flutter or myocarditis early in treatment, although uncommon, may occur.

Table 24.3 Side-effects of the traditional antipsychotics

Side-effects	Key features	Time of maximal risk	Interventions
CNS			
Extrapyramidal (EPS)			
Acute dystonic reaction	Painful muscle spasms in head, back and torso; can last minutes to hours, occur suddenly; causes fear	1 to 5 days	Administer antiparkinsonian drug quickly, respiratory support if needed, reassure and remain with patient
Akathisia	Restlessness, leg aches, person cannot stay still	5 to 60 days	Administer antiparkinsonian drug, change drug
Parkinsonism	Rigid, mask-like facial expression; shuffling gait; drooling	5 to 30 days; can recur even after a single dose	Administer DA agonist, support patient
Tardive dyskinesia	Results from prolonged use of traditional antipsychotics; stereotyped involuntary movements (tongue, lips, feet)	After months or years of treatment (worse on withdrawal)	Assess patients often, change to atypical drugs, no other treatment available
Neuroleptic malignant syndrome	Potentially fatal with hyperthermia, severe EPS, sweating, muscle rigidity, clouding of consciousness, elevated creatine phosphokinase	Weeks usually	Supportive therapy, cease all medications, treat with bromocriptine or dantrolene
Seizures	Traditional antipsychotics reduce seizure threshold, risk about 1% but greater with rapid titration or history of seizures	Early in treatment	May need to stop drug, observe patient, or manipulate drug dose
Other			
Sedation	May be beneficial in agitated patients, can be mistaken for cognitive slowing		Educate patient to avoid driving or operating machinery, rest periods, adjust dose
Photosensitivity	Skin hyperpigmentation		Avoid sun, wear protective clothing, sunscreen, sunglasses
Anticholinergic	Dry mouth, blurred vision, orthostatic hypotension, tachycardia, urinary retention, nasal congestion		Observe, educate patient, provide support where needed, may need to change drug
Endocrine	Weight gain, diminished libido, impotence, amenorrhoea, galactorrhoea		Educate patient, reduce caloric intake, may need to change drug

Table 24.4 Antiparkinsonians: action and side-effects

Name	Action	General side-effects (dose-related)
Benztropine mesylate	Antihistamine and sedating qualities, long-acting	(Anticholinergic) Dry mouth, dilated pupils, urinary hesitancy, constipation, blurred vision, nausea
Benhexol	Specific anticholinergic action Stimulant properties	Dizziness, hallucinations
Biperiden	Anticholinergic action	Euphoria, hyperpyrexia
Orphenadrine	Anticholinergic action	Delirium in older people

- *Clozapine*: a serious adverse effect is the potential for agranulocytosis, which occurs in approximately one to two per cent of patients. Precautions must be taken to ensure swift detection of this side-effect should it occur.
- *Risperidone*: insomnia, agitation, anxiety, headache, postural hypotension particularly at the commencement of treatment, drowsiness, weight gain, GIT upset, sexual disturbance and EPS.
- *Olanzapine*: drowsiness, weight gain, postural hypotension, peripheral oedema, EPS and anticholinergic side-effects (dry mouth, hypotension, tachycardia).

NURSE'S STORY: Antipsychotic drug side-effects

I remember talking to a young man about the side-effects he was experiencing as a result of taking a number of the traditional antipsychotics to treat his schizophrenia. The experiences he described made me aware of the serious impact these drugs can have on a person's life. For example, he described how the akathisia he experienced was so extreme that he felt it was no longer worth living. The choice between taking the drug, which he experienced extreme pressure to do, and experiencing the side-effects (especially akathisia, which was not resolved by any other treatment), or not taking the drugs and living with the symptoms of the illness, caused him a great deal of confusion and distress. He said there were many times when he considered suicide the only option, as he could see no way out of the predicament. He believed that living with the side-effects caused such a poor quality of life that it was possibly not worth being alive. Similarly, he also experienced suicidal thoughts when the symptoms of the illness were at its worst. He also told me how he believed the drug side-effects made him stand out from the crowd and be recognised by others as mentally ill. This also caused him a great deal of personal distress as he remembered times when he felt conspicuous due to the visible drug side-effects. He also recalled a time when he visited his sister's house, where he believed his drug side-effects caused the whole family embarrassment, as the side-effects drew people's attention to him and to his behaviour. This man's experience of the side-effects of psychotropic drugs made me realise the importance of listening to the patient's side of the treatment story and helped me to become more cognisant of the issues surrounding medication compliance.

- *Quetiapine*: mild somnolence, mild asthenia, dry mouth, limited weight gain, postural hypotension, tachycardia and occasional syncope.

Contraindications/precautions

Traditional antipsychotics—Caution should be taken in administering these drugs to older people and to medically ill or diabetic people. Safety in pregnancy and lactation is not clear. They are contraindicated in people with a known sensitivity to one of the phenothiazines as a cross-sensitivity is possible. People taking typical antipsychotics should avoid extremes of temperature.

Atypical antipsychotics: clozapine—People taking clozapine must be made aware of the potential risk of agranulocytosis and be monitored regularly. Because of the drug's link to agranulocytosis it is restricted to those who have not responded to at least two other antipsychotics (Treatment Protocol Project 2000). Clozapine can only be prescribed through the Clozaril Patient Monitoring System program. The patient's blood should be monitored weekly for 18 weeks and monthly thereafter. An immediate differential blood count must be ordered if the patient reports flu-like symptoms. If during treatment an infection occurs and/or the WBC count has dropped below 3500/mm^3, or has dropped by a substantial amount from baseline, a repeat WBC and differential count should be done. If the results confirm a WBC below 3500/mm^3 and/or reveal an absolute neutrophil granulocyte count of between 2000 and 1500/mm^3, the leucocytes and granulocytes must be checked at least twice weekly. If the WBC falls below 3000/mm^3 and/or the absolute neutrophil granulocyte drops below 1500/mm^3, clozapine must be withdrawn at once and the patient closely monitored. Care should be taken when using these drugs with older people.

Interactions

Traditional antipsychotics—Concurrent use with antidepressants, antihistamines and antiparkinsonian agents may result in additional anticholinergic effects. Antacids and antidiarrhoeals may disrupt absorption of the antipsychotic. Alcohol may cause additional CNS depression.

Atypical antipsychotics—Drugs known to have a substantial potential to depress bone marrow function should be avoided concurrently with clozapine. Atypical antipsychotics may enhance the effect of alcohol and other CNS depressants.

Box 24.6 Useful tools for assessing drug side-effects

LUNSERS

The LUNSERS (Liverpool University neuroleptic side-effect rating scale) is a useful tool for assessing side-effects. It is designed for self-administration but can also be a useful tool for nurses to help detect patient reactions to changes in treatment (Morrison et al. 2000). It can be accessed in the following journal article:

Day JC, Wood G, Dewey M & Bentall R 1995, A self-rating scale for measuring neuroleptic side-effects. Validation in a group of schizophrenic patients, *British Journal of Psychiatry*, 166, pp 650–3.

AIMS

The AIMS (Abnormal Involuntary Movements Scale) is a widely used tool for use with people on long-term antipsychotic medications. It is designed to assess for signs of tardive dyskinesia. It can be accessed in the following journal article:

Munetz MR & Benjamin S 1988, How to examine patients using the Abnormal Involuntary Movements Scale, *Hospital and Community Psychiatry*, 39, pp 1172–7.

Patient education

Traditional antipsychotics—The patient will need education about the drug side-effects and help with improving adherence. People taking typical antipsychotics should be careful in the sun and in extremes of temperature.

Atypical antipsychotics—Advice about having regular blood levels should be provided. Patients should be told the importance of seeing a doctor immediately for any flu-like symptoms while taking clozapine. Information on possible side-effects and drug interactions should be provided.

PRN (AS-NEEDED) ANTIPSYCHOTIC DRUG ADMINISTRATION

The need to reduce agitation, distress or aggression rapidly often results in the prescription and administration of a PRN (or as-needed) antipsychotic medication (Whicher, Morrison & Douglas-Hall 2002). Antipsychotics and benzodiazepines are the main classes of medications used in this way. Past research has shown that PRN psychotropic medications are prescribed for approximately seventy-five per cent of psychiatric inpatients and administered to approximately fifty per cent (Craven, Voore & Voiineskos 1987). These medications are usually administered orally or by intramuscular injection and, although prescribed by a doctor, are usually administered on the initiative of the nurse (Geffen

et al. 2002). Once a PRN regimen is instigated, it is usually administered about ten times per person and most often in the first few days of admission (Gray, Smedley & Thomas 1997). Generally, most PRNs are given in the first few days after admission and are most frequent in the evenings and at weekends (Fishel et al. 1994; Gray & Smedley 1996; McKenzie et al. 1999; Usher et al. 2001). When nurses give PRNs they are often required to make decisions about what to give from a range of medications, as well as the amount to give, and when to administer (Usher et al. 2003).

The drugs most often prescribed for PRN administration have been the traditional antipsychotics, in particular drugs like haloperidol. There is now evidence to suggest that the benzodiazepines are just as effective as the traditional antipsychotics in managing acute agitation and disturbed behaviour and should therefore be the drug of choice (Geffen et al. 2002; Usher & Luck 2004). However, examination of current practice indicates that this is not happening and that the traditional antipsychotics are being used predominantly for PRN management of psychotic disturbance (Geffen et al. 2002; Usher et al. 2001).

PATIENT COMPLIANCE/ADHERENCE

Adherence to the prescribed antipsychotic medication regimen is an ongoing problem for patients with schizophrenia. Failure to take medications as prescribed is often the cause of relapse and readmission to hospital. In fact,

NURSE'S STORY: Using PRN medication

I have worked in an inpatient mental health service for some time. I clearly remember working with Adam, a thirty-year-old man diagnosed with chronic schizophrenia who had been a client of the mental health service for the past ten years, and had had numerous admissions to hospital. Adam's admissions were usually precipitated by ceasing his medication, increased substance use, hostile behaviour towards others, damage to property including setting fire to clothes and furniture, and a deterioration in mental state with increased paranoid thinking and delusional beliefs related to the government.

During one particular admission, Adam was verbally aggressive towards staff. Adam would respond to his delusional beliefs and paranoid ideas, and this resulted in damage to property as he believed that certain items were harmful to him or had cameras hidden in them.

Adam didn't like taking medication, as he believed he didn't need it. He said he had experienced side-effects from haloperidol, chlorpromazine and zuclopenthixol decanoate. He had clear signs of increasing arousal prior to his violent outbursts: he would look agitated, and pace the unit and mutter to himself, and on occasions he would approach staff and be verbally abusive. The staff observed that Adam

would settle with PRN clonazepam and haloperidol. However, Adam began refusing the haloperidol. Some of the staff did not give PRN medication when he was pacing and agitated. There were a number of incidents where PRN was not given and Adam physically assaulted staff and property, resulting in the use of seclusion and intramuscular medication being administered.

I was concerned about this situation because I felt it just reinforced Adam's reluctance to take medication. I decided to talk with the staff about some strategies we could all use so that there was a consistent approach to Adam's need for PRN medication. I sat down with Adam and talked to him about his concerns and found that he was agreeable and willing to take PRN clonazepam, which was administered in liquid form. However, he was very clear that he wouldn't take haloperidol as he experienced quite a few side-effects from it. After discussion with his psychiatrist regarding the antipsychotic component of the PRN medication, the staff eventually managed to get Adam to agree to taking PRN medication by developing a trusting relationship with him and educating him about his medication regimen.

The authors acknowledge this contribution from Corianne Richardson, Clinical Nurse Specialist, Armadale Mental Health Service, Perth, Western Australia.

adherence to the antipsychotic medication regimen has been claimed as the single most important factor in deferring admission (Fernando et al. 1990). The issue of medication adherence is complex and multifaceted (Happell, Manias & Pinikahana 2002).

Causes of non-adherence are related to issues such as: drug side-effects, where the antipsychotic medication may have an adverse impact on the person's quality of life (Keks 1996) and may even cause more distress than the symptoms of the illness (Usher 2001); insight into the illness (Schwarz, Vingrano & Bezirogowan 1998); and lack of education about the medications (Coudreaut-Quinn et al. 1992). Against advice, people sometimes stop taking their medications and, because they do not relapse immediately, fail to see the connection between the medications and their health (Treatment Protocol Project 2000).

To help overcome lack of adherence with antipsychotic medication, a number of strategies have been explored (see Box 24.7). Evidence suggests that an active relationship between the nurse and the patient is essential for improving adherence (Bebbington et al. 1996; Vivian & Wilcox 2000). Other helpful strategies to aid adherence include education about the medications and their side-effects (Coudreaut-Quinn, Emmons & McMorrow 1992), frequent follow up and support (Phan 1992), and motivational interviewing (Kemp, David & Hayward 1996).

It appears that no strategy is sufficient on its own, and a mixed approach to adherence may in fact be the best approach. However, it is clear that adherence to the newer atypical antipsychotics is not such a problem (Davies et al. 1998), probably because many of their side-effects are less serious.

CASE STUDY: Non-adherence to psychotropic medications (Part A)

Tony was first diagnosed with paranoid schizophrenia five years ago. His symptoms were exacerbated by poor adherence to prescribed medications and 'self-medication' with cannabis. Despite it being objectively clear that cannabis use made him more paranoid, Tony felt that it helped him relax and was dismissive of education about harm-minimisation or abstaining.

The main hurdle to adherence with prescribed medication for Tony was denial. Tony did not accept his diagnosis; consequently, he did not accept his treatment. If we accept that a diagnosis of schizophrenia would provoke a sense of loss

(e.g. normalcy, altered levels of independence, re-evaluated life goals, decreased acceptance), we may be able to understand the denial as a component of grief. Tony certainly displayed other classic stages of grief, most notably anger (at his treating psychiatrist) and bargaining (with his community case manager re postponing or cancelling administration of depot medications).

Other contributing factors to Tony's non-adherence were: the illness itself—paranoia is a barrier to building trust and rapport with clinicians; lack of education/understanding about the illness and its treatment; and unwanted side-effects of prescribed medications.

CASE STUDY: Non-adherence to psychotropic medications (Part B)

A management plan was developed to address the factors contributing to Tony's non-adherence. Tony's outpatient care was assigned to a clinical nurse in the role of case manager. This nurse administered and monitored prescribed medications and worked to build a therapeutic alliance with him. When Tony was an inpatient, as frequently occurred during the first three years of diagnosis, he was assigned a primary nurse on the mental health unit, who collaborated with the case manager to provide continuity of care and another avenue for Tony to develop rapport.

Over time, Tony began to engage with his two primary carers, which provided an opportunity for education about his diagnosis and treatment options. In time, Tony became more accepting of the treating team as a whole, and would discuss medication issues freely with his treating psychiatrist.

As Tony's acceptance improved, medication options were no longer restricted to depot injections, and oral medications were trialled. Tony was very sensitive to traditional antipsychotics and developed extrapyramidal side-effects at

subtherapeutic doses. Trials of other atypical antipsychotic medications also had problems—poor symptom control and marked weight gain.

Twelve months ago a trial of clozapine commenced. It took four months to stabilise the dose at 450 mg nocte. In doing so, Tony's mental state also stabilised. He developed considerable insight into his condition and treatment, and has developed a good degree of acceptance.

Nine months later, with encouragement from the treating team, Tony undertook a trial of abstinence from cannabis. Tony says he has used cannabis only twice since. This hasn't been objectively checked through urine samples, but his case manager has noted further improvement in symptom control and better motivation to undertake activities of daily living and social interaction.

Tony has not required admission to the mental health unit for over eight months now. If he remains stable until the new year, his case manager intends to assist Tony in seeking work.

The authors acknowledge this contribution from Paul McNamara, CNC, Consultation Liaison Team, Cairns Base Hospital.

Box 24.7 Interventions to help with adherence to medication

- Get to know your patient well.
- Help your patient develop an understanding of why the medications have been prescribed.
- Spend time talking about medications and the decisions related to adherence.
- Ask about the side-effects being experienced and offer strategies to manage side-effects where possible.
- Help the patient discuss issues related to their medications with their doctor or nurse.
- Provide education sessions for family or significant others.

CRITICAL THINKING CHALLENGE 24.1

- Denial is a commonly used defence mechanism when a person is faced with issues they are not yet able to cope with on a conscious level. Discuss the concept of denial as a component of grief and loss in relation to the diagnosis of a chronic mental illness. How does the concept of denial differ from that of insight? In part A of the case study, how could the nurse manage Tony's non-adherence while recognising the importance of denial as a coping mechanism?
- Explore relevant strategies to address the other factors contributing to Tony's non-adherence, such as his paranoia, lack of education and understanding, and unwanted side-effects.

CRITICAL THINKING CHALLENGE 24.2

- In part B of the case study, Tony was trialled on atypical antipsychotics. How does this group of medications differ from typical antipsychotics? Identify the benefits and disadvantages of each of these drug groups.
- The incidence of EPS varies according to the particular antipsychotic medication used. Identify the various EPS and explore the most effective management for these.
- Tony was trialled on clozapine. What are the benefits and disadvantages of using this particular antipsychotic drug? Why is it not necessarily the first drug of choice for patients with psychosis?
- Cannabis is commonly used by patients with a mental illness. What are the reason(s) for this? What does the term 'self-medicating' mean? Explore the effect(s) of cannabis when a person has a psychosis.
- Critically analyse the strategies in the management plan used for Tony's non-adherence. In your opinion, was the plan successful? If so (or not), explain the reason(s) for this.

DEPOT PREPARATION OF ANTIPSYCHOTIC DRUGS

Depot antipsychotic preparations, introduced in the 1960s, are useful where there might be problems with compliance with oral medications, where the patient is unable to take oral medications, or if intestinal absorption is questioned. They are long-acting, injectable forms of the traditional antipsychotic drugs, produced mostly in decanoate esters dissolved in an oily base. When administered by deep intramuscular injection, the drug is de-esterified to release the active drug, which slowly diffuses into the circulation. The injections are usually given every two to four weeks (Therapeutic Guidelines: Psychotropic 2000) and generally the release of the drug must last at least one week to be considered a depot preparation (Dencker & Axelsson 1996). However, it is important to remember that a well-targeted nurse–patient relationship can help to promote medication adherence (Marland, Sharkey & Ward 1999) and that the patient has a right to be involved in choosing the route of administration of prescribed medications wherever possible.

Table 24.5 Depot antipsychotic drugs

Name	Route	Typical maintenance dosage
Zuclopenthixol decanoate	IM	200 to 400 mg every 2 to 4 weeks
Fluphenazine decanoate	IM	12.5 to 75 mg every 4 weeks
Flupenthixol decanoate	IM	20 to 80 mg every 2 to 4 weeks

PSYCHOTROPIC DRUG USE IN SPECIAL POPULATIONS

Pregnant and lactating women

The management of women who are pregnant or lactating poses a significant challenge for the mental health nurse. The prescription and administration of psychotropic drugs, if required during pregnancy and lactation, presents many risks to the unborn fetus or the newborn child. However, the consequences of untreated psychiatric disorders during pregnancy must be weighed against the risk of prenatal exposure to drugs, as antenatal psychological distress is known to be linked to premature labour, low birth weight, smaller head circumference and inferior functional assessments in the newborn (Viguera & Cohen 1998). The evidence of the teratogenic effects of psychotropic drugs is mixed, and their use during pregnancy can expose the fetus to an increased risk of congenital malformation. Drugs such as lithium, valproate and carbamazepine are known to have teratogenic effects in early pregnancy, as well as probable adverse effects on neonates late in pregnancy (Baldessarini & Tarazi 2001; Pinelli

, Viguera & Cohen 1998). Most antidepres-
ar to be safe during pregnancy. However, as
ssants and lithium are excreted in breast milk, at
mall quantities, their safety for newborns is not
ied (Baldessarini 2001).

ren

ugh psychotropic drugs have been used with chil-
n for several decades, the use of these drugs with
children should be carefully monitored. Children are
particularly vulnerable to the cardiotoxic and seizure-
inducing effects of high doses of tricyclic compounds.
Deaths have been reported in children after accidental
or deliberate overdosage with as little as a few hundred
milligrams of a tricyclic drug (Baldessarini 2001).
Therefore, the nurse must be particularly vigilant if working with children who are prescribed psychotropic drugs.

Older people

Particular care must be taken when psychotropic drugs
are considered for use with older clients. It is generally
considered that older people will experience more adverse
effects from psychotropic drug use, especially people over
the age of seventy, due to slower drug metabolism and
excretion. For example, benzodiazepines are more likely
to cause dizziness, which can lead to falls and serious
injury (Shupikai Rinomhota & Marshall 2000). Antidepressants in older people can be problematic and are
more likely to cause dizziness, postural hypotension,
constipation, delayed micturition, oedema and tremor
(Baldessarini 2001). It is important for mental health
nurses to be aware of the special problems these drugs
may pose when used with older patients and to be vigilant regarding supervision and monitoring of side-effects.
Polypharmacy may have dire consequences for this group
and should be avoided wherever possible.

CONCLUSION

This chapter has presented an overview of the issues related
to psychopharmacology, including the use of PRN psychotropic drugs, adherence with the drugs as prescribed,
and their use with special populations. To be effective practitioners, mental health nurses also need to be equipped
with knowledge that enables an understanding of the distinct drug indications, interactions, side-effects and precautions related to the four major psychotropic medication
groups (anti-anxiety, antidepressant, mood-stabilising and
antipsychotic). The skilled mental health nurse needs to
have a working knowledge of psychopharmacology, as well
as the related issues, as the administration of these drugs is
a common but important nursing intervention. The knowledge presented here will help to prepare the mental health
nurse to make well-informed treatment decisions and
engage in successful patient education. It will also help the
nurse to detect and manage side-effects from the psychotropic drugs, many of which can be harmful or even life
threatening.

EXERCISES FOR CLASS ENGAGEMENT

- In a small group discuss the legal and ethical issues that a
  mental health nurse needs to consider when administering
  psychotropic medications. In particular, consider the issues
  related to adherence within inpatient settings.

  As a group, outline what you believe are the important
  issues related to medication adherence How might your
  beliefs differ from those of others? Larger group discussion
  to follow.

- In small groups, debate and respond to the following
  questions.
  - How would you manage a situation where you were of
    the opinion that a patient was being prescribed and
    administered a toxic level of a drug?

- Describe how polypharmacy can be a problem for
  persons taking antipsychotic medications and for members of vulnerable groups, such as older people.
- Describe the signs of a tricyclic overdose and list those
  who might be at high risk of such an outcome.
- Anticonvulsant drugs are used in the management of
  people with bipolar disorders. Describe the action of
  these drugs and list their potential side-effects.
- Lithium is commonly used as a mood stabilising drug.
  Outline why it is important to obtain regular blood tests
  for people taking this drug and outline the therapeutic
  range and signs of lithium toxicity.
- The MAOIs, although used to treat depression, are no
  longer a popular choice. Outline the reasons why this is
  the case.

REFERENCES

Arana GW 2000, An overview of side-effects caused by typical antipsychotics, *Journal of Clinical Psychiatry*, 61 (suppl. 8), pp 5–13.
Baldessarini RJ 2001, Drugs and the treatment of psychiatric disorders:
depression and anxiety disorders. In: Hardman JG, Limbard LE &

Gilman AG (eds), *Goodman and Gilman's the Pharmacological Basis of
Therapeutics* (10th edn), McGraw-Hill, New York, pp 447–83.
Baldessarini RJ & Tarazi F 2001, Drugs and the treatment of psychiatric
disorders: psychosis and mania. In: Hardman JG, Limbard LE &

Gilman AG (eds), *Goodman and Gilman's the Pharmacological Basis of Therapeutics* (10th edn), McGraw-Hill, New York, pp. 485–543.

Ballanger J 2000, Benzodiazepine receptor agonists and antagonists. In: Sadock B & Sadock V (eds), *Comprehensive Textbook of Psychiatry* (7th edn), Lippincott Williams & Wilkins, Philadelphia.

Battaglia J, Moss S, Rush J, Mendoza R, Leedom L, Dubin W et al. 1997, Haloperidol, lorazepam, or both for psychotic agitation? A multi-center, prospective, double blind emergency department study, *American Journal of Emergency Medicine*, 15(4), pp 335–40.

Bebbington P, Brewin CR, Marsden L & Lesage A 1996, Measuring the need for psychiatric treatment in the general population: the community version of the MRC needs for care assessment, *Psychological Medicine*, 26(2), pp 229–36.

Craven J, Voore P & Voiineskos G 1987, PRN medication in psychiatric inpatients, *Canadian Journal of Psychiatry*, 32(3), pp 199–203.

Coudreaut-Quinn EA, Emmons MA & McMorrow MJ 1992, Self-medication during inpatient psychiatric treatment, *Journal of Psychosocial Nursing*, 30(12), pp 32–6.

Day JC, Wood G, Dewey M & Bentall R 1995, A self-rating scale for measuring neuroleptic side-effects: validation in a group of schizophrenic patients, *British Journal of Psychiatry*, 166(5), pp 650–3.

Davie A, Adena MA, Keks NA, Catts SV, Lambert T & Schweitzer I 1998, Risperidone versus haloperidol: a meta-analysis of efficacy and safety, *Clinical Therapy*, 20(1), pp 58–71.

Dencker JS & Axelsson R 1996, Optimising the use of depot antipsychotics, *Central Nervous System Drugs*, 6(5), pp 367–81.

Fernando ML, Velamoor VR, Cooper AJ & Cernovsky Z 1990, Some factors relating to satisfactory post-discharge community maintenance of chronic psychotic patients, *Canadian Journal of Psychiatry*, 35(1), pp 71–3.

Fishel AH, Ferreiro BW, Rynerson BC, Nickell M, Jackson B & Hannon BD 1994, As needed psychotropic medications: prevalence, indications and results, *Journal of Psychosocial Nursing*, 32(8), pp 27–32.

Garza-Trevino E, Hollister L, Overall J & Alexander W 1989, Efficacy of combinations of intramuscular antipsychotics and sedative hypnotics for control of psychotic agitation, *American Journal of Psychiatry*, 146(12), pp 1599–601.

Geffen J, Sorensen L, Stokes J, Cameron A, Roberts MS & Geffen L 2002, Pro re nata medication for psychoses: an audit of practice in two metropolitan hospitals, *Australian and New Zealand Journal of Psychiatry*, 36(5), pp 649–56.

Gray R & Smedley N 1996, Administration of PRN medication by mental health nurses, *British Journal of Nursing*, 5(21), pp 1317–22.

Gray R, Smedley N & Thomas B 1997, The administration of PRN medication by mental health nurses, *Journal of Psychiatric and Mental Health Nursing*, 4(1), pp 55–6.

Happell B, Manias E & Pinikahana J 2002, The role of the inpatient mental health nurse in facilitating patient adherence to medication regimes, *Australian and New Zealand Journal of Mental Health Nursing*, 11(4), pp 251–9.

Keks NA 1996, Minimizing the non-extrapyramidal side-effects of antipsychotics, *Acta Psychiatrica Scandinavia*, 389 (suppl.), pp 18–24.

Kemp R, David A & Hayward P 1996, Compliance therapy: an intervention targeting insight and treatment adherence in psychotic patients, *Behavioural and Cognitive Psychotherapy*, 24(4), pp 331–50.

Kingsbury SJ, Yi D & Simpson M 2001, Psychopharmacology: rational and irrational polypharmacy, *Psychiatric Services*, 52(8), pp 1033–6.

Marland GR, Sharkey V & Ward E 1999, Depot neuroleptics, schizophrenia and the role of the nurse: is practice evidence based?, *Journal of Advanced Nursing*, 30(6), pp 1255–62.

McKenzie A, Kudinoff T, Benson A & Archillingham A 1999, Administration of PRN medication: a descriptive study of nursing practice, *Australian and New Zealand Journal of Mental Health Nursing*, 8(4), pp 187–91.

Morrison P, Gaskill D, Meehan T, Lunney P, Lawrence G & Collings P 2000, The use of the Liverpool University neuroleptic side-effect rating scale (LUNSERS) in clinical practice, *Australian and New Zealand Journal of Mental Health Nursing*, 9(4), pp 166–76.

Munetz MR & Benjamin S 1988, How to examine patients using the Abnormal Involuntary Movements Scale, *Hospital and Community Psychiatry*, 39(11), pp 1172–7.

Nassir Ghaemi S, Manwani SG, Katzow JJ, Ko JY & Goodwin FK 2001, Topiramate treatment of bipolar spectrum disorders: a retrospective chart review, *Annals of Clinical Psychiatry*, 13(4), pp 185–9.

Phan TT 1992, Enhancing client adherence to psychotropic medication regimens: a psychiatric community trial, *Australian Journal of Mental Health Nursing*, 2(3), pp 94–104.

Pinelli JM, Symington AJ, Cunningham KA & Paes BA 2002, Case report and review of the perinatal implications of maternal lithium use, *American Journal of Obstetrics and Gynecology*, 187(1), pp 245–9.

Schwarz HI, Vingrano W & Bezirogowan P 1998, Autonomy and the right to refuse treatment: patient attitudes after involuntary medication, *Hospital and Community Psychiatry*, 39(19), pp 1049–54.

Shupikai Rinomhota A & Marshall P 2000, *Biological Aspects of Mental Health Nursing*, Churchill Livingstone, Edinburgh.

Therapeutic Guidelines: Psychotropic 2000, Therapeutic Guidelines Limited, North Melbourne, Australia.

Treatment Protocol Project 2000, *Management of Mental Disorders* (3rd edn), World Health Organization Collaborating Centre for Mental Health and Substance Abuse, Sydney.

Usher K 2001, Taking neuroleptic medications as the treatment for schizophrenia: a phenomenological study, *Australian and New Zealand Journal of Mental Health Nursing*, 10(3), pp 145–55.

Usher K & Happell B 1996, Neuroleptic medication: the literature and implications for mental health nursing, *Australian and New Zealand Journal of Mental Health Nursing*, 5(4), pp 191–8.

Usher K & Happell B 1997, Taking neuroleptic medications: a review, *Australian and New Zealand Journal of Mental Health Nursing*, 6(1), pp 3–10.

Usher K, Lindsay D & Sellen J 2001, Mental health nurses' PRN psychotropic medication administration practices, *Journal of Psychiatric and Mental Health Nursing*, 8(5), pp 383–90.

Usher K, Lindsay D, Holmes C & Luck L 2003, PRN psychotropic medications: the need for nursing research, *Contemporary Nurse*, 14(3), pp 248–57.

Usher K & Luck L 2004, Psychotropic PRN: a model for best practice management of acute psychotic behavioural disturbance in inpatient psychiatric settings, *International Journal of Mental Health Nursing*, 13(1), pp 18–21.

Viguera AC & Cohen LS 1998, The course and management of bipolar disorder during pregnancy, *Psychopharmacology Bulletin*, 34(3), pp 339–53.

Vivian BG & Wilcox JR 2000, Compliance communication in home health care: a mutually reciprocal process, *Qualitative Health Research*, 10(1), pp 103–16.

Whicher E, Morrison M & Douglas-Hall P 2002, 'As required' medication regimens for seriously mentally ill people in hospital (Cochrane Review), The Cochrane Library, Issue 3, Oxford: Update Software.

Glossary

KEN/FLEMING SC
NURSI
PETERBOROUGH, ONTARIO, CANADA

1600 West Bank Driv
Peterborough, ON Ca

Telephone (705) 748-10
Facsimile (705) 748-1088
E-mail cathygraham@tran
Web www.

Cathy Graham, B.Sc.N., M.Sc.
Lecturer

Activity groups: part of psychosocial rehabilitation programs where organised activities such as art, walking and discussion are designed to engage clients to construct a therapeutic milieu and to help with socialising techniques and imitative behaviour.

Acute dystonic reaction: one of the side-effects of traditional antipsychotic medication. Can include the patient having painful muscle spasms in the head, back and torso, which can last minutes or hours; these occur suddenly and can cause fear in the patient.

Adjustment disorder: an exaggerated emotional or behavioural response to significant life change or stressor such as a relationship break-up, bereavement, divorce or illness.

Adulthood: a series of cognitive, social, psychological and physical changes that occur after adolescence until the final stages of one's life.

Advanced practice: a level of nursing aimed at maximising the nursing contribution to health care and improving health outcomes.

Affect: the observable behaviours associated with changes in a person's mood, such as crying and looking dejected.

Ageism: the systematic stereotyping of and discrimination against people because of their age alone; making assumptions about how people are viewed throughout the lifespan.

Agenda setting: when the client is allowed to control the therapeutic relationship and the treatment regimen.

Aggression: actions or behaviours ranging from violent physical acts such as kicks or punches, through to verbal abuse, insults and non-verbal gestures. The overall feeling projected is an attempt to dominate.

Agoraphobia: anxiety about being in places or situations from which escape might be difficult (or embarrassing) or in which help might not be available.

Agranulocytosis: a blood disorder characterised by severe depletion of white blood cells, rendering the body almost defenceless against infection.

Akathisia: one of the side-effects of traditional antipsychotic medication; involves the person not being able to stay or remain still, being restless and suffering from leg aches.

Ambivalence: an individual's tendency to hold conflicting views and feelings such as love and hate, making meaningful decision-making difficult.

Amnesia: an inability to remember events from a particular period. There are a number of different amnesias, including localised amnesia, selective amnesia, generalised amnesia and systematised amnesia.

Anhedonia: loss of the feelings of pleasure previously associated with favoured activities.

Anorexia nervosa: a disorder characterised by a refusal to maintain minimal, normal body weight for age and height; an intense fear of gaining weight; disturbed perception of body shape and size and amenorrhoea in post-menarcheal females.

Anti-anxiety medication: medication used when anxiety for the individual becomes debilitating. Benzodiazepines are the drug of choice for short-term treatment of anxiety states.

Anticholinergic: side-effects of traditional antipsychotic medication, including dry mouth, blurred vision, orthostatic hypotension, tachycardia, urinary retention and nasal congestion.

Anti-depressant medication: medication that enhances the transmission of neurochemicals, particularly serotonin and norepinephrine, by blocking the reuptake of [...] mitters at the synapse, inhibiting their metaboli[...] ing and/or enhancing activity of the receptors. [...]

Antipsychotic medication: also known as [...] typical antipsychotics, these drugs were intr[...] 1950s and revolutionised the treatment of [...] Traditional antipsychotics are dopamine an[...] reduce the 'positive' symptoms of schizophrenia [...] the 'negative' symptoms.

Anxiety: a common human experience that is a n[...] felt in varying degrees by everyone; also a state [...] viduals experience feelings of uneasiness, apprehension and activation of the autonomic nervous system in response to a vague, non-specific threat.

Assertiveness: a communication skill that enhances one's interpersonal effectiveness and allows one the choice of how to respond to others. The assertive person protects the rights of each party and achieves goals without hurting others. This results in self-confidence and the ability to express oneself appropriately in emotional and social situations.

Attachment: the strong bond or connection one feels for particular people in one's life; usually associated with the primary bond between infant and mother, which can influence one's self-concept, relationships and life experiences.

Autism: an individual's tendency to retreat into an inner fantasy world, resulting in socially isolating or withdrawing behaviours and loss of contact with reality.

Avolition: loss of motivation resulting in impairment in goal-directed activities.

Behavioural theories: theories that emphasise the importance of the environment in shaping and changing behaviour in individuals.

Behavioural therapy: therapy used to determine what causes and maintains certain behaviours and to develop treatment plans with specific goals; identifies what will be done to achieve goals, how goal achievement will be measured and a timeline for goal achievement.

Biomedical model: a model based on the idea that normal behaviour occurs because of equilibrium within the body and that abnormal behaviour results from pathological bodily or brain function.

Biopsychosocial model of assessment: a comprehensive assessment of all aspects of information concerning the consumer—biological, psychological, sociological, developmental, spiritual and cultural information.

Bipolar disorder: a diagnosis outlined in DSM-IV-TR when a person has previously experienced at least one manic episode and a depressive episode.

Body image assessment: assessment of components of body image, including body image distortion, body image avoidance and body image dissatisfaction.

Body image avoidance: a disturbance of cognition and affect that leads to repetitive body checking and avoidance of social situations that provoke anxiety about the body.

Body image dissatisfaction: a disturbance of cognition and affect that leads to a negative evaluation of physical appearance.

Body image distortion: a disturbance of perception in which clients describe their body or parts of it as large or fat despite concrete evidence to the contrary.

Body mass index (BMI): a mathematical formula, based on the height and weight of an individual, which is used to help determine the degree of starvation.

Bulimia nervosa: a disorder characterised by binge-eating behaviour—eating much larger amounts of food than would normally be eaten in one sitting, and inappropriate, compensatory weight loss behaviours such as self-induced vomiting and purging.

Burnout: a syndrome in which health-care workers lose concern and feeling for clients/consumers under their care, becoming detached and distancing themselves from the client/consumer; characterised by emotional exhaustion, depersonalisation and decreased personal accomplishment.

Case management: assessing, planning, linking, monitoring and evaluating services with the client, with case loads shared among the multidisciplinary team.

Catastrophising: when a person feels inappropriate guilt and thinks of self as incompetent, faulty, unlovable and a failure.

Catatonia: a severe and debilitating condition with disorganisation of motor behaviour and inability to relate to external stimuli; one of the sub-types of schizophrenia.

Challenging behaviour: unusual or disturbed, maladaptive behaviours which can include: stereotypical or repetitive behaviours (e.g. body rocking); 'acting out' behaviours (e.g. yelling out); self-injurious behaviours (e.g. scratching at own skin); or aggression towards others.

Child and Adolescent Mental Health Services: comprehensive services including specialist assessment and treatment options, usually only available in main centres.

Child behaviour checklist: checklist used by many services in Australia; places stronger emphasis on general and specific behaviours and problems than on the categories of disorders as in DSM-IV-TR.

Childhood: the early years of life in which foundations are laid for future development and outcomes.

Circumstantiality: a disturbance in form of thought, in which speech is indirect and longwinded (adapted from Treatment Protocol Project 2000).

Clanging: a disturbance in form of thought, in which words are chosen for their sounds rather than their meanings; includes puns and rhymes (adapted from Treatment Protocol Project 2000).

Classification of mental disorders: classification enables information to be provided concerning the patterns of behaviour, thoughts and emotions of consumers.

Clinical supervision: a positive process that involves reflection of clinical interactions and interventions by one clinician to another more experienced clinician for support, professional development, education and development of clinical practice skills.

Code of ethics: guidelines for members of professional groups as to the nature of proper ethical conduct and their obligations to the public.

Coexisting disorder: having more than one disorder at the same time, most commonly a mental health disorder and a substance use disorder. Similar terms are co-morbidity and dual diagnosis.

Cognitive behavioural therapy (CBT): therapy that aims to help people develop more efficient coping mechanisms by equipping them with strategies that promote logical ways of thinking about and responding to everyday situations.

Cognitive restructuring: a collaborative nurse–client intervention that aims to monitor and reduce distressing negative cognitions (thoughts), especially in people who are depressed.

Collusion: when the client attempts to persuade individual staff members to endorse their way of behaving.

Community care: health services available from community mental health centres and emphasising the multidisciplinary team; includes services such as counselling, follow-up treatment, referrals and supported accommodation.

Co-morbidity: having more than one disorder at the same time, most commonly a mental health disorder and a substance use disorder. Similar terms are coexisting disorder and dual diagnosis.

Competency: when a patient can or should decide and/or be permitted to decide for themselves; beyond this point another or others will need to, or should, decide for the patient.

Competency skills: in order to protect the public, a specific framework that describes the expected skill base of all practitioners within a specific discipline is set by regulatory bodies and professional nursing organisations.

Compulsions: repetitive behaviours (e.g. hand washing, checking) or mental acts (e.g. praying, counting), the goal of which is to prevent or reduce anxiety or distress, not to provide pleasure or gratification.

Confidentiality: a primary principle of the therapeutic relationship; involves maintaining confidential information about a consumer within the treatment team.

Consumer: someone who has the lived experience of mental distress and who has received care from mental health professionals.

Containment: to provide a place of safety, the hospital and confinement can be seen as a refuge from self-destructiveness and an opportunity to reassure the client and others that illness will not overwhelm them.

Continuous care: long-term, ongoing, supportive care of clients with access to a range of services, usually commenced by committed staff and in the discharge planning process.

Coping: the way one deals with change, conflict and demands in life, which can be influenced by factors such as our feelings, thoughts, beliefs and values.

Counter-transference: the response of the therapist to the patient. Having strong feelings for the patient, either negative or positive, might be a cue that one is experiencing counter-transference.

Crisis: an event/s that changes one's day-to-day existence and creates a sense of one's life being out of control, feeling that one is vulnerable and that events are unpredictable; can involve a significant loss for the person involved.

Crisis intervention: involvement of assessment, planning, intervention and resolution of a crisis.

Cultural competence: a model developed from transcultural nursing to describe the role of culture in nurse–patient dynamics and to attempt to understand these cultural dynamics.

Cultural respect: allows the individual mental health nurse to value the contribution that culturally appropriate interventions can make to the therapeutic environment.

Cultural safety: goes beyond describing the practices of other ethnic groups to nurses learning about themselves in terms of their own attitudes and values in their own culture, rather than just learning about the cultures of their clients.

Cultural sensitivity: being informed about the 'legitimacy of difference' and allowing oneself to be open to self-exploration.

Culture: a body of learned behaviours that is used to interpret individual experience and shape individual behaviour, emotion and social responses.

Defence mechanisms: unconscious processes whereby anxiety experienced by the individual's ego is reduced.

Deinstitutionalisation: closure of major psychiatric hospitals and expansion of community-based care for consumers, including relocation of inpatient psychiatric beds into general hospitals.

Delirium: a syndrome that constitutes a characteristic pattern of signs and symptoms that reduce clarity of awareness and impair the client's ability to focus, sustain or shift attention; tends to develop quickly and fluctuates during the course of the day.

Delirium tremens (DT's): a major withdrawal syndrome in which the client presents with a number of complaints, which can include agitation, disorientation, high fever, paranoia, visual hallucinations, coarse tremors and seizures.

Delusion: false, fixed belief that is inconsistent with one's social, cultural and religious beliefs and cannot be logically reasoned with.

Dementia: a progressive illness that involves cognitive and non-cognitive abnormalities and disorders of behaviour; presents as a gradual failure of brain function. It is not a normal part of life or ageing.

Democratisation: creating an environment in which staff and clients feel free to express themselves without fear of rejection and to participate in decision-making to the extent of one's abilities.

Dependence: a maladaptive pattern of substance abuse leading to significant impairment or distress and manifested in tolerance, withdrawal and increasing consumption, to the point where obtaining the substance becomes the main focus for the individual; can be physical and/or psychological.

Depersonalisation: a sense of personal reality being lost or altered, of being estranged from oneself, as if in a dream, or that one's actions are mechanical or otherwise detached from the body or mind.

Depot antipsychotic medication: long-acting, injectable forms of traditional antipsychotic medication, used when the patient is unable to take oral medication, if intestinal absorption is questioned or when there might be a medication adherence or compliance problem.

Depression: a disorder characterised by depressed mood, with feelings of hopelessness and helplessness, lack of pleasure or interest, appetite disturbance, sleep disturbance and fatigue.

Derailment: a disturbance in form of thought, in which thoughts do not progress logically and ideas are unconnected, shifting between subjects; also known as loosening of association (adapted from Treatment Protocol Project 2000).

Derealisation: a phenomenon in which the person's sense of the object world is altered. The person might perceive objects to be bigger or smaller than they really are, or that once familiar objects now seem strange.

Detoxification: the process by which an alcohol- or drug-dependent person recovers from intoxication in a supervised manner so that withdrawal symptoms are minimised.

Developmental theories: theories that highlight the importance of the early months and years of one's life in laying a solid foundation for mental health and wellbeing in adulthood.

Dialectical behaviour therapy (DBT): similar to cognitive behavioural therapy but actively incorporates social skills training; moves between validation and acceptance of the person.

Disability: an individual's impairment in one or more areas of functioning.

Disability services: a variety of services for people with intellectual disabilities, including living at home with relatives, shared accommodation, group homes, community-based services, non-government organisation service provision and residential institutions.

Dissociation: being focused on one's own internal thoughts, and being unaware of the external environment. For example, daydreaming is considered a mild form of dissociation.

Distractible speech: a disturbance in form of thought, in which nearby stimuli cause repeated changes in the topic of speech (adapted from Treatment Protocol Project 2000).

DSM-IV-TR: *Diagnostic and Statistical Manual for Mental Disorders*, 4th edition (text revised), published by the American Psychiatric Association. This classification system assesses the patient across five domains, which help with treatment planning and outcome.

Dual diagnosis: having more than one disorder at the same time, most commonly a mental health disorder and a substance use disorder. Similar terms are coexisting disorder and co-morbidity.

Dual disability: having a co-morbid intellectual or developmental disability.

Dualism: a philosophical position derived from the Cartesian idea that there is a mind–body duality, the body being separate from the soul or moral features (mind).

Duty of care: the taking of reasonable care by a nurse to avoid acts or omissions which one can reasonably foresee would be likely to injure another.

Eating disorders: complex and serious disorders that involve physical, psychological, social, family and individual factors characterised by serious disturbance of eating behaviours; include anorexia nervosa, bulimia nervosa and eating disorders not otherwise specified.

Echolalia: a disturbance in form of thought, in which other people's words or phrases are echoed, often in a 'mocking' tone; not the same as repetition of the person's own words (perseveration) (adapted from Treatment Protocol Project 2000).

Egocentrism: focusing on oneself to a degree that other people's needs are beyond one's awareness.

Ego-dystonic: when a patient's symptoms are experienced as distressing to the individual.

Electroconvulsive therapy (ECT): the application of metal electrodes to the head, through which an electric current is delivered. The electrodes can be placed unilaterally or bilaterally. ECT remains a controversial intervention in psychiatry, although it is widely accepted as an effective intervention in the treatment of severe depression.

Empathy: observing, listening, understanding and attending; 'being' with the person physically, cognitively and emotionally, understanding their story, thoughts, feelings, beliefs and emotions.

Engagement: the process of establishing rapport with a client through interactions based on acknowledging and developing a relationship based on trust.

Ethical conduct: principles for the practice of ethical conduct by health professionals, including issues of autonomy, beneficence, non-maleficence and justice.

Ethnocentrism: the belief that our own cultural values constitute the human norm and that difference is deviant and wrong.

Externalising problems: problems that include antisocial or under-controlled behaviour, such as delinquency or aggression.

Extrapyramidal side-effects: side-effects of antipsychotic drugs on the extrapyramidal motor system; include acute dystonia, parkinsonism akathisia and tardive dyskinesia.

Family therapy: an approach to treatment that is based on the idea that when a family member has a problem, it usually involves the whole family. Family therapists aim to effect change in the entire family system.

Fear: a response to a known threat; manifests in the same way as anxiety.

Flight of ideas: a disturbance in form of thought, in which the person's ideas are too rapid for them to express, and so their speech is fragmented and incoherent (adapted from Treatment Protocol Project 2000).

Forensic patient: a person who has committed a crime while mentally ill and is remanded in custody in an approved mental health service, within a prison, remand centre or forensic psychiatric hospital.

Form of thought: the amount and rate of production of thought, continuity of ideas and language. Disturbances in form of thought include: circumstantiality, clanging, derailment (loosening of associations), distractible speech, echolalia, flight of ideas, illogicality, incoherence, irrelevance, neologisms, perseveration, tangentiality, thought blocking, thought disorder and word approximations (adapted from Treatment Protocol Project 2000, p 13). For descriptions of each, see individual entries in this glossary.

Fugue: in a long-term dissociative state; the person is unable to remember the past and may also be confused about their identity, unable to remember their name or their occupation.

Generalised anxiety disorder (GAD): excessive anxiety and worry concerning events or activities (apprehensive expectation), occurring more days than not for a period of at least six months, and the individual finds it difficult to control.

Geriatric Depression Scale (GDS): assessment too designed to assist in making a diagnosis of depression, referral for treatment, and to provide a baseline assessment with which to measure the outcome of treatments.

Gillick competence: the ability of young people to consent to medical treatment or seek medical consultation as seen in their cognitive ability to make an informed judgment to give consent for treatment.

Glasgow Coma Scale (GCS): a standardised system for assessing the degree of conscious impairment in the critically ill and for predicting the duration and ultimate outcome of coma, primarily in clients with head injury.

Grief: a natural process that can be experienced after loss, and can be an emotional response of distress, pain and disorganisation.

Group cohesion: an important component in creating a climate of support and involvement. Sharing among the staff and patients of daily duties and unit resources helps communalism and cohesion to occur.

Group therapy: the engagement of two or more people in therapy at the same time. Interactions with others in a group situation, especially people who come together with others who experience the same or similar difficulties, have been shown to have positive and beneficial effects.

Harm reduction: the guiding principle used to identify a range of strategies that target the consequences of drug use rather than the drug itself.

Hazardous substance use: a repetitive pattern of use that poses a risk of harmful physical and psychological consequences.

Health of the Nation Outcome Scales (HoNOS): designed in Britain, this scale is used to gather information concerning key areas of mental health and social functioning for service monitoring and outcome measurement.

Helping relationship: a therapeutic interaction facilitating exploration of responses following a major and significant personal loss leading to a client experiencing grief.

Holism: healing of the whole person by recognising the importance of the interrelationships between biological, psychological, social and spiritual aspects of a person.

Hope: a state of mind that anticipates positive expectations of personally meaningful goal achievement.

Hypochondriasis: a disorder in which the person is intensely preoccupied with their bodily functions and can report any of a wide range of symptoms. The client focuses on what the symptoms might signify and can misinterpret ordinary bodily functions as symptoms of a serious physical illness.

Hypomania: a form of elevated mood less severe than mania.

ICD-10-AM: *International Statistical Classification of Diseases and Related Health Problems*, 10th revision, published by the World Health Organization; provides a comprehensive listing of clinical diagnoses, each with its own numerical code.

Ideas of reference: belief that an insignificant or incidental object or event has special significance or meaning for that individual.

Identity: part of one's self-concept; develops over time and contributes to one's overall sense of self.

Illicit drugs: drugs that are classified as illegal.

Illogicality: a disturbance in form of thought, in which the conclusions reached in a person's speech are illogical (adapted from Treatment Protocol Project 2000).

Incoherence: a disturbance in form of thought, in which there is verbal rambling with no clear main idea.

Incongruent affect: a mismatch between a person's thoughts and their emotional expression in a given situation.

Informed consent: consent that is (among other requirements) voluntary and specific and comes from a competent person.

Insane: coming from the Latin word 'insana' meaning not of right mind; the equivalent Greek term is 'mania'.

Intellectual disability: see mental retardation. Consumers and disability service professionals in Australia prefer this term rather than mental retardation.

Internalising problems: problems that include inhibited or over-controlled behaviours, such as anxiety or depression.

Interpersonal therapy (IPT): therapy that targets relationships as a key factor in the contribution and maintenance of eating disorders.

Intoxication: a reversible state that occurs when a person's intake exceeds their tolerance and produces behavioural and/or physical changes.

Involuntary admission: compulsory or involuntary detention in an approved psychiatric institution in the best interests of the individual, for treatment that will alleviate the individual's symptoms of mental illness.

Irrelevance: a disturbance in form of thought, in which a person's replies to questions are not related to the topic being discussed (adapted from Treatment Protocol Project 2000).

JOMAAC: a client assessment tool based on observation of the client's judgment, orientation, memory, affect, attitude and cognition.

La belle indifference: 'beautiful indifference', where the client shows a marked indifference to or unconcern about their symptoms, even if the symptom is blindness or paralysis.

Learned helplessness: both a behavioural state and personality trait of one who believes their control over a situation has been lost. It can also relate to hopelessness and powerlessness — an inability to escape an intolerable situation, leading to the ultimate mode of adaptation: subjugation and acceptance.

Least-restrictive alternative: the option of least restriction for the individual (e.g. community-based care or institution-based treatment), with consideration of the person's level of autonomy, their acceptance and cooperation, and potential for harm to self and to others.

Lifespan: the sequence of events and experiences in a person's life from birth until death.

Limit setting: explaining to clients what behaviours are acceptable and what is unacceptable, and informing them of the consequences of breaking the rules; aims to offer the client a degree of control over their behaviour by setting firm, fair and consistent limits or rules.

Mad: a middle-English, pre-twelfth-century word which means a loss of reason and judgment.

Major depressive disorder: a condition involving seriously depressed mood and other symptoms defined by DSM-IV-TR that affect all aspects of a person's bodily system and interfere significantly with their daily living activities.

Malingering: the intentional production of symptoms in order to avoid some specific duty or responsibility; the incentive to become sick is clearly identifiable.

Mania: a state of euphoria that results in extreme physical and mental overactivity.

Medication adherence/compliance: the taking of medication for ongoing treatment of the client's illness. Failure to take medication is often the cause of relapse and readmission to hospital, and can be caused by factors such as: medication having an adverse impact on the patient's life; side-effects; insight into the illness and lack of education about the medication.

Mental health: a state in which an individual has a positive sense of self, personal and social support with which to respond to life's challenges, meaningful relationships with others, access to employment and recreational activities, sufficient financial resources and suitable living arrangements.

Mental health assessment and outcome measures: standardised measures in mental health for more reliable, valid and consistent measures of initial assessment and of change that occurs with treatment.

Mental health disorders: conditions in which an individual cannot cope and function as previously, causing considerable personal, social and financial distress and affecting health-care funding, implementation of service provision and community resources.

Mental health policy: health policy based on the World Health Organization (WHO) guiding principles of access, equity, effectiveness and efficiency for all people with mental health issues.

Mental health promotion: a population-health approach to mental health, which attends to the mental health status and needs of the whole population, emphasising a continuum of care from universal prevention to long-term, individual care with early intervention and treatment.

Mental illness: a condition of impairment and disorganisation of mental function for an individual.

Mental retardation: a disability typified by major limitations in intellectual functioning and in conceptual, social and practical adaptive skills, that originates before the age of eighteen.

Mental Status Examination (MSE): a semi-structured interview with a consumer to assess the person's current neurological and psychological status using several dimensions, such as perception, affect, thought content, form of thought and speech.

Mentoring: process aimed at promoting growth and development in clinicians by means of partnerships with other clinicians in the workplace, involving problem solving, feedback, support and relationship building.

Milieu: a physical environment including the social, emotional, interpersonal, professional and managerial elements that comprise a particular setting.

Milieu therapy: therapy that involves the environment in the treatment process, the participation of patients and staff in decision-making, the use of a multidisciplinary team, open communication and individualised goal-setting with patients.

Mini Mental Status Examination (MMSE): an abbreviated form of the Mental Status Exam; based on observable behaviour in a client assessment interview.

Mini Psychiatric Assessment Schedule for Adults with Developmental Disabilities (Mini PAS-ADD): an accessible assessment tool based on a life events checklist and the client's symptoms.

Misconceptions: misinformation and misunderstanding about the origins, course and treatment of mental health problems and mental disorders.

Motivational interviewing: basically an adaptation of the Socratic style of interviewing; proceeds from the assumption that change is produced collaboratively and cannot be imposed from outside.

Mourning: a process needed to help overcome grief, involving the person extricating themselves from their relationship with the deceased person (or object or part of their person).

Multidisciplinary team (MDT): a team of individuals from multiple disciplines, such as nurses, psychologists, psychiatrists, social workers and occupational therapists, working together to provide a holistic team approach to care.

Nature versus nurture debate: a continuing discussion concerning the effects of biological phenomena and inheritance (nature) and the individual's environment and experiences in the world (nurture) and whether both are vital, inseparable, interdependent components of personality development that influence human behaviour.

Negative symptoms of schizophrenia: tend to include signs and symptoms such as blunting of affect, avolition and anhedonia.

Neologisms: disturbance in form of thought, in which a person creates new words or expressions that have no meaning to anyone else (adapted from Treatment Protocol Project 2000).

Neuroleptic malignant syndrome: a rare disorder that resembles a severe form of parkinsonism with coarse tremor and catatonia, fluctuating in intensity, accompanied by signs of autonomic instability and stupor; risk of death is high.

Neuroleptic medication: see also antipsychotic medication; the term 'neuroleptic' is used to indicate the movement and posture disorder caused as part of the extrapyramidal side-effects of some antipsychotic drugs. 'Antipsychotic medication' is the preferred term, because the atypical antipsychotics have very little extrapyramidal action.

Neuropsychological disorders: disorders, such as schizophrenia, in which the origin of the psychological disturbance lies in the neurological structure and function of the brain.

Neurosis: a term of mainly historical interest that was used in reference to madness caused by nervous system disease. Since Freud's time, 'neurosis' has been used to refer to non-psychotic disorder characterised mainly by anxiety.

Non-government organisations: services that operate outside mainstream government authority and at a community level to support consumers and carers with a range of special needs, e.g. Association of Relatives and Friends of the Mentally Ill (ARAFMI).

Normalisation: a humanistic model of care in which people with an intellectual disability are given the same rights and opportunities as any other person, even if the support of appropriate services is needed.

Nurse practitioner: an advanced practitioner with a high degree of autonomy, who has extended education within a defined scope of practice and is licensed to practise within an extended role.

Observation: experienced staff maintain a continuous watchful presence in a non-threatening, non-intrusive manner to set reasonable limits on behaviour.

Obsessions: recurrent persistent thoughts, impulses, images that are intrusive and inappropriate and cause marked anxiety or distress in an individual.

Obsessive-compulsive disorder: recurrent obsessions or compulsions that are severe enough to be time-consuming or cause marked distress or significant impairment in an individual.

Panic attack: a discrete period of intense fear or discomfort in the absence of real danger.

Panic disorder: the presence of recurrent, unexpected panic attacks followed by concern about having another panic attack or significant behavioural change related to the attacks.

Parkinson's syndrome: one of the side-effects of traditional antipsychotic medication, with the person exhibiting a rigid, mask-like facial expression, shuffling gait and drooling.

Perseveration: a disturbance in form of thought, in which the individual persistently repeats the same word or ideas; often associated with organic brain disease (adapted from Treatment Protocol Project 2000).

Personality: expression of our feelings, thoughts and patterns of behaviour that evolve over time.

Personality disorder: a diagnosis that occurs when manifestations of personality in an individual start to interfere negatively with the individual's life or with the lives of those close to them.

Personality traits: aspects of our personality that make us unique and interesting and differentiate us from each other.

Pharmacokinetics: the study of the actions of drugs within the body, including the mechanisms of absorption, distribution, metabolism and excretion.

Positive symptoms of schizophrenia: tend to include signs and symptoms such as delusions, hallucinations and motor disturbance.

Preceptoring: a preceptoring relationship is usually based in the clinical environment and occurs when someone is new to an area (e.g. a new employee or student) and a preceptor is allocated. This is usually an experienced clinician who has been prepared for the preceptoring role, which involves guidance, helping to develop confidence and skills, and facilitates the new person becoming a member of the team.

Primary gain: results in relief from psychological pain, anxiety and conflict. For example, having physical symptoms gives legitimacy to feeling unwell.

Primary health care: strategies and interventions for reducing the prevalence and impact of mental health problems in the community; includes increasing detection, promotion, prevention, early intervention and effective treatment.

Professional boundaries: limitations that need to be agreed upon in therapeutic relationships between the client/consumer and the nurse. These boundaries define acceptable and expected behaviour for both the nurse and the client that ensure a 'safe' environment based on ethical practice.

Protective factors: a number of aspects that guard a person against mental health problems or mental illness; can include, for example, positive relationships, support from peers and a sense of humour.

Psychiatric diagnosis: a tool designed to describe psychiatric criteria for the behaviour of an individual for purposes of treatment and care.

Psychoanalytic theory: developed by Freud, this theory places a strong emphasis on the role of the unconscious in determining human behaviour. Mental illness is seen as a state of being fixated at a developmental stage or conflict that has not been resolved.

Psychoeducation: education concerning the mental health status and treatment given for the client's mental illness. It is aimed at promoting wellness and providing an opportunity for the young person to gain insight into their condition.

Psychosis: a condition in which a person has impaired cognition, emotional, social and communicative responses and interpretation of reality.

Psychotherapy: a form of therapy that is concerned with the nature of the human experience; has a number of interpersonal models with individual philosophy and set techniques, such as cognitive behavioural therapy, motivational interviewing and planned short-term psychotherapy.

Psychotropic medications: a collection of pharmacological agents in current psychiatric use: anti-anxiety sedatives, anti-depressants, mood-stabilising, neuroleptic and anti-psychotic drugs.

Reality confrontation: reflecting an individual's behaviour back to them; a form of giving information and sharing of feelings in an acceptable way.

Recovery: begins as soon as a person develops mental health problems; emphasises hope and positive mental health and wellness, and focuses on the person being able to live well with or without the illness.

Reflective practices: processes that allow the nurse to examine both their practice (actions) and the accompanying cognitions (thoughts) and affective meanings (feelings) in relation to his or her values, biases and knowledge, in the context of a particular situation.

Regulation: system whereby authorities set and monitor standards in the interests of the public and the professions, and maintain registers of individuals licensed to practise nursing.

Rehabilitation: working with mentally ill people to reintegrate them back into the community.

Relapse prevention: programs that aim to teach consumers a set of cognitive and behavioural strategies to enhance their capacity to cope with high-risk situations that could otherwise precipitate relapse.

Resilience: an individual's innate ability to achieve good outcomes in spite of adversity, serious threats and risks.

Resocialisation: re-establishing social support networks and peer support through group therapy and individual goal setting.

Risk assessment/management: identifying and estimating risk so that structured decisions can be made as to how best to manage a risk behaviour.

Risk factors: factors that influence adolescent development and can change ongoing development; can include, for example, school factors, poverty and peer friendships.

Risk/harm assessment: questioning a client about risk of harm to self, risk of harm to others, risk of suicide, risk of absconding and vulnerability to exploitation or abuse.

Rumination: repetitive and increasingly intrusive negative thoughts and ideas, which can eventually interfere with other thought processes.

Schizophrenia: a disorder characterised by major disturbance in thought, perception, thinking and psychosocial functioning; a severe mental illness.

Seclusion: method of managing difficult behaviour, based on the therapeutic principles of containment, isolation and decrease in sensory input; usually instigated when other methods, such as talking and medication, have failed.

Secondary gain: the attention and support provided by others for a physical illness; can involve any benefit other than relief from anxiety.

Self-awareness: the process of becoming aware of and examining one's own personal beliefs, attitudes and motivations and recognising how these may affect others.

Self-disclosure: to make knowledge about oneself known to others; to publicly divulge information about one's own life.

Self-harm: behaviour occurring along a continuum, from pulling one's own hair out, cutting, piercing, burning oneself, through to suicide. These behaviours are a mode of self-regulation for the client, and can be comforting and confirming in a world that is out of control from their perspective.

Self-help: listening to one's own self-wisdom; can also involve seeking assistance and support from others who have had similar experiences to learn coping skills, tap into resources and find useful information.

Set-point theory: argues that weight is largely stable over time and that changes to increase or decrease weight are opposed by the body's internal mechanisms.

Sociological theories: theories that examine the influence of societal factors on the behaviour of individuals.

Socratic questioning: a common technique for encouraging motivation, which helps the client to come to an alternative belief of their own.

Somatisation: a psychological process whereby anxiety or psychological conflict is translated into physical complaints, although no mechanism has been found.

Spiritual assessment: undertaking questions that can provide a deeper understanding of the patient, their social setting and possible origins of the problem. Questions concerning the client's concept of God, sources of strength and hope, religious practices and meaning and purposes in the client's life would be considered.

Splitting staff: an attempt by the client to split the treatment team by appealing to individual members, by sharing 'secrets' and suggesting that the staff member is the 'only one' who understands or is approachable.

Stage theories: theories developed from Darwin's work on evolution that are based on measuring and monitoring a person's individual development against a set of expected 'norms' as certain age milestones are achieved.

Standards of practice: standards that describe the expected performance of nurses providing mental health care; represent the commitment to accountability of mental health nurses. Mental health nursing standards of practice include a rationale and attributes for each standard, performance criteria and clinical indicators of practice.

Stigma: a notion that mental illness is something to be avoided, hidden away or shameful.

Strengths: a person's resilience, aspirations, talents and uniqueness; what a person can do and do well.

Stress: a psychological response to any demand or stressor; can be experienced as negative (distress) or positive. Individuals can respond differently to the same stressor.

Stress-diathesis model: a model used to understand how mental illness occurs; individuals are exposed to stressful events in the course of their lives and these events may precipitate symptoms in some people who have a predisposition to mental illness.

Stress management: managing the effects of the stress one is experiencing by changing the situation, increasing one's ability to deal with the situation, changing one's perception of the situation, and/or changing one's behaviour.

Substance abuse: the use of drugs or alcohol in a way that disrupts prevailing social norms; these norms vary with culture, gender and generations.

Sundowning effect: an increase in behavioural problems for the client, occurring in the evening hours and beginning around sunset.

Tangentiality: a disturbance in form of thought, in which the individual gives irrelevant or oblique replies to questions. The reply might refer to the topic but not give a complete answer (adapted from Treatment Protocol Project 2000).

Tardive dyskinesia: stereotypical involuntary movement of the tongue, lips and feet; results from prolonged use of traditional antipsychotics.

Telephone counselling: method of crisis counselling that usually involves a single session and affords anonymity to the caller at a time when the person may be feeling vulnerable. The counsellor helps the person cope with the crisis by working through feelings and problem solving.

The 'humours': the humoural theory was based on the belief that the body contained within it four humours—blood, phlegm, yellow bile and black bile—and disease developed when internal or external factors disturbed the balance of the humours and produced injurious effects such as mental illness.

Therapeutic alliance: the development of the trusting, beneficial and understanding partnership that needs to exist between the nurse and the client/consumer for a therapeutic relationship to develop.

Therapeutic community: an environment in which the emphasis is on normal functioning rather than on a psychiatric illness or disability. In this community, the people who are being treated are referred to as consumers or residents.

Therapeutic relationship: an enabling relationship that supports the needs of the patient; is based on rapport and differs from social and intimate relationships.

Thought blocking: a disturbance in form of thought, in which there are abrupt gaps in the individual's flow of thoughts; not caused by anxiety, poor concentration or being distracted (adapted from Treatment Protocol Project 2000).

Thought disorder: a disturbance of the form in which an individual expresses their thoughts (structure, grammar, syntax, logic), or sometimes the content of their thoughts (adapted from Treatment Protocol Project 2000).

Thriving: where a person is better off after an adverse situation than before; can be seen as a positive response to the adverse situation.

Transference: when a person transfers beliefs, feelings, thoughts or behaviours that occurred in one situation, usually in their past, to a situation that is happening in the present. Traditionally referred to the patient with unconscious feelings or beliefs about someone in their past transferring these feelings or beliefs onto the therapist.

Triage assessment: a process for decision-making that occurs when alternatives for acute care are being considered. A comprehensive assessment is undertaken, including the person's symptoms and current situation.

Victim: a person who has endured a form of physical and/or psychological or emotional harm at another's hand, e.g. a person who has suffered sexual assault, domestic violence and/or rape.

Violence: a serious physical attack where the intent is to cause harm to an individual or object.

Voluntary admission: admission of individuals, with their full permission, who require treatment in an approved mental health setting because of the severity of their mental illness, and also for individuals suffering from an acute episode of a mental illness.

Withdrawal: usually but not always associated with substance dependence. Most individuals going through withdrawal have a craving to re-administer the substance to reduce the symptoms. The development of a substance-specific syndrome due to the cessation of (or reduction in) substance use that has been heavy and prolonged.

Word approximations: a disturbance in form of thought, in which the individual strings words together in new and unconventional ways to create a particular meaning; often associated with organic brain disease (adapted from Treatment Protocol Project 2000).

Index